YO-EHB-508

Fifth Edition

Jonas's
Health Care Delivery in the United States

Anthony R. Kovner, PhD
with Contributors

with a Foreword by
Founding Editor **Steven Jonas**, MD, MPH

Springer Publishing Company
New York

362.10973
J69j

D

Springer Publishing Company, Inc.
536 Broadway
New York, NY 10012

First edition published, 1977
Second edition published, 1981
Third edition published, 1986
Fourth edition published, 1990

Cover design by Tom Yabut
Production Editor: Pamela Lankas

96 97 98 99 / 5 4

Library of Congress Cataloging in Publication Data

Jonas's Health care delivery in the U.S. / Anthony R. Kovner, editor. —5th ed.
    p. cm.
Fourth ed. published and cataloged under the title: Health care delivery in the United States.
Includes bibliographical references and index.
ISBN 0-8261-2078-4 (softcover); 0-8261-2079-2 (hardcover)
1. Medical care—United States.   I. Kovner, Anthony R.
II. Health care delivery in the United States. III. Title.
RA395.A3H395   1994
362.1'0973—dc20   94-31916
                                                          CIP

Printed in the United States of America

Contents

v

Foreword

This fifth edition of *Health Care Delivery in the United States* is the second to appear under the leadership of my friend and professional colleague, Dr. Anthony Kovner. When preparing for the fourth edition Dr. Ursula Springer (President of Springer Publishing Company) and I decided that the time had come to name a successor to me as the book's Editor, Dr. Kovner was my first choice for the post. Dr. Kovner has a thorough knowledge of health care delivery in the United States and a fine record of teaching, service, research, and publication in the field. He pledged at that time that he would continue the most important traditions of the book: comprehensiveness, an emphasis on description of things as they are, objectivity with a measured allowance for presentation of the authors' viewpoints, and readability. At the same time, he promised to bring in new blood and a fresh approach to the subject matter.

Dr. Kovner has succeeded admirably. His work has led to the results I had hoped for. The book has been freshened and refreshed, and of course appropriately updated. The quality has been maintained at a level with which I am proud to be associated. The annual sales rate has increased under his editorship. Thus it appears that our readers, who have purchased in excess of 150,000 copies of this book in the first 18 years of its existence have agreed with my assessment of Dr. Kovner's work.

An Old Chapter in Health Care Delivery

Having been associated with this book since its conception, I am impressed with how much things change in the health care delivery system (HCDS), yet how much they stay the same. There are many subjects covered in this Fifth Edition that were either nonexistent or not considered important enough for inclusion in the First Edition, published in 1977. These new subjects reflect both new problems and proposed solutions for them, and proposed new solutions to old problems. However, analysis reveals that most apparently new problems are but offspring of the major issues that the U.S. HCDS has faced for quite some time. In fact, the major issues have changed little if at all since at least 1932, if not earlier.

Dr. Kovner begins Chapter One of the Fifth Edition with the same quote from the *Final Report of the Committee on the Costs of Medical Care* (published in 1932) with which I began Chapter One of each of the first three editions of this book. Reading it is both instructive and depressing. It could have been written yesterday. Perhaps of most concern is the fact that in 1994 we are spending over 300 times what we spent in 1932, a multiplier that far exceeds the results of inflation during the period. But still, as the *Final Report* concluded, "many persons do not receive service which is adequate either in quantity or quality." (In 1989, when I wrote the Foreword to the Fourth Edition of this book, we were spending "only" 200 times what we spent in 1932.)

Now as then "the problem of providing satisfactory medical service to all the people of the United States at costs which they can meet is a pressing one." And, for all of the HCDS's achievements, there is still "a tremendous amount of preventable physical pain and mental anguish, needless deaths, economic inefficiency, and social waste." It is striking that these sentences from that 60-year-old report encapsulate the three principal problems upon which meaningful health care reform efforts of the 1990s focus: cost-containment; guaranteeing for all access to comprehensive health services; improving the content of the services that people do receive, with a special emphasis on prevention.

There have been enormous advances in both biomedical and epidemiological knowledge since 1932. Hundreds of billions of dollars of capital have been invested in biomedical research, the construction of hospitals and other health care facilities, and the training and education of millions of physicians, nurses, and other health care professionals. More than one *trillion* dollars are now spent every year *using* that capital base.

Much that is beneficial for the population is done. Yet, to repeat, the major problems remain. A significant minority of the population does not receive "medical service . . . which is adequate either in quantity or quality"; costs are ever more out of control; and there still is a tremendous amount of "preventable . . . pain . . . anguish . . . death . . . and . . . waste."

The New Chapter

The opening paragraph of the *Final Report* concludes that: "[T]hese conditions are . . . largely unnecessary. The United States has the economic resources, the organizing ability and the technical expertise to solve this problem." One must agree with that sentence. The experience with national health care reform that we shall have during the life of the Fifth Edition of this text will tell us if the second is in fact true.

We certainly have the economic resources. But do we have the organizing ability and the technical expertise? In the abstract, yes. Our nation is the only one to have put men on the moon. We created the most powerful military force the world has ever known. We developed marvelous systems for growing food and creating an abundance of consumer goods that benefit many, though certainly not all, of our people. The question still remains. Can we solve the listed health and health care problems?

In my view, the answer will be found in the political, not the policy, arena. We do have the organizing ability and the technical expertise to solve the problems we face. Our achievements in other realms prove it. But to bring our organizational abilities to bear in solving our long-standing health and health care problems requires major, wrenching changes in how the U.S. HCDS goes about its business. And many players in the HCDS simply don't want to change.

Persuading those players to change, using the force of law and regulation where necessary, is a political, not a policy, matter. Thus the central obstacles to be overcome if effective change is to be successfully made lie in the political, not the programmatic, realm. Making change in the end will require as much political will and muscle, accompanied by an effective sales and marketing plan for the product, as it will require a workable program that has the potential to actually solve the problems.

Will a national health care reform plan that will really lead to other than cosmetic change come out of the political cauldron in Washington? Will those same self-interested forces that opposed the conclusions of the *Final Report*, labeled them a "communist plot," and stopped the types of reform that virtually every other leading industrialized country was in the process of making at the time dead in its tracks, be successful once again? Will party political interests that have nothing to do *per se* with national health reform lead the nation into a functional dead-end on this issue? The answers to these questions will, primarily, determine what will happen to the structure and functions of the U.S. HCDS during the publishing term of this edition of *Health Care Delivery in the United States*.

All this being said, however, please note that this book is primarily descriptive, not prescriptive. Thus it serves the needs of readers both who simply want to know what the U.S. HCDS is like and how it works as of 1994, and who would use the descriptions provided to develop their own prescriptions for change. Before one can usefully say what might be or what ought to be, one must know what *is*. That is the need this book is intended to meet. The rest, dear reader, is up to you.

STEVEN JONAS, M.D., M.P.H.
Professor, State University of New York
*   at Stony Brook*
Founding Editor,
Health Care Delivery in the United States

Preface

Health Care Delivery in the United States is intended as an introduction for those studying to be clinicians or managers and for those who wish to know more about health care and how it is delivered in this country.

Deuschle noted in his preface to the first edition:

> The book is basically descriptive in nature, examining the various elements in the delivery system and elucidating their interactions; it succeeds in describing this labyrinthine system lucidly and comprehensively. It does not neglect the economic ramifications . . . nor the political controversies. . . . The book is up to date in terminology and thus will help meet the urgent need of health workers to communicate with one another and with the public at large.

The mission of this fifth edition is identical to that of the preceding four; we hope we have achieved a similar measure of success.

Since publication of the first edition in 1977, the book's contributors have tried to reflect the changing health care delivery system. Although some of the nomenclature has varied, all five editions have had chapters on the concept of health care, data, manpower, nursing, ambulatory care, hospitals, mental health, financing, government, planning, and control of quality. Long-term care has merited its own chapter since the second edition in 1981. Technology assessment and futures were first presented in the third edition and are in the fifth as well.

Included in the fourth edition for the first time were chapter-length discussions of governance and management, comparative health systems, and ethics. These are all major topics that are continued in the fifth edition.

This book is going to press in Autumn 1994, four years subsequent to the last edition. Despite the possibility of significant change coming out of Washington this year (probably more change has come from states, regions, and localities in adaptation to the Clinton initiatives) we decided to stick to a four-year cycle: because so much has changed since Spring 1990, and because it is impossible to predict now what will pass Congress and be signed by the President during 1994–1995. In any event, given historical patterns, change in the American health care delivery system over the next few years is likely to be more incremental than discontinuous.

As with earlier editions, we hope this book continues to add value for students and practitioners.

ANTHONY R. KOVNER, PH.D.
Professor, Robert F. Wagner Graduate
School of Public Service
New York University
New York, N.Y.

Acknowledgments

The editor wishes to acknowledge the prompt and effective effort of all chapter authors and the research assistance of Jacqueline Karali.

Contributors

H. David Banta is Senior Researcher with the Netherlands Organization for Applied Scientific Research (TNO) in Leiden, the Netherlands. He also does extensive consulting internationally in health care technology assessment and technological diffusion. He moved to the Netherlands in 1985 to direct a WHO-sponsored project on future health care technology and has remained in the country. He was previously Assistant Director of the Office of Technology Assessment, United States Congress and Deputy Director of the Pan American Health Organization (WHO for the Americas). Dr. Banta received his M.D. from Duke University and his M.P.H. and M.S. Hyg. degrees from Harvard University.

Charles Brecher is a Professor of Public and Health Administration at the Robert F. Wagner Graduate School of Public Service, New York University. He has a Ph.D. in political science from the City University of New York and serves as Research Director of the Citizens Budget Commission. He has pubished frequently in the fields of state and local politics and finance as well as health policy. His two most recent books, both published in 1993, are *Power Failure: New York City Politics and Policy since 1960* for Oxford University Press and *Managing Safety Net Hospitals: Cases for Executive Development* for the Health Administration Press.

Steven Jonas is Professor of Community and Preventive Medicine, School of Medicine, State University of New York at Stony Brook. The Founding Editor of *Health Care Delivery in the United States,* and author of Springer Publishing's short text, *An Introduction to the U.S. Health Care System,* he has authored/coauthored 5 books and more than 100 professional articles and book reviews on health policy, medical education reform, and the role and function of health-promotion/disease-prevention services in the health care delivery system. For the general public he has authored/coauthored four books and numerous articles on exercise, health, and nutrition. Dr. Jonas received his M.D. from Harvard and his M.P.H. from Yale. He is a past president of the Association of Teachers of Preventive Medicine, a Fellow of the American College of Preventive Medicine, an associate editor of *Preventive Medicine*, and Editor of the *Springer Series on Medical Education*.

James R. Knickman is Vice President of The Robert Wood Johnson Foundation. He oversees the Foundation's efforts in the evaluation field and in health services research. Prior to joining the Foundation staff, Dr. Knickman was a Professor at NYU's Robert F. Wagner Graduate School of Public Service and Director of the University's Health Research Program. His research has addressed a range of issues related to the delivery of health care in urban areas and on the financing of long-term care.

Lorrin M. Koran, Professor of Psychiatry at Stanford University Medical Center, is the Director of the Obsessive Compulsive Disorders Clinic and Chief of the Psychiatric Consultation Service. His research interests include new drug treatments for obsessive compulsive and depressive disorders, and characteristics of the mental health services delivery system. Dr. Koran has served as Special Assistant to the Director of the National Institute of Mental Health. He received his M.D. from Harvard Medical School.

Anthony R. Kovner is Professor of Health Policy & Management at the Robert F. Wagner Graduate School for Public Service at New York University. He has been a senior manager in two hospitals, a nursing home, a group practice, and a neighborhood health center, as well as a senior health care consultant of a large industrial union. An organizational theorist by training, his research interests include health services management and governance. He has edited three textbooks and written two books and numerous articles on health services management, hospital governance, community benefit programs and rural health care. Dr. Kovner has been a senior program consultant for the Robert Wood Johnson Foundation and the W. K. Kellogg Foundation. He received his M.P.A. from Cornell University and his Ph.D. in public administration from the University of Pittsburgh.

Christine Tassone Kovner is Associate Professor, Division of Nursing, School of Education at New York University. She has worked as a public health nurse, a home-care coordinator, and as a director of staff development at a small acute-care hospital. Her research interests are nursing resource use and the cost of nursing care. She earned her baccalaureate from Columbia University, MSN from the University of Pennsylvania and PhD in nursing from New York University.

Roger Kropf, Associate Professor of Public and Health Administration at the Robert Wagner Graduate School of Public Service, New York University, is a specialist in health planning and management information systems. He is the author of *Service Excellence in Health Care Through the Use of Computers*, published by the American College of Healthcare Executives, which examines how computers and telecommunications technology can improve patient and physician satisfaction with health care services. He is also the senior author of *Strategic Analysis for Hospital Management*, which examines strategic planning in hospitals and how management information systems can be used to improve decision-making. Professor Kropf received a Ph.D. from the Maxwell School of Citizenship and Public Affairs at Syracuse University.

Robert S. Lawrence is the Director of the Division of Health Sciences at the Rockefeller Foundation and Adjunct Professor of Medicine at New York University. He was the Director of the Division of Primary Care at Harvard Medical School from 1974 to 1991 and chief of medicine at the Cambridge Hospital from 1980 to 1991. Earlier he served as medical director of a rural neighborhood health center network affiliated with the University of North Carolina. For most of his career he has taught medical students and residents ambulatory care and preventive medicine. He chaired the U.S. Preventive Services Task Force from 1984 to 1989 and received his A.B. and M.D. from Harvard University.

Andrew P. Mezey is Professor of Pediatrics and an Associate Dean at the Albert Einstein College of Medicine, and previously the Medical Director of the Bronx Municipal Hospital Center, a member hospital of the New York City Health and Hospitals Corporation. From 1967 to 1979 he was in the private practice of pediatrics in Hartsdale, New York. From 1979 to 1989 Dr. Mezey was the Director of Pediatrics at the Bronx Municipal Hospital. He received his M.D. degree from New York University School of Medicine in 1960 and his M.S. (Management) degree from the Wagner School of Public Service at New York University in 1992. He is a coauthor of "Primary Care Pediatrics: A Symptomatic Approach", on the editorial board of the American Academy of Pediatrics book "Caring for Your Baby and Young Child: Birth to Age 5", and a coeditor of the journal "Emergency and Office Pediatrics". He was recently appointed to the New York State Board of Midwifery.

Hila Richardson is the Study Director for A Healthy New York City Project based at the Center on Addiction and Substance Abuse (CASA) at Columbia University. Previously, she was Senior Assistant Vice President for Long-Term Care at the New York City Health and Hospitals Corporation, and before that, Associate Director of the Rural Hospital Program, a national demonstration sponsored by the Robert Wood Johnson Foundation and based at New York University's Program in Health Policy and Management. Dr. Richardson also was on the staff of the Institute of Medicine and has held several nursing positions. She has held teaching positions at the University of Virginia School of Nursing, Columbia University School of Public Health, and New York University School of Graduate Public Administration. Dr. Richardson received a B.S. in Nursing from the University of Virginia, an M.P.H. from Johns Hopkins University, and a Dr.P.H. from Columbia University.

Victor G. Rodwin is Director of the Office of International Programs and an Associate Professor of Health Policy and Management at the R. F. Wagner Graduate School of Public Service, New York University. Professor Rodwin is a specialist in the comparative analysis of health care systems and policy. He is the author of numerous articles and books: *The Health Planning Predicament: France, Quebec, England and the United States* (University of California, 1984); *The End of An Illusion: The Future of Health Policy in Western Industrialized Nations* (with J. Kervasdoué and J. Kimberly, University of California Press, 1984); and *Public Hospitals in New York and Paris* (with C. Brecher, D. Jolly and R. Baxter, new York University Press, 1992). Professor Rodwin holds an MPH in health care administration and a Ph.D. in city and regional planning from the University of California at Berkeley.

Edward S. Salsberg is the Director of the Bureau of Health Resources Development in the New York State Department of Health. The Bureau is responsible for health professions planning and policy development for the State Department of Health. Prior to his present position, he held a variety of positions with the New York City Health Services Administration and New York State Department of Health. Mr. Salsberg holds a Masters Degree in Public Administration from New York University and a Bachelors Degree in political science from the State University of New York at Stony Brook.

Dena J. Seiden is bioethicist at both St. Clare's Hospital and Elmhurst General Hospital in New York City, and principal of Medical Ethics Consulting Services, also in New York. She has worked as consulting ethicist to Kaiser-Permanente Health Plan, the Harvard Community Health Plan and St. Luke's Roosevelt Hospital Center. She teaches ethics at the R. F. Wagner Graduate School of Public Service at New York University, the New School for Social Research and Marywood College, PA. She is a former health care manager with 13 years of experience. Dr. Seiden received her doctorate in ethics at Union Theological Seminary in 1991.

Steven S. Sharfstein is currently President and Medical Director at The Sheppard and Enoch Pratt Hospital and Clinical Professor of Psychiatry at the University of Maryland. He spent 13 years with the National Institute of Mental Health, where he was Director of the Mental Service Programs and also held positions in consultation liaison and behavioral medicine on the campus of the National Institutes of Health. From 1983 to 1986 he was Deputy Medical Director of the American

Psychiatric Association. He has written on a wide variety of clinical and economic topics and has published more than 95 professional papers, 24 book chapters, and 9 books, including (as coauthor) *Madness and Government: Who Cares for the Mentally Ill?*, a history of the federal community mental health centers program. Trained in psychiatry at the Massachusetts Mental Health Center from 1969 to 1972, Dr. Sharfstein also received an M.P.A. from the Kennedy School of Government in 1973.

Anne M. Stoline is currently a Staff Psychiatrist at The Sheppard Pratt Hospital. Her research interest is health care policy and financing. She has co-authored numerous articles and papers and has presented at several symposiums. She received her M.D. in 1988 from Johns Hopkins School of Medicine.

Kenneth E. Thorpe is currently Deputy Assistant Secretary on Health Policy in the Department of Health and Human Service. He is currently on leave as an associate professor at the School of Public Health University of North Carolina at Chapel Hill. He has served as consultant to the Rand Corporation and the Subcommittee on Health Insurance for the New York State Council on Health Care Financing, where he aided in the development of New York's new hospital payment system. His primary research interests include evaluations of the impact of public policies on hospital and nursing home behavior. Recent projects include an evaluation of the cost and access implications of alternative hospital payment methodologies in New York's (Medicare) waiver program and the impact of DRG payment on hospital readmission rates, as well as his ongoing research evaluating the RUG-II nursing home payment system in New York. Most reccently, his research has focused on the effects of proposed employer health insurance mandates and expansions of Medicaid. He received his M.A. in public policy analysis from Duke University and his Ph.D. from the Rand Graduate School.

Beth C. Weitzman, Associate Professor of Public and Health Administration, at the R. F. Wagner School of Public Service, New York University. She teaches courses in quality assessment, community health and medical care, and statistics. Her research interests focus on urban policies affecting poor families, particularly in regard to health care utilization. She is currently working on a longitudinal study of homeless families, funded by the National Institute of Mental Health. Professor Weitzman recently completed an assessment of the impact of employment-based health insurance on working poor and immigrant families. She has worked both as a researcher for the New York City public school system and as an evaluation consultant. She holds an M.P.A. and Ph.D. from New York University.

Permissions

Table 4.3 is adapted from Jonas, Etzel, and Baransky, "Educational programs in U.S. medical schools," *The Journal of the American Medical Association 270* (9), September 1, 1993; Appendix II, *270* (9), September 1, 1993; and Crowley *258* (8), August 28, 1987. Reprinted with the permission of the publisher, Chicago, IL.

Figure 4.4 is adapted from Randlet, R. D., Overview of positions in residencies, *The NRMP Dictionary: 1993*, © 1992. Reprinted with the permission of The National Residency Matching Program, Washington, DC.

Table 4.4 is adapted from *The Journal of the American Medical Association 270* (9), September 1, 1993, Appendix II. Reprinted with the permission of the publisher, Chicago, IL.

Table 4.5 is adapted from Roback, Randolph, Seidman, and Bradley, *Physician Characteristics and Distribution in the U.S.*, Table EE, p. 12, © 1993. Reprinted with the permission of the American Medical Association, Chicago, IL.

Table 4.6 is adapted from Roback, Randolph, Seidman, and Bradley, *Physician Characteristics and Distribution in the U.S.*, Table A-17, p. 33, © 1993. Reprinted with the permission of the American Medical Association, Chicago, IL.

Table 4.7 is adapted from Roback, Randolph, Seidman, and Bradley, *Physician Characteristics and Distribution in the U.S.*, © 1993. Reprinted with the permission of the American Medical Association, Chicago, IL.

Table 4.8 is adapted from Roback, Randolph, Seidman, and Bradley, *Physician Characteristics and Distribution in the U.S.*, Table A-2, p. 18, © 1993. Reprinted with the permission of the American Medical Association, Chicago, IL.

Table 4.9 is adapted from Mulhausen and McGee, "Physician need: An alternative projection from a study of large, prepaid group practice," *The Journal of the American Medical Association 261* (13): 1930–1934, April 7, 1989. Reprinted with the permission of the publisher; and from Roback, Randolph, Seidman, and Bradley, *Physician Characteristics and Distribution in the U.S.*, © 1993. Reprinted with the permission of the American Medical Association, Department of Physician Data Services, Chicago, IL.

Figure 4.6 is adapted from Gonzalez and Martin, *Socioeconomic Characteristics of Medical Practice*, Figure 5, p. 71, © 1993. Reprinted with the permission of the American Medical Association, Chicago, IL: Center for Health Policy Research.

Figure 4.7, Table 4.10 are adapted from Gonzalez and Martin, *Socioeconomic Characteristics of Medical Practice*, Figure 17, p. 141, © 1993. Reprinted with the permission of the American Medical Association, Chicago, IL: Center for Health Policy Research.

Table 8.1 is from "Medicare-Certified Home Health Agencies." Reproduced by permission of the National Association for Home Care, 1992, from *Basic Statistics About Home Care*, 1992. Not for further reproduction.

Table 10.3 is adapted from Hay/Huggins Company, 1992, as abridged in *Medical Benefits 10* (1), January 15, 1993. Reprinted with the permission of Panel Publishers, Charlottesville, VA, A Division of Aspen Publishers, Inc.

Table 10.4 is adapted from Gruber, Shadle, and Polich, "From movement to industry: The growth of HMOs," *Health Affairs 7* (3), p. 198, Summer 1988. This article is reprinted with the permission of *Health Affairs*, 7500 Old Georgetown Road, Suite 600, Bethesda, MD 20814, 301-656-7401.

Table 11.1 is adapted from "Percentage change in medicare inpatient expenses, hospital staffing, and hospital volume, 1980–1987." *National Panel Survey, Annual Report to Congress.* Reprinted with the permission of the American Hospital Association.

Fifth Edition

**Jonas's Health Care Delivery
in the United States**

1

Introduction

Anthony R. Kovner

The State of Health Care Delivery in the United States

In the third edition of this book, Jonas cites a study of health care delivery made over 60 years ago, which summarized its findings in these terms:

> The problem of providing satisfactory medical service to all the people of the United States at costs which they can meet is a pressing one. At the present time, many persons do not receive service which is adequate either in quantity or quality, and the costs of service are inequitably distributed. The result is a tremendous amount of preventable physical pain and mental anguish, needless deaths, economic inefficiency, and social waste. Furthermore, these conditions are . . . largely unnecessary. The United States has the economic resources, the organizing ability and the technical expertise to solve this problem. [Committee on the Costs of Medical Care, p. 2]

This statement is applicable to the health care delivery system and to President Clinton's health care agenda in the United States today.

If this is the problem, what then should we do about it, and would the remedy be worse than what we have? According to Easterbrook (1987),

> The U.S. approach costs more than other systems, but it also produces the most sophisticated care; an outcome which should not be dismissed as coincidental. Of the socialized nations only Canada is thought to have medicine equal to ours, and its conversion from an enterprise system is most recent. European socialized approaches are possible in part because the money-hungry American system produces break-throughs others can buy or duplicate. [p. 74]

Although many would disagree with the above statement, according to a 1987 Cambridge Report nationwide survey;

While Americans appear to be satisfied with the performance of their health-care system, two out of three say they would favor national health insurance funded by tax dollars. At the same time, however, they appear unwilling to pay what a program might realistically cost. Fewer than 20% say they would be willing to spend more than $50 a year in higher taxes or insurance premiums to help pay for care for people who can't afford it. [Pokorny p. 3]

Others, like Abramowitz (1988), argue that government should promote market competition:

United States health care delivery over the next five to ten years will see tremendous competition, resulting in wider choices for consumers, declining profit margins for virtually all providers, and tottering market shares for traditional providers. The times will increasingly favor managed fee-for-service medicine incorporating preadmission certification, and HMOs and PPOs will proliferate. These trends will eventually shrink excess capacity eliminating marginal providers and causing cost growth to steadily grow, at the same time enabling the quality of health care to rise—assuming of course that the "right" providers leave the market. [Abramowitz, p. 42]

Halvorson (1993) concludes that "our system does exactly what we pay it to do," and a dollar spent on health care is a dollar earned by Americans. The above quotations suggest that (1) the United States has serious problems of cost, access, and quality of health care; (2) how serious these problems are depends on who is answering the question: most of the poor, minority, and rural Americans or most of the rest, which is the majority of the population; (3) how we can solve these problems and the consequences of different approaches is a matter for dispute among the informed (as well the uninformed); moreover, many Americans are indifferent to and uninformed about these matters. Others are perfectly well satisfied with health care the way that it is.

How well the country is doing in health care delivery depends on the standard we wish to compare ourselves against, as well as how we define health.

How healthy is a country where, with 4 to 5% of the world's population, we consume 50% of the world's cocaine? In 1989 alone, approximately 375,000 Americans were born addicted to drugs, mainly cocaine and heroin (Gergen, 1989). Americans possess an estimated 60 million handguns and 120 million long guns and kill each other at a rate of around 19,000 per year, mostly with handguns. American prisons hold more than a million convicted prisoners. Three thousand of every 100,000 black American males are in prison (Wicker). One-fifth of all high-school pupils drop out each year, and various studies claim that millions of Americans, ranging from 23–84 million are functionally illiterate. According to Kozol (1985), 25 million adults cannot read well enough to understand a warning label on a medicine bottle, and 22% of adults are unable to address a letter correctly.

These are not problems usually addressed by a nation's health care delivery system. And yet who can deny that drugs, crime, and illiteracy result in disease, and in the expenditure of millions of dollars that could be reduced if our nation's drug, crime, and literacy rates were the same as those of other developed countries.

On the other hand Americans consume a great deal of health care, much of which is medically unnecessary. Interventions such as physician office visits do not always result in predictable measurable improvements in health status. Does this mean we should make fewer physician and emergency room visits? Not necessarily.

The infant death rate and life expectancy are two common standards for comparing a population's health status. In 1960 the U.S. mortality rate for infants under 1 year of age was 26.0 per 1,000 live births (U.S. Bureau of the Census, 1988). In 1990 the rate had decreased by over half to 9.1 (OECD, 1991). The infant mortality rate in Japan was 4.6 deaths per 1,000 live births (OECD, 1991).

With regard to life expectancy, women live longer than men. In the United States in 1960 life expectancy was 66.6 years for men and 73.1 years for women. By 1990 life expectancy had risen to 72.0 years for men and 78.8 years for women (OECD, 1991). In Japan in 1990 the average life expectancy for men was 75.9 years, 81.9 years for women (OECD, 1991).

On the expenditure side, in 1960 Americans spent $27 billion on health care, which was 5.3% of our gross national product (U.S. Bureau of the Census, 1988). In 1990 we spent $675.0 billion, which was 12.4% of our GNP (OECD, 1991). Japan's health expenditures were $195.4 billion or 6.5% of the GNP in 1990 (OECD, 1991). For 1990, approximately $2,566 per year was being spent for health care for each American, while the Japanese, in 1990, were spending $1,113 for each person (OECD, 1991). And over 35 million Americans lack health insurance, while all Japanese have some form of health insurance.

Do these figures mean that health care for most Americans is not as good as that for most Japanese? Not necessarily. The figures say nothing about the quality of health care, its distribution, its appropriateness, or the way in which care is given. One's answer also depends on how "good health care" is defined. Is emphasis placed on access to care, utilization of care, preventable death and disability, or on perceptions of how care is given by clinicians in organizations? Quality of care also has to do with the standard against which care is measured. Are we comparing the quality of care for all Americans to that of Japanese in 1995? Are we comparing the quality of health care for all Americans in 1995 to that in 1960? Or are we comparing the quality of care used by white Americans in 1995 to that used by black Americans? Different answers will be given to ratings of quality depending on which specific question is asked.

Harris and Associates have surveyed Americans, Britons, and Canadians on these matters. According to their 1988 poll, Americans are significantly less happy with their health care system than either the British or Canadians are with theirs (Blendon, 1989). Only 54% of Americans report being "very satisfied" with their last physician encounter, compared with 73% of Canadians and 63% of British. And only 57% of Americans who were hospitalized in the 12 months prior to the survey say they were "very satisfied" with their hospital stays. This compares to 71% for Canadians and 67% for British. The majority of Americans say they would prefer a system like the Canadian health care system to the one they currently have.

In analyzing the results of the Harris survey, Blendon (1989, p. 7) concludes that

> a new (or perhaps newly recognized) climate of public opinion about health care is taking shape in the 1990s . . . of Americans say they want a fundamental break with their current health care policies and a much more central role played by the federal government in remedying America's health problems.

Blendon is discussing two different questions. First, how satisfied are insured Americans with the health system? Second, how dissatisfied are the more than 35 million Americans who lack adequate health insurance? Prior to the 1988 Harris survey, it was commonly accepted that Americans, if they had adequate health insurance, were more or less satisfied with the system, particularly in contrast to the British. Those lacking health insurance have been dissatisfied for many years, but they have lacked the political power to bring about change.

To what extent are the significant differences that exist among Americans confined to the health sector? Aren't there similar inequities between poor black and most white Americans in education, housing, income, and consumption in general? Why aren't more Americans more concerned about these kinds of inequities, and when, if ever, will we become more concerned? How will we become more concerned if we don't know about the seriousness of the problems? Thirty-six million American adults read below the eighth-grade level, and 45% of Americans never read books. In addition, 46% of black children are below the poverty line (Conn & Silverman, 1991).

This book will not authoritatively answer questions such as (1) who should pay for the care of the nation's uninsured poor; (2) who should pay for extended nursing home care or in-home care for elderly patients; (3) how should health care costs be controlled; and (4) how should quality of care be assured. These are "value" questions, not "fact" questions. Reasonable men and women presented with the same facts on these issues will come up with different answers. Reasonable people may also differ on whether these issues need to be resolved now or in the near future, on what will be the consequences of not doing anything significantly different, and on the consequences of implementing an Option A versus an Option B, C, or D.

This book does present the elements of the health care delivery system, and it analyzes how they function. We describe the people who use health care and the people who provide health care, as well as the organizations in which they work. We examine how different parts of the health care delivery system function, and we discuss assessment of the current and future health care delivery system.

What Is Health Care, and Who Is Served?

The United States had a population of more than 253 million Americans in 1991. The population resides in an area greater than 3.6 million square miles. So we are one of the largest countries in the world, based on either population or area. Unlike that of most European and other developed countries, the American population is heterogeneous—that is, we are made up of people from a wide variety of cultures, races, and ethnic groups, and we are dispersed over a large land mass. This has implications for the types of health care and the ways in which they should be provided. For example rural Eskimos in Alaska, middle-class working people in the suburbs, and blacks who live in our large cities have differing needs in different geographic situations.

In Chapter 2 the many definitions of health and disease are discussed, including their biological, psychological, and social components. Health has its personal and community aspects. And health care can be viewed as a right or as a privilege.

In Chapter 3 we present the principal quantitative measures used to describe the health and illness of the population. Vital statistics are routinely compiled on births, deaths, sickness and health status, and utilization of care by populations. Data concerning health and health care are expressed in terms of numbers and rates. They include demographic characteristics, sickness and health status, and utilization of health services.

Who Provides Health Care in What Kinds of Organizations?

Health care is provided by doctors and nurses and by more than 200 different occupational groups, ranging from physical therapists to lab technicians. Chapters 4 and 5 examine the professionals, particularly physicians and nurses, who provide most of the care. Health care is increasingly being provided in larger and more complex organizations, which are governed and managed. Chapters 6 through 9 examine four leading types of health care organizations: ambulatory care, hospitals, long-term care, and mental health. Some of these types of organizations overlap. For example, health maintenance organizations (HMOs) commonly provide inpatient hospital care, ambulatory care, and mental health services. Mental health organizations and hospitals commonly provide inpatient and outpatient care.

What Are Some Important Ways of Analyzing the Health Care System?

An important way of analyzing the health care sector is by looking at how services are financed. This includes how much money is spent on health care, what the money buys, where the money comes from, and how the money is paid out. Chapter 10 looks at these areas; Chapter 11 examines cost containment. Containing health care costs has been an important national problem for at least 30 years. To ameliorate this problem, we must first understand the factors accounting for increasing costs and then review efforts to control costs, which so far have focused on the hospital. It may then be possible to learn what has succeeded, what has failed, and why.

The government's role in health care is more extensive than that of financing and containing costs; government agencies also regulate providers and provide health services directly. Federal, state, and local governments have different and overlapping health care roles. These are examined in Chapter 12.

Planning is important for health care organizations and is addressed in Chapter 13. As with financing, planning can be analyzed at the various governmental or institutional levels. Techniques for planning health care include measuring health status, analyzing consumer preferences, and measuring and evaluating utilization. Quality control and technology assessment, covered in Chapters 14 and 15, respectively, are concerned with the benefits of health care, sometimes in relationship to their costs. Technology assessment includes evaluating efficacy, safety, and cost-effectiveness by identifying, testing, synthesizing, and disseminating results. The computerized axial tomography (CAT) scanner and the electronic fetal monitor are two technological developments that have been thoroughly assessed in this way.

The quality of care is increasingly being measured as we learn more about the relationship between medical and other interventions and related health outcomes. The quality of health care comprises the patient's health status and attitudes to care and the structures, processes, and outcomes of care. Simply defining what is meant by high-quality care does not guarantee its implementation. Approaches to assuring quality health care include licensing, accreditation and certification, and review of care by organizations such as Professional Review Organizations (PROs) that target inappropriate utilization relative to agreed-upon standards of care. How are policy and administrative decisions made in health care organizations? Chapter 16, "Governance and Management," explores this question by focusing on the role, structure, and function of governing boards and the role, function, and training of health care organization managers.

Chapter 17 looks at health systems in other countries. There is a large literature on the comparative analysis of health care systems, but Americans have rarely attempted to draw lessons from the experience of other countries. This, however, shows signs of changing as Americans have recently looked to the Canadian system with regard to containment of costs. Canada has adequate health insurance for all high levels of health status and has achieved notable success in controlling the growth of health care costs. And of course, other countries can and do learn from the American experience, for example, in the area of quality assessment and assurance.

Health care ethics, addressed in Chapter 18, is a relatively recent academic discipline. Among the major topics in health care ethics are informed consent, do-not-resuscitate orders, forgoing of life-sustaining systems, treatment of multiply handicapped newborns, abortion, confidentiality, allocation of scarce resources, equity of access, and issues relating to the care of AIDS patients.

What Is the Present and Future of Health Care Delivery in the United States?

The authors of this book present the reader with the facts and issues in 18 chapters. In Chapter 19 we review these facts and ask you to consider what should be done to alter health care delivery in the United States in the years ahead. We hope that you will care about these issues, discuss them, and work with us to retain the best in the American system while creating better ways to deliver good-quality health care at reasonable costs to all Americans.

References

Abramowitz, K. S., "The Future of Health Care in America." *MGM Journal*, July/August 1988, p. 42.

Blendon, R. J., "Three Systems: A Comparative Survey." *Health Management Quarterly, 11*(1), 2, 1989.

Committee on the Costs of Medical Care, *Medical Care for the American People.* Chicago: University of Chicago Press, 1932. Reprinted, Washington, DC: USDHEW, 1970.

Conn, C., & Silverman, I. (Eds.), *What Counts—The Complete Harper's Index.* New York: Henry Holt, 1991.

Deuschle, K. W., "Foreword." In S. Jonas (Ed.), *Health Care Delivery in the United States* (pp. x–xi). New York: Springer Publishing Co., 1977.

Easterbrook, G., "The Revolution." *Newsweek*, January 26, 1987, pp. 40–74.

Gergen, D. R., Remember the Drug War?" *US News and World Report*, December 18, 1989, p. 84.

Halvorson, George C. (1993). *Strong Medicine.* New York: Random House, p. 229.

Iglehart, J. K., "Japan's Medical Care System." *New England Journal of Medicine, 319*(17), 1166, 1988.

Kozol, J., *Illiterate America*, Garden City, NY: Doubleday 1985, pp. 4, 8–9.

Lapham, L., Pollan, M., & Etheridge, E., *The Harper's Index Book.* New York: Henry Holt, 1987.

OECD (Organization for Economic and Community Development), 1991. *OECD Health Data*. Paris: OECD.

Pokorny, G., "Report Card on Health Care." *Health Management Quarterly, 10*(1), 3, 1988.

U.S. Bureau of the Census, *Statistical Abstract of the United States* (108th ed.), Washington, DC: U.S. Government Printing Office, 1988.

Wicker, T., "The Iron Medal," *The New York Times*, January 9, 1991, p. A21.

2

Health and Health Care

H. David Banta and Steven Jonas

Introduction

In 1787, Thomas Jefferson wrote:

> Without health there is no happiness. And attention to health, then, should take the place of every other object. The time necessary to secure this by active exercises should be devoted to it in preference to every other pursuit. I know the difficulty with which a strenuous man tears himself from his studies at any given moment of the day; but his happiness, and that of his family depend on it. The most uninformed mind, with a healthy body, is happier than the wisest valetudinarian [person in poor health] (Foley, p. 402).

In our own era, George Sheehan, the "Running Doctor," put it in a slightly simpler way (1989, p. 24):

> Health makes for the happy pursuit of happiness and gives us a longer time to do it.

It seems a truism that the purpose of health care is to promote health. Yet most observers of the U.S. health care system would agree that it has been almost exclusively concerned with the diagnosis and treatment of disease, not with the protection and promotion of health. In that regard, it is noteworthy that the education of health professionals, physicians in particular, focuses almost exclusively on physical pathology and derangements of biophysiologic functioning, rather than health and its maintenance (Jonas, 1978; Millis, 1971).

It is doubtless easier to care for disease than to promote good health. Moreover, such activities as health education lack the drama associated with the high-technology crisis-care so often observed in university hospitals. One must also recognize that our knowledge and understanding of the psychological and social components necessary if the interventions for the promotion of health and prevention of disease is to be most effective, are limited.

Nevertheless, the growth of self-care and alternative systems of care (Eisenberg, et al., 1993; Wolinsky, 1988, Chap. 10), which often stress the incorporation of good health habits into one's everyday life (Wallis, 1991), indicates considerable discontent with the present patterns of health care practice in regard of health promotion/disease prevention. As Freymann (1989) has said, ". . . health is a natural state, and the key to maintaining it lies in lifestyle and the environment."

In the run-up to the introduction of the Clinton health care reform package in 1993, in public statements Hillary Rodham Clinton and others paid a good deal of attention to the importance of including a comprehensive set of preventive services as part of the benefit package in any program finally adopted and implemented. It remains to be seen if those good intentions will be played out in practice.

What are Health and Disease?

Definitions

Historical Development. Health, disease, and illness are terms we use often without thinking about precise definitions. It is easy to think of health as simply being the lack of disease, and of illness and disease as being interchangeable terms. In fact, health and disease are not simply opposites, and disease and illness do not mean the same thing (Kass, 1981; Wolinsky, 1988, Chap. 4).

The Greeks made a philosophical distinction between the concepts of health and disease. As the medical historian Sigerist (1970, p. 57) said:

> The [ancient Greek] physicians had an explanation for health. Health, they believed, was a condition of perfect equilibrium. When the forces or humors or whatever constituted the human body were perfectly balanced, man was healthy. Disturbed balance resulted in disease. This is still the best general explanation we have.

This was the view of the followers of the Greek Goddess of *health*, Hygeia, daughter of Apollo, the supreme healer (Durant, 1939, pp. 342–348). The Greek physician Hippocrates, for whom is named the present professional oath that many medical school graduates take, focused his own teaching on health promotion. For the individual, the teaching addressed such elements as exercise, nutrition, and achieving the "Greek mean," that is, moderation in all things. For the population as a whole, the teaching addressed public health measures, to the extent they were understood at the time. The Romans continued the Greek "Hygienic" approach to health, stressing especially its public health aspects.

However, the followers of the Greek God of *medicine*, Asklepios (a son of Apollo), concentrated on disease and miracle cures. With the collapse of civilization that accompanied the gradual disintegration of the Roman Empire and the eventual rise of Christianity, the idea of disease was given a preferential place. The Greek idea of health as a perfect balance had little meaning to the masses of the Dark and Middle Ages, and even the Renaissance and Enlightenment periods, living as they did in poverty, sickness, and oppression. Magic, miracle cures, and religious salvation became the focus of what attention to health there was.

In our own era, even after the development of scientific medicine, the idea of an approach to health based on curing, even of miracle cures (think of the term "medical miracle" as it is applied to the latest surgical intervention) has persisted. It is still a seductive dream. Cures are sought that can compensate, not for unknown or misunderstood causes of illness, but for well-known abuses of the body the individual and society have themselves perpetuated—correcting at a stroke the effects of cigarette smoking, or of breathing polluted air, or of working in an unhealthy workplace over a period of years.

Health. Webster's Unabridged Dictionary reflects the age-old conflict over the relationship between health and disease. It defines health first as "physical and mental well-being," but then continues, "freedom from defect, pain, or disease." Disease, too, Webster's defines ambiguously: "uneasiness or distress," and more sweepingly, "any departure from health." Adding to the confusion, what we often call "health statistics" are in fact disease statistics, and health care is most often disease care. Furthermore, the word "health" is sometimes used as an adjective when health is not the focus of that use. Jago (1975) listed 43 examples of such use, including "health status," "health center," and "health worker," which in practice most often mean, respectively, "sickness status," "disease treatment center," and "disease care worker."

The World Health Organization (WHO) defined health as a (1958, p. 459):

> . . . state of complete physical, mental, and social well-being, and not merely the absence of disease or infirmity.

This definition has been criticized as being utopian (Dubos, 1971; Kass, 1981). A more functional definition is that proposed by Kass, namely, "the well-working of the organism as a whole" (p. 4).

Other definitions of health have stressed life functioning, seeing health as the "state of optimum capacity for effective performance of valued tasks" (Parsons, 1958, p. 168) or as "personal fitness for survival and self-renewal, creative social adjustment, and self-fulfillment" (Hoyman, 1967, p. 189). The 1988 *Consensus Statement on Exercise, Fitness, and Health* defined health as (Bouchard et al., 1988, p. 6):

> . . . a human condition with physical, social, and psychological dimensions, each characterized on a continuum with positive and negative poles. Positive health is

associated with a capacity to enjoy life and to withstand challenges; it is not merely the absence of disease. Negative health is associated with morbidity and, in the extreme, with mortality.

Taking into account all of these different approaches to a definition of health and the many others not quoted here, a useful functional definition of health is perhaps as follows:

A state of well-being, of feeling good about oneself, of optimum functioning, of the absence of disease, and of the control and reduction of both internal and external risk factors for both disease and negative health conditions.

(A risk factor is some environmental element, personal habit, or living condition which increases the likelihood of developing a particular disease or negative health condition at some time in the future.)

Health status indicators have been developed to measure functioning as an outcome of health care (Kaplan et al., 1976; Mc Peek et al., 1977; Mushkin & Dunlop, 1979; see also Chapters 3 and 13, Fourth Edition. Many have been proposed; none broadly accepted. A comprehensive review of health status indicators was published by McDowell and Newell (1987) in the mid-1980s.

Health and Dying. Interestingly enough, none of the definitions of health presented above see death as the natural endpoint of life. But some consider that how one comes to terms with death and suffering must be a part of one's health. As Sheehan (1989) said (pp. 230, 233):

Death makes the everyday magical, the ordinary unique, the commonplace one-of-a-kind. . . . Once I accept death, I center on the present. . . . To have a death worth dying, you must have a life worth living.

And what would a "life worth living" be, according to Sheehan? "The normal life," he said (p. 3), "is one of continual expansion." And, he went on (p. 5):

Life is not a skill sport. . . . It is a game that anyone can play and play well.. . . The diligent use of our allotted life span is the secret of the successful life.

But as the boundaries of what we called "life," (not always "successful life" in the Sheehan sense) are stretched ever further with tubes and wires by modern, hi-tech, organ-focused medicine, it becomes increasingly important to take into consideration that part of health that sees dying at a certain time as well as living in a certain way. Considering the argument that death must be part of a definition of health, some people surveyed find some states of life worse than death (Williams, 1988) (see also the section below on the "Kevorkian situation").

Disease and Illness. A classic medical dictionary, Blakiston's, took a precise, functional approach to defining disease (1956):

> . . . a failure of the adaptive mechanisms of an organism to counteract adequately the stimuli and stresses to which it is subject, resulting in a disturbance in function or structure of any part, organ, or system of the body.

Recall that Webster's Unabridged Dictionary called disease "uneasiness or distress" and "any departure from health." The Random House Unabridged Dictionary is much more precise (Flexner, 1987):

> . . . a disordered or incorrectly functioning organ, part, structure, or system of the body resulting from the effect of genetic or developmental errors, infection, poisons, nutritional deficiency or imbalance, toxicity, or unfavorable environmental factors; . . . .

Whatever its definition, however, disease is a biomedical concept, a state of being that a health care worker finds. Illness, on the other hand, is a state of being that the ill person feels. As Cassell said (1976, p. 48):

> . . . let us use the word "illness" to stand for what the patient feels when he goes to the doctor and "disease" for what he has on the way home from the doctor's office. Disease, then, is something an organ has; illness is something a man has.

Illness has social and psychological as well as biomedical components. One can have a disease without feeling ill, as in asymptomatic hypertension; and one can surely be ill without being diseased. As it is for the most part practiced in the United States, medicine still has trouble incorporating these concepts into its ethic.

Some progress has been made, however, with the gradual adoption of the Parsons' (1951) "sick role" concept (Wolinsky, Chap. 5). It was the first modern approach to extending our understanding of "nonhealth" beyond the biomedical model, relating disease/illness to social roles. For Parsons:

> . . . the sick role has four components: 1) the nonresponsibility of the individual for his or her condition, 2) the exemption of the sick individual from normal task and role obligations, 3) the recognition that being sick is undesirable and one should want to get well, and 4) the obligation to seek out competent help.

USA Disease Profile: Changes Over Time

There have been some remarkable improvements in population health levels in the United States since 1900. (For a fuller consideration of health and disease data, see Chapter 3.) Unfortunately, the most readily available and verifiable data are for mortality, not morbidity. Furthermore, as noted above there are not as yet any generally accepted direct measures of health itself. Thus, for long-term historical analysis of health levels, we are forced to rely on mortality data.

Between 1900 and 1990 in the United States, both the overall (crude) death rate and infant mortality rate fell, while life expectancy from birth rose (see Table 2.1). While crude mortality declined by 50% during that period, the infant mortality rate declined by about 90%. In fact, the major portion of the decline in the crude mortality rate is due to the remarkable drop in mortality that occurred generally in the younger age groups in the population.

Table 2.2 shows the 1990 age-specific mortality rates as percentages of the 1900 age-specific mortality rates. The death rate for the 1- to 4-year-old age group in 1990 was less than 3% of the rate in 1900, whereas for people over age 85 in 1990 it was close to 60% of the 1900 rate. Note too the large gap in percentage improvement between the 15-to-35 age group and the 45-to-65 age group.

This evidence that life expectancy improvements over time are primarily due to declines in the death rates of the younger age-groups is corroborated if one looks at mortality data in another way. Table 2.3 shows the average number of years of

TABLE 2.1 Mortality Rate, Infant Mortality Rate, and Life Expectancy from Birth, U.S., 1900–1990

Year	Crude mortality rate (per 1,000 pop.)	Infant mortality rate per 1,000 live births(a)	Life expectancy from birth (in years)
1900	17.2	(99.9)	47.3
1920	13.0	85.9	54.1
1940	10.8	47.0	62.9
1960	9.5	26.0	69.7
1970	9.5	20.0	70.9
1980	8.8	12.6	73.7
1990	8.6	9.1	75.4

(a) Data available only from 1915

Sources: Data for 1900–1960 derived from R. D. Grove and A. M. Hetzel, Vital Statistics Rates in the United States, 1940–1960 (National Center for Health Statistics, U.S. Dept. of Health, Education and Welfare, 1968), Tables 38, 51, and 53. Data for 1970 are from *Health United States, 1979* (National Center for Health Statistics), Tables 8, 9, and 10. Data for 1980 are from *Health United States, 1983* (National Center for Health Statistics), Tables 9, 10, and 11. Data for 1990 are from *Monthly Vital Statistics Report,* Vol. 41, No. 7, "Advance Report of Final Mortality Statistics, 1990," pp. 2–3, and *Monthly Vital Statistics Report,* Vol 40, No. 13, "Annual Summary of Births, Marriages, Divorces, and Deaths, 1991," p. 8.

TABLE 2.2   Age-Specific Mortality Rates, U.S., 1900 and 1990

Age group (years)	Age-specific mortality rate (per 1,000 pop.)		1990 rate as % of 1900 rate
	1900	1990	
1–4	19.8	0.5	2.5
5–14	3.9	0.2	5.0
15–24	5.9	1.0	17.0
25–34	8.2	1.4	17.1
35–44	10.2	2.3	22.6
45–54	15.0	4.8	32.0
55–64	27.2	12.0	44.1
65–74	56.4	27.1	48.0
75–84	123.3	63.1	51.2
85 and over	260.9	153.3	58.8

Source: Statistical Abstract of the United States, 1974 (Bureau of the Census, U.S. Dept. of Commerce, 1974), Table 83, and *Monthly Vital Statistics Report*, Vol. 40, No. 13, "Annual Summary of Births, Marriages, Divorces, and Deaths, 1991, Table 2.

TABLE 2.3   Average Remaining Lifetime in Years at Specified Ages, U.S., 1900 and 1990, and Percentage Change Between 1900 and 1990

Age in years	Life expectancy		Years difference	% change
	1900	1990		
0	47.3	75.4	28.1	59.4
5	55.0	71.2	16.2	29.5
15	46.8	61.3	14.5	31.0
25	39.1	51.9	12.8	32.7
35	31.9	42.6	11.0	34.5
45	24.8	33.4	8.6	34.7
55	17.9	24.8	6.9	38.5
65	11.9	17.2	5.3	44.5
75	7.1	10.9	3.8	53.5
85	4.0	6.1	2.1	52.5

Source: Statistical Abstract of the United States, 1971, 1974, 1978, and 1993 (U.S. Bureau of the Census, Dept. of Commerce, 1971, 1974, 1978, and 1993, Table 117).

life remaining at specified ages in 1900 and in 1990 and the percentage change in life expectancy at specified ages between those two years. The percentage increase in life expectancy is a large one.

Further, in 1990 one could expect to live 28.1 years longer from birth than one could in 1900. However, upon reaching age 65, one could expect to live only 5.3 years longer than one could have in 1900. Tables 2.2 and 2.3 thus indicate that the most important factor in the fall in the crude mortality and the rise of life expectancy from birth is the decrease in the infant mortality rate. If many more individuals survive the first year of life and then live into their 60s and 70s, the overall life expectancy of any one group of such fortunate infants is going to rise.

The leading causes of death changed significantly between 1900 and 1990. In 1900, the ten leading causes of death by diagnosis were, in order, influenza and pneumonia, tuberculosis, gastritis, heart disease, stroke, personal injury, chronic nephritis, cancer, "diseases of early infancy," and diphtheria (USNOVS, 1950, Table 2.26). In 1990, the ten leading causes of death by diagnosis were heart disease, cancer, stroke, personal injury, chronic obstructive pulmonary disease, pneumonia and influenza, diabetes mellitus, suicide, chronic liver disease and cirrhosis, and human immunodeficiency virus infection (MVSR, 1990, Table 6).

In 1990 the top ten causes of death by major contributing factor were: tobacco use, diet and activity patterns, ethyl alcohol use, microbial agents, toxic agents, firearms, sexual behavior, motor vehicle operation, and illicit drug use (McGinniss & Foege, 1993). In 1900, three of the five leading killers by diagnosis were infectious diseases. In 1990, none of the top five were infectious diseases. But for each of the leading killer diagnostic categories in that year, cigarette smoking and/or alcohol abuse was a major risk factor.

Determinants of Health

Biological/Environmental Factors. Health is obviously dependent upon biological factors. Genetic endowment of the individual is the starting point, and the importance of genetics may have been underestimated in recent years. For example, a number of studies have demonstrated that there is a genetic basis for alcoholism (Reich, 1988). Those who contract lung cancer from smoking cigarettes may well have a genetic predisposition for the disease. The essential point is that the interaction between genetic factors and the environment in producing individual disease is enormously complex, and much research is needed to fully elucidate the relationship.

Health is certainly to a large extent the result of the complex interaction of the soma with the environment (Berkman & Breslow, 1983, see esp. Chap. 3; Burnett, 1971). The environment includes physical surroundings, social factors (largely beyond the control of the individual), and personal lifestyle. We now know beyond question that such risk factors as diet, air and water pollution, occupational hazards, and cigarette smoking are critical in the genesis of chronic disease. For example, epidemiological studies indicate that the occurrence of about 90% of cancers is attributable to environmental factors such as cigarette smoking, diet, sexual behavior, occupational exposure, and sunlight (Thomas, 1992, Table 47-5).

The Role of Medicine in Improving Health Levels Over Time. In 1857 the tuberculosis death rate in Massachusetts was 450 per 100,000; by 1890, the rate had fallen to 250; by 1920, to 114; and by 1938, to 35.6 (Sigerist, 1970, p. 46). Yet the first specific antituberculosis therapy was not in general use until after 1938. This is convincing evidence that the prevalence of a disease can decline dramatically without effective medical care, apparently related to environmental factors.

An analysis of falling death rates and increasing population size since 1841 in England and Wales has shown that these changes considerably preceded the introduction of any effective direct medical intervention. Death rates in England and Wales fell from about 22 per 1,000 in 1841 to around 6 per 1,000 in 1971. In a seminal study, McKeown (1976, pp. 93–94) concluded that 92% of the death rate decline between 1848 and 1901 and 73% of that between 1901 and 1971 resulted from a reduction in the number of deaths from infectious diseases. Most of this reduction was due to a drop in the tuberculosis death rate that paralleled the one occurring in Massachusetts at the same time.

In England and Wales as in Massachusetts, death rates from respiratory tuberculosis fell steadily from 1838, although effective chemotherapy for the disease was not available until 1948. This is not to say that effective treatments should not be sought. After 1948, the decline in the tuberculosis death rate did accelerate, indicating an effect of chemotherapy. However, in the 1990s the tuberculosis incidence rate in the United States rose. This occurred as an apparent concomitant of Acquired Immunodeficiency Syndrome (AIDS) and intravenous drug use. The increase is at least in part the result of the incomplete application of preventive measures during the preceding 30 years when the disease might have been virtually eradicated in the United States, not any failure of treatment *per se.*

McKeown (1976) also examined the death rates for bronchitis, pneumonia, and influenza, which, after tuberculosis, were the major causes of mortality in the infectious disease era. The death rates for these conditions was little affected by the introduction of antibiotics. As was the case with tuberculosis, those deaths had dropped significantly before their discovery. Rather, McKeown concluded, improvement in nutrition over the period 1750–1950 was the most important influence on the improving health levels that occurred during that time. (The first element in that improvement was simply an increase in the *amount* of food generally available, due to the improvement in farming techniques, the development of the first bulk transportation system, the canals, and possibly the climatic warming trend that occurred just before the beginning of that period.)

McKeown estimated that hygienic measures, such as improvement in water supplies and sewage disposal, were responsible for about one-fifth of the reduction. Moreover, he stated (p. 94):

> With the exception of vaccination against smallpox, whose contribution was small, the influence of immunization and therapy on the death rate was delayed until the 20th century, and had little effect on national mortality trends before the introduction of sulphonamides in 1935. Since that time it has not been the only, or [even] the most important influence.

Since the mid-1970s in the United States, there have been significant declines in the heart disease, stroke, personal injury, and nontobacco-related cancer death rates (McGinnis, 1993). It appears that these are the result of preventive measures such as improved early detection and treatment of hypertension, reduction in driving-while-intoxicated-related trauma, increased use of automobile seatbelts, the lowering of dietary fat and cholesterol, and the decline in cigarette smoking among adults. Nevertheless, the unmet opportunities for health promotion/disease prevention to improve the health of the American people remain legion.

Psychological Factors in Health

The biomedical model of health and disease has been challenged over the years. For example, as Engel (1981) said, this model (p. 591):

> . . . assumes disease to be fully accounted for by deviations from the norm of measurable biological variables. It leaves no room within its framework for the social, psychological and behavioral dimensions of illness.

Yet, as he also said, treatment directed at a biochemical abnormality does not necessarily restore health. This is because of discrepancies between the physical measurements and the psychological and social variables. Parsons' sick role model (1951) discussed briefly above, and its more modern variants as developed by Freidson and others (Wolinsky, 1988, Chaps. 4, 5), also has bearing on this concept.

Although there is much disagreement as to just what constitutes mental health and mental illness, derangements in psychic functioning have been shown to cause physical health problems, including death (Friedman, 1990). For example, a large body of research has demonstrated the effects of bereavement (Osterweis, Solomon, & Green, 1984), leading Engel to ask, "Is grief a disease?" His answer is, "Yes, if the grieving person is functioning badly" (p. 601).

At the same time, the health care provider's behavior and "the relationship between patient and physician powerfully influence therapeutic outcome for better or for worse. These constitute psychological effects which may directly modify the illness experience or indirectly affect underlying biochemical processes" (Engel, 1981, p. 599). As Friedman noted (1990, pp. 4, 8):

> . . . the relationship between personality and disease is not a simple one. People are complex, dynamic organisms [that] are constantly facing new environments, growing and aging, and striving to maintain health. Understanding the relationship between personality and disease necessitates a sophisticated appreciation of the relevant issues. . . . In brief, [however], there is evidence that patterns of negative emotions are associated with illness, and there is evidence to deem it physiologically plausible that personality would play a causal role in disease.

Social Factors in Health

Since health and illness are defined functionally, as noted, sickness can be seen not only as a biological phenomenon but also in terms of a social role that carries with it certain rights and obligations (Brown, 1989, pp. 142–145). However, even when a person has brought an illness upon themselves—as in a careless self-induced personal injury or lung cancer caused by cigarette smoking—they are not assumed to be solely responsible for the process of getting well. Going beyond the individual to society as a whole, it is by now clear that social factors have a very significant impact on disease and health (Brown, 1989, Section One). Although much remains to be learned, the science of *social epidemiology* (Wolinsky, 1988, Chap. 1) has elucidated the relationship between many social characteristics, such as nationality, social class, race, employment status, occupation, behavior patterns, and geography, and states of health and illness.

The Role of the Health Care Delivery System

What Health Care Is. Health services have been defined as (1) those services delivered by personnel engaged in medical occupations, such as physicians and nurses, plus other personnel working under their supervision; (2) the physical capital, such as hospitals, in which services are provided; and (3) the other goods and services, from drugs to medical information systems, used by the personnel in the facilities to provide the services (Fuchs, 1966). Taking a less functional, more outcome-oriented viewpoint, Weinerman defined the health services system as (1971, p. 273):

> All of the activities of a society which are designed to protect or restore health, whether directed to the individual, the community, or the environment.

However they are defined, health and health care services may generally be divided into two broad categories: personal and community. Personal health care services deal directly with individuals for the maintenance of health or the control or cure of illness. Community health services are directed toward population groups. They include such services as: the provision of pure drinking water, sanitary sewage disposal, solid waste disposal; food, milk, and drug control and inspection; fluoridation of water; and control of air and noise pollution.

A number of health services—which can be called "combined" services—have aspects of both community and personal health services. Mass immunization programs protect each immunized individual and also protect the community as a whole, by a phenomenon called "herd immunity." This is especially the case for diseases caused by obligatory human parasites like the now-eradicated smallpox virus. Other such combined community and individual services include tuberculosis and venereal disease case-finding and treatment programs, which while helping infected individuals also gradually reduce the total number of sources of infection for healthy persons, thereby contributing to community health.

If health care is in part aimed at improving or assisting social functioning, it must grapple with societal as well as individual health problems. Perhaps overstating the case somewhat, Virchow, the great German pathologist who as a youth fought on the barricades against Bismarck's authoritarian Prussian government, described his profession in these words (Sigerist, 1970, p. 93):

> Medicine is a social science and politics is nothing else but medicine on a large scale.

Goals and Objectives for Health Promotion/Disease Prevention. In 1979, the United States Public Health Service published *Healthy People: The Surgeon General's Report on Health Promotion and Disease Prevention* (USDHEW, 1979). As the then Secretary of Department of Health, Education, and Welfare, Joseph Califano, said (p. vii):

> . . . the purpose of this Report is to encourage a second public health revolution in the United States. . . . This document is properly optimistic about our growing scientific knowledge and about the possibility of setting clear measurable goals for public health action.

The *Report's* opening chapter states (p. 3):

> It is the thesis of this report that further improvements in the health of the American people can and will be achieved—not through increased medical care and greater health expenditures—but through a renewed national commitment to efforts designed to prevent disease and to promote health.

The *Report* then set specific health objectives in 15 "priority areas" for intervention, ranging from family planning and toxic agent control to smoking cessation.

They were arranged in three categories: Health Promotion, Health Protection, and Preventive Services.

In 1991, the Department of Health Human Services published the second iteration of this work, *Healthy People 2000: National Health Promotion and Disease Prevention Objectives* (USDHHS, 1991). In his foreword to *Healthy People 2000*, Dr. Louis Sullivan, then Secretary of Health and Human Services, said (p. v):

> . . . health promotion and disease prevention comprise perhaps our best opportunity to reduce the ever-increasing portion of our resources that we spend to treat preventable illness and functional impairment. . . . We would be terribly remiss if we did not seize the opportunity presented by health promotion and disease prevention to dramatically cut health care costs, to prevent the premature onset of disease and disability, and to help all Americans achieve healthier, more productive lives.

Dr. Sullivan pointed out that illnesses related to cigarette smoking—a both preventable and treatable drug addiction—"cost our health care system more than $65 billion annually" [as of 1989], that AIDS, which in ten years came from nowhere to be in the top ten killers nationally, "is an almost entirely preventable disease," and that alcoholism and drug abuse other than cigarette smoking, both significantly preventable, together cost the society over $100 billion annually in treatment costs, premature death, personal injury, crime, and lost productivity.

Continuing the emphasis of the original report, *Healthy People 2000* sets three "overarching goals" (p. 43): increase the span of healthy life for Americans, reduce health disparities among Americans, achieve access to preventive services for all Americans. To reach these goals, the number of "priority areas" for intervention was expanded to 22, grouped in the same intervention categories as presented in the 1979 *Report*, plus a new one for data collection (Table 2.4).

Examples of objectives for the year 2000 include (pp. 91–125): reduce coronary heart disease deaths to no more than 100 per 100,000 people; reduce deaths caused by unintentional injuries to no more than 29.3 per 100,000 people; increase years of healthy life to at least 65 years.

Reviewing the top ten causes of death by diagnosis in the U.S. as of 1990, heart disease, cancer, stroke, personal injury, chronic obstructive pulmonary disease, pneumonia and influenza, diabetes mellitus, suicide, chronic liver disease and cirrhosis, and human immunodeficiency virus infection (MVSR, 1990, Table 6), and the top ten causative factors of death (McGinniss & Foege, 1993) it can be seen by an examination of the priority areas that the full implementation of the described interventions would have a very significant positive impact upon the health status of the American people.

Progress toward achieving the objectives is summarized each year in the annual publication *Health United States* (USDHHS, 1992). To consider the scientific basis of many common health promotive/disease preventive measures, "An

TABLE 2.4 National Health Promotion and Disease Prevention Objectives Priority Areas, Grouped by Category

Health Promotion

1. Physical activity and fitness	5. Family Planning
2. Nutrition	6. Mental Health and Mental Disorders
3. Tobacco	7. Violent and Abusive Behavior
4. Alcohol and other drugs	8. Educational and Community-Based Programs

Health Protection

9. Unintentional injuries	12. Food and drug safety
10. Occupational safety and health	13. Oral health
11. Environmental health	

Preventive services

14. Maternal and infant health	18. HIV infection
15. Heart disease and stroke	19. Sexually transmitted diseases
16. Cancer	20. Immunization and infectious diseases
17. Diabetes and chronic disabling conditions	21. Clinical preventive services

Surveillance and Data Systems
22. Surveillance and data systems

Source: USDHHS, *Healthy People 2000* (see reference list), p. vii.

Assessment of the Effectiveness of 169 Interventions" used for personal health promotion/disease prevention efforts was carried out by the U.S. Preventive Services Task Force. Its first report, the *Guide to Clinical Preventive Services*, was published in 1989 (USPSTF, 1989). Publication of the second edition is expected in 1995.

The Task Force approached the area of prevention as all health services should be analyzed. What is the evidence of effectiveness? Is the evidence convincing that the intervention should be made part of the standard package of services? Alternatively, should unproven procedures be allowed, even encouraged, to be widely diffused, as if often the case in the curative medical sector? While we strongly support broad recognition of the importance of preventive services, we agree with the Task Force that they should be proven to be of benefit before they are broadly offered. The Task Force did identify a number of common preventive interventions that are not effective, or probably not effective, underlining the importance of this point.

Reviewing the status of the *Healthy People 2000* project as of the summer of 1993, the Office of Disease Prevention/Health Promotion of the U.S. Public Health Service concluded (*Prevention report*, 1993, p. 1):

For some objectives, trends are going in the wrong direction; for others no changes are reported. For a number of objectives, substantial progress has occurred, with a few targets having been achieved.

Obviously, the general approach works, but much remains to be done. It is to be hoped that whatever system for national health care reform is finally adopted in the United States, significant attention to the achievement of the established health promotion/disease prevention objectives will be provided for (McGinniss, 1989).

Health and High-Tech Medicine: Areas of Conflict. As the US health care delivery system has developed, it has concentrated with an ever-increasing emphasis on high-tech, hospital-based, acute disease care, whether at the beginning, in the middle, or at the end of life. In addition to the missed opportunities for prevention cited above, super high-technology interventions themselves have produced negatives. Consider the following story (Jonas, 1993, [c]).

> Several weeks ago, my friend Harry's wife died. This lady was in her early 70s. The ultimate cause of her death will not be found recorded on her death certificate. For want of better phraseology, it is best described as "fear-of-what-the-doctors-and-the-hospitals-might-do-to-me-if-I-get-really-sick-and-lose-control-of-my-own-destiny."
>
> About 20 years ago Harry's wife had a heart valve replaced, a true miracle of modern medicine. Early in the spring of 1993, Harry's wife needed some dental surgery. She was told that it was essential for her to take anti-biotics both before and after the dental work. Having some fears about that, she failed to do so.
>
> Developing an infection following the dental work, she again failed to take the anti-biotics. The artificial valve and her remaining natural main valve both became infected. She finally went on medication, but by this time it was too late. Both valves decompensated. Told she would need a pacemaker, and possibly a replacement of her remaining natural valve, she refused both interventions and died soon thereafter.
>
> Why did this otherwise healthy, hale, and hearty woman refuse treatment, all along the line, even of prophylactic antibiotics? Because, Harry told me, she was scared of what modern, invasive, high-tech medicine might do to her if she got really sick and went totally under its control. She was deathly afraid of ending up in a hospital, attached to tubes and wires, with no quality of life, and worse yet, no say in what was being done to her.
>
> "I really thought we would have a few more years together," Harry told me sadly. "What a tragedy," I thought. "It was fear of what my profession might do *to* her, not happy anticipation of what it might do *for* her, that seems to have deprived you and your wife of those years."

Or consider the case of Michigan's Dr. Jack Kevorkian, labelled "Dr. Death" by the media (Jonas, 1993 [a]). He made a practice of assisting suicides by terminally ill people, at their request, of course. In 1993, the Michigan State Legislature passed a law specifically aimed at preventing Dr. Kevorkian from doing that. One important question is whether a licensed physician should be able to help a fully competent, adult patient, commit suicide. But the broader issue is *why* there were so many people who *wanted* Dr. Kevorkian's help.

Why does the health care delivery system routinely substitute its wishes and judgement for that of the patient and keep people alive, but in great pain and/or great disability, in many cases forcing them to spend money which cannot in any way buy them health, but which will disappear into the pockets of the health care providers rather than being available to the patient's surviving family members? *Why* has so much time and money been spent figuring out ways to keep people alive at the ends of their lives, so little spent in figuring out how to help people make life healthier and happier during the bulk of it? *Why* is a physician who decides to treat indefinitely when there is no hope of recovery *and* the patient wishes so mightily that he or she would just stop, any more practicing good medicine than the Dr. Kevorkians of this world?

The Caring Function. Health professionals sometimes become so involved in delivering technology-driven services that they neglect one of medicine's traditionally most roles, caring for people. As Sigerist (1970, p. 93) said:

> Disease, then, is a biological process. . . . But this process takes place in man, and thus always involves the mind. . . . Disease, a destructive process that threatens life, may destroy only a few cells that can easily be replaced, but it may destroy the entire organism and with it the individual. For this reason, man suffers and is afraid: disease reminds him that he is mortal, that he must die sooner or later, and if the illness is serious, it may be very soon. . . . Elementary fears, age-old views, come from the depth of the unconscious, breaking through the thin crust of education.

Although care has a long history, it is little spoken of in today's technological world of medicine. However, there are studies that support the importance of care. It has been shown that patients who demonstrate acceptance—measured by a scale including trust in the surgeon, optimism about the outcome, and confidence in their ability to cope—healed faster in a trial involving eye surgery (Frank, 1975). Caring itself can be an effective method of therapy (Haggerty, 1979; Mechanic, 1974, pp. 129–130). As noted earlier in this chapter, there is extensive evidence that psychological and social supports affect medical outcomes.

The Value We Place on Health

It is commonly felt among health professionals that all possible services should be provided by the health care system. But are people willing to support health services to that extent? Health is certainly an important value, but it is not the only value. Achilles recognized this in the Iliad:

> Either, if I stay here and fight beside the city of the Trojans, my return home is
> gone, but my glory shall be everlasting; but if I return home to the beloved land of
> my fathers, the excellence of my glory is gone, but there will be a long life left for
> me, and my end in death will not come to me quickly (Homer, 1951, p. 209).

Achilles chose to stay and die. The modern analogue might be the skydiver or
skier who intentionally takes a risk for the sake of the thrill derived from the sport.
To the extent that the public is aware of risk factors, one could say that the person
who smokes cigarettes, eats saturated fats, or refuses to wear seat belts is deciding that other values are more important than good health.

Society can invest more in justice, beauty, or knowledge, in the same way as it
invests in health (Fuchs, 1974). Health economists deal with the problem of limited resources for such investments by speaking of marginal benefit and marginal
cost. Is the added benefit of a day in the hospital, for example, worth the added
cost? What are our values and priorities? Every physician confronts conflicting
values each day in practice. A person may continue to indulge in unhealthy behavior, even though knowing the risks, because the values of the person make
that behavior more important than theoretical future health consequences. Such
problems can be dealt with only by active, public intervention in matter that society generally considers personal.

It may not be necessary to intervene actively in affecting values and behavior
in all cases. Workplaces can be engineered for safety. Beef can be produced with
less saturated fat. Air bags can be installed in all cars. Cigarettes can be made that
are safer; in fact, the amount of tar and nicotine in the average cigarette has been
reduced approximately 25% over the past 20 years. Although the balance between
public health and personal freedom is difficult to attain, society cannot afford to
be passive in the face of mounting evidence of risk factors that can in many cases
be controlled. Some interventions are necessary to protect the public, as when
vaccination was made compulsory, over the objections of a vocal minority.

As Sigerist (1970, p. 102) said:

> The people's health is the concern of the people themselves. They must be enlight-
> ened in matters of health. They must want it and take an active part in its adminis-
> tration. And since the protection of health is a task of great magnitude, the people
> will endeavor to fulfill it collectively through the state and its organs. That is why
> health is a primary concern of the people and of government.

What Needs to be Done

Producing Health; Containing Disease. Four primary elements determine
health and disease: human biology, environment, lifestyle, and health care
(Lalonde, 1974). To be healthy, one needs both a good external environment, such
as a healthy food supply, decent housing, productive employment opportunities,

and control of external disease-causing factors, and a good internal environment, such as is created by eating a balanced diet, exercising regularly, not smoking cigarettes, controlling drug and alcohol use, maintaining a positive self-image, managing stress in a healthy way, and so on. As noted above, as the United States struggles with health policy reform, these issues need to be considered equally with cost and access.

Much of the current discussion about national health insurance and health care delivery system reform is based on the premise that the two basic problems requiring solution are those of access and cost (Jonas, 1993 [b]). Once they are taken care of, so conventional wisdom goes, everything else will be fine. That is the original premise on which the first stage U.S. national health insurance system was likely to be designed (before the advent of the debate stimulated by the submission of the original Clinton Health Plan). That premise is in fact incorrect, which is why the first stage US-NHI plan may not work as predicted and may not produce significant improvements in health care in the United States, except to the extent that it provides coverage for the currently uncovered.

Why is that so? Because the *underlying* problems of the US health care delivery system are *not* access and cost. Those are simply outcomes of in-built and long-standing system difficulties. The underlying problems are rather those of access *to* what and expenditures *for* what. If the money the American people are spending on health care bought the kind of health and health care product it easily could buy, then: (a) we all would be among the healthiest people in the world (which by certain common counts of mortality, at least, we are not [USBOC, 1993, Table 1376]); and, (b) there would probably be little concern about the amount of money being spent.

Most proposals on the table in 1993 would attempt to contain cost increases by controlling the supply of funds. However, only certain ones, like the Clinton Health Plan (1993), begin to get at *why* the U.S. health care system is so expensive, or its failure to meet the health and health care needs of the American people.

Primarily, the U.S. system is so expensive not because of its administrative arrangements (although if one set out to design a more expensive administrative system, this would be difficult to devise) [Woolhandler et al., 1993]). Rather, the system is so expensive because of what it does and doesn't do in the *practice of medicine* and the *delivery of health care*, e.g., spending billions on "saving" low birth-weight babies with high-tech machines, spending little to reduce the incidence of low birth-weight babies, spending billions to prolong unhealthy life at the end of the life span, spending little to help people live healthy lives to the end of it, spending billions on expensive testing, spending little on communicating the results of those tests and other vital health promoting/disease preventing information and attitudes to patients.

To correct the fundamental illogic of this approach, the way doctors practice medicine and the way they are paid has to be changed, the way hospitals deliver services and the way they arc paid has to be changed. Unless the adopted alternative for U.S. national health reform, be it "managed care" or "managed competition" or "tax incentives and medical savings accounts," even "Canadian-style," is made to directly address the practice of medicine, the delivery of health services by institutions, biomedical research, and health sciences education policy, the *health* and *health care* of the American people will not be significantly improved. To do that, major changes will have to be made in each of these arenas (hopefully by incentive, not by direction), beginning with changing the primary orientation of each to one that puts much more emphasis on health.

Unfortunately, with a few exceptions reform proposals have paid relatively little attention to the content of care and the technology of care (see Chapter 15). The fact is that relatively few interventions in health care have been clearly shown to be of benefit (Banta & Luce, 1993; Brook & Lohr, 1985). Brook and Lohr (1986) estimated that in the United States from 30 to 50% of expenditures support services that produce little or no demonstrable benefit.

Recently, a proposal has been made to change medical education itself to an "evidence base" (Evidence-Based Medicine Working, 1992). The proposal acknowledges that medicine traditionally has included and excluded the use of interventions based on the personal experience of faculty, and the latter have used authority more commonly than science to convince their students to follow their precepts. Clinicians, however, can be taught to be skeptical of unsupported authority and to seek good clinical evidence before using various interventions. Changes in access to information, such as those promoted by the U.S. National Library of Medicine (which is moving to include technology assessment in its indexing systems) can support such changes in education.

Patients also need to be informed of the uncertainties in health care practice. How many patients would accept major surgery if they were told that experts disagreed as to whether or not it was effective in that circumstance?

Summary and Conclusions. As we conclude this chapter, it is important to emphasize once again that treating disease is not the same as creating health. Different people define health differently, but virtually all agree that health is more than the absence of disease. Definitions of health differ among people, cultures, and age groups. The U.S. "health care delivery system" as now constituted is mis-named: it focuses primarily on disease treatment rather than health promotion and maintenance. Given the health and disease profile of the American people, it should be obvious that in any reformed health care delivery system, significantly more attention should be paid to disease prevention and health promotion than is presently given.

But health should not be seen as some fixed end point that will be reached if only we try hard enough to get there. Rather it should be seen as a process of life. Dubos, for example, saw health as a mirage that will continue to recede just beyond reach, and he believes that this is a good thing (1971, p. 278):

Human life implies adventure, and there is no adventure without struggles and dangers. . . . Attempts at adaptation will demand efforts, and these efforts will often result in failure. . . . Disease will remain an inescapable manifestation of his struggles. While it may be comforting to imagine a life without stresses and strains in a carefree world, this will remain an idle dream. Man cannot hope to find another Paradise on earth because Paradise is a static concept while human life is a dynamic process.

But within that limitation, as documented in *Healthy People 2000* (USDHHS, 1990) there is much that can be done and much that remains to be done to improve the health of our population. This goal can be achieved through the application of health promotive/ disease-preventive measures, the use of which is based in existing knowledge, science, and technology, with the resulting assurance that the services are effective and cost-effective.

A remaining question is, however, who is to decide what "cost-effective" means and is? Who is to say that the benefits and risks are worth the costs? Eddy (1991) has argued that only patients, whether present or future, can make such determinations, since they are the ones who receive the benefits, take the risks, and pay the costs. In the health care reform movement of many countries, including the United States, defining a basic benefit package available to all citizens is a central element of change. Should not the citizens themselves have a strong voice in determining the nature of the benefit package? Freymann (1989) has argued that the public's paradigm for health care has changed to value disease prevention and health promotion. Such a change needs to be reflected in the composition of health care itself.

References

Banta, H. D. & Luce, B. R., *Health Care Technology and its Assessment in International Perspective*, Oxford, England: Oxford University Press, 1993.

Berkman, L. F. & Breslow, L., *Health and Ways of Living: The Alameda County Study*, New York: Oxford University Press, 1983.

Blakiston's New Gould Medical Dictionary, 2nd Ed. New York: Blakiston Division, McGraw-Hill, 1956.

Bouchard, C., et al., (Eds.) *Exercise, Fitness, and Health*, Campaign, IL: Human Kinetics Books, 1988.

Brook, R. & Lohr, K., "Efficacy, Effectiveness, Variations, and Quality," *Medical Care*, 23, 710–722, 1985.

Brook, R. & Lohr, K., "Will We Need to Ration Effective Health Care?," *Issues in Science and Technology*, 3, 1–10, 1986.

Brown, P. (Ed.), *Perspectives in Medical Sociology*, Blooming, CA: Wadsworth Publishing Co., 1989.

Burnett, M., *Genes, Dreams, and Realities*. New York: Basic Books, 1971.

Cassell, E., *The Healer's Art*. Philadelphia: Lippincott, 1976.

Clinton, W. J., *Health Security: The President's Report to the American People,* Washington, DC: The White House Domestic Policy Council, 1993.

Dubos, R., *Mirage of Health.* New York: Harper & Row, 1971.

Durant, W., *The Life of Greece*, New York, Simon and Schuster, 1939.

Eddy, D., "What Care is 'Essential?' What Services are 'Basic?'" *Journal of the American Medical Association, 265*, 783–88, 1991.

Eisenberg, D. M. et al., "Unconventional Medicine in the United States," *New England Journal of Medicine, 328*, 246–52, 1993.

Engel, G., "The Need for a New Medical Model: A Challenge for Biomedicine." In A. Caplan, H. T. Engelhardt, & J. McCartney (Eds.), *Concepts of Health and Disease* (pp. 589–607). Reading, MA: Addison-Wesley, 1981.

Evidence-Based Medicine Working Group, "Evidence-Based Medicine," *Journal of the American Medical Association, 268,* 2420–2425, 1992.

Flexner, S. B. (Ed.), *The Random House Dictionary of the English Language, 2nd Edition Unabridged*, New York: Random House, 1987.

Foley, J. P. (Ed.), *Jeffersonian Cyclopedia: A Comprehensive Collection of the Views of Thomas Jefferson* (Vol. I). New York: Russell and Russell, 1967.

Frank, J., "Mind-Body Interactions in Illness and Healing." Paper Presented at the May Lectures, "Alternative Futures for Medicine," Airlie House, Airlie, VA, April 4, 1975.

Freymann, J. G., "The Public's Health Care Pardigm is Shifting: Medicine Must Swing with It," *Journal of General Internal Medicine*, 313–319, 1989.

Friedman, H. S., *Personality and Disease*, New York: Wiley, 1990.

Fuchs, V., "The Contribution of Health Services to the American Economy." *The Milbank Memorial Fund Ouarterly, 44*, 65, 1966.

Fuchs, V., *Who Shall Live?* New York: Basic Books, 1974.

Haggerty, R., "The Boundaries of Health Care." In D. S. Sobel (Ed.), W*ays of Health* (pp. 45–60). New York: Harcourt, Brace, Jovanovich, 1979.

Homer, *The Iliad.* Translated by R. Lattimore. Chicago: University of Chicago Press, 1951.

Hoyman, H., "The Spiritual Dimensions of Man's Health in Today's World." In D. Belgum (Ed.), *Religion and Medicine.* Ames, IA: Iowa State University Press, 1967.

Jago, J., "'Hal'—Old word, new task: Reflections on the words' 'Health' and 'Medical.'" *Social Science and Medicine, 9*, 1, 1975.

Jonas, S., *Medical Mystery: The Training of Doctors in the United States.* New York: W. W. Norton, 1978.

Jonas, S., "On Dr. Kevorkian" Commentaries, WBT-AM, Charlotte, NC, May 11, 1993, (a).

Jonas, S., "On National Health Insurance, I, II," Commentaries, WBT-AM, Charlotte, NC, May 17 and July 19, 1993, (b).

Jonas, S., "Harry's Wife Died," Commentary, WBT-AM, Charlotte, NC, August 16, 1993, (c).

Kaplan, R. M., Bush, J., & Berry, C., "Health status: Types of validity and index of well-being." *Health Services Research, 11*, 478, 1976.

Kass, L., "Regarding the end of medicine and the pursuit of health." In A. Caplan, H. T. Engelhardt, & J. McCartney (Eds.), *Concepts of Health and Disease, Interdisciplinary Perspectives* (pp. 3–30). Reading, MA: Addison-Wesley, 1981.

Lalonde, M., *A New Perspective on the Health of Canadians.* Ottawa, Canada: Government of Canada, 1974.

McDowell, I., & Newell, C., *Measuring Health: A Guide to Rating Scales and Question-naires*, New York: Oxford University Press, 1987.

McGinniss, J. M., "Prevention in 1989: The State of the Nation," *American Journal of Preventive Medicine, 6,* 1–5, 1990.

McGinniss, J. M. & Foege, W. H., "Actual Causes of Death in the United States,"*Journal of the American Medical Association, 270,* 2207–2212, 1993.

McKeown, T., *The Role of Medicine: Dream, Mirage, or Nemesis.* London: The Nuffield Provincial Hospitals Trust, 1976.

McPeek, B., Gilbert, J., & Mosteller, F., "The End Result: Quality of Life." In J. Bunker, B. Barnes, & F. Mosteller (Eds.), *Costs, Risks, and Benefits of Surgery* (pp. 170–175). New York: Oxford University Press, 1977.

Mechanic, D., *Politics, Medicine, and Social Science.* New York: Wiley, 1974.

Millis, J., *A Rational Policy for Medical Education and Its Financing.* New York: The National Fund for Medical Education, 1971.

Mushkin, S., & Dunlop, D.,*Health: What Is It Worth?* New York: Pergamon Press, 1979.

MVSR: *Monthly Vital Statistics Report*, Vol. 41, No. 7, "Advance Report of Final Mortality Statistics, 1990."

Osterweis, M., Solomon, F., & Green, M., (Eds.), Bereavement, Reactions, Consequences and Care. Washington, DC: National Reading Press, 1984.

Parsons, T., *The Social System*, New York: The Free Press, 1951.

Parsons, T., "Definitions of Health and Illness in the Light of American Values and Social Structure." In E. Jaco (Ed.),*Patients, Physicians, and Illness.* Glencoe, IL: The Free Press, 1958.

Prevention report, (U.S. Public Health Service), August-September 1993.

Reich, T., "Biologic-Marker Studies in Alcoholism," *New England Journal of Medicine, 318,* 180, 1988.

Sheehan, G., *Personal Best,* Emmaus, PA: Rodale Press, 1989.

Sigerist, H., *Medicine and Human Welfare.* College Park, MD: McGrath Publishing Co., 1970.

Thomas, D. B., "Cancer," Chap. 47 in Last, J. M. and Wallace, R. B., Eds.,*Maxcy-Rosenau-Last: Public Health and Preventive Medicine*, Norwalk, CN: Appleton-Lange, 1992.

U.S. Bureau of the Census, *Statistical Abstract of the United States: 1993* (113th edition.) Washington, DC: 1993.

U.S. Department of Health, Education, and Welfare, *Healthy People: The Surgeon General's Report on Health Promotion and Disease Prevention*, Washington, DC: DHEW (PHS) Pub. No. 79-55071, 1979.

U.S. Department of Health and Human Services, *Healthy People 2000: National Health Promotion and Disease Prevention Objectives*, Washington, DC: DHHS Pub. No. [PHS] 91–50213, 1991.

U.S. Department of Health and Human Services,*Health United States 1991, and Prevention Profile*, Washington, DC: DHHS Pub. No. [PHS] 92–1223, 1992.

U.S. National Office of Vital Statistics, *Vital Statistics of the United States, 1950, Vol. 1,* Washington, DC: 1950.

United States Preventive Services Task Force, *Guide to Clinical Preventive Services*, Baltimore, MD: Williams and Wilkins, 1989.

Wallis, C., "Why New Age Medicine is Catching On," *Time,* Nov. 4, 1991, p. 68.

Weinerman, E. R., "Research on Comparative Health Service Systems." *Medical Care*, *9*, 272, 1971.

Williams, A., "Economics and the Rational Use of Medical Technology." In F. F. H. Rutten, & S. J. Reiser (Eds.), *The Economics of Medical Technology* (pp. 109–120). New York: Springer-Verlag, 1988.

Wolinsky, F. D., *The Sociology of Health*, Belmont, CA: Wadsworth Publishing Co., 1988.

Woolhandler, S., et al., "Administrative Costs in U.S. Hospitals," *New England Journal of Medicine, 329*, pp. 400–403, 1993.

World Health Organization, *The World Health Organization: A Report on the First Ten Years*, Geneva, Switzerland, 1958.

3

Population Data for Health and Health Care

Steven Jonas

Introduction

Quantitative description and analysis provide the basic means for understanding the nature and health status of the population the health care delivery system serves and of the system's operations. Because of the nature of most data gathering and reporting on the one hand, and book-writing and publishing on the other, most of the data presented in this chapter will be 2- to-4 years out of date by the time this book is published. Thus, the utility of the numbers presented is found not in their description of current reality at the time the book is being read. Rather, the specific data presented should be viewed as examples of *how* numbers are and can be used to better understand the health care delivery system.

It happens that virtually all the numbers presented are from sources that are published on a regular, usually annual, basis. Thus the diligent reader can fairly easily find the most recent data for the descriptor in question, should that be necessary.

Quantitative Perspectives

Overview

There are three major quantitative perspectives on health and health care services from which a population can be viewed. First are the simple *numbers* of people and what are called their *demographic* characteristics (from the Greek "describing the people). Among the important demographic characteristics are: age, sex, marital status, geographic location, and such social characteristics as ethnicity, income, education, employment, and measures of social class.

Second are the health and sickness status of the population. Given the current level of sophistication of data gathering and analysis, it is much easier to characterize the latter than the former. The ill-health status of the population is described by measures of mortality (death) and morbidity (sickness). Mortality and morbidity may be counted for the population as a whole. In this case the numbers or rates are defined as *crude*. Alternatively, mortality and morbidity may be counted by cause, or by demographic characteristics used in describing segments of the population (e.g., age, sex, ethnicity).

The third quantitative perspective for viewing a population is *utilization of health services*: who uses how many of what kinds of services, when, and where. Utilization can be measured from two points of view: that of the consumer and that of the provider. For example, physician/patient encounters can be reported in terms of how many visits the average patient makes to the physician each year. The same set of events can be reported in terms of how many patient visits the average physician provides each year. An excellent review of patient-perspective utilization research has been carried out by Hulka & Wheat (1985).

When one knows how many and what kinds of people there are, what their health and sickness status is, and their service utilization levels, one has fairly well quantitatively characterized a population's health and health care status. The system's operations are fairly well quantified by the provider-perspective data recording the same events.

Numbers and Rates

Population, health status, and utilization data all can be presented in two forms: numbers and rates. A *number* is simply a count of conditions, individuals, or events. A *rate* has two parts, a numerator and a denominator. The numerator is the number of conditions, individuals, or events counted. The denominator is a (usually) larger group of conditions, individuals, or events from among which the population described by the numerator is drawn.

It is customary to give a rate as applying during a particular time period. For example, one could determine that 1,000 deaths occurred in a particular population during a year. This *number* of deaths becomes a *rate* if one counts the whole population, finds that number to be 100,000, and then says that the mortality *rate* is 1,000/100,000, per year. The rate can be expressed as a percentage (in this case, 1%), or as a rate per thousand (in this case, 10), or any other formulation that is useful.

The multipliers for rates are usually given in powers of 10. The magnitude of the denominator is usually chosen to make the rate a number of reasonable size. Thus, the less frequent the event being counted by the numerator, the larger the denominator. For example, crude death rates for a whole population, all causes, are usually given as per thousand population. Cause-specific mortality rates are usually presented as per 100,000 or even as per 1,000,000. This is done so the rate's numerator will not appear as a fractional number.

Both denominators and numerators can be fairly specific. In discussing deaths from lung cancer caused by cigarette smoking, for example, a rate can be determined for the number of deaths per year from lung cancer in males over age 45 who have smoked 2 or more packs of cigarettes per day for 20 years or more (the numerator), per all males over 45 who have smoked 2 or more packs of cigarettes per day for 20 years or more (the denominator). Usually, however, the units of the numerator and the denominator in health indices are different. For example, in cause-specific mortality rates, the unit for the numerator is deaths by cause, while the unit for the denominator is persons.

Although rates are usually fractions, occasionally they will be whole numbers. For example, in measuring total morbidity in a population, one may find that the number of diagnosed disease conditions is greater than the number of people. The rate then is usually given with a denominator of 1. For example: "In the population of a central African city there are 2.5 disease conditions per person." This usage also occurs in utilization rates. For example: "The annual physician-visit rate in the United States is about 5.6 per person." Rates are especially useful for measuring and describing changes over time, in everything from deaths to per capita health care expenditures.

Health care service utilization rates constitute a special group of rates, not usually presented in terms of numerators and denominators. For example, hospital-specific admission rates are commonly presented simply as a number per unit of time, as follows: "In 1989, the admission rate for hospital Y was 1,000 per month." This formulation is used because the sizes of the populations served by most institutional and individual providers are not known.

The Purposes of Quantification

Description. There are two major purposes for quantification of health care delivery system events. First, quantification *describes* the numbers and characteristics of the population being served. Demographic characteristics such as geographic location (do many people live near marshes inhabited by malaria-carrying mosquitoes?) and age distribution (are there many infants and/or old people?) may well provide some indication of the population's relative disease risks.

Disease-specific mortality and morbidity rates highlight the major clinically apparent health and illness problems in the population. The infant mortality rate gives some indication both of general health levels and the availability of medical care. The distribution of crude and disease-specific mortality and morbidity rates by place, age, sex, ethnic group, and social class shows which population subgroups are being affected by what diseases.

As noted, utilization data quantify how the population uses the health care delivery system. Utilization of health services can be quantified both from the consumer's perspective, for example, how many times the average person sees a physician per year, and from the provider's perspective, for example, how many patient visits the average physician provides in a year.

Consumer-perspective data can be presented as the overall, or "crude," numbers and rates, or it can be subdivided according to various demographic characteristics of the population. For example, the crude average annual per-person physician visit rate described just above can also be reported by the age, sex, and geographic distribution characteristics of the total group of patients making the visits. Provider-perspective utilization data can also be subject to demographic analysis. For example, one can determine the average number of visits provided annually by physicians according to their age, practice location, and specialty.

In summary, quantification describes, for example, how many of what kind of people are at risk, what kinds of diseases and ill health conditions they have, how those problems are distributed in the population, and who goes where for how many of what kinds of health services, delivered by which types of providers.

Program Planning. The second purpose of quantification in health care delivery is for *program planning*, which might be done by a hospital, a health services network, a city health services administration, or a private physician. Descriptive data can reveal the existence of problems. Then, if there is the interest, the will, and the money to do something about them, data can also be used to help design solutions, first by clearly defining the unmet need that has to be met. In other uses of data for health services program planning, service projections for the proposed new program defined by data are essential for calculating cost estimates. Once new programs are under way, data are necessary for evaluating their effects and effectiveness.

Thus data are required for logical program planning, as they are in most fields of human endeavor. However, it must be remembered that data in themselves are not sufficient for effective and useful planning. Before the use of data has any real meaning for planning, the agencies and institutions in charge must first make a policy decision to undertake program planning. They must agree to make their planning data-based. (It is too often not, in the real world.) Then they must decide to implement a suitable plan, once arrived at. Data for planning mean nothing unless planning is done using it and planned programs are implemented when needed.

To illustrate the use of data for planning, let us take the hypothetical case of program and then physical planning for a medical school hospital located in a suburban/semirural area. The university trustees for the medical school have already decided that this hospital is to be designed so that it can help meet the health care needs of the community as well as serving the educational and research needs of the medical school. (The three functions of any medical school, in theory at least, are patient care [service], teaching, and research.) It is to be hoped, of course, that the subprograms for carrying out each of these three functions can be coordinated in a positive way so that all will be benefited.

The first step in rationally planning for a new medical school hospital would be to delineate a proposed service area. One would count population, determine population density, examine modes of transportation, and evaluate existing health care resources, particularly the more complex and sophisticated ones already in place. Some data-based questions to be asked are:

- How many people are there, and where are they located?
- What are the age, sex, and marital status distributions?
- What are the social class and ethnic makeups?
- What is the sickness and health profile?
- How is the population size and composition changing over time?
- What are the existing health care resources, and how are they used?
- What do existing providers see as their needs?
- How do they view the new facility, and how will they relate to it?

The answers to these and many other similar questions define the health and health care needs of the population to be served. They also characterize the existing health care resources. These and other data are essential to identifying and quantifying both the met and the unmet health and health care needs of the population. The data also afford the opportunity to make intelligent decisions on facility design, location, services and service priorities, space allocation, administrative structure, community relations, staffing and personnel policies, teaching and research programs, capital cost, expense budget, and the other myriad details that confront the health services program planner.

Amalgamating, classifying, and analyzing all these data are the bases for rational program planning. In general, one can say that intelligent decisions in health services planning depend on intelligent use of health and health care data. Unfortunately that does not always happen in the United States.

A particular problem with health and health care data occurred during the early 1980s. The Reagan Administration sharply reduced federal data-gathering and -analysis activities (Mundinger, 1985). This meant that less information was published, especially on population characteristics such as health status. Moreover, the publication of data was increasingly delayed.

The reader of this chapter will notice that certain data—census and vital statistics, for example—are reasonably up to date, in relation to the book's publication date. However, other data are some years behind (and further behind than they were formerly). Certain classes of data presented in previous editions of this book are now simply unavailable. It may be possible to remedy this situation in the context of national health care reform. Health care program planning in the United States is discussed further in Chapter 13. Now let us turn to a consideration of certain classes of data in some detail.

Population

Number

The Constitution of the United States requires that a census of the nation be taken at least once every 10 years (USBOC, 1993, p. l). The original purpose of the census was to provide the basis for the apportionment among the states of seats in the House of Representatives of the U.S. Congress. A census has been carried out every 10 years since 1790. Although every effort is made for completeness, the Census Bureau has estimated that in 1990 it undercounted by between 1% and 2%, ranging from 4.5% for American Indians to 0.7% for whites (USBOC, 1993, p. 1).

In addition to the decennial censuses, the Census Bureau makes interim estimates on various parameters, based on information gathered from population samples and a variety of other sources. The estimated U.S. resident population as of July l, 1992 was 255,082,000 (USBOC, Table 2). In addition, there were about 400,000 U.S. citizens (including military servicepeople), living abroad.

Births, deaths, immigration, and emigration are the four factors producing change in population size. During the 1970s and 1980s, the population growth rate averaged about 1.0% per year (USBOC, 1993, Tables 2, 4). During the 1960s the population had grown at the rate of about 1.3% per year. The decline in rate of growth resulted primarily from a decrease in the birth rate. It is projected that the population growth will likely decline further, to 0.5% per year by 2040. Nevertheless, the "mid-range" population size projection for that year is about 364 billion, an increase of about 43% over the 1992 population. The bearing on health services need and utilization of such matters as population size and growth rate should be obvious.

Demographic Characteristics

In 1990 79.3% of the U.S. population lived in what are called *metropolitan statistical areas* (MSAs, variously also referred to, with slightly different definitions, as standard metropolitan statistical areas, SMSAs and consolidated metropolitan statistical areas, CMSAs) (USBOC, 1993, Table 38). The figures for 1960 and 1980 were 63% and 78%, respectively.

The Federal Office of Management and Budget, an agency of the Executive Branch, is charged with defining the term "Metropolitan Statistical Area" (USBOC, 1993, p. 916). The definition has changed over time. As of 1990 an MSA included at least, (1) one city with a population of 50,000 or more, or (2) a Census Bureau-defined urbanized area of at least 50,000 inhabitants and a total MSA population of at least 100,000 (75,000 in New England). In addition, the county (or counties) containing the central city, as well as adjacent counties that have at least 50%

of their population in the urbanized area surrounding the city are included. Out-lying "commuting counties" may be included as well if they meet certain require-ments.

As of 1991, it was estimated that the U.S. population was 48.8% male, 83.6% nonblack, and had a median age of 32.8 (31.9 for males, 34.3 for females) (USBOC, Table 13, 14). The median age was up from 28 in 1970. In 1991, 28.6% of the population was under 20; 12.6% was age 65 and over, up from 9.8% in 1970. In 1992, about 60% of males and 61% of females 18 and over were married, con-trasting with 74% and 70%, respectively, in 1970 (USBOC, 1993, Table 59). In 1990, about 3.3 million Americans were inmates of institutions, with 1,115,000 in prisons and jails, 1,772,000 in nursing homes, and 104,000 in juvenile institu-tions (USBOC, 1993, Table 85). Almost 200,000 lived in emergency shelters for the homeless.

Social-class status is often thought to be a valuable parameter by which to cross-tabulate population, health/illness, and utilization data (Dutton, 1989)[1]. However, unlike the British government, for example, the U.S. government has not devel-oped a "social class" index by which it cross-tabulates its demographic data. Thus we are forced to use ethnicity and income as rough indicators of social class. This is unfortunate, because social class is determined not simply by income, but by a combination of several factors, including education, employment, and dwelling place, as well as income. A great deal of such information is in fact collected by the government, but an index has not been created.

The information presented so far in this chapter comes from the "Population" section of the *Statistical Abstract of the United States: 1993* (USBOC). Additional information necessary to develop a comprehensive profile of the population is

TABLE 3.1 Demographic Characteristics, United States Population, 1988–1992, with Selected Comparisons for 1970

Characteristic	Year	
	1988–1992	1970
Number (millions)	255 (1992)	203
Percentage of population living in an MSA	79 (1990)	69
Percentage male	49 (1991)	49
Percentage white	84 (1991)	87
Median age	32.8 (1991)	28
Number of persons living in instuitutions (millions)	3.3 (1990)	2.1
Marriage rate (per thousand)	9.7 (1988)	10.6
Divorce rate (per thousand)	4.7 (1988)	3.5

Sources: USBOC, *Statistical Abstract of the United States: 1971*, Tables 14, 15, 21; *1993*, Tables 2, 13, 14, 38, 85, 140. Washington, D.C.: U.S. Government Print-ing Office, 1971, 1993.

contained in the "Vital Statistics," "Education," "Social Insurance and Human Services," "Labor Force, Employment, and Earnings," and "Income Expenditures, and Wealth" sections of the same publication.

Vital Statistics

How They Are Collected

In public health, the "vital statistics" are classically defined as data on births, deaths, marriages, and divorces (USBOC, 1993, p. 71). In the United States, primary responsibility for collecting these data lies with the states, usually through a state's Department of Health or its equivalent. Not all states collect all categories of data (although all states have collected birth and death data since 1933). The states generally publish at least some of the data they collect on a regular basis. Where possible, state health departments rely on county and other local health departments to do the actual counting and then transmit the results to the state level. The states in turn send their results to the Federal National Center for Health Statistics. The District Government for Washington, DC, carries out primary data collection for that city.

The first vital statistic to be collected in the United States on an annual basis was mortality data. In 1990, 10 states and the District of Columbia became the first "death registration states," carrying out that task and forwarding the results to the federal government (USBOC, 1993, p. 71). Until 1946, the Census Bureau assembled the vital statistics at the national level. From 1946 to 1960, the work was performed by the Bureau of State Services of the U.S. Public Health Service. Since 1960, the National Center for Health Statistics, USDHHS, has carried out the function.

Beginning in 1915, 10 states and the District of Columbia formed a "birth registration area," collecting birth data on an annual basis. Fetal deaths have been counted annually since 1922. Since 1933, the birth and death registration area has included all of the states and the District of Columbia. A "marriage registration area" was first formed in 1957. By 1993 it included 42 states, the Virgin Islands, Puerto Rico, and the District of Columbia. The "divorce registration" area was established in 1958. By 1987 it covered 31 states and the Virgin Islands.

The National Center for Health Statistics calculates vital statistics rates. They are based upon the actual number of persons counted by the Census Bureau on April 1 of each decennial year, as well as the midyear estimates made for other years. Cause-specific mortality data are classified according to the *International Classification of Diseases, Ninth Revision, Adapted for Use in The United States* (NCHS, 1979[a]), the so-called ICDA. The ICDA-9-Clinical Modification (ICDA-9-CM) is an extension of the ICDA-9, which all hospitals in the U.S. receiving federal funds are required to use.

Natality

In 1992, about 4.08 million babies were born in the United States, a decline of 1% from 1991 (MVSR, 1993, p. 2). The annual birth rate rate was 16.0 live births per 1,000 population, up from the lowest rate recorded in recent years, 14.6 in 1975–1976 (USBOC, 1993, Table 91), but down from the provisional rate for 1991 of 16.3. Until the turn-around in 1975–1976, the birth rate had been steadily dropping from a post-World War II high of 25, achieved in 1955, the peak year of the so-called "baby boom."

The "fertility rate" is defined as the number of births per 1,000 women aged 15–44. For 1992, provisionally it was 69.2 (MVSR, 1993, Fig. 1). That was down from the post-World War II high of 123 in 1957, but up slightly from the low of 65 recorded in 1976. If the death rate were to remain stable over a long period of time and there were no immigration, with this birth rate the U.S. population would gradually decrease over time.

Mortality

Crude Death Rates. Mortality data are rather neatly reported. As noted, there is one primary reporting authority, usually the local health department or, where none exists, the state health department acting in its place. Death is a well-defined event in the vast majority of cases, although with recent developments in medical technology, legal, ethical, and religious, as well as biomedical, disputes do arise as to just what the definition of "death" is (President's Commission, 1981; Wikler & Weisbard, 1989). Because both hospitals and funeral directors are legally required to report all deaths, with rather serious penalties for failure to comply, we can assume that most deaths are reported.

For 1991 the crude death rate (total deaths per 1,000 population) in the United States was 8.5 (USBOC, 1993, Table 91). This compares with a rate of 9.6 for 1950, 9.5 for 1960, 9.5 for 1970, and 8.8 for 1980. Mortality is relatively high during the first year of life, drops to a relatively low level until the mid-40s, and then begins to climb again (USBOC, 1993, Table 118–119). Males have a higher mortality rate than females at all ages. Thus, as the average age of the population increases, the female/male ratio increases as well. Although the crude death rate for nonwhites is lower than for whites, the age-specific death rates for nonwhites are higher than for whites at all ages until 85. The crude death rate is lower for nonwhites because the nonwhite population is younger.

Much data on differential death rates by the basic demographic variables of age, color, and sex can be found in the *Monthly Vital Statistics Report, Vital Statistics of the United States,* special studies published in the NCHS publication *Vital and Health Statistics*, Series 20, as well as the *Statistical Abstract*.

Cause-specific Mortality. Determination of the cause of death has presented some problems from time to time. In most cases it is left up to the physician to certify that the patient is dead. Physicians have varying diagnostic styles, opinions, and abilities. Furthermore, there have been changes in the technical definitions of causes of death over time.[2] As an example of the potential difficulty, consider the question, is the cause of death in a patient who dies from a heart attack that resulted from the complications of diabetes mellitus, diabetes or coronary artery disease? The reporting authorities do have rules covering most of these instances. Most physicians follow them, but problems do occasionally crop up.

In 1991 the 10 leading causes of death by diagnosis (excluding the diagnostic categories of "symptoms and ill-defined conditions" and "all other diseases") were heart disease, cancer, stroke, personal injury, chronic obstructive pulmonary disease, influenza and pneumonia (primarily pneumonia), diabetes mellitus, other infectious and parasitic diseases (including AIDS), suicide, and homicide and legal intervention (USBOC, 1993, Table 126).

By contrast, in 1970, the 10 leading causes of death by diagnosis were heart disease, cancer, stroke, personal injury, pneumonia and influenza, "certain conditions originating in the perinatal period," diabetes mellitus, cirrhosis of the liver, suicide, and congenital anomalies (USBOC, 1993, Table 126), with the rates for heart disease, stroke, and personal injury being considerably higher at that time, the rates for cancer and chronic obstructive pulmonary disease being considerably lower. Further, by 1991, AIDS and murder had taken the places of cirrhosis of the liver and fatal conditions associated with pregnancy and childbirth in the "top ten."

In certain areas we are making progress then. However, in others we are not. In the modern United States, most deaths are caused by chronic diseases or conditions (such as personal injury) in which environmental factors play a major causative role. To make the mortality data picture more useful for truly understanding what is going on and for program planning, in 1993 McGinniss and Foege took a different approach to identifying the causes of death in the United States.

They went beyond the classic lists of death-associated diagnoses to the identification of the external (nongenetic) factors known to be causally associated with the identified diseases. After an exhaustive review of the literature covering the period 1977–1993, McGinniss and Foege (1993) were able to attribute approximately half of all deaths occurring in 1991 to the following 10 factors: tobacco use (400,000 deaths annually), diet and activity patterns (300,000), alcohol use (100,000), microbial agents (90,000), toxic agents (60,000), firearms (35,000), sexual behaviors (30,000), motor vehicle use (25,000), and use of "illicit drugs," primarily heroin and cocaine (20,000).

The picture arising from the McGinniss/Foege analysis is particularly helpful in planning public health programs to prolong life, especially healthy life. Using it, one can focus on changeble human behaviors, that is, cigarette smoking, eating, physical activity, using machines, rather than classical, diagnostically related "disease prevention" for heart disease, cancer, and stroke, let us say. The former, focussing on the here and now, have much more relevance to the otherwise healthy patient than do the latter, which concern an event that may or may not happen, in the future.

Infant Mortality. The *infant* mortality rate is the number of deaths under the age of one year among children born alive, divided by the number of live births. As was pointed out in Chapter 2, infant mortality appears to be related to a variety of socioeconomic, environmental, and health care factors. Some authorities (Morris, 1964, pp. 56ff., 267; Rosen, 1958, p. 342) have considered it to be a fairly sensitive indicator of general health levels in a population. In 1992, the infant mortality rate in the United States was 8.5 per 1,000 live births (*MVSR*, 1993, p. 7), the lowest ever recorded in the United States. The rate has been declining steadily since 1940, when it was 47 (Grove & Hetzel, 1968, Table 38). In fact, the infant mortality rate has been falling since it was first recorded in this country at 99.9 in 1915.

The most striking feature of the U.S. infant mortality rate is, however, that while it has consistently fallen over the years, the rate for blacks has just as consistently remained about double the white rate (USBOC, 1993, Table 121). Detailed examinations of the relationships among ethnicity, other factors, and infant mortality are contained in *Vital and Health Statistics* (NCHS, 1992, Series 22), and a publication of the Office of Health Resources Opportunity (1979, pp. 35–39).

A classic study of factors related to infant mortality is the work of Kessner (1973) sponsored by the National Academy of Sciences. It found that in 140,000 births in New York City, with the infectious diseases that formerly took the lives of many infants in the main under control, "generally, adequacy of [health] care . . . is strongly and consistently associated with infant birth weight . . . and survival" (Kessner et al., p. 1). Kessner and his co-authors also concluded from their study that (pp. 2–3):

> the survival of infants of different ethnic groups varies widely; . . . there is consistent association between social classes as measured by the educational attainment of the mothers and infant birth weight and survival; . . . within categories of mothers' educational attainment, there are consistent trends relating the adequacy of care . . . to infant survival; . . . there is a gross misallocation of services by ethnic group and care when the risks of the women are taken into account.

Over 20 years later, the results of this study appear to be valid still.

Marriage and Divorce

In 1992 the marriage rate stood at 9.3 per 1,000 population (*MVSR*, 1993, Table D), down from 10.6 in 1970 (USBOC, 1993, Table 140). The divorce rate, which had stood at 3.5 per 1,000 population in 1970 (USBOC, Table 126), was 4.8 in 1992, over 50% of the marriage rate. Detailed analyses of birth, marriage, and divorce statistics can be found in the *Vital and Health Statistics Series 21*, "Data on Natality, Marriage and Divorce," as well as in *MVSR* itself.

Morbidity

Definitions

Morbidity refers to sickness, illness, and disease. Like mortality, morbidity data can be expressed in both numbers and rates. It can be cross-tabulated with the broad range of demographic characteristics. Morbidity data are extremely important in characterizing the health status of a population. Because many diseases and conditions of ill health widely prevalent in the population do not appear in mortality figures, alone they are not adequate for that purpose. This is particularly so in a country like the United States, in which communicable disease, with a few notable exceptions such as AIDS, is not a major cause of death.

Morbidity data can be reported in terms of both *incidence* and *prevalence*. *Incidence* is the number of new cases of the disease in question occurring during a particular time period, usually a year. *Prevalence* is the total number of cases existing in a population during a time period, or at one point in time (in which case it is known as *point-prevalence*).

The list of significant nonfatal causes of ill-health in the United States includes: arthritis, low-back pain, the common cold, influenza, nonfatal injuries, dermatitis, and mild emotional and sexual problems. There are other diseases that may kill but do so rarely in relation to their prevalence. Included in this category are sexually-transmitted disease (STD) other than Acquired Immune Deficiency Syndrome (AIDS), duodenal ulcer, and gall bladder disease. Morbidity data highlight not only the important diseases and the patterns of their distribution in the population. They also illustrate how they affect people in terms of limitation of activity.

Counting and reporting morbidity is not nearly as simple as reporting mortality, however. What is meant by the term "sickness," and when is a person "sick?" Who decides? The physician? The patient? The problems of perception of illness and of the sick role were referred to in the previous chapter. Furthermore, while the law requires that all deaths be reported, only certain categories of sickness, the infectious diseases, must be reported. The list appears in a weekly publication of the Centers for Disease Control and Prevention of the United States Public Health Service called *Morbidity and Mortality Weekly Report.* Among the 34 such diseases only 5 can be considered significant in the United States: AIDS, gonorrhea, viral hepatitis, syphilis, and tuberculosis. Clearly there are no reporting requirements for many disease categories that are important.

It is known that physicians fail to report certain diseases, even when legally required to do so. Some private physicians will not report venereal disease in private patients, on the grounds of "avoiding embarrassment." Tuberculosis reporting, other than from institutions, is inhibited by the possible economic consequences for the patient. For example, some employers automatically fire persons with tuberculosis. (Although the disease is one of low infectivity, it is commonly thought to be highly contagious, even by some health professionals.) Many physicians fail to report cases of the common childhood viral infections because they consider them to be "inconsequential."[3] The reporting of both AIDS and seropositivity for the Human Immunodeficiency Virus (HIV) is an extremely complex and controversial subject (Bayer, 1991; Dickens, 1988; Walters, 1988).

Data

Turning to the data itself, for mortality there is only one possible source—and it isn't the patient. For morbidity, it is obvious that both providers and patients can be data sources; as a result, quite different pictures of the same reality can be obtained. Providers can report morbidity by diagnostic categories and also by patient chief complaints; that is, what the patient reports to the physician as being the problem. However, patients don't usually come to a physician saying "I think I've got diabetes mellitus, Doc," but rather something like, "Doc, I've been feeling kind of weak, I'm drinking a great deal of water, and urinating a lot. Do you think maybe something's wrong?" It is up to the physician to characterize the problem and make a diagnosis, which he or she then can report. Patients can also report chief complaints directly to data gatherers, as in a population survey.

From a chief complaint profile for a population, obtained from either source, a partial picture of morbidity patterns can be drawn. One advantage of deriving information directly from patients is that certain patients with certain types of illnesses will never come to medical attention. Thus morbidity surveys that gather information only from providers will not give a complete picture.

In the United States, morbidity data are published on a regular basis by the National Center for Health Statistics (NCHS), and, for the reportable communicable diseases, the Centers for Disease Control and Prevention (in the *Morbidity and Mortality Weekly Report*). From the NCHS, the data sources include the Health and Nutrition Examination Survey (HANES), the Health Interview Survey (HIS), the Hospital Discharge Survey (HDS), and the National Ambulatory Medical Care Survey (NAMCS). The results of these surveys are published periodically in both *Vital and Health Statistics* and *Monthly Vital Statistics Report*. Together these activities constitute the National Health Survey (NCHS, 1963). Series 1 of *Vital and Health Statistics* contains the general methodological and historical accounts of the whole endeavor. Detailed descriptions of all the surveys can be found in Appendix I of *Health United States 1992* (NCHS, 1993).

Considering some examples of morbidity data, in 1991 the incidence of acute conditions was 192 per 100 persons per year, about the same as it was in 1986, but up from 172 per 100 in 1990 (NCHS, 1992, Series IV, pp. 3–4). Most common were respiratory conditions (including the common cold and influenza) (101 per 100), injuries (24 per 100), infective and parasitic diseases (18.5 per 100), and digestive system conditions (6.6 per 100).

Persons sought medical attention for these conditions about 63% of the time. Acute conditions were associated with about 733 days of restricted activity per 100 persons per year, leading to about 314 days in bed due to illness per 100 persons. For persons 18 and over, there were about 315 workloss days per 100, while for youths aged 5 to 17, there were about 411 school loss days per 100.

About 14% of the population experienced limitation in all activity due to chronic conditions (NCHS, 1992, Series IV, p. 6). The major chronic conditions causing limitations in activity in 1991 were (in descending order of frequency) sinusitis, arthritis, deformity or orthopedic impairment, hypertension, hearing impairment, heart disease, and chronic bronchitis (NCHS, 1992, Series IV, Table 57).

The Hospital Discharge Survey (HDS) reports on morbidity and mortality occurring in hospitals. This is an example of provider-perspective data. It affords a rather accurate illness profile of those patients in hospitals. It must be remembered, however, that the overwhelming majority of ill persons do not require hospitalization. Thus the morbidity profile of the population as a whole does not match that seen in hospitals. The results of the HDS are published in *Vital and Health Statistics*, Series 13, and in *Advance Data* from *Vital and Health Statistics*, published on an irregular basis.

The HDS is carried out on a sampling basis in nonfederal, short-stay hospitals (hospitals with six or more beds and an average length of stay of 30 days or less). In 1991, about 52% of the 31.1 million discharges that occurred from those hospitals were accounted for by four diagnostic groups: diseases of the circulatory system, 17%; "supplementary classifications" (primarily females with deliveries), 13%; diseases of the digestive system, 11%; and diseases of the respiratory system 10% (*Advance Data*, 1993 [a], Table 5). The five most common specific diagnoses are females with deliveries; heart disease; malignant neoplasm (cancer); pneumonia, all forms, and fractures, all sites.

The National Ambulatory Medical Care Survey (NCHS, 1974a, 1974b) was developed in the 1970s as a component of the National Health Survey. It is a continuing survey of private, office-based Federal physicians practicing in the United States (*Advance Data*, 1993 [b]). The data are collected using a stratified random sample of all office-based allopathic and osteopathic physicians in the contiguous United States, excluding anesthesiologists, pathologists, radiologists, and physicians engaged primarily in teaching, research, and administration. In the early 1990s, the data were being reported primarily by specialty.

In the NAMCS, morbidity data are collected from two perspectives: (1) the patient's reason for coming to the office and (2) the physician's diagnosis. For example, in 1989–1990, the 5 leading patients' reasons for coming to the offices of general surgeons were: lump or mass in breast; stomach pain, cramps or spasms; hernia of abdominal cavity; skin lesion, and suture insertion/removal. (*Advance Data,* 1993 [b], Table 7). The 5 leading physicians' diagnoses were: benign mammary dysplasias, inguinal (the groin area) hernia, other disorders of the breast, malignant neoplasm of the female breast, disease of the sebaceous gland (on the skin) (*Advance Data,* 1993 [b], Table 9).

Health Status and Health Behaviors

In 1979, the Office of the Assistant Secretary for Health (OASH) of the U.S. Department of Health and Human Services published the first national health status report, *Healthy People: The Surgeon General's Report on Health Promotion and Disease Prevention* (OASH). Subsequent to it, the Office of Disease Prevention and Health Promotion (ODPHP), part of OASH, published *Promoting Health and Preventing Disease: Objectives for the Nation* (ODPHP, 1980). For dealing with 15 major diseases and conditions that can be prevented using existing knowledge and techniques 216 objectives were established. The 15 were grouped into three sets of five: "Preventive Health Services" for such conditions as high blood pressure and sexually transmitted disease, "Health Protective Services" for such problems as toxic agent control and occupational safety and health, and "Health Promotion Programs" to deal with such conditions as cigarette smoking and sedentary lifestyle.

Implementation plans were published in 1983 (ODPHP, 1983), *Prospects for a Healthier America* in 1984 (ODPHP, 1984), and *A Midcourse Review* in 1986 (ODPHP, 1986). In 1990, the U.S. Public Health Service published the next comprehensive update, *Healthy People 2000* (USPHS, 1991). This document provides the public health planning guide for the 1990s.

In support of this effort, in 1985 the National Center for Health Statistics carried out a Health Promotion/Disease Prevention (HP/DP) Survey as part of the ongoing HIS (NCHS, 1988). The HPDP Survey was repeated in 1990. Results are published in *Vital and Health Statistics* Series 10, *Advance Data,* and *Morbidity and Mortality Weekly Report* (reporting data from the related Behavioral Risk Factor Surveillance System).

Key findings include (NCHS, 1993, Tables 64–72): in 1990–1991, about 25% of people 18 or older regularly smoked cigarettes, about 20% of persons 20 and over had an elevated serum cholesterol, 14% of men and 3% of women drank more than one ounce of alcohol per day, and fewer than 5% of adults exercised regularly at an intensity level high enough to reduce the risk of heart disease. About 25% of the population 18 and over could be classified as overweight, close to 30%

do no leisure-time physical activity, about 60% wear an automobile seat-belt regularly, about 70% of women 40 and over have had at least one clinical breast examination and a mammogram, and over 90% of women 18 and over have had a uterine cervix Pap smear (Siegel, et al., 1993, Tables 1–8). Note that this "risk factor" approach to morbidity has much in common with the McGinnis-Foege (1993) approach to classification of causes of death.

By 1993, the Healthy People project had expanded its scope to set National Health Promotion and Disease Prevention Objectives for dealing with 19 diseases and health behaviors (NCHS, 1993, pp. 234–384): physical activity and fitness, nutrition, tobacco use, alcohol and other drugs use, family planning, mental health and mental disorders, violent and abusive behavior, unintentional injuries, occupational safety and health, food and drug safety, oral health, maternal and infant health, heart disease and stroke, cancer, diabetes, HIV, sexually transmitted disease, immunization and infectious disease. Objectives were also established for educational and community-based programs, clinical preventive services, and surveillance and data systems. A total of 520 objectives and sub-objectives were established for the 22 designated areas.

Utilization of Health Care Services

Introduction

We come now to the third health data perspective: how the population uses the health care delivery system. We have pointed out that in quantifying utilization of health services, the same series of events can be counted either from the patient's or the provider's perspective. The results of the two types of counts are not always the same. Thus, when discussing utilization one has to be careful to distinguish the two approaches.

It should be noted that reliable utilization data is regularly reported only for services provided by licensed M.D.s and D.O.s (Doctors of Osteopathic Medicine) in licensed allopathic (M.D. staffed) and osteopathic hospitals, and by licensed dentists. In the United States there is an unknown amount of "alternative therapy" provided by such healing disciplines as chiropractic, naturopathy, homeopathy, acupuncture/acupressure therapy and its variants, and "holistic health practitioners," among many others. These practitioners do not report utilization, they are not surveyed, and much of their service is not reimbursed by insurance companies.

However, although regular utilization statistics are not collected, a sampling survey estimated that about a third of all adults use at least one alternative therapy, with an average annual visit rate of 19 (Eisenberg et al., 1993). This means that (for 1990 at least) there were more visits made to alternative therapists (425 million) than to primary care physicians (388 million).

Ambulatory Services

As we have noted, the HIS provides patient-perspective data for the utilization of ambulatory services. According to the HIS, in 1991 there were about 5.6 physician contacts per person (NCHS, 1993, Table 78). Of these, about 59% took place in a physician's office, 14% in a hospital outpatient department (including an emergency room), and 12% on the telephone, 3% in the home, and 12% in other locations. Females averaged 6.3 visits per year, while males averaged 4.9. Whites averaged 5.8 visits, while blacks averaged 5.2. Persons in families with an income of $14,000 or less averaged 6.8 visits per year. Persons in the Western geographic region averaged the most visits, 5.9.

There are several sources for provider data on the utilization of ambulatory services. The most comprehensive is the National Ambulatory Medical Care Survey, described briefly above, reported upon most commonly in *Advance Data*. In addition to morbidity data, the NAMCS provides data on visits by age, race, sex, geographic region, metropolitan/nonmetropolitan living area, type of physician, and duration of visit. The other major source of provider-perspective ambulatory service utilization data is the AHA's annual publication *Hospital Statistics*, published each summer.

Utilization of Hospital Services

Turning to utilization of hospital services, the HDS (described briefly above) reported that for 1991 there were about 31.1 million discharges from such hospitals, (excluding newborn infants). These patients used about 199 million inpatient days of care (with an average length of stay of 6.4 days) for a total of about 34.2 million discharges (*Advance Data,* 1993 [a], p. 1). Other classes of data provided by the HDS are utilization according to various hospital characteristics, morbidity (discussed previously), and an analysis of surgery.

NCHS also provides patient-perspective hospital utilization data through the HIS. NCHS points out that, because of "differences in collection procedures, population sampled, and definitions," the results from the HIS and the HDS are not entirely consistent (NCHS, 1979(b), p. 1). For 1991, the HIS reported significantly fewer discharges from short-stay hospitals than did the HDS: about 22.2 million discharges, 89 per thousand population, with an average length of stay of 6.6 days (NCHS, 1993, Table 83).

Hospital utilization data is also published in the American Hospital Association's *Hospital Statistics*. For AHA-registered hospitals, it contains a voluminous amount of data on bed size, admissions, occupancy rate, average daily census, and fiscal parameters, according to hospital type, size, ownership, geographic location, and the like (see also Chapter 7). Certain provider-perspective hospital utilization data also appear in *Health: U S*

Conclusion

In the United States, much data concerning the population, its health, and how it uses the health care delivery system are collected and published. As noted just above in the case of hospital utilization, not all of these data are consistent with one another. This lack of consistency may result in part from a lack of coordination of data-collection efforts. Furthermore, there is the obvious gap between the provider perspective and the patient perspective on the counts of events. One initiative of the proposed Clinton Health Plan of 1993 was to significantly improve health and health services data collection and analysis.

There have been criticisms of the Federal statistical collection, reporting, and analysis system over a period of many years. A 1979 study by the Office of Technology Assessment found "federal data collection activities . . . to be overlapping, fragmented, and often duplicative" (p. iii).[4] In brief, the report recommended that a "strengthened coordinating and planning unit within [HHS]" be established that "would embody three basic characteristics: sufficient authority to impose decisions on agencies; the necessary statistical and analytical capabilities to conduct activities requiring technical expertise and judgement; and adequate resources to build a viable core effort" (p. 55). This recommendation has not yet been followed.

Regardless of the problems with the system, however, we do know a great deal about health, disease, and illness in the United States, and about the functioning of the U.S. health care delivery system. There are gaps in our knowledge, to be sure; some of them would have been filled if the provisions of the National Health Resources Planning and Development Act (P. L. 93-641, Sect. 1513, b, l) relating to data had been carried out. They were not. These requirements called for the mandatory national collection of data on (1) population health status, (2) health care delivery system utilization, (3) effects of the health care delivery system on health, (4) health care delivery resources, and (5) environmental and occupational exposure factors relating to health.

It may well be that as part of any national health care reform measure, these data reforms will be instituted. However, given whatever problems there may or may not be with the available health and health care data, we need to remember above all that data mean little unless they are put to proper use.

Notes

1. A detailed discussion of this very important subject area, with an extensive bibliography, is presented in *The Health Gap*, edited by Robert Kane, M.D. (New York: Springer Publishing Co., 1975). See also Office of Health Resources Opportunity, *Health Status of Minorities and Low Income Groups* (DHEW Pub. No. HRA 79-627) (Washington, D.C.: U.S. Government Printing Office, 1979), and Alcena, V., *The Status of*

Health of Blacks in the United States of America, Dubuque, IA: Kendall/Hunt Publishing Co., 1992.

2. For a detailed discussion of this problem, see "Estimates of Selected Comparability Ratios Based on Dual Coding of 1976 Death Certificates by the Eighth and Ninth Revisions of the International Classification of Diseases," *MVSR*, 28 (11) (Suppl., February 1980).

3. For example, we can estimate that just before the introduction of the measles vaccine in the mid-1960s, the measles reporting rate was around 10%. Almost all children get measles before their fifth birthday. There were about 4,000,000 births the U.S. at that time, but only 400,000 cases of measles were reported annually. Since, on the average, 4,000,000 children were getting the disease each year, the reporting rate was about 10%.

4. This report will still be valuable to students of the Federal data system and its users. It not only described data collection activities and the way they were organized and supervised, but also presented and analyzed all of the statutory authorities that establish those existing at the time (which happen to be almost all of those still in use.)

References

Advance Data, "1991 Summary: National Hospital Discharge Survey," No. 227, March 3, 1993 (a).

Advance Data, "Office Visits to General surgeons 1989–90, National Ambulatory Medical Care Survey," No. 228, March 2, 1993 (b).

Bayer, R., "AIDS: The Politics of Prevention and Neglect." *Health Affairs,* Spring, 1991, p. 87.

Dickens, B. M., "Legal Rights and Duties in the AIDS Epidemic." *Science, 239,* 580, 1988.

Dutton, D. B., "Social Class, Health, and Illness," Chap. 2 in Brown, P. ed., *Perspectives in Medical Sociology*, Belmont, CA: Wadsworth Publishing Co., 1989.

Eisenberg, D. M., et al., "Unconventional Medicine in the United States," *New England Journal of Medicine, 328,* 246–52, 1993.

Grove, R. D., & Hetzel, A. M., *Vital Statistics Rates for the United States: 1940–1960.* Washington, DC: NCHS, 1968.

Hulka, B. S. & Wheat, J. R., "Patterns of Utilization: The Patient Perspective," *Medical Care, 23,* 438, 1985.

Kessner, D. M., et al., *Infant Death: An Analysis by Maternal Risk and Health Care.* Washington, DC: Institute of Medicine, National Academy of Sciences, 1973.

McGinniss, J. M., & Foege, W. H., "Actual Causes of Death in the United States," *Journal of the American Medical Association, 270,* 2207–2212, 1993.

Morris, J. N., *Uses of Epidemiology.* Baltimore, MD: Williams and Wilkins, 1964.

Monthly Vital Statistics Report, "Annual Summary of Births, Marriages, Divorces, and Deaths: United States, 1992, *41,* September 28, 1993.

Mundinger, M. N., "Health Service Funding Cuts and the Declining Health of the Poor." *New England Journal of Medicine, 313,* 44, 1985.

National Center for Health Statistics, "Origin, Program and Operation of the U.S. National Health Survey," *Vital and Health Statistics*, Series 1, No. 1, August, 1963.

National Center for Health Statistics, *International Classification of Diseases, Ninth Revision, Adapted for Use in The United States.* Hyattsville, MD, USGPO, 1979(a).

National Center for Health Statistics, *Health Resources Statistics: Health Manpower and Health Facilities, 1976–77*, DHEW Pub. No. (PHS) 79-1509, Hyattsville, MD: 1979(b).

National Center for Health Statistics, "Health Promotion and Disease Prevention, U.S., 1985," *Vital and Health Statistics*, Series 10, No. 163, 1988.

National Center for Health Statistics, "Infant Mortality Rates: Socioeconomic Factors," *Vital and Health Statistics,* Series 22, No. 14, 1992.

National Center for Health Statistics, "Current Estimates from the National Health Survey, 1991," *Vital and Health Statistics*, Series 10, No. 184, 1992.

National Center for Health Statistics, "National Ambulatory Medical Care Survey: Background and Methodology: United States—1967–1972." *Vital and Health Statistics*, Series 2, No. 61, April 1974(a).

National Center for Health Statistics, "The National Ambulatory Medical Care Survey: Symptom Classification." *Vital and Health Statistics*, Series 2, No. 63, May 1974(b).

National Center for Health Statistics, *Health United States 1992 and Healthy People* 2000 Review, Hyattsville, MD: US Public Health Service, DHHS Pub. No. (PHS) 93-1232, 1993.

Office of the Assistant Secretary for Health, *Healthy People: The Surgeon General's Report on Health Promotion and Disease Prevention*, DHEW Pub. No. (PHS) 70-55071, Washington, DC: USGPO, 1979.

Office of Disease Prevention and Health Promotion, *Promoting Health/Preventing Disease: Objectives for the Nation.* Washington, DC, USGPO, 1980.

Office of Disease Prevention and Health Promotion, "Public Health Service Implementation Plans for Attaining the Objectives for the Nation, *Public Health Reports*, Sept.–Oct., 1983 (Suppl.).

Office of Disease Prevention and Health Promotion, *Prospects for a Healthier America.* Washington, DC: USGPO, 1984.

Office of Disease Prevention and Health Promotion, *The 1990 Health Objectives for the Nation.* Washington, DC: USGPO, 1986.

Office of Health Services Opportunity, *Health Status of Minorities and Low Income Groups* (DHEW Pub. No. HRA 79-627). Washington, DC: USGPO, 1979.

Office of Technology Assessment, *Selected Topics in Federal Health Statistics.* Washington, DC: USGPO, 1979.

President's Commission for the Study of Ethical Problems in Medicine and Biomedical and Behavioral Research, *Defining Death.* Washington, DC: USGPO, 1981.

Rosen, G., *A History of Public Health.* New York: MD Publication, 1958.

Siegel, P. Z., et al., "Behavioral Risk Factor Surveillance, 1991: Monitoring Progress Toward the Nation's Year 2000 Health Objectives," *Morbidity and Mortality Weekly Report*, Vol. 42, No. SS-4, August 27, 1993.

USBOC: U.S. Bureau of the Census, *Statistical Abstract of the United States: 1993* (113th edition). Washington, DC, 1993.

USPHS: United States Public Health Service, *Healthy People 2000: National Health Promotion and Disease Prevention Objectives*, DHHS Pub. No. (PHS) 91-50213, Washington, DC: USGPO, 1991.

Walters. L., "Ethical Issues in the Prevention and Treatment of HIV Infection and AIDS." *Science, 239*, 537, 1988.

Wikler, D., & Weisbard, A.J., "Appropriate Confusion Over 'Brain Death.'" *Journal of the American Medical Association, 261*, 2246, 1989.

4

The Health Care Workforce

Edward S. Salsberg and Christine Kovner

Introduction

The health workforce is the infrastructure of the health care delivery system. Even with major technological advances, it is the health worker who ultimately determines the availability, quality, and cost of health services. Any effort to reform or improve health services or control costs must consider the supply, distribution, use, and education of the health workforce. Conversely, any change in financing, organization, or technology will also impact on health personnel.

The health care workforce is diverse. It includes many of our society's most educated and highest paid professionals, such as physicians and researchers. It includes a wide range of care givers, from nurses to therapists. It includes millions of skilled technicians who work in hospitals, laboratories, and other settings; and it includes millions of semi-skilled workers, such as aides, clerks, and housekeeping staff. Large numbers of managers, administrators, analysts, lawyers, computer operators, and insurance sales personnel also work in health care organizations.

The health care industry is large and fast growing. Health services are labor intensive. This is true whether the services are provided in hospitals, in nursing homes, or in physicians' offices. In 1992, more than 11 million people, approximately 10% of the nation's total workforce, were employed in health or health-related settings and jobs (U.S. Department of Labor, Labstat Series Report, June, 1993). For comparison, in 1990, there were 1.7 million people employed in elementary, secondary, postsecondary education, and vocational settings in America (U.S. Department of Labor, Outlook 2005, May, 1992).

As health care expenditures rise, so too does employment in health care. Despite efforts over the years to control the rise in health care expenditures, health care employment has consistently grown at a faster rate than the rate of employment in the American economy. From 1975 through 1990, employment in health facilities grew from 4.1 million to 7.8 million, or more than 90%. During the same period, employment in the rest of the economy grew less than 40% (U.S. Department of Labor, May 1992). Even in national recessions, health care employment has risen sharply.

Health care reform may eventually slow the growth of jobs in health care, and it will certainly have a major impact on the number, types, and locations of health professionals who are needed. However, the aging of the population, expansion of insurance coverage, new technologies, and efforts to address specific health problems, such as high rates of infant mortality, will all contribute to the need for health personnel. The Federal Bureau of Labor Statistics has projected that health care employment will continue to rise at an annual rate twice that of the general economy between 1990 and 2005 (U.S. Department of Labor, 1992).

At the same time, pressure to contain costs, the expansion of managed care systems, growing expectations for higher quality care, and other changes in the health care delivery system will contribute to changes in the mix of workers, where and how they practice, and the skills they will need. One recent national commission, the Pew Health Professions Commission, has called for major reform in the education of health professionals to assure that they are better prepared to meet the challenges of the changing needs of the health care delivery system (Shugars, O'Neil & Bader, 1991; O'Neil, 1993).

This chapter provides an overview of the health care workforce—who the workers are, where they work, and some major issues and trends likely to impact on health workers. Physicians play a central role in the health care delivery system. For most people, physicians are the entry point into the health care system and the gatekeeper determining which services are provided. A major portion of this chapter, therefore, is devoted to the supply, distribution, education, and use of physicians. The chapter also provides an overview of additional health care practitioners including: dentists, podiatrists, chiropractors, optometrists, physician assistants, allied health workers, public health workers, and pharmacists. Chapter 5 provides details on nurses, who comprise the single largest category of personnel within the health workforce.

Health Care Employment

Health care employment can be viewed in two ways: by where health personnel work, or by occupation. Health sector employment includes large numbers of health professionals and others who support their work. Persons trained as health care professionals or who provide health-related services work in many settings in addition to hospitals and nursing homes. For example, physicians teach at medical schools; nurses work in school health offices; pharmacists work for the pharmaceutical firms; and nurse aides work assisting the frail elderly in their homes.

TABLE 4.1   1990 National Health Workforce in Health and Non-Health Settings

	Health settings	Other settings	Total
Health Diagnosing	504,754	78,866	583,620
Health Assessing	1,731,209	503,512	2,234,721
Health Technicians	1,371,956	418,587	1,790,543
Health Service	1,495,469	440,493	1,935,962
Home Health	158,811	231,721	390,532
Other Health Occupations	200,713	179,581	380,294
Health Support Occupations	3,464,588	N.A.	3,464,588
Total	8,927,500	1,852,760	10,780,260

Category Explanation:
Health Settings include hospitals, nursing homes, doctors offices, and others.

Health Diagnosing includes Dentists, Optometrists, Physicians, and Podiatrists.

Health Assessing and Treatment includes RNs, other therapists, Physician Assistants, Pharmacists, and others.

Health Technicians include LPNs, EMTs, and most other technicians.

Health Service includes aides, assistants, ambulance attendance, and others.

Health Support Occupations include primarily administrative and management support staff, and others.

Source: U.S. Department of Labor, Bureau of Labor Statistics, Industry Occupation Matrix, 1990.

Table 4.1 shows the number and types of health personnel who work in various settings. Although 85% of the health workforce worked in health settings (facilities), nearly two million worked in other settings. Figure 4.1 shows the health workforce distribution by practice setting.

Employment by Setting

Table 4.2 shows health sector employment growth by major type of health facility for the years 1982 through 1992 (U.S. Department of Labor, 1993). Hospitals continue to employ more people than any other health care setting. During this period, the overall workforce grew about 39%, whereas the hospital workforce grew 17%. This reflects the efforts to shift health care services away from more costly institutional settings to ambulatory care settings and other efforts to contain health care costs. Figure 4.2 graphically depicts this growth relative to a 1980 base of 100.

TABLE 4.2 National Health Workforce in Health Industry Setting (In Thousands)

Year	Total, all health industries	Offices of physicians	Offices of dentists	Offices of other practitioners	Nursing/ personal care facilities	Hospitals	Medical & dental labs	Home health care
1982	6940.1	887.2	384.2	121.0	1066.9	4143.7	109.5	—
1983	7101.0	933.5	407.0	134.5	1106.0	4151.4	111.5	—
1984	7199.9	977.2	425.3	149.3	1147.2	4085.2	115.2	—
1985	7349.2	1028.2	439.4	165.3	1197.5	4953.2	119.1	—
1986	7567.0	1081.4	457.7	181.5	1244.6	4076.8	126.6	—
1987	7846.8	1139.1	469.6	198.1	1282.6	4194.7	135.0	216.1
1988	8158.0	1199.5	483.5	220.7	1310.6	4346.4	146.2	243.7
1989	8537.2	1267.9	499.9	247.9	1355.7	4512.9	158.3	290.6
1990	8886.6	1338.2	512.9	276.5	1415.4	4621.0	166.2	344.5
1991	9252.5	1404.5	527.6	304.4	1492.6	4724.7	172.7	401.6
1992	9612.8	1472.7	541.9	327.3	1542.8	4849.3	181.0	

Average Annual Rate of Change (Percentage)

1982–1987	2.5	5.1	4.1	10.4	3.8	0.3	4.3	—
1987–1992	4.1	5.2	2.9	10.6	3.8	2.9	6.0	16.8
1982–1992	3.3	5.2	3.5	10.5	3.8	1.6	5.2	—

Source: U.S. Department of Labor, Bureau of Labor Statistics, Labstat Series Report, June 7, 1993.

FIGURE 4.1 National Health Workforce Distribution by Practice Setting in 1992

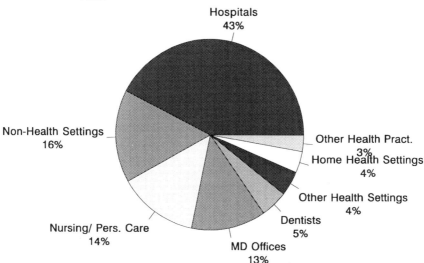

Source: U.S. Department of Labor, Bureau of Labor Statistics, Labstat Series Report, June 1993. U.S. Department of Labor, Bureau of Labor Statistics, Industry Occupation Matrix, 1990.

Hospitals

Hospital admissions and the average length of stay for hospitalized patients have fallen since the early 1980s. At the same time, hospital employment has continued to grow, leading to an increase in staff-to-bed ratios. In addition, the skill mix (ratio of higher skilled to lower skilled workers) of hospital workers has been consistently increasing. One example is the use of more registered nurses, as the severity of patient illness has increased (Berliner, 1987; Pope & Schneider, 1992).

Figure 4.3 shows the major types of workers employed in various settings, including hospitals. Although administrative support is the largest category of personnel, registered nurses comprise the single largest category of direct care providers.

Most observers believe that hospital employment growth will continue to be moderate over the next decade. This reflects continuation of trends to move services out of inpatient settings, the expansion of managed care, and other cost containment strategies. However, historically, hospitals have shown great resilience and flexibility, and it may be that hospitals will continue to evolve and take on

FIGURE 4.2 Growth Trends in Health Practice Settings

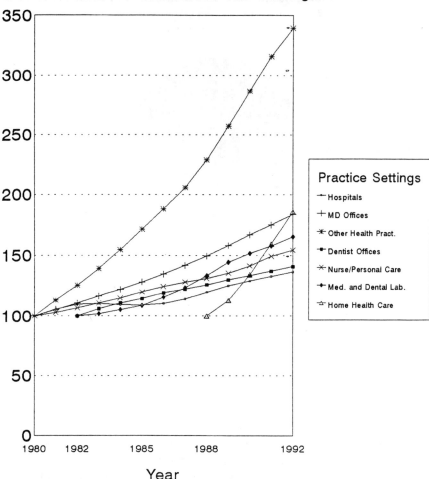

Year

Index year is 1980 for all settings, except Dental Offices and Medical and Dental Labs indexed 1982 and Home Health indexed 1988. The index year for each is set equal to 100.
Source: U.S. Department of Labor, Bureau of Labor Statistics, Labstat Series Report, June 1993.

new roles, such as sponsors of ambulatory care services and managed care programs. This would lead to continued growth in the number of hospital employees. The Bureau of Labor Statistics predicts that hospital employment will be among the slowest growing areas of the health sector between 1990 and 2005—however, even this growth is projected to be 50% higher than for the general

FIGURE 4.3   **Health Workforce in Selected Health Industry Settings Given as Percentage of Distribution**

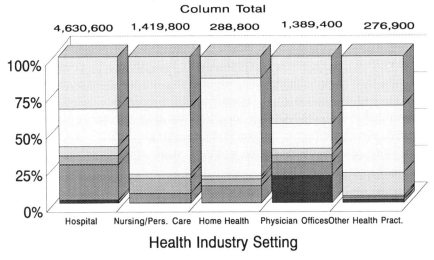

Column Total

| 4,630,600 | 1,419,800 | 288,800 | 1,389,400 | 276,900 |

Health Industry Setting

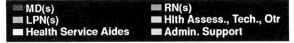

MD(s)
LPN(s)
Health Service Aides
RN(s)
Hlth Assess., Tech., Otr
Admin. Support

Source: U.S. Department of Labor, Bureau of Labor Statistics, Industry Occupation Matrix, 1990.

economy (U.S. Department of Labor, 1992). In any case, cost and competition may lead to major shifts in the mix of hospital workers, to a growing use of contracts for services and part-time employees to limit costs. The continued growth in the use of technology is likely to require more educated and sophisticated workers in the hospital of the future.

Nursing Homes and Home Health Agencies

Over two million Americans work in nursing homes, home health agencies, and other settings providing long-term care services to the elderly or chronically ill. As the baby boom generation ages and people live longer, there will be a sharp increase of those over 75 and even over 85 in the decades to come. This will lead to the need for a wide range of additional health and health-related long-term care workers. Currently, nursing homes use a lower skill mix than hospitals, reflecting the nursing home focus on maintenance. Figure 4.3 provides a profile of the long-term care workforce.

With the effort to contain costs, including shifts to the least intensive level of care, it is expected that the number of home health workers will increase very rapidly over the coming years—four times the rate of growth in the general economy. The need for nursing home workers will also increase, but more slowly (U.S. Department of Labor, 1992). The shifting of patients with greater health care needs to nursing homes and home care will lead to increased employment of skilled professionals in these settings.

Health Practitioner Offices

Private physician and dentist offices and other ambulatory care settings, such as clinics and health maintenance organizations, employ large numbers of workers. With the exception of offices of dentists, employment in these settings has been growing rapidly and is expected to continue to grow for the foreseeable future. In addition to the increased number of workers required as services shift from inpatient to outpatient care, many new technologies, such as diagnostic procedures, are available on an ambulatory basis.

Physician Education and Training

Historically, physicians have been the leaders of the health services delivery system. Their decisions determine the use of most health services, such as care provided by other professionals, return visits, laboratory services, hospital use, and home health services. Medicine is among the highest paid and most respected professions in America (Ginzberg, 1993). Physician training takes 11 to 13 years beyond high school. Policy discussions related to health care reform, increasing access, cost containment and improving quality all include discussions of the supply, distribution, and education of physicians. This section provides an overview of these areas as they relate to physician education.

There are two types of physicians: allopathic (M.D.) and osteopathic (D.O.). Allopathic medicine is "a system of medicine based on the theory that successful therapy depends on creating a condition antagonistic to or incompatible with the condition to be treated" (Slee & Slee, 1986). Osteopathic medicine "emphasizes a theory that the body can make its own remedies, given normal structural relationships, environmental conditions, and nutrition. It differs from allopathy primarily in its greater attention to body mechanics and manipulative methods in diagnosis and therapy" (Slee & Slee, 1986).

Undergraduate Medical Education

There are 126 allopathic medical schools in the United States, most of which are part of academic medical centers that include tertiary hospitals and medical complexes. These medical schools graduated 15,554 physicians in 1992 (Jonas, Etzel, & Baransky, 1993). In addition, there are 15 osteopathic schools, which graduated 1,537 physicians in 1992 (American Association of Colleges of Osteopathic Medicine, 1992). Of the 126 allopathic schools, 76 (60%) are publicly sponsored medical schools.

Medical school is the first formal step in the professional education of physicians. Medical school usually requires four years following baccalaureate education. The first two years are usually didactic, that is instruction taught in the classroom; and the second two years are primarily clinical experience. Usually, medical students in their third and fourth years receive training in different specialties. Nationally, medical students spend about 13 weeks in internal medicine, 7 weeks in pediatrics, 7 weeks in obstetrics-gynecology, 6 weeks in family practice, 9 weeks in general surgery, and 6 weeks in psychiatry (Jonas, Etzel, & Baransky, 1993).

Numerous questions have been raised regarding the adequacy and appropriateness of the traditional medical education model. The current process is lengthy, costly, and has produced an overabundance of specialists and too few primary care physicians. Medical schools have also been criticized for not encouraging physicians to practice in inner-city or rural areas, for overemphasizing high-tech tertiary care, for emphasizing organ systems rather than the whole patient, and for not educating more underrepresented minorities.

As a result of these criticisms, there has been a major reassessment of medical school curricula, and many schools have modified or are considering modifying the traditional curriculum (Jonas, Etzel, & Baransky, 1993). In some cases, medical schools are coordinating their education with colleges and graduate training programs to shorten the education process. In other cases, schools are beginning clinical training earlier in the education process, and many are providing more experience and training outside of acute care hospitals.

Medical School Enrollment

Medicine is a highly sought profession, and applications far exceed available slots. This is despite high tuition and length of the education. There was concern in the late 1970s and 1980s about declining applicants to medical schools. Table 4.3 highlights enrollment trends. The number of applicants to medical school dropped nearly 40% from a high of 42,600 in 1974 to 26,700 in 1988–1989. However, the downward trend in applicants ended in 1988–1989, and applica-

TABLE 4.3 Allopathic Medical School Enrollment

Academic year	Number of applicants	Applicant/ acceptance ratio	First year enrollment	Graduates	Percentage of women graduates	Percentage of underrepresented minority graduates
1971–72	29,172	2.4	12,361	9,551	8.9	N.A.
1981–82	36,727	2.1	17,320	15,824	25.0	7.7
1986–87	21,232	1.8	16,779	15,836	32.1	9.7
1992–93	37,410	2.1	17,001	15,554	38.2	11.5

Source: Jonas, Etzel, & Baransky. "Educational Programs in U.S. Medical Schools," *Journal of The American Medical Association,* 270:9, September 1, 1993.

Journal of The American Medical Association, Appendix II, 270:9, September 1, 1993.

Crowley, *Journal of The American Medical Association,* 258:8, August 28, 1987.

U.S. Department of Health and Human Services, *Minorities and Women in the Health Fields,* June, 1990, Table 13, p. 37.

tions are again rising. Although not identified in Table 4.3, there were an estimated 42,000 applications for 17,000 first-year slots in 1993 (Jonas, Etzel, & Baransky, 1993).

While medical school graduations have been relatively stable, between 15,000 and 16,000 since 1980, female graduates have continued to increase. As indicated in Table 4.3, female graduations have risen from 8.9% in 1971–1972 to 38.2% in 1992–1993. This has implications for the health care system, as female physicians have different specialty and practice patterns than male physicians.

Despite extensive concern expressed over the past several decades regarding the low percentage of minority physicians, there has been little growth in underrepresented minority enrollment in medical schools. In 1982, 7.7% of the medical school graduates were black, Native American, and Hispanic; and in 1992–1993, they represented 11.5% of graduates (Crowley, Etzel & Shaw, 1987; Jonas, Etzel, & Baransky, 1993). According to the 1990 census, 22% of Americans were black, American Indians, and Hispanic; and the percentage is expected to increase in future years. This underrepresentation in medicine is important not only in terms of social equity, but also because of the potential impact of cultural sensitivity on the outcomes of care.

An issue of growing concern for faculty, students, and policymakers is the rise in medical school tuition and student debt. Tuition in private medical schools more than doubled from an average of $9,300 per year in 1981 to $18,900 in 1990. Tuition in public medical schools has nearly tripled, increasing from $2,500 in 1980 for in-state students to $7,205 in 1992 (Jolin et al., 1992). Scholarship funding did not keep pace with this rise in tuition. While tuition more than doubled, scholarship support went up only 36%. For example, the Federal Government's National Health Service Corps, which provided about 1,900 new service-conditioned scholarships in 1979–1980, has provided fewer than 100 new awards per year since 1982. The mean debt of graduating medical students increased from $21,051 in 1982 to $55,859 in 1992 (Jolin et al., 1992). This level of debt may discourage medical students from choosing primary care specialties and from going into underserved areas.

Government policies on medical education have evolved over the years. From the early 1960s until the late 1970s, federal and most state policies were designed to increase the number of physicians. During this period, the Federal Government provided construction grants and subsidies to expand medical educational capacity, as well as scholarships and low-interest loans to students. States supported the development of many medical schools. The number of medical schools grew from 89 in 1966–1967 to 126 in 1980–1981. During this same period, the number of medical school graduates more than doubled from 7,743 to 15,667 per year. In 1980, the Graduate Medical Education National Advisory Council (GMENAC) concluded that medical education capacity had grown too much and that the country would face a surplus of physicians (GMENAC, 1980)—which would be costly, inefficient, and endanger patient care. An oversupply could lead to physicians providing unnecessary services, or to a loss of skills if physicians were not able to maintain a minimum level of activity.

Despite the potential for an oversupply of physicians, there are serious geographic and specialty maldistribution problems. There are too few physicians in rural and poor urban communities, and in primary care specialties. Policymakers hoped that by increasing the number of physicians throughout the 1970s, the marketplace would eventually correct this distribution without government intervention. However, while the increase in the number of medical graduates did lead to some dispersal of physicians into underserved areas, most of the additional physicians chose subspecialties, and most located in urban areas (AMA, 1993a). Attempting to address distribution problems by producing additional physicians is inefficient and usually ineffective.

Graduate Medical Education

Medicine is the only profession where graduation from professional school is not sufficient for entry into active practice. In all states, to be licensed as a physician, to practice independently, and to be recognized by the profession as fully prepared, a physician must complete at least some supervised practical clinical experience through graduate medical education, known as residency training. Until the early part of the Twentieth Century, most physicians went directly from medical school to clinical practice. In response to the 1910 Flexner Report, a period of a year or two of internship was established to provide physicians with practical experience (Flexner, 1910). Following this internship, most physicians practiced as generalists, providing a full range of services to their patients. As medicine became more complex and the number of physicians grew, specialization occurred. Following medical school, most physicians choose a specialty. Specific training then occurs in this area. Figure 4.4 shows the number of years needed for major specialty credentialing. After specialty training, a physician may choose to "subspecialize. For example, after training in internal medicine, a physician can choose additional training and subspecialize in cardiology.

The vast majority of allopathic medical school graduates (92% in 1992–1993) participate in the National Residency Match Program (NRMP) to select a residency program. In their senior year, medical students assess and evaluate residency training programs. This usually includes interviews at specific programs. Each March residency programs submit, in order of preference, the list of medical students the program would like to have in their program; simultaneously, students submit their ranked preferences. The respective preference lists are then compared and matched by a computer. Both medical students and residency programs are then notified of their match. Students who participate must agree to abide by the computer match (NRMP, 1992).

Osteopathic graduates are required to do a 1-year osteopathic internship after

FIGURE 4.4   Overview of Positions in Residencies

The various types of residencies are diagrammed in the figure below. The length of each bar is the period of years of training required for certification by the various Specialty Boards. These are unofficial assignments derived from published materials and are offered only for information. Consult the current *Directory of Graduate Medical Education Programs Accredited by the Accreditation Council for Graduate Medical Education* (the "Green Book") for the official requirements.

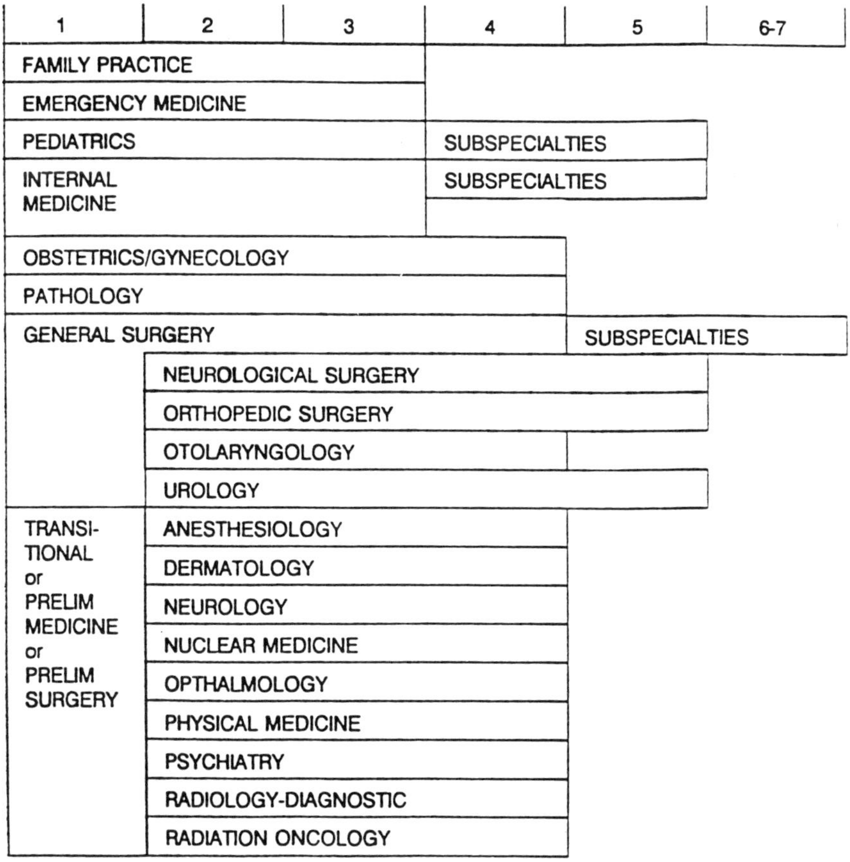

1	2	3	4	5	6-7
FAMILY PRACTICE					
EMERGENCY MEDICINE					
PEDIATRICS			SUBSPECIALTIES		
INTERNAL MEDICINE			SUBSPECIALTIES		
OBSTETRICS/GYNECOLOGY					
PATHOLOGY					
GENERAL SURGERY				SUBSPECIALTIES	
	NEUROLOGICAL SURGERY				
	ORTHOPEDIC SURGERY				
	OTOLARYNGOLOGY				
	UROLOGY				
TRANSI-TIONAL or PRELIM MEDICINE or PRELIM SURGERY	ANESTHESIOLOGY				
	DERMATOLOGY				
	NEUROLOGY				
	NUCLEAR MEDICINE				
	OPTHALMOLOGY				
	PHYSICAL MEDICINE				
	PSYCHIATRY				
	RADIOLOGY-DIAGNOSTIC				
	RADIATION ONCOLOGY				

Many specialties indicated as starting at the PGY-2 now offer categorical tracks which include the first year.

NRMP Directory: 1993. Washington, D.C.: National Residency Matching Program, 1992, p. vi.

completion of medical school. Most then enter an osteopathic or allopathic residency position before entering practice.

The Residency Experience

Traditionally, residency training has been a grueling and intense experience involving long hours and low pay. This has not changed much over the past several decades. According to the AMA, the average resident worked 72 hours per week, with many residents working more than 100 hours per week in 1987 (Silberger, 1988). In 1992, the mean salary for a first-year resident was $29,700. Residents care for patients in the evening and on weekends when few other physicians are available. As a consequence, most residents must work every few nights in addition to their daytime activities. Many residents regularly work shifts of greater than 24 consecutive hours, and many moonlight to supplement their income (Martini, Carlos, & Grenholim, 1993). The long hours may be changing as concerns are raised regarding the impact on both patients and residents. In 1991, New York State, the state with the most residents, established a limit of 80 hours per week, limited the number of consecutive hours of work, and required a minimum time off each week. Other states are also considering imposing similar limits.

The vast majority of residency training takes place in large teaching hospitals. These hospitals offer residents an opportunity to see a wide range of patient conditions; and, in many cases, these hospitals are where medical schools and their faculty are located. Although the primary purpose of graduate medical education is physician education, residents are an excellent source of low-cost medical personnel for hospitals. Not only is the pay low for long hours of work, but the Medicare method of reimbursing hospitals provides major financial benefits to hospitals that use residents (PPRC, 1993). There is no support from Medicare or other payors for training that occurs outside of hospitals.

The concentration of training in large teaching hospitals has been criticized as resulting in the overuse of high-cost technology and inpatient services (COGME, 1992; PPRC, 1993). With the shifting of more services to ambulatory care settings, the shortage of primary care physicians, and the surplus of subspecialists, there is a growing effort to provide more training in ambulatory settings to better prepare physicians and encourage them to practice primary care. This shift has not been easy to accomplish because of the fiscal disincentives. Training in ambulatory care settings also reduces practitioner productivity more than in the hospital setting.

The Growth of Residency Programs and Specialties

In 1992, there were 7,065 residency programs accredited by the Accreditation Council for Graduate Medical Education (ACGME) (JAMA, 1993). The ACGME is a private national body that oversees the accreditation of allopathic residency programs. Its governing board includes representatives from the American Board of Medical Specialties, the American Hospital Association, the American Medical Association, the Association of Amcrican Medical Colleges and the Council of Medical Specialty Societies. In each specialty, a Residency Review Committee (RRC) establishes standards and assesses individual residency program performance against those standards.

In 1992, there were 19,794 first-year residents in ACGME accredited residency programs, a number substantially higher than the 15,554 graduates of U.S. allopathic medical schools. Nearly 25% of first-year residents (4,870) were graduates of foreign medical schools, and approximately 4% were graduates of osteopathic medical schools (JAMA, 1993).

Throughout the 1980s, there was a sharp increase in the total number of residents and specialty areas in which physicians could train. As indicated in Table 4.4, the number of residents increased nearly 30% from 69,142 in 1982 to 88,620 in 1992 (JAMA, 1993). During this same period, the number of first-year residents rose only about 4% from 18,972 in 1982 to 19,794 in 1992. The rapid growth in the number of residents in all years reflects the sharp increase in the number of residents going on to subspecialty training. Between 1987 and 1992, the number of ACGME approved subspecialties grew from 47 to 82. In 1992, in response to this rapid growth, the ACGME declared a one-year moratorium on the accreditation of new subspecialties (Martini, 1992).

The number of subspecialty residents grew at a substantially higher rate than primary care residents. As indicated in Table 4.4, between 1982 and 1992, the number of internal medicine residents grew by almost 12%, whereas the number in acciedited internal medicine subspecialty programs grew from 0 to 7,400 in the same time period (JAMA, 1993). Although there was some limited subspecialty training in 1982, there were no accredited programs. This growth in residency training positions is expected to contribute to an increase of over 200% in the number of practicing internal medicine subspecialists between 1978 to 1998, while the general population is expected to grow by about 19%. As a result, it is estimated that the number of adults for each internal medicine subspecialist will drop from 7,225 to 2,995 (Kletke, Shleiter, & Tarlov, 1987). Despite the concern with likely surpluses in most subspecialties, more than half the physicians in internal medicine residency programs choose to subspecialize (Martini, 1992).

The growth in residency positions and subspecialties was acceptable when there was a perceived shortage of physicians and increased specialization was viewed as improving quality and a necessary component of medical advances. However, as concerns grow about the potential negative aspects of an oversupply of specialists and the shortage of primary care physicians, there is a growing consensus that change is needed in the specialty distribution and the central role played by residency training (Wennberg et al., 1993).

TABLE 4.4 Residency Training

Specialty	First year-residents			All residents			
	1982	1992	Percentage of change (82–92)	1982	1992	Percentage of change (82–92)	Percentage female in 1992
Anesthesiology	537	371	–30.9	3,369	5,297	57.2	21.7
Dermatology	10	18	80.0	789	861	9.1	50.4
Emergency medicine	132	474	259.1	885	2,115	139.0	25.4
Family practice	2389	2069	–13.4	7,040	6,976	–0.9	37.3
Internal medicine	6319	7369	14.0	17,185	19,191	11.7	30.6
IM subspecialties	0	0	0	0	7,403	—	28.8
Neurosurgery	40	45	12.5	621	703	13.2	6.8
Neurology	60	40	–33.3	1,276	1,308	2.5	26.2
Obstetric & gynec.	1052	1043	–.9	4,702	4,843	3.0	49.9
Ophthalmology	27	13	–51.9	1,553	1,584	2.0	24.1
Orthopedic surgery	231	347	50.2	2,733	2,843	4.0	6.0
Otolaryngology	81	49	–64.2	1,001	1,071	7.0	14.6
Pathology	530	435	–17.9	2,437	2,418	–0.8	40.0
Pediatrics	1865	2103	12.8	5,720	6,680	16.8	58.9
Pediatric subspec.	0	0	0	104	1,208	1,061.5	37.9
Physical med & rehab.	93	82	–11.8	624	970	55.4	34.2
Plastic surgery	0	0	0	365	441	20.8	14.7
Psychiatry	931	954	2.5	4,235	4,879	15.2	44.0
Child psychiatry	0	0	0	528	643	21.8	47.8
Radiology-diagnos.	358	384	7.3	3,155	4,005	26.9	26.2
Surgery-general	2805	2550	–9.1	8,064	7,995	–0.9	15.7
Urology	64	70	9.4	1,041	1,003	–3.7	6.5
Transitional year	1381	1390	0.6	0	1,458	—	26.3
All	18,972	19,794	4.3	69,142	88,620	28.2	30.0

Source: Journal of American Medical Association, 270:9, September 1, 1993, Appendix II.

Women in Residency Training

As indicated in Table 4.4, women are far more likely to go into those specialties generally considered primary care. While women made up 30% of all residents in 1992, they constituted 37% of the residents in family practice, 59% in pediatrics, and 50% in obstetrics. On the other hand, they represented only 16% in surgery and 6% in orthopedic surgery (JAMA, 1993).

International Medical School Graduates

Foreign medical school graduates, referred to as international medical school graduates (IMGs), are eligible to apply for residency training if they pass specific examinations testing medical knowledge and English proficiency and meet other conditions. Because of the concern with shortages in the 1950s and 1960s, immigration requirements for physicians were reduced. In 1992, 20% of all residents were foreign medical school graduates. However, discussions on limiting the supply of physicians are focusing on policies on residency slots, which would likely limit the number of IMGs in residency training. For example, the National Council on Graduate Medical Education and the Physician Payment Review Commission have recommended that the total number of residency slots in the U.S. be limited to the number of U.S. medical school graduates plus 10% (COGME, 1992; PPRC, 1993). The reduction of the number of IMGs in training could create problems for many inner-city hospitals that rely on IMG residents to provide services.

Approximately one-third of IMGs in training in the U.S. are on exchange visas allowing them to learn American medical care and requiring them to return to their native countries (JAMA, 1993). The remainder are immigrants planning to stay in the U.S.

Cost and Financing of Medical Education and Residency Training

In 1991–1992, the nation's 126 allopathic medical schools reported expenditures of $22 billion, of which $6 billion was for instruction, $5 billion for research, $5 billion for services, and $2 billion for support (Krakower, 1993). During the 1980s medical school expenditures tripled, in part attributable to a sharp increase in faculty-to-student ratios (Ginzberg, Ostow & Dutka, 1993). It is difficult to estimate the actual cost of medical education, as medical centers produce a variety of products. For example, faculty teach as well as provide patient care. However, one estimate of instruction costs per student was $68,000 per year in 1990–1991 (Ginzberg, Ostow, & Dutka, 1993).

Although student tuition covered only a small share of education costs, rising tuition has contributed to rising student debt, as has the termination of a number of federal scholarship and subsidized loan programs. Although physicians can anticipate higher than average incomes once they begin practice, the very lengthy period for education and for residency training with its relatively low salaries, combined with most loans coming due in the second year of residency training, may discourage medical students from choosing primary care. One recent survey found that higher debt had a significant impact on career decisions by medical students (Ginzberg, Ostow, & Dutka, 1993).

Medicare, which pays about 38% of all hospital costs nationally, reimburses hospitals with residency programs for direct and indirect costs. Direct costs include the costs of salaries, fringe benefits, and facility overhead for residents and their faculty. Indirect costs include the higher costs associated with patient care in teaching hospitals. Some of the costs reflect sicker, higher-need patients than those in the average nonteaching hospital, and some costs may reflect the use of additional services (e.g., diagnostic tests), which are part of the residents' education. One estimate of the total direct and indirect costs for GME for all payors (Medicare, Medicaid, private insurance, etc.) is more than $13 billion per year or $184,400 per resident (Mullan, Rivo, & Politzer, 1993).

The current system of financing GME has been criticized for a variety of reasons in addition to high cost. First, because Medicare and other payors reimburse hospitals generously for resident training, this payment encourages hospitals to develop residency programs and to use residents as a cost-effective source of medical care, even if additional physicians are not needed in the community. Second, because Medicare and other insurers reimburse graduate medical education in hospitals and not in ambulatory care settings, training in ambulatory care settings is discouraged. Finally, the whole community benefits from the education and training of physicians. Adding the costs for training into the rates of only teaching hospitals that provide the training makes them uncompetitive in a managed care environment where HMOs and other plans contract with hospitals based in part on their costs.

As a result of these concerns, major organizations, such as the Council on Graduate Medical Education and the Physician Payment Review Commission, have recommended changes in the financing and organization of residency training. The suggested changes include: limiting total funding for GME, providing reimbursement for training in ambulatory care settings, and developing a central national fund to spread the costs of GME and the development of a national commission to determine the number and mix of residency positions (COGME, 1992; PPRC, 1993; O'Neil, 1993).

Physician Supply and Distribution

The adequacy of the supply and distribution of physicians and the appropriate government role in these issues has been debated for years. The government's role was historically referred to as "manpower policy." In the 1980s, government let the marketplace determine how many of what types of professionals to educate. In the early 1990s, it became clear that the marketplace was probably ineffective and, at least, inefficient in preparing the numbers and types of physicians needed by Americans. The number of specialists rapidly increased and continued to concentrate around large urban academic medical centers. With the growing discussion of national health care reform, attention once again turned to the adequacy of the supply and distribution of physicians and whether the nation's health care goals can be achieved without more explicit government policies related to physician supply (Kindig, Cultice, & Mullan, 1993). This new discussion is referred to as "workforce planning" (Mullan, 1992; Rivo & Satcher, 1993).

Total Physician Supply

In 1992, there were approximately 687,000 physicians in the U.S. Of these, 500,092 (73%) were graduates of U.S. allopathic schools; 34,050 (5%) were graduates of U.S. osteopathic schools; 8,571 (1%) were graduates of Canadian medical schools; and over 144,000 (21%) were graduates of foreign medical schools (American Medical Association, 1993a; U.S. DHHS, September 1992). As shown in Table 4.5, 82% of the allopathic physicians are patient care providers. The majority of these physicians are in office-based practice, which includes solo and group practice, as well as other ambulatory care settings, such as HMOs.

The number of patient care physicians more than doubled between 1970 and 1992. One common way of viewing physician supply is as a ratio of the number of physicians there are for each 100,000 people. The physician-to-population ratio, as shown in Table 4.6, increased from 125 patient care physicians per 100,000 people in 1970 to 204 in 1992, or about 80%. Another way of relating physician supply to population is the number of people for each physician. This dropped from 798 to 489 during the same period.

Geographical Distribution

The supply of physicians is not evenly distributed across the U.S. The majority of physicians are concentrated in urban areas around tertiary care medical centers. The geographic distribution of physicians reflects a variety of factors. Many physicians practice in areas near where they trained, which tends to be in urban academic medical centers. Some specialties require a hospital or tertiary care center for practice. Other physicians are also involved in teaching at academic medical centers.

The geographic distribution of physicians in the U.S. is of concern in both urban and rural areas. Many rural counties have a serious problem with access to physi-

TABLE 4.5　Distribution of Allopathic Physicians by Activity in 1992

	Number	Percentage
Patient Care	535,220	82.0
Office-Based Practice	389,364	59.6
Hospital-Based Practice	145,856	22.3
Residents	86,468	13.2
Clinical Fellows	7,128	1.1
Full Time Staff	52,260	8.0
Other Professional Activity	42,888	6.6
Medical Teaching	7,983	1.2
Administration	14,923	2.3
Research	16,367	2.5
Other	3,615	0.6
Not Classified	16,589	2.5
Inactive	55,656	8.5
Address Unknown	2,709	0.4
Total	653,062	100

Source: American Medical Association, *Physician Characteristics and Distribution in the U.S.*, 1993, table EE, p. 12.

cian services. As shown in Figure 4.5, as county population decreases, so too does the ratio of physicians to population. The lower physician-to-population ratio in most rural areas reflects, in part, the need for a minimum population base required to support a physician practice and to maintain skill levels for certain specialties. However, primary care physicians should be available to all people.

TABLE 4.6　Patient Care Physicians in the U.S. 1970 to 1992

	Patient care physicians	Physicians per 100,000 civilians	Civilian population per physician
1970	252,778	125	798
1975	285,345	135	741
1980	358,420	159	629
1985	426,721	180	555
1990	487,796	198	505
1992	520,216	204	489

Note: Nonfederal allopathic patient care physicians.

Source: American Medical Association, *Physician Characteristics & Distribution in the U.S.*, 1993, Table A-17, p. 33.

FIGURE 4.5   Physicians per 100,000 Rate, by Type of Area, 1989

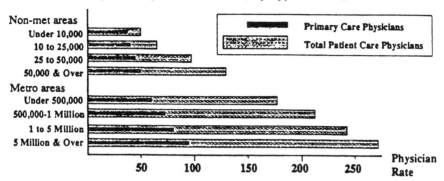

Source: U.S. Department of Health and Human Services. *Health Personnel in the United States Eighth Report to Congress: 1991.* Resources and Services Administration, September 1992. (DHHS Pub. No. HRSPOD 92-1).

Doubling the total U.S. physician supply has led to some dispersal of physicians to rural areas, but the vast majority of new physicians locate in urban areas. From 1970 to 1992, the supply of allopathic physicians grew by 299,635 in metropolitan statistical areas, an increase of 116%. During the same period, the number of physicians in nonmetropolitan areas went up 30,179, an increase of 70% (American Medical Association, 1993a). About one out of eleven new practitioners went into nonmetropolitan areas. Serious access problems remain in rural areas (National Rural Health Association, 1992). In 1992, there were 146 counties in the nation without a single active physician (American Medical Association, 1993a).

Problems of access to care in urban areas differs from those in rural areas. For most urban dwellers, hospitals and even major academic medical centers are within reasonable distances. However, large concentrations of low-income populations in the inner city lack access to primary care physicians and overuse hospital emergency departments or hospital specialty clinics for their basic care. In 1992, there were nearly 2,200 urban and rural areas that were classified by the federal government as "Health Professional Shortage Areas" or HPSAs. In total, these areas needed about 4,500 additional physicians to adequately serve their respective populations (Rivo & Satcher, 1993).

Gender and Nationality

One of the most striking recent changes in the physician supply in the U.S. has been the steady growth in the number of female physicians. As shown in Table

4.7, the percentage of female patient care physicians grew from 6.5% in 1970 to 18.6% in 1992. This trend will continue as the number of women in medical school continues to increase. In 1992–1993, nearly 42% of new medical students were women (Jonas, Etzel, & Baransky, 1993). Female physicians are more likely to go into primary care specialties and to work on regular schedules in salaried positions, making them more amenable to practice in managed care settings.

Table 4.7 also shows that the growth in the number of International Medical Graduates has been steady, although far less dramatic than for women. This growth is likely to continue for several years, as international medical school graduates were nearly 25% of first-year residents in the U.S. in 1992 (JAMA, 1993). Proposals under consideration to limit the number of residency positions would significantly decrease the percentage of IMGs in practice in the U.S.

Specialty Distribution

Table 4.8 presents the number of allopathic physicians in selected specialties from 1970 to 1992. Although the three specialties with the greatest number of physicians are considered primary care (internal medicine, family practice, and pediatrics), other specialists comprise 65% of all practicing physicians. The number of other specialist physicians is growing far faster than the number of primary care physicians. This growth is significantly different from most other countries, such as Canada, Great Britain, and Germany, where more than 50% of physicians are in primary care specialties (PPRC, 1993).

As indicated in Table 4.8, the rapid increase in physicians between 1970 and 1992 has not been evenly spread among specialties. One study has calculated that

TABLE 4.7 Female and IMG Physicians

Year	Fed/non-fed total patient care physicians	Fed/non-fed female patient care		International medical graduated (IMG)	
		Number	Percentage	Number	Percentage
1970	278,535	18,362	6.5	48,191	17.3
1975	311,937	24,345	7.8	61,416	19.7
1980	976,512	39,969	10.6	72,935	19.4
1985	448,820	64,424	14.4	95,362	21.2
1990	503,870	86,376	17.1	106,515	21.1
1992	535,220	100,024	18.6	118,531	22.1

Note: Federal and Nonfederal allopathic physicians.

Source: American Medical Association, Physician Characteristics and Distribution in the U.S., 1993.

TABLE 4.8 Allopathic Physicians by Specialty 1970–1992

Specialty	1970	1980	1990	1992	Percentage of change (70–92)
Total Physicians	334,028	467,679	615,421	653,062	95.5
Anesthesiology	10,860	15,958	25,981	28,148	159.2
Cardiovas. Disease	6,476	9,823	15,862	16,478	154.4
Dermatology	4,003	5,660	7,557	7,912	97.7
Diagn. Radiology	1,968	7,048	15,412	17,253	776.7
Emergency Medicine	0	5,669	14,243	15,470	—
Family Practice	0	27,530	47,639	50,969	—
Gastroenterology	2,010	4,046	7,493	7,946	295.3
General Practice	57,948	32,519	22,841	20,719	−64.2
General Surgery	29,761	34,034	38,376	39,211	31.8
Internal Medicine	40,153	70,013	98,349	109,071	171.5
Neurology	3,074	5,685	9,237	9,742	216.9
Obstetrics/Gyn.	18,876	26,305	33,697	35,273	86.9
Ophthalmology	9,927	12,974	16,073	16,433	65.5
Orthopedic Surgery	9,620	13,996	19,138	20,640	114.6
Otolaryngology	5,409	6,553	8,138	8,373	54.8
Pathology	10,283	13,402	16,170	17,005	65.4
Pediatrics	18,332	28,803	40,893	44,881	144.8
Psychiatry	21,146	27,481	35,163	36,405	72.2
Radiology	10,524	11,653	8,492	7,848	−25.4
Urological Surgery	5,795	7,743	9,372	9,452	63.1

Note: Total Federal and Nonfederal physicians.

Source: American Medical Association, Physician Characteristics and Distribution in the U.S., 1993, Table A-2, p. 18.

between 1978 and 1998, internal medicine subspecialists will increase by 206%, whereas general internists will grow by only 77% (Kletke et al., 1987). Surveys of graduating medical students indicate that interest and intentions to go into specialties other than primary care is not only continuing but increasing (Petersdorf, 1993).

Future Growth and Future Needs

The increase in the number of physicians and the physician-to-population ratio raises several serious concerns. First, the lack of primary care physicians in many communities will prevent access to needed services and deter effective implementation of health care reform. Second, an excess supply of specialists will contribute to higher costs and unnecessary services. Third, many specialist-trained physicians may be displaced by the changes in the health care system, and these specialists will provide primary care services that they are not appropriately educated to provide.

The Graduate Medical Education National Advisory Committee (GMENAC), after extensive study of the practice of different specialties and the medical needs of the nation, estimated the nation's needs in each specialty. The GMENAC report of 1980 was the first major report suggesting the nation would have a surplus of physicians (GMENAC, 1980). Table 4.9 presents the GMENAC recommendations, the staffing used at several large prepaid group practices, and the current national physician-to-population ratios. Although the GMENAC recommended 191 physicians per 100,000 and HMOs used 111 per 100,000, it is estimated that the nation already had 220 patient care physicians per 100,000 in 1992, with the number growing rapidly. Although the GMENAC recommendations have been questioned and debated—with some arguing the numbers are too high and others that they are too low—they remain the most systematic and comprehensive assessment of the supply and demand for physicians.

Physician Practice Patterns

Because HMOs use far fewer physicians than more traditional fee-for-service care, there is growing concern that health care reform and increased enrollment in managed care arrangements will lead to a surplus of physicians in many nonprimary care specialties. This has led to a number of proposals to reduce the number of specialists and to retrain existing specialists (Mullan, 1993; Wennberg et al., 1993).

According to the American Medical Association (American Medical Association, 1993b), in 1991, physicians worked on average 59 hours per week; this reflected a modest but steady increase over the prior ten years, from 57 hours per week in 1982. Within those 59 hours, on average, 53 were devoted to patient care activities. This too has increased steadily from 1982, when it was 51 hours per week. In 1991, physicians worked on average 47 weeks per year (American Medical Association, 1993b).

The distribution of direct patient hours among such activities as office visits, surgery, hospital rounds and other visits, varies considerably among specialties. Although specialists spend the majority of their time providing care in the office, the amount of time is highest for general/ family practitioners and pediatricians. Obstetricians/gynecologists, who provide more hours of patient care per week than the other specialties, spend the same percentage of their time in providing hospital services as surgeons.

The average visits per week per doctor declined from 1983 to 1992, from 123 to 115. This includes a drop in hospital round visits from 33 in 1983 to 21 in 1992,

TABLE 4.9   Comparison of Physician to Population Ratios (per 100,000)

	HMOs[1]	GMENAC[2]	U.S. active 1992
Family and General Pract.	10.3	25.2	27.1
General Internal Medicine	23.8	28.8	38.8
General Pediatrics	14.9	15.1	16.2
Osteopathic	—	—	6.2
Subtotal Primary Care	49.0	69.1	88.3
Obstetrics/Gynecology	10.7	9.9	13.3
General Surgery	5.8	9.7	14.8
Psychiatry	3.8	19.5	12.9
Anesthesiology	3.6	9.1	10.6
Dermatology	2.3	2.9	2.9
Emergency Medicine	4.9	5.5	5.8
Gastroenterology	1.5	2.7	2.8
Neurological Surgery	1.5	3.4	3.3
Ophthalmology	2.9	4.8	6.4
Orthopedic Surgery	3.9	6.2	7.9
Urological Surgery	2.2	3.2	3.6
Otolaryngology	2.3	3.3	3.2
Pathology	1.7	6.5	5.4
Radiology	4.4	8.9	9.3
Other physicians	0.0	26.7	29.7
Total Patient Care Phys.	111.2	191.4	220.2

Explanation:
[1]HMO figures reflect 1983 data for seven large HMOs.
[2]GMENAC figures reflect the recommended physician to population ratios developed by the Graduate Medical Education Advisory Committee.
Sources:

HMO and GMENAC data from: Mulhausen, Robert and McGee, Jeanne. "Physician Need: An Alternative Projection From a Study of Large, Prepaid Group Practice." *Journal of American Medical Association*, 261:13:1930–1934, April 7, 1989.

U.S. Active, except for the osteopathic numbers, were taken from: American Medical Association. *Physician Characteristics and Distribution in the U.S.* Roback, Gene, Randolph, Lilliam, Seidman and Bradley (Eds.). Chicago, IL: Department of Physician Data Services, 1993. This data source includes residents in the counts.

The osteopathic numbers in U.S. Active were taken from: American Association of Colleges of Osteopathic Medicine, *1992 Annual Statistical Report*, Rockville, Maryland, June 1992.

reflecting the increase in services being provided on an ambulatory basis. As indicated in Figure 4.6, the average number of visits and their location varies significantly by specialty, ranging from 102 for surgeons to 138 for general and family practitioners. The vast majority of all physician visits occur in physician offices (American Medical Association, 1993b).

Physician Income

Physicians are among the highest paid professionals in the U.S., and their income through the 1980s grew faster than any other profession (Pope & Schneider, 1992). Figure 4.7 indicates the average and median net income after expenses but before taxes for some of the major specialties. Of particular interest is the much lower level of net income for primary care physicians.

FIGURE 4.6   Distribution of Average Total Patient Visits per Week, by Specialty, 1992

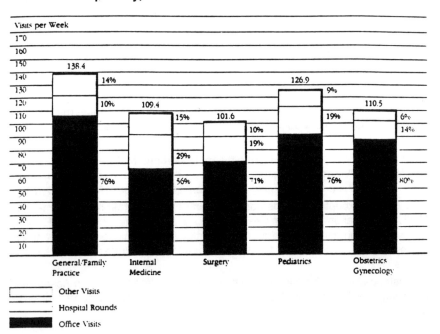

Source: American Medical Association. *Socioeconomic Characteristics of Medical Practice.* Gonzalez and Martin (Ed). Chicago, IL: Center for Health Policy Research, 1993, Figure 5, p. 71.

FIGURE 4.7   Average and Median Physician Net Income (in Thousands of Dollars) after Expenses before Taxes, by Specialty, 1991

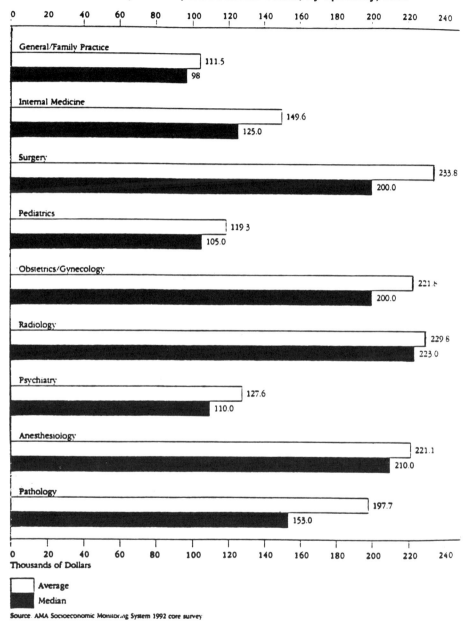

Source: American Medical Association. *Socioeconomic Characteristics of Medical Practice.* Gonzalez and Martin (Ed). Chicago, IL: Center for Health Policy Research, 1993, Figure 17, p. 141.

In response to concerns regarding the growing disparity between the incomes of subspecialists and primary care physicians and the increased awareness of the need for more primary care physicians, Congress enacted major changes in 1989 in the way Medicare fees would be determined. After extensive study, a reimbursement method called Resource Based Relative Value Scale, or RBRVS, was developed. Under this methodology, physician fees are determined based on the time, effort, and knowledge required for a specific service. The methodology attempts to recognize, through increases in reimbursement, the importance and value of time spent with the patient on assessment and diagnosis and to reduce the fees paid for specific procedures, such as surgical procedures. The net result is intended to moderate the income of most subspecialists, especially surgical subspecialists, and increase relative income for primary care physicians. The reimbursement methodology is being phased in over five years, beginning in 1992 (Colby, 1992).

In order to encourage physicians to practice in underserved areas, Congress authorized higher Medicare fees for physician service areas designated as Health Professional Shortage Areas. Although Medicare only represents a portion of physician revenues, these changes provide additional income to physicians in those underserved areas.

Urban/Rural

Practice patterns also vary between urban and rural settings. As indicated in Table 4.10, physicians in nonmetropolitan areas work more hours per week overall and on patient care and provide significantly more visits per week. Fees are also lower in nonmetropolitan areas. While professional expenses and net income in larger metropolitan areas are significantly higher than nonmetropolitan areas for all physicians in those areas, this appears to reflect, at least in part, the different mix of specialties in the different areas. When family practice is considered alone, family practitioners in less urbanized areas had higher office expenses and higher net income after expenses. This reflects the provision by nonmetropolitan family practitioners of 43.5% more visits but charges of 38.8% less (for an office visit with an established patient). The net result is that rural family practitioners actually made 15.6% more than their urban counterparts.

Physician Workforce Issues

The Council on Graduate Medical Education (COGME) was authorized by Congress in 1986 to advise the federal government and the Congress on issues related to the supply, distribution and use of physicians. The Council issued its third report with specific findings and recommendations for physician workforce reform (COGME, 1992). The following is a brief summary of the Council's findings and recommendations:

TABLE 4.10 Urban and Rural Practice Patterns

All Physicians

Setting	Hours per week in profession	Patient care hours	Patient visits per week	Mean fee patient office	(In Thousands)	
					Professional expenses	Net income before taxes
Nonmetro	62.7	57.8	148.5	$34.24	$156.9	$150.4
Metro < 1 million	59.5	54.0	121.0	$43.41	$168.2	$174.8
Metro > 1 million	57.6	51.0	102.9	$51.90	$171.2	$170.4

Family Practitioner

Setting	Hours per week in profession	Patient care hours	Patient visits perweek	Mean fee patient office	(In Thousands)	
					Professional expenses	Net income before taxes
Nonmetro	63.1	58.2	173.3	$30.15	$158.0	$123.8
Metro < 1 million	58.3	52.5	135.1	$36.69	$136.2	$108.4
Metro > 1 million	55.9	50.6	120.8	$41.85	$150.3	$107.1

Sources: American Medical Association. *Socioeconomic Characteristics of Medical Practice.* Gonzalez, Martin (Ed). Chicago, IL: Center for Health Policy Research, 1993.

Findings of the Council on Graduate Medical Education

1. The Nation has too few generalists and too many specialists.
2. Problems of access to medical care persist in rural and inner-city areas despite large increases in the number of physicians.
3. The racial/ethnic composition of the Nation's physicians does not reflect the general population and contributes to access problems for underrepresented minorities.
4. Shortages exist in the specialties of general surgery, adult and child psychiatry, preventive medicine, and among generalist physicians with geriatrics training.
5. Within the framework of the present health care system, current physician-to-population ratio in the nation is adequate. Further increases in this ratio will do little to enhance the health of the public or to address the Nation's

problems of access to care. Continued increases in this ratio will hinder efforts to contain costs.

6. The Nation's medical education system can be more responsive to public needs for more generalists, underrepresented minority physicians, and physicians for medically underserved rural and inner-city areas.

7. The absence of a national physician workforce plan, combined with financial and other disincentives are barriers to improved access to care (COGME, 1992).

Quality Improvement

The quality of health care is discussed in depth in Chapter 14. The discussion in this chapter will focus on quality issues particularly related to physician practice. Quality of medical care historically has been promoted through licensure, accreditation, and certification, and controlled by physicians.

Freidson (1973) states that autonomy is a characteristic of a profession. The profession of medicine maintains its claim to autonomy because:

> First, the claim is that there is such an unusual degree of skill and knowledge involved in professional work that nonprofessionals are not equipped to evaluate or regulate it. Second, it is claimed that professionals are responsible—that they may be trusted to work conscientiously without supervision. Third, the claim is that the profession itself may be trusted to undertake the proper regulatory action on those rare occasions when an individual does not perform his work competently or ethically. (p. 137)

Historically, physicians have maintained that they and they alone determine the quality of their practice. Over the last 20 years, physicians have seen increased public concern with quality and increased government control over the practice of medicine. This includes state agencies that discipline physicians for unethical or unsafe practice and reimbursement procedures that restrict payment unless certain guidelines are followed.

Government Regulation

As Freidson (1973) points out, "The foundation of Medicine's control over its work is thus clearly political in character, involving the aid of the state in establishing and maintaining the profession's preeminence" (p. 23). Ultimately, medicine is not autonomous, for physician practice is controlled by government.

Much of current government regulation is based on the premise of finding the "bad apple." Rather than assuming that most physicians are professionals with the best interest of their patients in mind, government regulation assumes that physicians will try to get around "the systems." Thus, systems need to identify those physicians who do not practice high-quality care and regulations promulgated to restrict their practice. On the other hand, Continuous Quality Improvement proposes that attention be focused on health care systems and continuously improving patient care. Whether this approach will be effective is not clear.

Government's primary method of medical quality assurance is licensure. Physicians are licensed by states; and licensure requires graduation from medical school, graduate medical education, and passage of an examination. Although the specific number of years of graduate training needed for licensure varies by state and by whether the physician is a graduate of a U.S. or foreign medical school, some graduate training is needed for licensure in all states.

As early as 1760, New York passed a physician license act. However, by the Civil War, there were no longer licensure laws in effect in any state (Jones, 1993). In 1873, the first modern physician practice act was passed by Texas; and by 1912, all states had licensure laws (Jones, 1993). Some states routinely grant licensure to physicians who are licensed in other states. Others, such as Florida, require a physician to retake the licensing exam. Some states require continuing education for relicensure, others do not. Licensure is seen by some as setting minimal safe criteria for safeguarding the welfare of the public and is seen by others as a way to restrict entry into practice and to restrict the scope of practice of nonphysicians.

In addition to formal licensure, government also exerts considerable control over the practice of medicine through requirements for and monitoring of a variety of financing systems, such as Medicaid and Medicare. It is a rare physician who does not receive payment through one of these systems, and thus a rare physician who is not subject to their regulations.

Practice Guidelines

Practice guidelines denote standard practice for particular problems or diagnoses. They usually identify appropriate tests, pharmaceuticals, and procedures for a specific medical problem or diagnosis. These guidelines may be developed by an individual physician in private practice and followed by ancillary staff or by groups of physicians who practice together, such as those working in HMOs, with the expectation that all physicians in the group will follow the protocol unless a well-documented reason is given. In recent years, the federal government through the Agency for Health Care Policy and Research (AHCPR) has developed and continues to develop suggested practice guidelines for selected medical problems. Examples include those developed for acute pain management and urinary incontinence (U.S. DHHS, February, 1992; and U.S. DHHS, March, 1992).

It is expected that these guidelines will improve the quality of medical care.

Some physicians argue that they are "cook book" medicine and do not take into account differences in individual patients. Critics also contend that medical care is constantly changing, and such protocols do not allow physicians to take into consideration the latest clinical experiences and research findings. Supporters contend that such guidelines protect the public from both over and under use of medical care.

Malpractice

Under the tort system in the United States, patients are permitted to sue physicians and others for personal injury. Malpractice is seen as an important protection for the public against physician error. Many argue that the threat of malpractice forces physicians to practice "defensive medicine." That is, physicians order additional and often unnecessary tests and procedures to protect themselves from potential malpractice suits. Malpractice premiums for physicians are about 5% of their revenue, or more than $7 billion annually. It is estimated that defensive medicine adds about $25 billion annually to the nation's health bill ("Care: How We Got To This Mess," October 4, 1993).

Other Credentialing

Another way to promote quality is through certification and accreditation. Each specialty establishes standards for physicians seeking to be "Board Certified." This includes, at a minimum, satisfactory completion of an accredited residency program and passage of an exam. It may also include several years of practice and completion of a minimum number of specific procedures. In some specialties, such as family practice, a physician must periodically pass an exam or demonstrate continuing competency. Board certification provides professional recognition within a specialty and sets minimum qualifications for practice as a Board Certified physician. This is an important example of the self-regulation of the medical profession by physicians.

Another approach to promoting high quality of care is through the regulation of health facilities, including requiring that they monitor the physicians who practice in their facility. For example, the Joint Commission on Accreditation of Health Care Organizations (JCAHO) requires that hospitals and other facilities monitor physicians who practice in their facilities. The JCAHO requires hospitals to set criteria for staff privileges. For example, the hospital's medical by-laws may state that only "board eligible" or "board certified" surgeons may conduct surgery. They may further state that only physicians with certain training or experience, as evaluated by the hospital's medical board, may perform certain complex procedures. In this way, although all physicians in the same state may have the same license, physicians are restricted by health facilities in the types of care they can provide. Unlike licensure, which is usually for life, health facilities are expected to monitor performance on an ongoing basis.

Ginzberg (1990) suggests that the medical establishment has experienced an erosion of power in recent years, which it can regain if the medical profession can achieve consensus on a range of issues. Among the critical issues he identifies are the supply of physicians and new medical technology. In addition, physicians must assure the public that they are concerned with and ready to do something about the quality and cost of medical care.

Organized Medicine

The American Medical Association (AMA) is a national group organized in 1846 (Jones, 1993) made up of state and territorial associations and county groups. A physician is not directly a member of the AMA, rather the physician joins a county association. These county members vote representatives to the state association. These representatives then elect members to the National House of Delegates. A Board of Trustees, elected by the House of Delegates, then governs the AMA. Full-time staff support the work of the AMA.

The AMA plays several important roles. In order to be licensed as a physician, states require that the student graduate from an approved medical school. Approved schools are those approved by the Liaison Committee on Medical Education, a joint committee of the AMA and the Association of American Medical Colleges (AAMC). Thus, the AMA is influential in controlling access to licensure.

In addition to its role in accreditation, the AMA is best known for its role in the politics and economics of medicine. Historically, the AMA has been opposed to a variety of payment mechanisms. As early as 1920, the AMA formally opposed any compulsory health insurance (Jones, 1993). Although states control the practice of medicine, states have looked to the AMA and state medical societies for advice.

Although in the early 1970s about 70% of physicians were members of the AMA (Pear, 1993), only about 271,000 physicians (40%) were members of the AMA in 1992 (Daniels & Schwartz, 1994). Although the AMA is still a powerful organization, other physician groups are increasing in power.

The National Medical Association (Daniels & Schwartz, 1994) is the professional society for black physicians. With membership of about 14,500, it has councils in areas such as maternal and child health, medical education, and sections on the major medical specialties.

In addition to the general medical societies, there are numerous specialty societies. They range from the American Academy of Pediatrics, with 38,000 members, to the American Association of Neuropathologists, with 660 members (Backus, 1992). According to Jones (1993), there are 12,200 medical organizations, boards, and groups in the U.S.

The American Board of Medical Specialties approves specialty boards to set specialty training guidelines and evaluate candidates. There were 24 specialty boards approved as of 1993. In addition to these boards, there are numerous additional boards that are not approved (Jones, 1993).

Jones (1993) describes the American Association of Medical Colleges (AAMC) as an association representing the American medical schools, Canadian medical schools, major teaching hospitals, VA centers, and academic and professional societies. The association accredits U.S. medical education programs, provides testing services, and manages the National Residency Matching Program.

Although the power of organized medicine is diffused by the sheer number of medical organizations, it continues to exert substantial influence over health care in the United States. However, as the health care system evolves and the country moves toward health care reform, the power of organized medicine may be further reduced.

Other "Doctors"

In addition to physicians, there are a variety of other health workers educated in graduate programs beyond the baccalaureate who use the title "doctor." These "doctors" (e.g., dentists, podiatrists, chiropractors, and optometrists) tend to specialize in specific areas of the body. Each of these professions include their own body of knowledge, professional association, and educational requirements.

Based on data from the Department of Health and Human Services (U.S. DHHS, September 1992), in 1990, there were approximately 149,000 Doctors of Dental Science (DDS), a 46% increase since 1970. The ratio of dentists to 100,000 population, 59.5, was at an all time high in 1990. Dentists, like other health care professionals, are increasingly specializing. About 18% of dentists were specialists in 1990. Unlike medicine, which has opportunities for all medical school graduates in GME, only about 75% of dental school graduates who would like advanced training in general dentistry are accepted because of limited training slots. The ratio of dentist-to-population varies widely by geography, with the Northeast having the highest ratio. Approximately 9.5% of dentists are female and 2.6% black. The percentage of female dentists will increase significantly in coming years. In 1990, more than 34% of new dental students were women (U.S. DHHS, 1992). In addition to dentists, there are dental hygienists, dental assistants, and dental laboratory technicians, all of whom work with or for dentists.

Podiatric Medicine practitioners diagnose, treat and prevent abnormal foot conditions. Educated at one of the seven Podiatric Medicine schools in the U.S., they perform surgery and prescribe and administer pharmaceuticals. Licensed by individual states, they deliver a wide range of medical and surgical services. According to estimates from the U.S. Department of Health and Human Services (1992), there were about 12,500 practitioners in 1991.

Doctors of Chiropractic treat problems of the body's structural and neurological systems. Chiropractors are educated in 4-year programs, which follow at least 2 years of undergraduate education. According to the U.S. Department of Health and Human Services (1992), of the nation's 17 chiropractic schools, 14 were accredited by the Council on Chiropractic Education (CCE). These programs include both a clinical and lecture component, and their graduates are eligible for licensure in all 50 states. In 1989, there were approximately 45,000 licensed chiropractors. About 87% were male, and 76% practiced in communities with fewer than 250,000 people.

Doctors of Optometry are licensed to diagnose and provide some eye treatment. In some states, they are licensed to prescribe a limited range of pharmaceuticals. According to the U.S. Department of Health and Human Services (1992), there were about 26,000 practicing optometrists in the U.S. in 1990. Educated at one of the 16 schools of optometry, students have 4 years of professional training following 3 or 4 years of undergraduate school. Although there were only 3,800 active female optometrists, their numbers are expected to increase, as approximately one-half of new students are female. Optometrists perform some of the same activities that are performed by Ophthalmologists (physicians with residency training in ophthalmology). Optometric services are generally less costly than services of Ophthalmologists. As state government increases the scope of practice of optometrists, there is likely to be more discussion about the overlapping roles and the appropriateness of each vision care practitioner performing the same service.

Physician Assistants

Physician Assistants (PAs) are educated and prepared to work under the direct supervision of physicians to help the physicians carry out their responsibilities. Regulation of PAs varies from state to state. Supervision does not mean on-site supervision, and in most states the amount of delegation to a PA is a decision between the physician and the PA.

Several factors are creating a demand for additional PAs. Efforts to expand access and contain costs have focused increased attention on PAs who have demonstrated the ability to provide high quality, effective services as an extension of physicians (U.S. DHHS, September, 1992). Although the majority of PAs work in primary care, a growing number are working effectively in medical and surgical subspecialty areas. This has increased the competition for the available PAs. In addition, with increasing pressure to reduce the number of hospital residents (to slow the growth of specialists), the use of PAs to provide the services now provided by residents is likely to increase (Physician Payment Review Commission, 1993).

Physician Assistant Education

The first PA educational program was established by Duke University Medical Center in 1965. PA education was developed, in part, to allow an opportunity for medics who had gained clinical experience in the Vietnam War to practice in the health care system. In 1971, with the passage of the Comprehensive Health Manpower Act, federal financial support became available and contributed to the rapid expansion of programs. From 1971 to 1975, 38 programs were established (Oliver, 1993). By 1992, there were 59 programs in 28 states that were accredited by the American Medical Association's Committee on Allied Health Education and Accreditation (CAHEA). In 1993, approximately 1,500 PAs graduated from PA programs across the country (Oliver, 1993).

PA programs are located in a number of academic settings and offer a variety of credentials. Most programs are 24 months long. The average cost to educate a PA student in 1993 was estimated to be $7,045 per year (Oliver, 1993). Seventy-one percent of the students received financial aid.

More than half the 1992 entering PA students already had a bachelor's degree or higher. Most students entered with extensive experience in the health field. The mean number of months of health care experience for entrants was 55.6 (Oliver, 1993). In 1992, more than 55% of new students were over the age of 27 (Oliver, 1993).

Practicing Physician Assistants

In 1993, there were more than 23,000 PAs practicing in the U.S. According to the American Academy of Physician Assistants, in 1993, 55% of the newly graduating PAs were women, and overall, 42% of practicing PAs were women (Willis, 1993b). Blacks and Hispanics represent 6.7% of practicing PAs. As a relatively new profession, a high percentage of PAs are just beginning their professional career. Approximately 25% of PAs have been in practice 3 years or less. Thus, even without the anticipated increase in the number of PA programs, the number of practicing PAs would increase for many years at the current level of graduations, because most PAs are not expected to retire for many years.

Specialty and Practice Location

PAs work in a wide variety of settings and specialties. The largest concentration of PAs work in family practice (33%). There was concern from 1985 through 1989, when the percentage of new graduates going into family practice, internal medicine, and pediatrics dropped steadily from nearly 55% to 42%, but the percentage bottomed out in 1989 and then rose to 52% in 1992 (Oliver, 1993). The second largest concentration, with 25.4% of PAs, is surgery This suggests the possibility that as the effectiveness and efficacy of PAs is demonstrated in more and more specialty areas, PAs may be drawn away from primary care.

PAs work in a wide array of practice settings. Twenty-six percent work in physician group practices. Although 28% work in hospitals, over one-quarter of these are in hospital outpatient clinics. Over one-third of all PAs are in towns with fewer than 50,000 people, and more than half of these (17%) are in towns of fewer than 10,000 people. Slightly less than one-third are in cities with more than 500,000 people—a sharp difference from the distribution of physicians (Willis, 1993a). For this reason, PAs continue to be viewed as a logical provider for addressing underservice in rural areas.

As demand for physician assistants has increased, so too have their salaries. According to Willis (1993b), the American Academy of Physician Assistants reports that from 1991 to 1992, the average salary for a full-time PA (nongovernmental) rose by $5,000 to $53,500 per year. New graduates were receiving $40,000 to $45,000 starting salaries. Salaries were reported to be higher on the east and west coasts and for surgical PAs (Willis, 1993b).

Allied Health Personnel

The Committee on Allied Health Education and Accreditation, of the American Medical Association, which oversees nearly 3,000 educational programs, defines allied health as "a large cluster of health care related professions and personnel whose functions include assisting, facilitating, or complementing the work of physicians and other specialists in the health care system, and who choose to be identified as allied health personnel" (U.S. DHHS, 1992, p. 177). Although this is a general definition, it allows for occupations to be added and subtracted as the health care system evolves.

Allied health occupations are among the fastest growing in health care. The U.S. Department of Health and Human Services, Bureau of Health Professions, estimates that there were approximately 1.8 million allied health personnel in the U.S. in 1990 (U.S. DHHS, 1992). Unlike medicine, women dominate most of the allied health professions, representing between 75 to 95% of most of the occupations. The following briefly describes some of the major occupations usually included under the allied health rubric.

Clinical Laboratory Personnel

Clinical laboratory workers perform a wide array of tests on body fluids, tissues, and cells to assist in the detection, diagnosis, and treatment of diseases and illnesses. The generalist medical technologist is the most common and most recognized laboratory practitioner, but there are several other major specialties, including blood bank technology (the preparation of blood for transfusion), cytotechnology (the study of body cells), hematology (the study of blood cells), histology (the study of human tissues), microbiology (the study of microorganisms), and clinical chemistry (the analysis of body fluids).

The American Society of Clinical Pathologists, which certifies and registers laboratory personnel, had registered 184,000 technologists and 43,200 technicians in 1990. Technologists are baccalaureate prepared and perform more complex analyses and have greater responsibility than technicians, who have an associate's degree or certificate. Most technologists and technicians work in hospitals. About 75% of clinical laboratory personnel are women (Institute of Medicine, 1989). Only a few states directly license laboratory personnel.

Diagnostic Imaging Personnel

Originally referred to as x-ray technicians and then as radiologic technologists and technicians, this field is now more appropriately referred to as "diagnostic imaging," as it continues to expand to include nuclear medicine technologists, radiation therapists, sonographers or ultrasound technologists, and magnetic resonance technologists. These personnel use a variety of imaging technologies to help in the diagnosis of injuries, diseases, or conditions. Approximately 122,000 diagnostic imaging personnel were employed in 1990 (U.S. DHHS, 1992). This number has been growing as the field has diversified and new imaging technologies have been developed.

Educational requirements vary by area of specialization and within many of the areas. For example, in radiography (x-ray technicians), sonography, radiation therapy technology, and nuclear medicine technology, education programs range from 1 to 4 years and grant a certificate, an associate's degree, or a bachelor's degree. Two-year associate's degrees are the most common (Institute of Medicine, 1989).

Dietetic Personnel

Dieticians are trained in nutrition and are responsible for providing nutritional care to individuals and for overseeing nutrition and food services in a variety of settings ranging from hospitals to schools. The American Dietetic Association (ADA) estimated that they had 58,800 active members working as dietitians in 1990 (U.S. DHHS, 1992). According to a 1984 study, 97% of the ADA's members were women (Institute of Medicine, 1989).

As of 1990, 26 states had laws governing the practice of dietetics, with a baccalaureate being the basic education requirement (U.S. DHHS, 1992). Dietetic technicians work with dieticians to help them carry out their responsibilities. Most dieticians work in hospitals.

Emergency Medical Personnel

Emergency medical technicians (EMTs) are responsible for providing a wide range of services on an emergency basis for trauma and other emergency situations, including the transport of such patients. There are three levels of EMTs—basic, intermediate, and paramedic—with the paramedic requiring the most education and providing the most advanced services. There is a 110-hour national EMT basic training course. Paramedics require additional education. Paramedics carry out a wide range of advanced procedures, including starting intravenous infusions, tracheal intubation, and defibrillation under remote medical supervision.

All 50 states have some form of certification procedure, although the exact requirements vary significantly by state. According to DHHS (September, 1992), there were approximately 100,000 EMTs, including paramedics, in 1990 (U.S. DHHS, September, 1992). Most EMTs are volunteers, particularly in rural areas where they play a major role in providing health services. Volunteer EMTs often work for volunteer rescue squads and fire departments.

Given their training and experience, hospitals in several parts of the country have begun to use paramedics in the emergency room to supplement existing staff. This has been met by resistance from nursing organizations (Institute of Medicine, 1989).

Medical Record Personnel

Collecting, maintaining, and managing medical information has become more critical as care has become more complex and as insurers and government have increased their monitoring of the cost and quality of services. Overseeing medical information to assure that it meets the medical, administrative, and legal requirements is the responsibility of medical record administrators, medical record technicians, and medical record coders. It was estimated that there were nearly 70,000 medical record personnel employed in the U.S. in 1990 (U.S. DHHS, 1992).

Medical record administrators generally have a bachelor's degree or a post-bachelor's certificate. Medical record technicians generally have an associate's degree, and medical record coders are generally taught on the job. More than 90% of students in medical record training programs are women (U.S. DHHS, June, 1990). While the demand for medical records personnel is expected to rise, the growing use of computers and the anticipated eventual development of an electronic medical record is likely to lead to a need for more highly educated personnel. On the other hand, efforts to simplify administrative requirements and to reduce processing costs may reduce demand for some medical records personnel.

Occupational Therapy Personnel

Occupational therapists (OTs) help individuals with physical or mental disabilities to learn skills necessary to perform daily tasks, diminish or correct pathology, and promote and maintain health. Occupational therapists enable individuals to live as independently and productively as possible. These therapists help their patients develop or redevelop the skills needed to perform daily activities like dressing, cooking, bathing, and eating. Occupational Therapy Assistants work under the supervision of OTs and help carry out treatment regimens developed by OTs.

Occupational therapists are registered by the American Occupational Therapy Association (AOTA) if they graduate from an accredited educational program and pass the AOTA certification examination. In addition, in 1990 35 states licensed OTs. Most accredited education programs offer a bachelor's degree, although some offer a post-bachelor's certificate or a master's degree as a first professional degree in OT. Occupational therapy assistants require a two-year associate's degree, and can then become certified by the AOTA as a certified occupational therapy assistant (COTA).

Occupational therapists and occupational therapy assistants work in a variety of settings, including rehabilitative and psychiatric hospitals, schools, and in private practice. The American Occupational Therapy Association estimated that in 1989 there were 37,600 OTs—of which about 25% were self-employed—and nearly 8,000 COTAs (U.S. DHHS, 1992). Approximately 95% of OTs are women (Institute of Medicine, 1989). OTs and COTAs are projected to be among the most rapidly growing occupations through the year 2005, according to the Federal Bureau of Labor Statistics (U.S. Department of Labor, 1992).

Physical Therapy Personnel

Physical therapists (PTs) evaluate and treat patients to improve functional mobility, reduce pain, maintain cardiopulmonary functioning, and limit disability. Physical therapists treat movement dysfunction resulting from accidents, trauma, stroke, fractures, multiple sclerosis, cerebral palsy, arthritis, and heart and respiratory illness. PTs work in a wide variety of settings, including hospitals, rehabilitation facilities, home health agencies, and nursing homes. Physical therapist assistants (PTAs) work under the direction of PTs and help carry out the treatment plans developed by PTs.

All states require that PTs be licensed. Graduation from a program accredited by the American Physical Therapy Association (APTA) and passage of a licensing exam are prerequisites for licensure. Accredited programs include bachelor's degree programs, and for individuals with bachelor's degrees in other fields, post-bachelor's certificate programs and two-year master's degree programs. A two-year associate's degree is required to become a PTA. According to the Bureau of Labor Statistics (BLS), there were approximately 88,000 jobs for physical therapists in 1990 (U.S. Department of Labor, 1992). Approximately 75% of all PTs are women (Institute of Medicine, 1989).

Physical therapists practice more independently than most allied health personnel occupations. Most states allow physical therapists to evaluate patients without medical referral. A growing number of PTs, now more than 22%, are going into private or group practice (U.S. DHHS, 1992). PTs can receive direct reimbursement from many insurers, including Medicare. Shortages of PTs already exist in many settings and in many parts of the country. These shortages are expected to worsen because the demand for physical therapy services is expected to continue to rise rapidly as the nation ages and the need for rehabilitation services increases. The BLS (U.S. Department of Labor, 1992) predicts that the number of PT jobs will increase by 76% between 1990 and 2005, the fifth highest of all occupations.

Respiratory Therapy Personnel

Respiratory therapy personnel evaluate, treat, and care for patients with breathing disorders. They work under the direction of qualified physicians and provide such services as emergency care for stroke, heart failure and shock, and treat patients with emphysema and asthma. They also treat patients who have received anesthesia because it depresses breathing, and respiratory therapy can help prevent the development of respiratory illness. According to the BLS (U.S. Department of Labor, 1992), there were about 60,000 respiratory therapy jobs in 1990, 90% of which were in hospitals. These jobs include both therapists and therapy technicians. Almost 40% of respiratory therapists are men, an unusually high percentage for an allied health occupation (Institute of Medicine, 1989).

Respiratory therapists are licensed in some states. The AMA's Committee on Allied Health Education and Accreditation accredits respiratory therapy programs that are at least 2 years in length and lead to an associate's or baccalaureate degree. Respiratory therapy technicians, also known as inhalation therapy technicians, who work under the direct supervision of respiratory therapists, require completion of a training program that is usually 1 year in length (Institute of Medicine, 1989). The demand for respiratory personnel is expected to grow substantially over the coming years (U.S. Department of Labor, 1992).

Speech–Language Pathology and Audiology

Speech–language pathologists and audiologists identify, assess, and provide treatment for individuals with speech, language, or hearing problems. Speech-language pathologists study human communication, and audiologists are experts on hearing impairments. Audiology practice is licensed in 39 states and speech-language pathology in 38 states (U.S. DHHS, 1992). About one-half the jobs for these occupations are in schools. Many also work in hospitals, facilities for the disabled, hearing centers, and in private physician offices. Unlike other allied health occupations, speech-language pathologists and audiologists are not exclusively or even primarily in the medical field, as the field developed initially in the education sector.

The American Speech-Language-Hearing Association (ASHA) estimated that there were approximately 86,700 active practitioners in the field in 1988, of whom nearly 90% were female (Institute of Medicine, 1989). Most states require a master's degree in speech-language pathology or audiology to become licensed.

Other Health Care Workers

In addition to physicians, nurses, and allied health personnel, there are a variety of other health care practitioners. Space does not permit a thorough discussion of each of these workers, but several examples will be given.

Pharmacists have traditionally prepared pharmaceutical prescriptions, however their role has expanded in some areas to include counselling about pharmaceuticals and drug interactions. According to the U.S. Department of Health and Human Services (1992), pharmacists are educated in 74 schools, which offer a five-year baccalaureate degree and/or 6-year Doctor of Pharmacy. Most graduates receive a baccalaureate degree. Advanced training is available in residency programs. Areas of specialization include nuclear pharmacy, pharmacotherapy, and nutrition support. The U.S. DHHS (1992) reports that there were about 161,900 pharmacists in the U.S. in 1990, an increase of 44% since 1970. Approximately 29% of pharmacists are women, and about 11% are minorities. The proportion of women pharmacists is expected to increase dramatically. Pharmacy technicians assist pharmacists with activities not requiring the judgment of a pharmacist.

Public Health Personnel include a variety of health workers. Whereas most health practitioners work with individual patients, public health workers are concerned with the health of entire communities and population groups. Many work in state and local health departments. The U.S. DHHS (1992) estimates that in 1989, there were approximately 500,000 professionals working in public health. Of these, a substantial proportion were educated in a specific clinical discipline, such as nursing, medicine, or other professions discussed in this chapter. Some public health professionals are graduates of the nation's 24 accredited Schools of Public Health (U.S. DHHS, 1992). In 1989, these schools had an enrollment of 10,000 students. Their graduates are prepared in such areas as epidemiology, nutrition, health education, environmental health, health administration, and health policy. Other schools also prepare students in these areas.

Conclusion

The rapid changes in the health care delivery system promoted in part by the possibility of health care reform, will undoubtedly lead to changes in the roles of health professionals and their relationships. Managed care and managed competition will require greater collaboration among health professionals. It will also mean greater supervision and management of health professionals by nonhealth professionals. Some health professionals may resist this inevitable oversight as an intrusion on their professionalism. New relationships and even a new definition of professional may need to be developed.

Health care reform may also require greater government workforce planning as recommended by the Council on Graduate Medical Education and the Physician Payment Review Commission. An adequate supply and distribution, geographically and by specialty, is essential to an effective and efficient health care system. This may require more active government policies influencing the education and training of practitioners especially physicians.

The provision of health care in the late twentieth and early twenty-first centuries will require the cooperation and coordination of the many health workers currently providing health care, those who will be educated in these health careers in the future, and will likely include health care workers educated in new careers. There are large areas of overlap in the care provided by health professionals. Physicians, nurses, and physical therapists all work with patients in performing range-of-motion exercises. Physicians, nurses, and pharmacists all teach patients about medications and their side effects. Nurses and respiratory therapists teach and supervise patients in deep breathing exercises following surgery. It is not surprising that patients in hospitals complain because they cannot tell who is who—everyone is wearing a white uniform or lab coat, or more recently, any health worker might be wearing street clothes.

Most health care professionals today are educated in their own professional schools, in health facilities, and divisions of colleges and universities. Few health professionals currently take any courses together, nor do many even share the same faculty. In many cases, students in a variety of professions receive their clinical training in the same institutions. However, there is rarely any shared clinical teaching or learning. The Pew Charitable Trusts Commission on the Health Professions (O'Neil, 1993) suggests that in the future, health care professionals, to be effective in providing care, should share much of their initial academic health experiences. If most health professionals take pathophysiology, why shouldn't they take it together? Others suggest that there should be a core health curriculum for health professionals, with specialization into physical therapy, respiratory therapy, or imaging occurring at the upper division in the undergraduate curriculum.

It seems clear that as health care moves from the hospital to the community, even more coordination of patient care and cooperation among health providers will be required. It is also likely that any one of a variety of health professionals will be the primary care giver or coordinator of care. The training and profession of this primary care giver or coordinator will vary depending on the health problem of the clients.

References

American Association of Colleges of Osteopathic Medicine (AACOM). *1992 Annual Statistical Report*. Rockville, MD, 1992.

American Medical Association. *Physician Characteristics and Distribution in the U.S.* Roback, Gene, Randolph, Lilliam, Seidman, & Bradley (Eds.). Chicago, IL: Department of Physician Data Services, 1993 (A).

American Medical Association. *Socioeconomic Characteristics of Medical Practice.* Gonzalez & Martin (Eds.). Chicago, IL: Center for Health Policy Research, 1993 (B).

Backus, K. (Ed.), *Medical and Health Information Directory*, 6th Edition. Detroit: Gale Research, 1992.

Berliner, H. S., *Strategic Factors in U.S. Health Care: Human Resources, Capital and Technology*. Westview Press: Boulder & London, 1987.

"Care: How We Got to This Mess." *Newsweek*, 22:14:31–35. October 4, 1993.

Colby, D. C., "Impact of the Medicare Physician Fee Schedule." *Health Affairs*, Fall 1992, pp. 216–226.

Council on Graduate Medical Education. *Third Report—Improving Access to Health Care Through Physician Workforce Reform: Directions for the 21st Century*. U.S. Department of Health and Human Services, Human Resources Services and Administration, October 1992.

Crowley, A., Etzel, S., & Shaw, C. H., "Graduate Medical Education in the United States." *Journal of the American Medical Association*, 258:8:1031–1040, August 28, 1987.

Daniels, P. & Schwartz, C. A. (Eds.), *28th Encyclopedia of Associations*, 1994. Washington, DC: Gale Research. Vol. 1, Part 2.

Flexner, A., *Medical Education in the United States and Canada*. New York: The Carnegie Foundation for the Advancement of Teaching, 1910. Reprinted, Washington, DC: Science and Health Publications, 1960.

Freidson, E., *Profession of Medicine*. New York: Dodd, Mead & Company, 1973.

Ginzberg, E., Ostow, M., & Dutka, A., *The Economics of Medical Education*. New York: Josiah Macy Jr. Foundation, March, 1993.

Graduate Medical Education National Advisory Committee (GMENAC). *Report of the Graduate Medical Education National Advisory Committee to the Secretary*. Washington, DC: U.S. Department of Health and Human Services, September 1980.

Institute of Medicine. *Allied Health Services: Avoiding Crisis*. Washington, DC: National Academy Press, 1989.

Jolin, Jolly, R., Krakower, J., & Beran, R., "U.S. Medical School Finances." *Journal of the American Medical Association*, 268:9:1149–1155, September 2, 1992.

Jonas, H., Etzel, S., & Baransky, R., "Educational Programs in U.S. Medical Schools." *Journal of the American Medical Association*, 270:9:1061–1068, and 1083–1090, September 1, 1993.

Jones, S. R., "Organized Medicine in the United States." *Annals of Surgery*, 217:5:423–429, 1993.

Journal of the American Medical Association, Appendix II, 270:9:1116–1122, September 1, 1993.

Kindig, P., Cultice, J., & Mullan, F., "The Elusive Generalist Physician: Can We Reach a 50% Goal?" *Journal of the American Medical Association*, 270:9:1069–1072, September 1, 1993.

Kletke, P., Shleiter, M., & Tarlov, A., "Changes in the Supply of Internists: The Internal Medicine Population from 1978 to 1998." *Annals of Internal Medicine*, 107:1:93–100, July 1987.

Krakower, J. Y., Jolly, R., & Beran, R., "U.S. Medical School Finances." *Journal of the American Medical Association*, 270:9:1085–1091, September 1993.

Martini, C. J., "Graduate Medical Education in the Changing Environment of Medicine." *Journal of the American Medical Association*, 268:9:1097–1105, September 2, 1992.

Martini, C. J., & Grenholim, G., "Institutional Responsibility in Graduate Medical Education and Highlights of Historical Data." *Journal of the American Medical Association.* 270:9:1053–1060, September 1, 1993.

Mullan, F., "Missing: A National Medical Manpower Policy." *The Milbank Quarterly*, 70:2:381–386, 1992.

Mullan, F., Rivo, M., & Politzer, R. M., "Doctors, Dollars, and Determination: Making Physician Work-force Policy." *Health Affairs*, 12:138–151, Supplement, 1993.

National Rural Health Association. *Study of Models to Meet Rural Health Care Needs through Mobilization of Health Profession Education and Services Resources.* Rockville, MD: U.S. Department of Health and Human Services, Health Resources and Services Administration, June 1992.

NRMP Directory: 1993, Washington, DC: National Residency Matching Program, 1992.

Oliver, D. R., *Ninth Annual Report on Physician Educational Programs in the United States, 1992–1993.* Iowa City, IA: Association of Physician Assistant Programs, June 1993.

O'Neil, E., *Health Professions Education for the Future: Schools in Service to the Nation.* San Francisco, CA: The Pew Health Professions Commission, 1993.

Pear, R., "A.M.A. Rebels Over Health Plan in Major Challenge to President." *New York Times*, 143:49,470:A1,A22, September 30, 1993.

Petersdorf, R., "Primary Care-Medical Students; Unpopular Choice." *American Journal of Public Health*, 83:3:328–330, March 1993.

Physician Payment Review Commission, (PPRC). *Annual Report to Congress 1993.* Washington, DC, 1993.

Pope, G., & Schneider, J., "Trends in Physician Income." *Health Affairs*, pp. 181–193, Spring 1992.

Rivo, M. L., & Satcher, D., "Improving Access to Health Care Through Physician

Workforce Reform: Directions for the 21st century. *Journal of American Medical Association*, 270:9:1074–1078, September 1, 1993.

Shugars, D. A., O'Neil, E. H., & Bader, J. D. (Eds.), *Practitioners for 2005, and Agenda for Action for U.S. Health Professional Schools*. Durham, NC: The Pew Health Professions Commission, 1991.

Silberger, A., Thran, F., & Marder, W., "The Changing Environment of Resident Physicians." *Health Affairs*, pp. 121–133, Supplement 1988.

Slee, V. M., & Slee, D. A., *Health Care Terms*, 2nd Ed. St. Paul, MN, Tringa Press, 1986.

U.S. Department of Health and Human Services. *Acute Pain Management: Operative or Medical Procedures and Trauma*. February, 1992.

U.S. Department of Health and Human Services. *Health Personnel in the United States Eighth Report to Congress: 1991*. Resources and Services Administration, September 1992. (DHHS Pub. No. HRSPOD 92-1).

U.S. Department of Health and Human Services. *Minorities and Women in the Health Fields*. Washington, DC: Bureau of Health Professions, Health Resources and Services Administration, June 1990. (DHSS Pub. No. HRADV 90-3).

U.S. Department of Health and Human Services. *Urinary Incontinence in Adults*. March, 1992.

U.S. Department of Labor. "Labstat Series Report." Bureau of Labor Statistics, June 12, 1993.

U.S. Department of Labor. *Outlook 2005*. Bureau of Labor Statistics, B.L.S. Bulletin 2402, May 1992.

Wennberg, J., Goodman, D., Nease, R. L., & Keller, R., "Finding Equilibrium in U.S. Physician Supply." *Health Affairs*, pp. 89–103, Summer 1993.

Willis, J. B., "Barriers to PA Practice in Primary Care and Rural Medically Underserved Areas." *Journal of the American Academy of Physician Assistants*, 6(6)418–422, June 1993a.

Willis, J. B., "PAs in 1993 . . . The Majority Continue to Practice Primary Care." Alexandria, VA: American Academy of Physician Assistants, 1993b.

5

Nursing

Christine Kovner

This chapter presents an overview of the nursing profession. After a brief history of nursing, the chapter looks at how nursing is defined in law and by professional nurses. The various educational programs for nurses are described, as well as the levels of practice. Finally, current issues in nursing are analyzed within the context of the health care system. "Nurse" is a generic term that is applied to a variety of practitioners from nurses' aides and assistants to nurse researchers with Ph.D.s. The focus of this chapter will be the professional registered nurse and the licensed practical nurse.

Historical Perspective

Aiken (1983, p. 408) points out four factors from nursing's history that influence nursing today:

1. Nursing developed as an occupation supportive of physicians.
2. Nurses work primarily in bureaucratic institutions.
3. Nurses are predominantly female.
4. Nursing's early educational history was linked to religious orders, with expectations of service, dedication, and charity.

Although English, Florence Nightingale (1820–1910) had a profound influence on American nursing. She advocated formal training for nurses and an administrative order for the hospital, with the matron (head nurse) as head (Rosenberg, 1987). After her success in decreasing the death rate of soldiers serving in the Crimean War, Nightingale opened a training school at St. Thomas's Hospital in England. The first training program in the United States was begun in 1872 at the New England Hospital for Women and Children in Boston. Training schools increased from 15 in 1880 to 1,105 by 1909, all under the direction of hospitals. Nursing students provided much of the care in these institutions. Married women and those over 30 were excluded, along with divorced women (Kelly, 1987). Nurses were treated as subservient to both physicians and hospital administrators. According to Rosenberg (p. 236), until the 1920s the nurse's status was somewhat above that of domestic servant. However, Wilkerson (1985) suggests that public health nurses were "disciplined and well bred" (p. 1155) and "associate or co-worker of the physician" (p. 1157). In the early 1920s soul searching and reform were beginning. Prior to World War I, Presbyterian Hospital, in conjunction with Teachers College, Columbia University, developed a 5-year combined college-diploma program.

Early nursing leaders include Lillian Wald, public health nursing leader and founder of the Henry Street Settlement; Mary Mahoney, the first black nurse to graduate from a nurse training program; Annie Goodrich, the first dean of the U.S. Army School of Nursing; Adelaide Nutting, the first nurse to receive a professorship at Columbia Teacher's College; and Mary Breckenridge, founder of the Frontier Nursing Service. These early American leaders paved the way for today's nurses.

What Is Nursing?

Nursing includes caring for a newborn moments after birth and monitoring the blood pressure of a person brought into the emergency room following an auto accident. It is teaching the diabetic how to inject insulin and advising a senator on how to finance and organize home care services for the elderly. It is identifying the strengths of a family facing the knowledge that both mother and father have AIDS and convincing illegal aliens that being treated for tuberculosis at the government clinic will not jeopardize their status in this country. And it is adjusting the tubes and drips of the person in the ICU. But what is the legal definition of nursing? How do academic theoreticians define nursing? How do nurses themselves define it?

The American Nurses Association (ANA) (1980) suggests that authority for nursing is based on a social contract between society and the profession. It is further suggested that the legal authority for nursing (nurse practice acts) stems from this social contract, rather than the other way around.

Legal Definition

The ANA's (1981) suggested nursing practice legislation defines professional nursing as

... services requiring substantial specialized knowledge of the biological, physical, behavioral, psychological, and sociological sciences and of nursing theory as the basis for assessment, diagnosis, planning, intervention, and evaluation in the promotion and maintenance of health; the casefinding and management of illness, injury, or infirmity; the restoration of optimum function; or the achievement of a dignified death. Nursing practice includes but is not limited to administration, teaching, counseling, supervision, delegation, and evaluation of practice and execution of the medical regimen, including the administration of medications and treatments prescribed by any person authorized by state law to prescribe. [p. 6]

For example, in New York State a registered professional nurse is defined as

... diagnosing and treating human responses to actual or potential health problems through such services as casefinding, health teaching, health counseling, and provision of care supportive to or restorative of life and well-being, and executing medical regimens prescribed by a licensed or otherwise legally authorized physician or dentist. A nursing regimen shall be consistent with and shall not vary from any existing medical regimen. (NY Education Law Article 139 Section 6902, 1989)

New York differentiates professional nursing from practical nursing, defining the later as "performing tasks and responsibilities ... under the direction of a registered professional nurse or licensed or otherwise legally authorized physician or dentist" (NY Education Law Article 139 Section 6902, 1989). In some states nurses (or certain categories of nurses) may prescribe pharmacologic agents or deliver a baby; in other states they may not. In addition, some states require continuing education for license renewal.

Nursing is usually defined as diagnosis and treatment of human responses. However, each state has its own legal definition because regulation of the practice of nursing is a state responsibility. The registered nurse is sometimes called a registered professional nurse. The legal term for the practical nurse is sometimes licensed practical nurse or licensed vocational nurse. Under a state board of nursing each state licenses people to practice as registered nurses and defines what this practice is. As nursing developed in the United States, practitioners called themselves nurses. By 1923 legislation was enacted in all states for voluntary registration (Bullough, 1975). The first mandatory licensing law went into effect in New York State in 1947. It required that, with certain exceptions, only licensed professional nurses could legally use the title Registered Nurse.

Currently Maine and North Dakota require a baccalaureate degree to become a registered nurse. All other states accept graduation from 4-, 3-, or 2-year programs. All states require that potential registered nurses attend an approved nursing program and take a national licensing exam, the National Council Exam for Registered Nurses (NCLEX-RN), developed by the National Council of State Boards of Nursing. In 1992, of the 49,134 first-time candidates educated in the United States and its territories taking the exam almost 90% passed.

In fiscal year 1990, 7,415 nurse immigrants entered the U.S.—an increase from 4,063 who entered in 1988. The majority (57%) came from the Phillipines (U.S. Department of Health and Human Services, 1992) of the 6,244 took the license exam in February 1991, with only 52% passing.

Theoretical Definition

A classic definition of nursing is that of Virginia Henderson (1966), who states:

> The unique function of the nurse is to assist the individual (sick or well), in the performance of those activities contributing to health or its recovery (or peaceful death) that he would perform unaided if he had the necessary strength, will, or knowledge. And to do this in such a way as to help him gain independence as rapidly as possible. [p. 15]

The ANA (1980) proposes that nursing is concerned "with human responses to actual or potential health problems" (p. 8). Nurses do not treat the underlying health problems. The underlying health problems are usually diagnosed and treated by physicians. Some examples of human responses that are the concern of nurses are:

1. Self-care limitations.
2. Impaired functioning in areas such as rest, sleep, ventilation, circulation, activity, nutrition, elimination, skin, sexuality, and the like.
3. Pain and discomfort.
4. Emotional problems related to illness and treatment, life-threatening events, or daily experiences, such as anxiety, loss, loneliness, and grief.
5. Distortion of symbolic functions, reflected in interpersonal and intellectual processes, such as hallucinations.
6. Deficiencies in decision making and ability to make personal choices.
7. Self-image changes required by health use.
8. Dysfunctional perceptual orientations to health.
9. Strains related to life processes, such as birth, growth and development, and death.
10. Problematic affiliative relationships. [ANA, 1980, p. 10]

Nursing care is based on theory that is both derived from other disciplines and developed by nurses. "The aims of nursing actions are to ameliorate, improve, or correct conditions to which those practices are directed, to prevent illness and to promote health" (ANA, 1980, p. 12). A distinguishing characteristic of nursing is that it includes nurturing to provide comfort—generative nurturing to develop new behaviors and protective nurturing involving surveillance. *Generative* implies newly developed, and *protective* implies monitoring (ANA, 1980, p. 18). Nurses encourage people to be responsible for their own health, and they work with patients to achieve mutually desirable outcomes.

There are many conceptual models and theories currently used and studied in nursing. Fawcett (1989) proposes that nursing is concerned with four concepts: patient, nurse, environment, and health. These four concepts are viewed differently in various models.

Orem (1980) proposes that nursing is helping the patient with self-care. When the patient is unable to provide self-care, this role is assumed by the nurse. She states five methods to help others:

1. Acting for or doing for another.
2. Guiding another.
3. Supporting another (physically or psychologically).
4. Providing an environment that promotes personal development in relation to becoming able to meet present or future demands for action.
5. Teaching another. [p. 61]

Rogers, another popular nursing theorist, describes the person as an energy field, having no real boundaries. She proposes that the energy field of each person is in constant interaction with the environment, which is itself an energy field that is everything outside the human field. Wellness and illness are not differentiated within this model; rather, they are value judgments of society. Rogers differentiates nursing from other professions in that nursing's central concern is unitary human beings and their environments. Rogers indicates that the goal of nursing is promotion of health (Fawcett, 1989).

These two examples of nursing theory indicate what is either nursing's greatest strength or its greatest weakness—the diversity of opinion on what it is. It is a strength that nurses are open to new ideas and are not stagnant in a traditional view of nursing. Such an attitude will aid nurses in adapting to changes in the health care delivery system and creatively responding to clients' needs. But a problem with diversity is the lack of a cohesive voice for nursing. However, it can be said that nursing differs from medicine in its focus on the whole person. When a nurse takes a person's blood pressure, the focus is the entire person, whereas a physician's focus in the same situation would tend to be on the cardiovascular system.

Education of Nurses

One of the most confusing aspects of nursing is the variety of educational programs for educating nurses. Unlike medicine, which has consistent educational requirements, nursing offers the student a number of options. The practical nurse can attend programs in high schools, hospitals, junior colleges, or vocational schools.

Likewise, the registered nurse can attend a 2-year college program, a 3-year hospital-based (diploma) program, a 4-year college program, a 2-year master's degree program, or a nursing doctoral (N.D.) program. State boards of nursing accept all of these programs as appropriate preparation for the licensing exam.

Licensed Practical Nursing (LPN/LVN)

The practical nurse provides direct patient care under the supervision of a registered nurse. The National League for Nursing (1993b) estimates the number of practical-nurse programs at 1,069. Programs are primarily in technical or vocational schools, junior colleges, hospitals, and secondary schools. Enrollment in 1991 was 56,762 an increase of 7.6% over 1990. Graduates in 1991 numbered 38,100 an increase of 7.6% from 1990, maintaining an upward trend that began in 1989, but which is substantially lower than graduation numbers in the 1970s and 1980s which were 40,000–45,000 per year. The typical program takes about 1 year and includes basic courses in physical and social sciences, and simple nursing procedures.

Registered Professional Nursing

During 1992 there were 1,484 basic educational programs for registered nurses in the United States, at the following educational levels: (1) associate degree (848); (2) baccalaureate degree (501); (3) diploma (135); (National League for Nursing, 1993a). In addition there were programs at the graduate level to prepare students for professional licensure. Enrollments in professional nursing programs continue to rise. Total enrollments were 257,983 in 1992, an 8.6% increase from 1991. Graduations from professional nursing programs rose 11.9% (to 72,230) over the same period. This increase is still well below the recent high of 80,132 in 1984. Minorities comprised about 15.4% of enrollees in 1992; however, men comprised 11.1% of enrollments (National League for Nursing, 1993a).

Accreditation standards do not specify specific course requirements. Consequently, curricula vary widely from school to school, and transfer of nursing course credits is extremely unlikely. The first associate degree program was begun in 1952 (Anastas, 1984). The typical associate degree program requires basic liberal arts courses such as English and sociology. In addition, science courses such as anatomy and physiology are required. Nursing courses usually include fundamentals of nursing (clinical skills), maternal and child health, and care of the acutely ill hospitalized adult patient. Practical experience is gained by practicing skills in the campus laboratory and care of patients in institutional settings such as hospitals. The nurses enrolled in associate degree programs are educated to be direct providers of care at the patient bedside. The programs are 2 academic years to 2 calendar years in length.

The typical diploma program is similar to the associate degree program, though usually under the auspices of a hospital. Often students are required to take liberal arts courses at a local college, and they receive college credit that can later be transferred to other colleges. The practical-experience sessions are usually longer than in the associate degree program, and the entire course takes about 3 years, with an emphasis on acute care (hospital-based) nursing. Diploma graduates who go to college often are not able to transfer the credits earned in the diploma program because until recently most of these were not degree-granting institutions.

The curriculum of the baccalaureate program is similar to that of liberal arts programs in other fields. Because the program is at least 8 semesters long, the student takes more courses than in either the associate or the diploma program. Students take liberal arts courses such as English, math, and psychology and are required to take science courses such as microbiology, anatomy, and physiology. In addition, approximately half of the credits are usually in nursing courses. The organization of these courses varies from school to school. Some schools organize curricula developmentally and have courses devoted to care of infants, children, adults, and older people. Others base the curriculum on the relative health of populations and offer courses on prevention, episodic care, continuous care, and critical care. In addition, students learn to read and interpret research. Nurses are prepared to work in community settings and leadership positions as well as in acute-care settings. They are generalists who can provide care to individuals, groups, and families. Graduates are also prepared for advanced education in nursing.

Another opportunity for education in nursing is the external degree program, such as that offered by the Board of Regents of New York State. In 1971 an associate degree program was begun, followed by a baccalaureate degree program in 1976. Students obtain either degree by completing equivalency testing in liberal arts, sciences, and nursing. Students also must complete a practical exam. The program's philosophy is that what the person knows, rather than how the information was acquired, is what matters. California's state education system has a similar program. Graduates of these programs are eligible for state licensure (Anastas, 1984).

Graduate Education

Nursing degree programs at the master's and doctoral level concentrate on nursing courses, with the assumption that the nurse baccalaureate graduate has had the basic liberal arts and science courses or will be required to make them up. Historically, specialists in nursing were educated in specialized hospitals or became specialists based on clinical practice with a particular type of patient. In the 1950s colleges and universities began offering programs for specialty education. By the 1960s postgraduate education for clinical practice specialization was in universities (ANA, 1980, pp. 21–22). The focus of these programs is expert competence. Functions of specialists include the following:

- Identification of populations or communities at risk.
- Direct care of selected patients or clients in any setting, including private practice.
- Intraprofessional consultation with nurse specialists in different clinical areas and with nurses in general practice.
- Interprofessional consultation and collaboration in planning total patient care for individual and groups of patients, and in planning and evaluating health programs for population groups at risk related to the specialty or the public in general.
- Contribution to the advancement of the profession as a whole and to the specialty field (ANA, 1980, p. 26).

Master's Degree Programs. People with a baccalaureate degree in another field can earn a master's degree to prepare them for professional practice. Registered nurses with baccalaureate degrees can earn master's degrees in advanced clinical practice, teaching, and nursing administration/management. Within these three broad areas students usually focus on a nursing content area such as adult health, maternal-child health, psychiatric-mental health, or community health. Specific programs include everything from nursing informatics (computers) to home health care management to geriatrics to pediatric nurse practitioner. Most students choose to focus on advanced clinical practice (49%). Adult Health/ Medical Surgical is the most popular clinical area (National League for Nursing, 1993b).

In 1991 there were 236 programs offering a master's degree in nursing, an increase of 85 in the last decade. In 1991 there were 26,308 students enrolled in master's degree programs. This was a dramatic increase over the 3,531 students enrolled in 1967. Only 23.6% were full-time, however, reflecting a steady decrease from the 68% full-time in 1972. This may relate to the decrease in federal funding for graduate education in nursing. The number of graduates per year increased slightly to 6,555 over the 5-year period from 1986 to 1991. About 10% were from minority groups (National League for Nursing, 1993b).

Doctoral Programs. Nurses also earn doctoral degrees in nursing. There are three types of degrees offered. The N.D. (doctor of nursing) is similar to the M.D., that is, it is the first professional degree, building on the earlier liberal arts or scientific education and preparing the student to take the state licensing exam to practice as a registered nurse. The D.N.S. and D.N.Sc. are professional doctorates that prepare the nurse for advanced clinical practice. The Ph.D. is a research degree, with requirements similar to the Ph.D. in other fields; extensive preparation in a narrow field and a dissertation. In 1991 there were 56 doctoral programs in nursing in the United States, having grown from five programs in 1967. In 1991 a record 2,765 RNs were enrolled in these programs, and 355 graduated from these programs (National League for Nursing, 1993b).

The National League for Nursing (NLN) (1993b) estimates that in 1992 about 19,548 nurses worked full-time in nursing education. Ninety-three percent of full-time faculty have graduate degrees, and 41% of those in baccalaureate and higher-degree programs have doctorates. Men continue to be underrepresented: only 2.3% of the full-time faculty are male (p. 217). Less than 10% of full-time faculty were members of ethnic minority groups (p. 200). The percentage of minority faculty is less than the percentage of minority students in nursing programs.

Nurse Practitioners

Nurse practitioners are registered nurses with training beyond their basic education, usually prepared to provide primary care; they were first educated at the University of Colorado in 1965. They are prepared in areas such as care of children or the elderly, women's health, and the like.

Government Aid for Nurse Education

During World War II, money was provided for nurse education. Later, the Nurse Training Act of 1964 provided money for direct support of students to increase the supply of nurses. The Health Manpower Act of 1968, Title II, provided additional aid. The Nurse Training Act of 1971 provided money for categories of advanced practice. Federal aid for basic nursing education was at its peak of $102.5 million in 1976 (New York State Department of Health, 1989). For Fiscal year 1993, the Federal appropriation for nursing education was $60.2 million. The funds were primarily for graduate education. States provide substantial amounts of money for support of nursing programs, primarily in operational support of state colleges and universities.

Careers in Nursing

The concentration of RNs varies from a high of 1,167 employed per 100,000 population in Massachusetts to a low of 442 per 100,000 population in Louisiana

(U.S. Department of Health and Human Services, 1992). There are approximately 2.2 million licensed registered nurses in the United States. About 1.85 million are employed (a 14% increase over 1988) an estimated 82.3% of work force participation rate in 1992. These nurses work in settings that vary from hospital bedside to occupational and industrial settings to elementary schools. About 66% of nurses work in hospitals. Unemployment is approximately 0.9% (Division of Nursing, 1993).

About 31% of nurses actually employed in nursing work part-time, usually half-time (Division of Nursing, 1993). Of those licensed nurses not actively nursing in 1988 approximately 23% work in nonnursing jobs, and 69% are not looking for work. Many of those who were not working were over age 50 or had children living at home (Secretary's Commission on Nursing, 1988).

Of the working nurses, about 67% work as staff nurses, 12% as supervisors or head nurses, 5% as administrators, and 0.2% as researchers. The remainder work as consultants, instructors, nurse specialists or clinicians, anesthetists, in private duty, or in other areas. Of the approximately 550,000 practical nurses (ANA, 1987, p. 104), 59% work in hospitals, 23% in nursing homes, 3% in community health, 9% in ambulatory care, and 7% in other settings.

Nursing Roles

Staff nurses typically work in direct patient care, where they provide nursing care to individuals who may be acutely ill, as in a hospital; chronically ill or recovering from illness, as in a home setting; or well but requiring preventive care, as in a health department or health maintenance organization (HMO). Supervisors or head nurses direct the care given by other nurses and nursing aides or other health workers. They may also provide direct care. Nurse managers manage a group of nurses. Nurse specialists or clinicians are generally experts in a narrow area of nursing, such as ostomy care or patients with pain. They provide care to patients, act as role models for nursing staff, and often serve as resource people for staff nurses. Consultants are often self-employed and provide a variety of services both to individual nurses and organizations. Instructors teach nursing in either health care settings or educational settings. They may teach in schools of nursing, provide orientation to new nurses, teach specialized classes, or conduct programs for nurse's aides. Researchers investigate nursing problems, such as how to decrease pain in patients following surgery. Private-duty nurses generally care for one patient for a large block of time (e.g., 8–12 hours a day) over several days to months. Public health nurses plan and provide care for groups of patients, usually prevention and education. Nurse practitioners usually provide primary care and usually work in ambulatory care facilities.

Career Options

Historically, the major focus of nurses has been the care of the sick in institutions, particularly hospitals. Although most nurses still work in hospitals, the focus of nursing is moving away from that of dependent worker with a focus on illness to independent practitioner with a focus on health. Porter-O'Grady (1986) proposes that the role of the nurse will shift from one in which responsibility for the care and safety of the patient is defined by the institution to one that focuses on health, with responsibility determined by the client. He suggests that functions will move from direct care dominated by the physician to team interaction focused on prevention. For many nurses this transition has already occurred.

Nurses have flexible options for the nature of their work, the hours they work, and the settings in which they work. Most people think of the nurse as the person in white caring for a patient in the hospital; and although the majority of nurses have such jobs, many nurses work in other settings. Nurses work on a fee-for-service basis with clients who have mood disturbances, they deliver babies, and they work for government agencies developing policies for health care in certain geographic or political areas. Nurses teach schoolchildren about health, provide family planning services, administer intravenous nutritional therapy to people at home, and serve as patient advocates.

The typical staff nurse in a hospital spends his or her day caring for 6 to 10 patients. Nurses act as care integrators as well as caregivers (McClure & Nelson, 1982). As care integrators, nurses manage communication and coordination of activities of other care providers. These hospital nurses are the one type of health care provider who is with the patient 24 hours a day. Nurses provide direct care, which may include personal care such as bathing and help with toileting. Nurses administer medications and treatments, from intravenous fluids to dressing changes. Nurses teach the patient about his or her illness and about treatments that may be needed, and nurses assist patients to assume life-style changes that will improve their health. Nurses organize patient care across hospital departments, including radiology and laboratory. Nurses are usually the first persons to recognize an emergency and mobilize others to respond.

Another type of nurse manages a home care agency that provides nursing care to patients in their homes. She or he hires staff, assumes the financial responsibility for the agency, and serves as its manager. The nursing care must be coordinated so that the patient is getting the right care at the right time. In addition, nurses supervise the care provided by home health aides. They are responsible for the quality of care provided and for assuring that all government and accreditation regulations are met.

The nurse providing direct patient care in such an agency performs many of the same functions as those of the hospital nurse. There is, however, a greater focus on the patient (and family) assuming responsibility for the care. The nurse teaches the family along with providing the care. Nurses at home provide intravenous therapy, change dressings, administer medications, supervise respirators, and help families cope with the death of a loved one.

Nurse researcher's spend their day reviewing journals, collecting and analyzing data, and writing reports on research. They usually have a doctorate. Areas of research of interest to nurses include nursing practice, such as decision making and validating the efficacy of nursing practice; nursing education, such as learning strategies and methods to assess competence; and the administration, organization, and delivery of nursing services, such as the cost-effectiveness of nursing services and delivery models (Welch, 1988).

Public health nurses usually work for a government agency and typically see clients in a clinic setting, trace contacts of communicable disease patients, and provide community education. They may work in a school or an immunization clinic. They may design community education programs to prevent adolescent pregnancies or to decrease the spread of AIDS. Their focus is truly prevention and education to promote the health of a community.

Advanced Practice Nurses

Advanced practice nurses are registered nurses with additional education and clinical experience. According to Sharp (1993) they include: Nurse practitioners, Certified Nurse Midwives, Clinical Nurse Specialists and Certified Nurse Anesthetists. There are approximately 25,000 to 30,000 nurses working as nurse practitioners in the U.S. They have from 2 to 4 years of education and clinical training in addition to the education received to become a registered nurse. Most have a master's degree and 36 states require national certification to practice. Advanced practice nurses conduct patient assessments, diagnose and treat people usually in primary care settings.

The approximately 5,000 Certified Nurse Midwives in the U.S. have about one and one-half years of post registered nurse education, increasingly in master's degree programs. They provide pre-, intra-, and post-partum care, provide family planning services, and routine gynecological care. They work in hospitals, clinics, private practice and homes. There is formal support for their practice from the American College of Obstetrics and Gynecology, the physician specialty group (Safriet, 1992, p. 162).

Clinical Nurse Specialists of whom there are about 40,000 are master's prepared nurses who have specialized education and experience in a particular area such as mental health. The 25,000 Certified Registered Nurses Anesthetists have 2 to 4 years of postbaccalaureate education and provide anesthesia care. Advanced practice nurses tend to have higher incomes and be more independent than many other nurses. They tend to work in geographic areas where and with populations with whom physicians do not work (Sharp, 1993).

Collective Bargaining

Nurses are organized in the work setting by professional organization, under the auspices of state nurses' associations, and by traditional trade unions. The ANA argues that it is appropriate for nurses to organize to improve both working conditions and the quality of care, although others argue that union membership is unprofessional. The issue of striking to improve conditions has long divided the nursing community: Some say that a strike is legitimate to attain improved conditions, and others argue that in a life-and-death profession such as nursing patient care should not be jeopardized under any circumstances.

In 1974 the Taft-Hartley Act was amended to make nonprofit health facilities subject to National Labor Relations Board ruling. This means that nurses can join unions without fear of retribution. In 1992 about 16% of working registered nurses belonged to collective bargaining associations. An additional 3.1% were covered by collective bargaining units. These additional nurses worked in facilities covered by collective bargaining agreements, but were not members of the organizing group (Daniel Hecker, personnal communication, 1993). The average salary of registered nurses increased 33% from $28,383 in 1988 to $37,738 in 1992. (Division of Nursing, 1993).

Organized Nursing

The ANA is the national professional organization for nurses. Founded in 1897, its members are not nurses but state or territorial nurses associations. The so-called tri-level system is composed of individual nurses who may join local and/or district nurses associations. These in turn are usually organized by city or county into state associations. Delegates from the state associations meet annually at a national convention to set policy for the ANA.

The ANA also offers voluntary certification exams in a variety of nursing specialty areas, such as community health nursing, mental health nursing, and nursing administration. It serves as a lobbying association for nursing, its headquarters are in Washington, DC.

The NLN, founded in 1893 and unrelated to the ANA, serves as the accreditation body for schools of nursing. Its subsidiary Community Health Accreditation Program (CHAP) accredits home health agencies. Membership is open to agencies, nurses, and nonnurses, although most members are in the nursing profession.

Sigma Theta Tau International is the honor society for nursing. An international organization located in St. Louis, its primary purpose is to foster scholarship in nursing. Membership is by election and restricted to those nurses who meet its academic and community service criteria.

In addition to the general organizations described above, nurses belong to numerous specialty groups. The groups tend to have as a focus the specialty area or site of practice for nurses. The first such organization was the American Association of Nurse Anesthetists (Kelly, 1987). Examples of other organizations include the American College of Nurse Midwives, the National Nurses Society of Addictions, the National Black Nurses Association, and the Society for Nursing History.

The National Institute for Nursing Research is part of the National Institutes of Health (NIH). Prior to its establishment, funding for nursing research was under the auspices of the Division of Nursing in the Health Resources and Services Administration. The purpose of the center is to conduct "a program of grants and awards supporting nursing research and research training related to patient care, the promotion of health, the prevention of disease and the mitigation of the effects of acute and chronic illnesses and disabilities" (Merritt, 1986). Funding for 1993 was $48.2 million. The primary focus is support of extramural research. Organized nursing viewed authorization of the Institute as a milestone in the acceptance of nursing as a research-based profession.

Issues for the 1990s

The major issues for the 1990s are those of the health care industry in general: the cost and quality of health care. Nurses are being asked to provide high-quality care at a cost that society is willing to pay.

Cost of Care

The federal government's attempt to control health care costs through a prospective payment system based on diagnostic-related groups (DRGs) had an impact on nurses. Over time DRGs have decreased lengths of hospital stays and increased intensity of care required by patients, early patient discharge, and cost-consciousness (Mitchell & Dibbles, 1988). The introduction of DRGs forced nurses to analyze the cost of nursing care. Initially, there were fears that nurses would be fired as length of stay decreased along with patient census. Although there was some early evidence of a decreasing need for nurses, this situation quickly changed because the patients who remained in the hospital were sicker. In addition, the AIDS epidemic has countered some of the expected decrease in the need for nurses. Since hospitals are no longer reimbursed by Medicare on a cost basis, there is an increased push to isolate nursing costs so that attempts can be made to decrease them. Hospital nurses are the managers of patient care and play a vital role in allocating the hospital's resources. The nurse knows how the patient is progressing, where the patient should be at what time, and where the patient is going next.

Under expert nursing care length of stay can be decreased and the patient discharged to well-organized care at home.

JCAHO requires now using acuity systems to measure the need for nursing care. Nurses use checklists to identify patient care needs. Results of the scoring are then translated into nursing hours required, and appropriate staffing is determined. Proprietary systems have been developed and sold, and many hospitals use systems developed for their special needs. Some have criticized the systems for their lack of validity, arguing that much of what nurses do cannot easily be quantified into mechanical tasks. These and other efforts are probably a result of the increased pressure on hospitals to use nursing resources efficiently.

Although RNs as a percentage of total labor in hospitals increased from 18% in 1962 to 23% in 1990, labor as a percentage of total per day expenses in 1962 decreased from 66.5% to 54.4% over the same period (Prescott, 1993).

Entry Into Practice

In 1965 the ANA voted to (1) move toward the baccalaureate degree as the minimum educational requirement for licensure as a registered nurse and (2) require technical nurses to be prepared in 2-year college programs. In 1976 the New York State Nurses Association recommended that the state pass legislation to establish these two levels of nursing. This legislation has never been passed. In 1983, after years of debate, the NLN issued a statement of support for this proposal. As of 1992 only two states, North Dakota and Maine, require the baccalaureate degree for professional nurses' licensure. This requirement was achieved by regulation of the North Dakota Board of Nursing rather than by legislation, as proposed in New York. This issue has divided the nursing community and pitted nursing against organized medicine and hospitals.

The argument for the proposal suggests that in the complex health care system 4 years of college is the minimal amount of education necessary to prepare nurses for practice. In addition, nursing is the only one of the major health professions (M.D., D.D.S., O.T., P.T.) that does not require at least a bachelor's degree. Proponents argue that nurses educated at the baccalaureate level provide better care. A study by Johnson (1988) that synthesized results of 139 studies found significant differences in communication skills, knowledge, problem-solving ability, teaching, and professional role between the baccalaureate-educated nurses and those educated in either a diploma or an associate-degree program: baccalaureate nurses perform these functions at a higher level than graduates of either diploma or associate degree programs. The groups did not differ on autonomy and leadership behaviors.

Those who argue against the proposal suggest that graduates from both diploma and 2-year programs provide a fine level of care and may be even better at skills such as giving injections than those with baccalaureate education. They also argue that a 4-year education is more costly to society than a 2- or 3-year education and that requiring a baccalaureate degree further restricts entry into the nursing field. Intuitively, it seems to make sense that nurses who have a thorough grounding in the basic sciences, the social sciences, and the humanities will be better able to adapt to a changing health care environment and provide better care to patients than nurses with less education.

Independent Practice

Most working nurses are employees rather than independent practitioners. A phenomenon of the 1980s and early 1990s was a movement toward independent practice, defined as self-employment. Independent practice falls into three areas: private duty, individual fee-for-service practice, and group practice. It is interesting to note that in the late 19th century most nurses were independent practitioners employed by people to care for family members at home. The popularity of that type of practice waned, although there have always been nurses employed by families to care for sick members either at home or in the hospital. Such nurses contract with the patient to provide a set amount of care for a set fee.

Nurses in the mental health area are in the forefront of independent fee-for-service practice and, increasingly, nurses in other areas, such as geriatric care and cardiac patient care are providing nursing on a fee-for-service basis. For example, nurses provide care to patients who have cardiac problems, assisting the client to change life-style patterns and providing education and comfort. In this broad category are nurses who act as consultants to other nurses in areas such as setting up educational programs, organizing nursing services, or carrying out evaluation projects.

A major obstacle to independent practice is lack of benefit coverage or third-party reimbursement for nursing services. Since so much of health care is now reimbursed by third-party payers, consumers may be reluctant to purchase nursing services on a fee-for-service basis and not be reimbursed when they can receive a similar service from a physician and obtain reimbursement. For example, if a patient is recovering from surgery and has a wound that must be observed for signs of infection and healing, this can be done by either a nurse or a physician. If the patient sees the physician, the service is usually reimbursed by the third-party payer; if the patient sees a nurse for the service, it is usually not reimbursed.

If this same patient is homebound and has Medicare coverage, a visit by the nurse from a home health agency is reimbursed (as long as a physician orders the care), whereas the patient who is not homebound and visits the nurse in his or her office will not receive reimbursement. It is understandable that insurers do not want to increase the number of providers who are able to authorize service. There is also some sense to not encouraging another group of fee-for-service practitioners besides physicians. Nevertheless, the cost-benefit of reimbursement for more expensive medical care and not for nursing is difficult to appreciate.

In response to what some would argue is an irrational reimbursement system, community nursing centers have been proposed. Based on the HMO concept, a group of nurses would agree to provide nursing care for a defined population for a set reimbursable fee. Federal legislation has funded the study of four such centers.

Many home care nurses work in a form of independent practice. They contract with an agency to provide patient care at a specific price per visit. Although these nurses are not directly paid by the patient or the insurer, they have many of the advantages of a fee-for-service practitioner. They are able to work as much as they like and earn more money by seeing more patients. If they are efficient and can complete their work quickly, they earn more money for fewer hours of work. They generally do not have the advantages of institutional employment, such as health benefits, vacation days, and guaranteed work even when demand is slow.

Organized nursing and individual nurses are working to change the regulations for reimbursement. This is a slow and tedious process done on a state-by-state basis. For example, New York State now has "Third Party Reimbursement" requiring insurance companies to provide reimbursement for nursing care if requested by the insured group. This has had a nominal effect on reimbursement because most purchasers see payment to nurses as additive, not substitutive, so paying nurses as independent health practitioners would add to health costs and premiums. The ideal law, according to nurses, would require insurance companies to reimburse for any health care services currently covered that can be provided by a nurse.

Advanced Practice Nursing and Primary Care

As discussed earlier, advanced practice nurses practice in a variety of settings. Legal limitations on such practice vary considerably from state to state. Numerous studies support the position that nurse practitioners provide health care equal in quality to that provided by physicians and at substantially less cost. This difference in cost is in part a reflection of the substantially lower costs to educate a nurse practitioner as compared to a physician.

Safriet (1992) points out that over 63,000 registered nurses are educated as nurse practitioners, well in excess of the number who practice. She attributes this difference to the regulatory constraints imposed by states. Examples include regulations or statutes limiting care practitioners can provide and restrictive reimbursement policies. In many cases when nurse practitioners are reimbursed, it is at a rate less than that provided to physicians who provide the same care with the same outcomes.

Safriet (1992) describes practice as prevention, diagnosis, prescription, and treatment and says that states have used a variety of approaches to expand the scope of practice for nurse practitioners, including revision of the Nurse and Medical Practice Acts. In addition to roles and title variations in different jurisdictions, restrictions on practice vary. They fall into two general areas: the relationship between the nurse practitioner and physician (e.g., formal practice relationships, written practice protocols, and physician supervision) and restrictions on site of practice (e.g., to rural areas, to clinics only).

State regulations on nurses prescribing pharmaceuticals are inconsistent. In Oregon, nurse practitioners can prescribe pharmaceuticals, with no conditions of physician oversight (Safriet, 1992). In some states (Oregon, Washington, Alaska, and Montana) advanced practice nurses can prescribe without physician collaboration or authorizations, while in other states the nurse must have a practice arrangement with a physician. Some states limit prescriptive authority to central sites, to formularies, or to specific drugs (Carson, 1993).

Reimbursement continues to be a restriction on practice. As of 1992, 25 states required mandatory reimbursement in some form (Safriet, 1992). Medicaid mandates direct Medicaid reimbursement of Pediatric and Family Nurse Practitioners (PNPs and FNPs) and Midwives. Of 47 states responding to a federal study 41 allow FNPs and PNPs to bill directly (Physician Payment Review Commission, 1993). In 1988, Midwifery care became a covered Medicare service. Gynecologic care is excluded. Nurse practitioner care is covered if the NP works in collaboration with a physician, and meets practice site restrictions (Safriet, 1992).

The issues for the 1990s will likely focus on scope of practice, prescriptive authority, and reimbursement. If the United States moves to a systems where financial barriers to health care are removed, the use of advanced practice nurses, especially nurse practitioners and nurse midwives will likely expand. It remains to be seen what physician reaction will be.

Nursing Supply

The supply and demand for nurses continues to be an issue in health care. During the early 1990s various approaches were implemented to balance supply and demand. Interventions included increasing the supply by recruiting more people into nursing and improving retention, thereby increasing supply; and decreasing the demand by having nonnurses perform activities usually performed by nurses and/or using technology in performing those activities.

Specific solutions to increasing the supply of active workers included raising starting salaries and increasing salary progression. In addition, many organizations decreased the number of nonnursing tasks performed by professional nurses in the hope of creating an environment in which nurses could nurse and including nurses in the governance of the health care organizations.

Attempts to increase the number of new entrants to the field have included the above-identified changes to improve the appeal of nursing positions and specific actions aimed at encouraging people to pursue a career in nursing. These included improving the image of nursing and increasing scholarships. Many organizations provided scholarships for nonprofessional staff, such as nurses aides and dietary workers, to attend nursing school.

Concurrently, health care organizations reorganized to decrease the demand for nursing. Approaches included: case management, work redesign, and use of technology among others. Case management has as its goal the prudent use of health resources, including nursing. Redesign interventions vary from nurse-nurse assistant partnerships to rethinking the components of care required by patients during an episode of illness. An example of technology is the increased use of computerized information systems to improve communication and decrease paper work.

Nursing and Health Reform

As of October 1993 President Clinton's Health Reform Proposal became public. Nurses have been actively involved in the development of the plan. Early reports suggested that nurses will have a major role in a proposed reformed health care system. There will likely be a greater focus both on primary care and health promotion, areas in which nurses have long had experience and in which they are recognized as providing excellent care. There are major questions about how a revised health care system will effect the supply and demand for nurses. Some say more nurses will be required under universal health insurance. Others say that although there will be fewer financial barriers to health care, people with increased access to primary care and health promotion will require less nurses in acute care hospitals. In any event, there will likely be an increase in the need for advance practice nurses such as nurse practitioners.

A recent report of the Pew Health Professions Commission (1993) suggests changes for nursing education to prepare nurses to work effectively in the future. Suggestions include differentiating nursing roles and changing regulations to reflect these roles, involving faculty in clinical practice, using interdisciplinary teaching, practice and research; and increasing focus on community-based patients.

In many ways nursing exemplifies a cyclical or spiral nature of the world with repeating patterns. Initially nurses were self-employed and responsible directly to patients; today's nurses again want to be self-employed and responsible to their clients. In earlier days nursing care was primarily provided at home. Today there are many in nursing who think this is where nursing should take place. At times the nurse has been a team leader, coordinating and providing patient care, and supervising LPNs and aides. Then, in the 1970s primary care—the nurse providing all of the care for a group of patients—was the vogue; and now there seems to be some movement toward hiring aides and assistants for the nurse. The nurse began as handmaiden to the physician; one circle that will surely not be redrawn is a return to that condition. Nurses will continue to work in an interdependent relationship with physicians in a variety of settings such as the acute-care hospital. Some nurses will continue a dependent relation when they work in a physician's office or in the operating room. But many nurses will move into areas of prevention and health promotion and work independently of physicians. Nursing has achieved independence; it remains to be seen how many nurses will choose this option.

References

Aiken, L. In D. Mechanic (Ed.), *Handbook of Health Professions*, pp. 407–431, New York: Free Press, 1983.

American Nurses Association. *Nursing Association Policy Statement*. Kansas City, MO: ANA, 1980.

American Nurses Association. *The Nursing Practice Act: Suggested State Legislation*. New York: ANA, 1981.

Anastas, L. *Your Career in Nursing*. New York: National League for Nursing, 1984.

Bullough, N. "Barriers to the Nurse Practitioner Movement: Problem of Women in a Women's Field." *International Journal of Health Services*, 5, 225, 1975.

Carson, W. Gains and challenges in prescriptive authority. *The American Nurse, 25*(6), 19, 20, June, 1993.

Division of Nursing, Bureau of Health Professions, Health Resources and Services Administration. "The March 1992 National Sample Survey of Registered Nurses." July, 1993.

Fawcett, L., *Analysis and Evaluation of Conceptual Models of Nursing* (2-nd Ed.). Philadelphia: F. A. Davis, 1989.

Hecker, D., U.S. Department of Labor, Bureau of Labor Statistics, Office of Employment Projections, 1993.

Henderson, V., *The Nature of Nursing*. New York: Macmillan, 1966.

Johnson, J., "Differences in the Performance of Baccalaureate, Associate Degree, and Diploma Nurses: A Meta-analysis. *Research in Nursing & Health*, 11, 183, 1988.

Kelly, L. Y., *The Nursing Experience*. New York: Macmillan, 1987.

McClure, M. L., & Nelson, M. J., Trends in Hospital Nursing in L. H. Aiken (Ed.) *Nursing in the 1980s: Crisis, Opportunities, Challenges*, pp. 59–73, Philadelphia: Lippincott, 1982.

Merritt, D., "The National Center of Nursing Research." *Image, 18*(3), 84, 1986.

Mitchell, M., & Dibbles, S., Acute Care Nursing: Impact of DRGs. In *Impact of DRGs on Nursing*. Washington, DC: Health Resources and Services Administration, pp. 5–31, (NTIS HRP-09071799), 1988.

National Council of State Boards of Nursing, Inc. *1992 Annual Report*. 676 North St. Clair, Chicago, IL, 1992.

National League for Nursing. *Nursing Data Source 1993. Vol. I. Trends in Contemporary Nursing Education*. New York: National League for Nursing Press, Publication No. 19-2526, 1993a.

National League for Nursing. *Nursing Data Review 1993*. New York: National League for Nursing Press, Publication No. 19-2529, 1993b.

New York State Department of Health. *Final Report of the New York State Labor-Health Industry Task Force on Health Personnel*. Albany: Author, 1989.

Orem, D. E. *Nursing: Concepts of Practice*. New York: McGraw-Hill, 1980.

Pew Health Professions Commission. (February, 1993). *Health Professions Education for the Future: Schools in Service to the Nation*. San Francisco, CA: Author, 1993.

Porter-O'Grady, T., *Creative Nursing Administration: Participative Management into the 21st Century*. Rockville, MD: Aspen, 1986.

Physician Payment Review Commission. Annual Report to Congress. Washington, DC: Author, 1993.

Prescott, P., Nursing an important compondent of hospital survival under a reformed health care system. *Nursing Economics, 11*(4), pp. 192–199, 1993.

Rosenberg, C., *The Care of Strangers*. New York: Basic Books, 1987.

Safriet, B., "Health Care Dollars and Regulatory Sense: The Role of Advanced Practice Nursing." *Yale Journal on Regulation*, 9(2), 149–220, 1992.

Secretary's Commission on Nursing. *Final Report. Secretary's Commission on Nursing Final Report*. Washington, DC: Department of Health and Human Services, December, 1988.

Sharp, N., Primary Care in Legislation and the Practice *Nursing Management. 24*(8) 20–23, 1993.

U.S. Department of Health and Human Services. *Health Personnel in the United States. Eight Report to Congress*. 1991. (DHHS Pub No HRS-P-00-92-1) Washington, DC: DHHS. September 1992.

Welch, C., "Conference Report: Directions for Nursing Research in New York State." *The Journal of the New York State Nurses Association, 19*(3), 16, 1988.

Wilkerson, K. B., "Public Health Nursing: In Sickness or in Health." *American Journal of Public Health*, 75, 1155–1157, 1985.

6

Ambulatory Care

Andrew P. Mezey and Robert S. Lawrence

Ambulatory care is personal health care provided to an individual who is not a bed patient in a health care institution. It includes all health services, other than community or public health services, provided to noninstitutionalized patients. Once the almost exclusive domain of physicians and dentists, ambulatory care now includes the services of public health nurses, nurse practitioners, physician assistants, social workers, optometrists, podiatrists, health assistants, and many others. Roemer (1981) provided the most comprehensive review of all features of this topic in *Ambulatory Health Services in America*. This chapter reviews the current organization of personal medical services provided in ambulatory settings but does not discuss mental health or rehabilitative services.

In 1990 the average person made 5.5 visits to a physician and spent 0.71 days in an acute-care hospital (709.5 short-stay hospital days per 1,000 population). Thus, 7.75 times more ambulatory care episodes than hospital days of care occurred (USDHHS, 1991, Tables 76, 84). This ratio is up from 4.7 in 1980, as the number of ambulatory visits increased from just under 5 per person and the number of hospital days declined sharply from 1,163 per 1,000 population in 1980 (USDHHS, 1982, Tables 35, 43). The unprecedented shifts away from inpatient care of the last decade have had enormous impact on the organization, staffing, and financing of ambulatory services in the United States. The number of Americans who reported a visit to a physician increased slightly from 75% in 1980 to 78.2% in 1990. A full 88.3% of the population had seen a physician in the past 2 years (USDHHS, 1991, Table 77 and 1987, Table 58). Meanwhile, the average length of stay in nonfederal acute-care hospitals decreased from 7.3 in 1980 to 6.4 in 1990 (USDHHS, 1982, Table 42 and 1991, Table 85). Most patient-physician contacts now take place on an ambulatory basis.

The rates of visits to physicians vary by age, gender, race, and socioeconomic status. About 93.6% of the very young (under 5 years) and 89.3% of the very old (75 years and over) have an annual visit with a physician; 73.3% of males and

82.9% of females report an annual physician visit; and 78.7% of whites and 77.5% of blacks saw a physician in 1990, compared with 75.4% and 74%, respectively in 1980 (USDHHS, 1991, Table 77 and 1982, Table 36). The narrowing of the gap observed between the races also occurred for differences of physician use by the rich and the poor. In 1964, 58.6% of those with a family income less than $14,000 reported seeing a physician; 70.2% of persons living in families earning more than $35,000 did so. By 1990, these rates had increased to 77.3 and 80.1, respectively (USDHHS, 1991, Table 77). The enactment of Medicaid and Medicare accounts for much of the increased use of physicians by lower-income groups.

Somewhat paradoxically, the number of physician visits per person is actually higher among lower income groups—those with less than $14,000 annual family income than among those with annual family incomes above $35,000; the reported rates are 6.3 and 5.7, respectively (USDHHS, 1991, Table 76). Thus, access—as measured by the percentage seeing a physician yearly—has improved for the poor but still lags; whereas utilization—as measured by the number of physician visits per person per year—is higher because there is more sickness among the poor (Wilensky & Berk, 1982). For the elderly poor, ambulatory visits actually decreased by 20% between 1982 and 1986, when the federal government reduced support for health services (R. W. Johnson Foundation, 1987).

In 1990, whites report 5.6 visits per year and blacks, 5.1 (USDHHS, 1991, Table 76). Although a larger proportion of blacks live in poverty (a condition associated with higher utilization rates), they experience more problems with access to physician services than do whites, who constitute the majority of poor people. The percentage of visits occurring in the hospital outpatient departments is almost double for blacks (24.3%) compared with whites (12.3%) (USDHHS, 1991, Table 76). Similar differences in hospital outpatient use exist by socioeconomic class. The inverse holds true for visits to doctors' offices and use of telephone contact with physicians when analyzed by race or socioeconomic status.

There are two major categories of ambulatory care. The dominant form is care provided by private physicians in solo, partnership, or private group practice on a fee-for-service basis. The other, growing dramatically in the last decade, is ambulatory care in organized settings that have an identity independent from that of the individual physicians practicing in it. This category includes managed care programs that, by the end of 1991, had enrolled over 110 million Americans, when one counts both health maintenance organizations (HMOs) and preferred provider organizations (PPOs). (MacLeod, 1993) Other forms of ambulatory health care delivery in this latter category are hospital-based ambulatory services, including clinics, walk-in and emergency services, hospital-sponsored group practices and health promotion centers; freestanding "surgi-centers" and "urgi- or emergi-centers"; health department clinics; neighborhood and community health centers (NHCs and CHCs); organized home care; community mental health centers; school and workplace health services and prison health services.

Different ambulatory care settings provide service for diverse groups in the population. Results in utilization and quality of services provided also differ by demographic group. A decade ago Dutton analyzed the impact of the major forms of ambulatory care on patients in Washington, D.C., in terms that apply today:

> Sources used primarily by the poor—hospital outpatient departments, emergency rooms, and public clinics—contained important structural and financial barriers, and had the lowest rates of patient-initiated use. The prepaid system, in contrast, maximized patient's access to both preventive care and symptomatic care, and did not seem to inhibit physician-controlled follow-up care. The results suggest some perverse effects of fee-for-service payment: patients, especially poor patients, appeared to be deterred from seeking preventive and symptomatic care, while physicians were encouraged to expand follow-up services. Moreover, services in fee-for-service systems were distributed less equitably relative to both income and medical need than in the prepaid system. (Dutton, 1979, p. 221)

Private Practice

Private practice remains the principal mode by which physicians provide services to patients in the United States. Only the licensure laws of the state limit the range of health care services that the physician can provide as an independent entrepreneur. The physician implicitly—and rarely in writing—contracts to provide these services to the patient in return for the payment of a fee, hence, the *fee-for-service* system.

Private practitioners care for patients on a fee-for-service basis in such settings as office space owned or leased by the physician, the patient's home or a bedded institution. When hospitalized under the care of his or her physician, the patient— or the patient's insurer—pays the hospital for all services other than physician care and pays the physician's fee directly. The physician remains a private contractor to the patient even in the hospital setting. Increasingly, physicians arrange for cross-coverage of ambulatory or hospitalized patients for nights, weekends, or holidays with other solo practitioners, or they form partnerships or group practices. Under these latter arrangements Medicare requires the covering physician to bill for services provided. Office billing arrangements follow the same pattern, although the distribution of practice income to the members of the group may use other systems to provide productivity incentives, reward longevity or partnership status, maintain the necessary specialty mix in the practice, or meet other goals set by the group.

As of 1989, 75% of the 468,902 nonfederal physicians in clinical practice were in office-based practice. Interns and residents in training comprised 17% of nonfederal practitioners. Full-time members of the hospital staff accounted for another 8.3%. Contrasting figures for the 20,359 federal physicians in 1989 are: 7.3% office-based practitioners among the 15,570 physicians engaged in patient care, 13.4% interns and residents, and 79% full-time members of a hospital staff (USDHHS, 1991, Table 98).

Data from the 1990 National Health Interview Survey show an increase in the proportion of physician visits made to a doctor's office, from 57.5% of all contacts in 1985 to 59.9% in 1990 (USDHHS, 1991, Table 76). Visits to hospital outpatient departments decreased slightly, from 14.7% to 13.7% during the same period. The remaining 26.4% of physician contacts in 1990 were by telephone (12.7%), patient's home (2.1%), and laboratory or clinic facilities located outside the hospital (11.6%). According to these patient interview data, just under 572 million visits to physicians in private offices or HMO practice occurred in 1990. The growth of HMO membership from just under 7 million in 1976 to 36.5 million by July 1991 (Parker et al., 1992) accounted for a significant portion of the decrease in traditional private-practice office visits.

Other statistics capture some of the interesting dynamics of private practice during the past decade. The number of office visits lasting 10 minutes decreased from 42.6% in 1985 to 41.3% in 1989. The proportion of visits generating a scheduled return visit also decreased slightly from 58.8% to 58.1% (USDHHS, 1991, Table 79). These changes held for both sexes and racial groups and some age groups. Those 15 and under had a slight increase (3%) in the proportion of visits lasting 10 minutes or less. Likewise, those 15 to 44, 45 to 64, 65 and over, 65 to 74, and 75 and over had slight increases (between 1% and 3%) in the proportion of visits generating a scheduled return visit.

Since first visits require more of the physician's time, it is possible that most or all of the decline in the number of short visits above was the result of the concomitant rise in proportion of first visits. The data are not definitive on this matter. Alternative explanations include an ever-more competitive health care market that encourages physicians to spend more time with their patients to increase patient satisfaction; the increase in the number of physicians relative to the patient population that allows more time per visit with fewer visits per physician; and the proliferation of employee benefit options with annual enrollment periods that raises the chance of the patient changing his or her physician because of changes in health insurance that increasingly emphasize managed care with closed panels of physicians.

Private practice is changing to compete with the HMOs and other forms of organized ambulatory care. One strategy is the development of women's health centers, special services marketed to women (Harrell & Fors, 1985; Wolinsky, 1986), or primary care centers staffed and run by women for women (Daily, 1986). Proponents of this strategy argue that women differ from men in the selection of health services. Offering services designed to appeal to these differences will provide a competitive advantage.

Practitioners have become more aware of the role of practice organization in growth or maintenance of practice size. Attention to all of the types of encounters that patients have with the practice improves the patient's experience with office staff, the billing procedure, and the medical office environment. One practice found high patient satisfaction with all major elements of the practice after paying special attention to these various encounter points (Tulli, 1987).

Some practitioners have adapted to competitive pressures by contracting for part or all of their practice with an HMO, a PPO, or an independent practice association (IPA). These arrangements, however, often change how physicians in private practice care for patients by limiting referrals to only the plan's consultants, by special data requirements, by termination agreements, and by requirements for compliance with state and federal laws. Since many practitioners sign up with several HMOs, PPOs, or IPAs, all with different forms, consultants, and agreements, life has become complicated for the physician in private practice.

With the arrival of freestanding emergency centers and surgi-centers some practices have responded with extended hours or increased walk-in services. One study compared two family practice groups using these adaptations with four freestanding emergency care centers (Chesteen, Warren, & Woolley, 1986). A total of 2,339 patient visits were examined, using data from both physicians and patients. Patient satisfaction with convenience and personal attention from the physicians and the cost of care were important in distinguishing the two forms of practice. The freestanding centers charged significantly more for their services ($45 vs. $27) but outperformed the family practices in convenience, time factors (waiting time, time spent with the physician, time to get an appointment, clinic location), and out-of-pocket costs. Patients judged the personal concern of the physician and the ability to see the same physician desirable attributes of the family practices.

Managed Health Care Organizations

Managed health care organizations provide for both the delivery and the financing of health care for their members (enrollees). These organizations take a variety of forms in how they deliver that care and in how they finance it. In addition, they are evolving, with the boundaries between older forms becoming blurred, and with new forms taking shape. If present trends continue, and it is likely that they will under current federal and state plans for health care reform, managed health care will become the predominant system for the delivery of health care in the United States before the end of the century. The driving force behind this growth is the belief that health care costs can be controlled by "managing" how health care is delivered.

All managed care organizations build on the foundation of the primary care provider (PCP). The term, primary care provider, generally means a family practitioner, general internist, or general pediatrician, but can also mean an obstetrician and gynecologist, or a nonphysician provider, such as a nurse practitioner, physician assistant, or midwife. This provider has the burden of limiting health care expenditures by limiting access to other providers of health care. Some have used the term "gate-keeper" to describe this function. Limiting referrals to specialists, and decreasing admissions to hospitals are the major means to control access to care. Incentives for the primary care provider to comply vary, depending on the type of managed care organization. The incentives may include bonuses or payments of fees that have been withheld. Wagner describes the types of managed care organizations and how they are organized as:

Health Maintenance Organizations. In classic indemnity insurance, the enrollee pays a premium to the health insurer, for which the health insurer contracts to pay for the health care that is delivered. In contrast, HMOs not only contract to pay for the health care of enrollees but to deliver the care to them also. There are five common models of HMOs: staff, group, network, independent practice association (IPA), and direct contract, with the primary differences being how the HMO relates to its participating physicians. Payment most often, but not necessarily, takes the form of a capitation fee. With capitation, the organization, be it a group practice or an individual physician, receives a monthly, prepaid, fixed fee for each covered individual or family. For that fee the HMO agrees to provide the services for which the contract calls. The organization attempts to provide those services to the individual at a cost lower than the fee paid. Thus, the incentives in HMO practices differ markedly from the incentives in fee-for-service practices. In a prepaid capitation system the provider profits by delivering less costly and less total services and by minimizing referrals to other providers, since the provider retains more of the prepaid fee by doing so. In a fee-for-service system, more money can be made by providing more services, and no financial risk accrues to the organization or to the individual physician by asking others to provide services since classic indemnity insurance will pay for them. The HMO hopes to persuade people to insure with them by offering similar health care services at a lower price, and by controlling those costs by having their providers manage care.

Preferred Provider Organizations. In PPOs, the organization contracts to provide health services for a set fee through the use of selected physicians. The physicians agree to the fee structure of the PPO in return for the PPO providing them with patients. These fees are generally lower than the physicians charge their non-PPO patients, but physicians are willing to accept the discounted rate because the increased volume will maintain or increase their revenue. In addition, physicians in PPOs usually incur no financial risk. Patients in PPOs are allowed to use providers outside the PPO, but must pay extra to do so. Physicians, in order to belong to the PPO, agree to abide by utilization management agreements. Therefore, should participating physicians wish to refer a patient to a specialist, they must first receive permission for the referral, and then refer to a specialist with whom the PPO has an existing arrangement. If participating physicians wish to admit a patient to the hospital, prior permission from the PPO must be obtained. Without these authorizations, the PPO will not pay for the service. Unlike in some

HMOs, in PPOs the patient can choose a non-PPO option but must pay extra to do so. The financial burden is placed on the patient rather than on the physician or the organization.

Point-of-Service Plans. Point-of-service plans combine features of classic HMOs with some of the characteristics of patient choice found in PPOs. Similar to the HMO model, the physician gets paid through a capitation or other risk-based model. Similar to the PPO model, a member of a point-of-service plan can choose to use a nonplan provider by paying extra. For example, the plan, under this option, may pay only 60% of nonplan provider charges rather than 100%. Thus, costs are kept down either by asking the patient to pay more or by making the provider act as a "gate-keeper," and enforced by placing a financial risk on the provider.

Hospital-Based Ambulatory Services

The hospital remains the institutional center of the U.S. health care system despite the enormous pressure in recent years to move the focus of care to the ambulatory setting. Inpatient services and revenues still drive the system. To a large extent the interest of hospital managers in improving ambulatory services reflects a desire to expand the patient base for their inpatient services. Thus, the outpatients are treated in anticipation of their eventually attaining inpatient status.

In the past, hospital-based ambulatory services meant services that were actually located in the hospital or on the hospital grounds. More recently, hospitals have aggressively sought to maintain their inpatient base by moving their ambulatory base away from the hospital. At the same time, especially in the case of some public hospitals that have expanded into rural areas and inner cities, expansion of clinics into the community improves access to health care for underserved populations. Tertiary care or academic medical centers have expanded into local communities and made affiliation agreements with hospitals in those communities. The local hospitals agree to care for the nontertiary, nonhighly specialized conditions and agree to refer patients for tertiary and specialized care to the medical center.

Outpatients present with problems ranging from life-threatening, acute illnesses requiring emergency services to chronic conditions calling on rehabilitative and social services. Patients with routine medical problems closely resemble patients seeking care in private practitioners' offices. Most hospitals provide two levels of ambulatory care: emergency services and outpatient clinic care. In many inner-city areas the hospital ambulatory services may be the only source of health care, and patients frequently present to emergency departments with routine medical problems. In recent years hospitals have organized "walk-in" clinics to provide a middle ground between true emergency visits and scheduled outpatient clinic visits.

Insurers have traditionally paid hospitals more reliably for emergency services than for clinic services. As a result, hospitals have been more effective in organizing emergency services. In 1991, approximately 93% of the nonfederal community hospitals in the United States (4,627) had emergency units (AHA, 1992–93, Table 12A). Emergency services are intended to care for acutely ill or injured patients—particularly those with life-threatening or potentially life-threatening problems requiring immediate attention, or personnel and equipment not found in private practitioners' offices—and to offer prompt hospitalization if needed.

In contrast, clinic services are provided by only two kinds of hospitals: (1) those located in areas where patients cannot or will not attend private practitioner's offices for more routine care, usually for economic reasons (Roemer, 1981); and (2) those that have teaching programs. About 87% of community hospitals (4,311 in 1991) have organized outpatient departments (AHA, 1992–93, Table 12A), up sharply from 49.4% (2,634) in 1984 (AHA, 1992–93, Text Table 8). These services for nonemergency problems compete with those offered by the private practitioner (economic considerations aside) whereas the emergency services that the office-based practitioner cannot provide do not. As hospitals expand their outpatient departments to increase their patient base, direct competition with private practitioners will continue to grow.

Hospital Clinics

Clinic services began growing in the voluntary hospitals in the latter part of the 19th century. By 1916, 495 hospitals had clinics, often serving both an educational and a charitable function (Roemer, 1975, 1981). Most were treated as the stepchild of the inpatient service, and physicians were often assigned to staff them as a duty in return for the privilege of hospitalizing their patients. From the beginning the clinics varied with the type of hospital (teaching vs. nonteaching, private voluntary vs. public). In community hospitals about 64% of outpatient emergency visits occurred in hospitals not affiliated with medical schools (AHA, 1992–93, Tables 3, 8). Most of the literature on hospital ambulatory care in the United States describes teaching hospitals, so a true picture of the typical unaffiliated hospital is not available.

Most hospital clinics continue to fulfill their role of providing care for the poor, although little free care remains. Those patients not covered by Medicare, Medicaid, or commercial insurance must usually pay according to a means-tested, sliding fee scale. Municipal hospitals serve the uninsured living within their jurisdiction. In some states a "free care pool" exists to help offset the costs of providing unreimbursed care. As the pressure on hospitals from HMOs and PPOs increases, more teaching hospitals have reorganized their clinics to function as group practices (Block, 1979). Goldberg et al. (1987) conducted a controlled trial of the adoption of a group practice model within the medical clinic of a teaching hospital. Randomization produced similar groups of patients and residents, and the clinic activity of 2,299 patients and 28 residents was monitored for 11 months. The group-practice clinics had 20% more visits per month than the control clinics, primarily because there were twice as many overflow sessions (20.2 vs 9.7 sessions per month). Patients spent 15% less time in completing scheduled visits in the group practice clinics. Regular users of the group-practice clinics had 7% more scheduled visits but 39% fewer walk-in visits. Continuity of care was not affected. The investigators concluded that the adoption of the group practice model for the medical clinic improved productivity, speeded up patient flow, and reduced unscheduled clinic visits.

The experiment also had important economic results. The hospital charges per patient were 26% lower in the group-practice clinics ($p = 0.003$). This difference was primarily the result of reduced inpatient charges that were 27% lower per hospitalized patient (Cohen et al., 1986). The mean length of stay among group practice patients was 8.3, compared to 10.5 for the control group ($p = 0.011$). Other hospitals have reorganized their clinics as components of an institution-wide HMO, some with satellite clinics set up to broaden the patient base (Nelson, 1972). The teaching hospital of the University of California at San Diego established an ambulatory clinic on the campus of its parent university several miles away to encourage faculty and students to seek care from medical school physicians and to use the teaching hospital for specialty and inpatient care (Selzer & Scholl, 1985). Montefiore Medical Center in the Bronx, New York has developed an ambulatory care network in the north Bronx and the adjacent suburban county of Westchester, expanding markedly a group practice previously located only at the hospital. The staff are all employees of the medical center, with referrals from the network for specialty care going to hospital-based clinics or to faculty practices, either at or adjacent to the medical center. Contractual agreements exist between the network and various HMOs (Foreman, 1993; C. Braslow, personal communication, 1993). The Johns Hopkins Medical Center in Baltimore Maryland, the Henry Ford Hospital in Detroit, Michigan, and the Rush-Presbyterian Medical Center in Chicago, Illinois, along with other organizations around the country, have developed or are developing, integrated systems in order to fulfill a social obligation—that of providing health services to a defined community—and to ensure that there are adequate numbers of patients to maintain the tertiary care base for their hospitals, to maintain their medical student and resident teaching programs, to maintain their clinical research base and to maintain their fiscal viability.

The machine that produces the energy to make these systems work is the expansion of ambulatory services into communities, often with the acquisition of other hospitals (Heyssel, 1990). Patients are enrolled into these systems through HMOs that may be owned totally by the system or through contracts with existing HMOs. The systems have had to shift their focus from the classical hospital focus—that of thinking only about keeping inpatient beds full—to providing the least expensive health care while attempting to keep beds full and turn them over quickly. This paradigm shift has produced investments in preventive services in an effort to reduce chronic illness and to reduce hospitalizations from preventable conditions. By expanding the ambulatory base there will be enough patients to maintain all the missions of the tertiary center while increasing revenues through the successful operation of managed health care organizations. These decisions were made in the 1980s based on the prediction of some economists that 70% of the U.S. population would belong to HMOs and PPOs by the early 1990s and that at least 10% of the acute care hospitals would have disappeared (Abramowitz; McManis & Hopkins, 1987; Sadowy & Wood, 1986). The recognition of academic medical centers and medical schools of their obligation to improve the health of the public, and not only to serve those who come to their doors reinforced these decisions (Showstack, Heyssel, & Foreman, 1992).

Most hospital organizations now include participation in a PPO, HMO, or alternative delivery system to take advantage of these organizations' ability to direct groups of patients to the hospital (Merz, 1986). Patients, physicians, and policymakers appear to have accepted the constraints on public payments for medical services. For employees the risks of rationed services and facilities appear inevitable (Mechanic, 1985) in return for affordable insurance premiums.

Ambitious strategies for expanding ambulatory care appear necessary for hospitals serving the inner city to survive. One example is the Lutheran Medical Center, serving a depressed Brooklyn neighborhood (Adams, 1988). The hospital, serving a population of 350,000 and providing more than 50,000 ambulatory visits per year, launched an aggressive program of community development that included the following:

1. Providing staff members to serve as resources and support staff for community groups.
2. Creating educational programs for the undereducated and underemployed residents of its service area.
3. Establishing a school health program.
4. Founding the country's largest federally supported neighborhood health center.
5. Contracting with the state of New York to provide health care for 10% less than the average cost for Medicaid patients.

New York City hospitals, with more than 10 million visits to outpatient clinics and emergency rooms each year, are under pressure to reduce the number of acute-care beds. Simultaneously, reduced Medicare reimbursement for graduate medical education squeezes them financially (Rogers, 1985). Hospital ambulatory services must expand and become more efficient if these institutions are to survive.

In 1992, New York State enacted a Medicaid Managed Care Initiative, mandating that, within 5 years, 50% of its Medicaid recipients be enrolled in managed care programs. To comply with this initiative, regions were set up to insure that 10% of those eligible were enrolled in the first year, 25% within 3 years, and 50% by the end of 5 years. HMOs and PPOs were required to enroll specific percentages of their membership into the Medicaid managed care program. The health policymakers in New York believed that increasing access to primary care services for Medicaid recipients would decrease health care costs. Primary care access to health care for the poor in New York is limited by low physician reimbursement by Medicaid for most medical conditions and surgical procedures (about 10% of usual charges). The exception is for services to pregnant woman and for children in some settings and for some procedures, where the fees paid range from 30 to 50% of usual charges.

Enrolling Medicaid patients in HMOs, would discourage emergency room use, and avoid hospital admissions resulting from a lack of access to primary care. These conditions, e.g., asthma and diabetes, are known as "ambulatory care sensitive," and are associated with much higher hospitalization rates in the low-income zip codes in New York City, when compared to high-income zip codes (Billings & Hasselblad, 1990). Since hospitals in New York City, including the 11 acute care hospitals and 6 diagnostic and treatment centers of the New York City Health and Hospitals Corporation that produce a total of 4.5 million ambulatory visits per year, have all shown a great interest in participating in the Medicaid Managed Care program, it is possible that hospital, as well as total, Medicaid health care costs decrease over time.

Clinic Organization and Staffing. The optimal organization of outpatient clinics to provide opportunities for teaching and research—especially in view of the current structure of medical education—is to have many disease-, organ-, or organ-system-specific clinics (Freymann, 1974 p. 255). The typical contemporary teaching hospital has three groups of clinics: medical, surgical, and others. The medical clinic group, which more and more commonly has a "general medical clinic" approximating the function of the general internist or a family practice unit, includes cardiology, neurology, dermatology, allergy, gastroenterology, and so on. Patients may stay in one or more specialty clinics for long periods if the general medical or family practice clinic is small or nonexistent; and specialty clinics admit patients directly, as walk-ins or on referral from the emergency room or inpatient service, rather than on referral from a general clinic. The surgical clinic group includes general surgery, orthopedics, urology, plastic surgery, and the like. Because surgical care is usually more episodic than is general medical care, patients are not as likely to remain in these clinics for long periods. The third group includes pediatrics and the pediatric subspecialties, obstetrics/gynecology and its subspecialties, and other specialties such as rehabilitation medicine.

A number of different types of physicians staff teaching hospital clinics: interns and residents, subspecialty fellows, full-time salaried attending physicians, voluntary (unpaid) attendings, and sessional (paid) physicians. Historically, when the number of full-time salaried physicians on staff was small, voluntary attending staff physicians were the main supervisors of the interns and residents, who actually saw the patients utilizing or using the clinics. This was true of both general and specialty clinics. With time, for both medical and surgical clinics, voluntary faculty found attending clinic less rewarding or too time-consuming, or felt less welcomed or appreciated, and ceased being of major importance in teaching clinics. They still come, but in less numbers and less frequently.

In the past, clinics in teaching hospitals stressed teaching, rather than patient care, as a priority. While this is often still the case, that view of the purpose of clinics is changing, even in specialty clinics. In medical specialty clinics, voluntary physicians have been replaced by full-time faculty and by subspecialty fellows. Though they need the learning experience, the physicians having completed a basic residency program, require much less supervision than interns and residents, are interested in long-term follow-up of patients, spend from 2 to 3 years in a training program, and generally go to the clinic on a regular basis during that period. Some even stay on as attending physicians after they complete their training. Thus, these clinics have become less dependent on residents and interns, with the result that continuity of care is maintained by the fellows and by the attendings.

In the general medical clinics the care of patients has changed also. Residency review committees for all basic primary care training programs require interns and residents to spend a significant portion of their training—approximately 10 to 20%—in continuity clinics. In these clinics the house staff follow their own panel of patients for the time they stay in training—usually 3 years. In clinic they are supervised by generalists, most often full-time in ambulatory care, who also have their own panel of patients for whom they provide primary care. While these physicians are interested in teaching and research, they do have a major commitment to patient care. Unfortunately, in most teaching hospitals the generalist physicians are less valued than are specialists. That equation may change in the 1990s. Voluntary physicians may attend general or specialty medical clinics; when they do, it is often to supervise medical students. In some clinics, especially the so-called walk-in clinics, sessional physicians may be hired to see patients. These physicians are often former trainees of the teaching hospital who are starting out in their own practices. Usually, they do no teaching in this setting.

Surgical clinics vary in their staffing, but still rely heavily on housestaff. Since there are many fewer house staff and many fewer attending staff in surgical subspecialty programs than in pediatrics, internal medicine, or family medicine, those patients that do require extended care in a particular surgical clinic may see the same physicians, be they attendings or housestaff, over long periods of time. The large volume surgical clinics generally do not require continuity of care, except for eye clinics. Ophthalmology has become an ambulatory specialty, both for medical and surgical conditions, so both residents and attendings are able to follow those patients that require continuity.

Most hospital outpatient departments are open all day on weekdays, but many individual clinics, particularly highly subspecialized ones, meet once or twice a week. Some teaching hospitals have more than 100 different specialty and subspecialty clinics. Thus, hospital-based physicians working in the usual hospital clinic can concentrate on diabetes, peripheral vascular disease, or stroke in their teaching and research. This can be an advantage for the physician who has a focus confined to a particular disease or condition. It also may be helpful to the patient who has a single disease problem of a rather complex or unusual nature.

Three kinds of patients face difficulties in using such clinics. First is the patient with an ordinary problem for which no specialty clinic exists. Second is the patient with a disease like uncomplicated diabetes. Attending the diabetes clinic, such a patient is likely to have to defer to a diabetic patient who has complications. Third is the patient with multiple problems. These patients, often elderly, may end up attending a different specialty clinic each day of the week, causing multiple trips to the hospital and preventing one physician from looking at the patient as a person rather than as a collection of diseased organs and organ systems.

Thus, the basic conflict in hospital ambulatory services is established. The needs of specialty-oriented providers conflict with those of the patients with either ordinary problems or with several different problems requiring the care of specialists. Attempts to resolve this conflict by providing group practice arrangements within the clinic have all the advantages described earlier. By their success, however, they threaten the very existence of the subspecialty teaching/research clinic. As hospitals become more responsive to community needs, in order to survive fiscally, the ambulatory clinics must provide more comprehensive services for most patients with common problems. As discussed below, educational reforms to improve the balance between generalists and specialists will also change the orientation of the physicians staffing these clinics (Jonas, 1978, Chapter 12). If teaching and research were oriented more toward an emphasis on the common rather than the uncommon and if hospitals defined their roles and responsibilities by community needs, the contradiction would resolve straightaway, and hospital clinics would be on the road to first-class status (Freymann, 1974, Chapter 18; Jonas, 1973).

The goal of organizing medical care in response to community needs is called community-oriented primary care, or COPC (Madison, 1983; Mullan, 1984; Mullan & Connor, 1982; Nutting et al., 1985; Rogers, 1982). The major elements of COPC are

1. The clinical practice of comprehensive primary medical care.
2. The use of applied epidemiology in practice planning.
3. Community involvement in program planning.
4. The use of data gathered in practice planning and organization.
5. A continuing surveillance of community health status and needs.

Parkland Memorial Hospital in Dallas, Texas has implemented a large community-oriented primary care (COPC) program, comprised of five health centers providing 110,000 visits annually, and serving six at-risk communities in Dallas County. In these areas, emergency room visits have decreased, teenage pregnancy rates in the Hispanic and African-American communities have fallen, and adolescent death rates have fallen (Smith, 1990). As part of a nationwide program sponsored by the Pew Charitable Trusts and the Rockefeller Foundation, entitled Health of the Public: An Academic Challenge, a number of medical schools and academic medical centers have undertaken to integrate population and clinical perspectives into their educational, research, and service programs (Showstack et al., 1992). The University of New Mexico offers an 8-week seminar to third year medical students in clinical epidemiology, health economics, and individual and population health promotion. The Johns Hopkins Medical Institutions link the clinical and public health sciences through its recently established Welch Center for Prevention, Epidemiology, and Clinical Research. Such initiatives exist at fourteen other academic health science centers.

All of these elements operate in a feedback loop. Any medical practice—solo, group, or hospital-based—can use the model. The principal problems are not conceptual; the ideas have been with us for many years. The problem is implementation.

Quality assurance requirements also influence the organization of ambulatory services. The University of Chicago Hospitals developed a system of clinic-based activity for all 60 of its clinics (Oswald & Winer, 1987). The staff developed indicators of quality of care to address both the servicewide and clinic-specific concerns. A single data collection and reporting instrument made it easier for hospital personnel to review and act on reports. The system appears to have improved care and encouraged better interdisciplinary cooperation in quality assurance activities. Other efforts to improve the quality of ambulatory services emphasize the medical record system (Barnett, 1984; Koster, Waterstraat, & Sondak, 1987). These include the advocacy of a standard outpatient medical summary to improve coordination among specialty clinics (Mak, 1987).

Because medical records are intended to assure continuity of care, with attention to applicable prior illness episodes, treatments, or laboratory data, some advocate the use of patient-carried records. Giglio and Papazian (1987) tested four types of patient-carried health records in a hospital outpatient department to determine the acceptability and use of the records. They estimated the costs and observed patient and physician reactions. A small record that fit in the patient's wallet was most acceptable, and the primary determinant of success was the physician's support of the process.

Hospital Emergency Services

Most U.S. hospitals provide emergency services, and over 93% of community hospitals have emergency departments (AHA, 1992–1993, Table 12A). These units serve several functions, from caring for the acutely ill or injured patient to providing walk-in services to less acutely ill patients. Many physicians on the hospital staff also use the emergency room as a setting to assess a patient with a problem that either may lead to inpatient admission or requires equipment or diagnostic imaging facilities not available in the physician's office. Increasingly, extended-care facilities such as nursing homes or chronic-disease hospitals may use the emergency services of an acute-care facility for evaluation of a patient with a sudden change in medical status. Emergency services also continue to function as the primary source of unscheduled admissions to the hospital, accounting for most hospital admissions in many inner city institutions (Kessler & Wilson, 1978; Schroeder, 1993). In 1993, over 75% of all admissions, and 90% of pediatric admissions at the Bronx Municipal Hospital Center (BMHC), a member hospital of the New York City Health and Hospitals Corporation, were through the Emergency Department (BMHC Finance Department Statistical Report, 1993). This percentage has remained stable over the years.

Two decades ago Weinerman et al. (1966, p. 1040) defined three categories of patients presenting themselves to emergency units:

1. *Nonurgent*: "Condition does not require the resources of an emergency service; referral for routine medical care may or may not be needed; disorder is nonacute or minor in severity."
2. *Urgent*: "Condition requires medical attention within the period of a few hours; there is a possible danger to the patient if medically unattended; disorder is acute but not necessarily severe."
3. *Emergent*: "Condition requires immediate medical attention; time delay is harmful to patient; disorder is acute and potentially threatening to life or function."

These terms derive from a professional perspective and are based on medical diagnoses. Most patients cannot make these distinctions and err in both over-intepreting and underinterpreting the gravity of symptoms. Most patients presenting to an emergency service feel that they need immediate attention, regardless of what the professional staff may think. Others know that they do not have an urgent or emergent problem. They simply use the emergency service because it is all that is available to them. A review done in the 1970s showed that the average distribution among patients using emergency services is about 5% emergent, 45% urgent, and 50% nonurgent (Jonas et al., 1976). The type and location of the hospital produce variations in these proportions (Torrens & Yedvab, 1970).

As discussed earlier, some hospitals have developed walk-in units to relieve the emergency services of the burden of the nonurgent patients and to respond to the competition from freestanding walk-in services or urgi-centers. With the organization of group practices in the outpatient clinics some hospitals have also provided "add-on" slots in the appointment schedule to accommodate the non-urgent patient demanding urgent attention. Financial incentives are forcing hospitals to make every effort to reduce the costly care of nonurgent patients in the emergency setting. These efforts include evening and weekend hours for walk-in units and after-hours telephone access for clinic patients. One study, however, found no difference in emergency service visits or hospitalizations between a group of patients randomized to telephone access to physicians, who in turn had access to computerized medical records, and control patients (Darnell et al., 1985).

Managed systems of care often require subscribers to get prior approval before authorizing emergency services, and unauthorized use may not be covered. As the role of provider and insurer become commingled, it is easier to design (and enforce use of) more efficient and less expensive methods of providing nonurgent care. Published studies are not yet available reporting the effectiveness and safety of these interventions designed to contain costs.

Staffing for Hospital-based Emergency Services. Dramatic changes in the staffing of emergency rooms have occurred in the past two decades. Teaching hospitals once relied almost exclusively on junior house officers (interns and assistant residents) to staff their emergency services with backup supervision by more senior house officers or staff members. Nonteaching hospitals either had physicians with staff privileges cover the emergency services in rotation or relied on "moonlighters" from residency programs of nearby teaching hospitals. Many teaching hospitals have now developed or are beginning to develop residency programs in Emergency Medicine, run by full-time board-certified emergency medicine specialists interested in academic careers. New York City hospitals find these programs particularly useful. Whereas residency programs in Internal Medicine in the city have declined in popularity with graduates of American medical schools, the Emergency Medicine programs have flourished. The New York Medical College recently established an academic department of Emergency Medicine, as has the University of Rochester. While most medical schools continue to resist such moves, the trend is likely to continue. Frictions also continue to exist between emergency departments and the other departments that previously dominated hospital emergency services. Most of this friction involves disagreements over who is best able to perform certain procedures, such as endotracheal intubation, pelvic ultrasound, or reductions of dislocated shoulders, and who has the right to admit the patient to a particular service, the Emergency Medicine attending or the attending on that service.

The nonteaching hospitals have also shifted to full-time emergency medicine specialists, frequently contracting with a physician group serving several hospitals in the area (Gersonde, 1971; Hannas, 1971). The hospitals that contract for coverage from an emergency medicine group are willing to pay a premium in return for reliable staffing.

Changes in organization and staffing are linked with efforts to classify the levels of emergency services provided (American College of Emergency Physicians, 1975; Harvey, 1984). Hospitals now compete for classification as comprehensive or designation as a regional trauma center to assure the flow of patients with a higher chance of requiring admission to the inpatient service after being stabilized in the emergency department.

Freestanding Emergi-centers and Urgi-centers

First established in Delaware and Rhode Island in 1973, freestanding ambulatory care facilities providing emergency services and urgent care for nonurgent patients now operate throughout the United States. Some, such as the emergi-center, have the same 24-hours-a-day, 7-days-a-week access that hospital emergency services provide. Others, so-called urgi-centers or "Doc in the Box," provide less comprehensive emergency services and are commonly open 12 hours a day, 7 days a week. These centers do not serve truly emergent patients, and most do not receive ambulance cases.

Two groups of patients find these centers attractive: those seeking the convenience and access of emergency services without the delays and other forms of negative feedback associated with using hospital services for nonurgent problems and those whose insurance treats emergi-centers preferentially compared with physicians' offices (Chesteen et al., 1986). Both hospitals and private practitioners feel the competitive pressures from these new centers. Hospitals have responded by sponsoring or buying emergi-centers and urgi-centers, and physicians have formed them. Several thousand of these facilities now exist. Precise data, however, are not available. There is no clear definition for the spectrum of services provided by an emergi-center. It can range from a group practice that has simply expanded hours and eased access for walk-in patients to hospitals with satellite services that are geographically separate but organizationally and administratively far from freestanding.

The National Health Interview Survey (USDHHS, 1991) does not report separately the use of emergi-centers. In 1990, an estimated 40.1% of physician contacts occurred in someplace other than the doctor's office (i.e., other clinics, emergency room or over the telephone) (USDHHS, 1991, Table 76). No data are available for the contacts with nurses, social workers, and other health professionals practicing in ambulatory settings.

As these centers have increased in number and become familiar to more patients, many have evolved to offer a combination of walk-in and appointment services. The appointment services initially provided follow-up for the presenting complaint. They have evolved into more comprehensive routine ambulatory services, especially among the urgi-centers. Many now market their services as having all of the advantages of the personal relationship with a primary care physician plus the convenience of expanded hours and short waiting times. In many geographic areas the chain-sponsored urgi-center is a convenient and economic method for a newly trained primary care physician to enter practice without the expense of acquiring an office and equipment. The flexible hours of employment are attractive to nurses and other health workers.

Other Emergency Medical Services

Emergency medical services extend beyond the hospital emergency department or the freestanding emergi-center to include other services provided to accident victims or individuals suffering acute, life-threatening illnesses such as acute myocardial infarction or stroke. The goals of these services are to preserve life and reduce disability by providing prompt treatment and transportation to comprehensive treatment facilities. The intended recipients of care are patients with emergent or urgent problems.

The emergency prehospital care for these problems requires a functioning emergency medical services system with 15 parts (Hoffer, 1979): provision of labor force, training of personnel, communications, transportation, facilities, critical-care units, use of public-safety agencies, consumer participation, accessibility to care, transfer of patients, standard medical-record keeping, consumer information and education, independent review and evaluation, disaster linkage, and mutual-aid agreements. A principal goal has been to provide for the whole nation a set of coordinated emergency care dispatch centers, using the uniform emergency telephone number, 911.

The crucial first step in providing emergency prehospital care is the existence of a high-quality ambulance service to provide first aid on site and during transit to a hospital emergency department (Gibson, 1973). Ambulance services have evolved from their origins as for-profit services set up by funeral directors. No consistent pattern of responsibility for providing ambulance services exists across communities. In many large cities the department of health and hospitals is responsible for either providing the service or contracting with qualified ambulance services for coverage. In smaller communities volunteer fire departments or ambulance services struggle to provide adequate care, and many deficiencies persist.

Death from traumatic injury is the leading cause of death in the United States in years of potential life lost (McGinnis, 1988–1989; Office of Disease Prevention, 1988), emphasizing the need to strengthen all links in the emergency services chain. In 1990, unintentional injuries among the population aged 1 to 64 cost approximately 2.5 million years of life (CDC, 1992). Although improving ambulance services across the country would prevent only a small percentage of this loss, the size of the problem is such that small gains translate into a large number of lives saved (National Conference on Cardio-Pulmonary Resuscitation, 1974).

Ambulance services must have adequate staff and organization to respond quickly to calls, using vehicles appropriately designed and equipped, and then take the patient to the hospital emergency department most appropriate for the patient's problem. A successful intervention depends on a series of functioning communication links between the patient and the ambulance service, between the dispatcher and the ambulance, and between the ambulance and the hospital (Gibson, 1973). Recently, the use of two-way radio and transmission of monitored data such as real-time electrocardiograms and vital signs has improved these links.

Gibson (1977) reviewed the policy issues in the development of emergency medical services that require adequate financing, personnel, equipment, and facilities—with strict standards for each—and the cooperation of professions, agencies, insitutions, and local government units to work together and coordinate their resources. Federal legislation has been important in setting standards and in providing resources for local emergency medical services to achieve these standards. The National Highway Safety Act of 1966 set performance criteria and required the states to submit emergency medical services plans. The Emergency Medical Services System Act of 1973 (P.L. 93-154) authorized $185 million over 3 years to states, counties, and other nonprofit agencies to plan, expand, and modernize their emergency medical services. Additional laws passed in 1976 (P.L. 94-573) and 1979 (P.L. 96-142) extended the act and expanded its scope. The Robert Wood Johnson Foundation helped greatly to develop the national emergency medical services system (R. W. Johnson Foundation, 1977).

P.L. 93-154 had several important requirements: rural areas applying for assistance received special consideration; applications coordinating local systems with statewide systems received preferential treatment; the emergency medical services were to organize "in a manner that provides persons who reside in the system's service area and who have no professional training or financial interest in the provision of health care with an adequate opportunity to participate in the making of policy for the system"; and emergency services were to be provided without prior inquiry as to ability to pay.

The modernization of services included changing the ambulance design from a vehicle patterned after a hearse to a light van with space and equipment to provide cardiopulmonary resuscitation (CPR) by an ambulance attendant while en route to the hospital. Many attendants are now licensed emergency medical technicians, trained to provide life-support services and acute management of trauma. Training requirements for licensure vary from state to state. In 1978 a national standard course of 185 hours was established (National Training Course). Most ambulance personnel have a rating of EMT-A that requires at least 81 hours of training, and many are EMT-Paramedics with more than 1,000 hours of training. With improved equipment and staff training, emergency medical services have increased survival rates for victims of traumatic injuries and acute medical conditions (Hoffer, 1979; Jacobs et al., 1984; Lewis et al., 1979; Montgomery, 1980; Roth et al., 1984; Sherman, 1979).

Other Hospital-Related Ambulatory Services

Competition has stimulated the development of a range of hospital-related ambulatory and other services. Hospitals now operate satellite ambulatory care facilities, nursing homes, health promotion programs, alcohol and drug treatment centers, freestanding ambulatory surgery centers, emergi-centers, urgi-centers, ambulance services, HMOs or IPAs, PPOs, doctors' office buildings, hospital-supply purchasing plans, health care management consultancy, office building management, real estate development, progressive care retirement communities, insurance company management, and hotel/restaurant/resort management (Ermann & Gabel, 1985). A 1985 national survey of hospital chief executive officers asked about plans to expand or add services. Of the top 10 services in the list, 5 are exclusively ambulatory services, and the others each have a significant ambulatory part. They are (with percentages of hospitals planning to add or expand each) home health service (75.6%), in-house outpatient surgery (74%), PPO (62%), wellness and health promotion (57%), outpatient diagnosis (55.2%), HMO (41.1%), cardiac rehabilitation (40.3%), oncology (39.8%), general rehabilitation (37.5%) and substance-abuse control (31.5%) (Moore, 1985).

The freestanding ambulatory surgery center is an important new development. In 1990 more than 8.5 million males and 14.5 million females had surgical procedures in nonfederal short-stay hospitals (USDHHS, 1991, Table 86). Approximately 40% of the procedures could be done in an ambulatory setting (Olson, 1982) without the patient staying overnight in a hospital bed, and each year the shift from inpatient to ambulatory surgery increases. Economic pressures, improved technology, and third-party payers contribute to this change (Berryman, 1987) as the patient base shifts to less costly settings. The acceptance of these changes by patients and surgeons has advanced the growth of outpatient surgery.

The facilities may be either in the hospital—in some instances using space from delicensed inpatient units—or freestanding. In 1983 approximately 370,000 procedures were performed in surgi-centers, and in 1984 there were about 300 such surgi-centers in the United States. Including ambulatory surgery done in hospitals themselves, about 5 million ambulatory procedures, or 24% of all surgical procedures, were done in 1983 (Shannon, 1985). Third-party payers now require that certain procedures be done on an ambulatory basis unless there is documented evidence that it would be unsafe for the patient. Patient satisfaction and quality of care seem to be good, and new centers continue to appear (Goodspeed & Earnhart, 1986). One study found that physician supply and insurance demand were more important than competition among hospitals in the development of ambulatory surgery centers and alternative forms of service delivery (Chirikos & White, 1987). Another found that facility-fee reimbursement is adequate to maintain a high-quality surgical facility if the Accreditation Association for Ambulatory Health Care grants accreditation and Medicare approves licensure (McDonald, 1987).

Freestanding diagnostic imaging centers have experienced a parallel growth in recent years and present an economic challenge to hospitals offering outpatient imaging and radiology services. These new facilities require expensive equipment and must rely on referrals from other physicians to succeed. This creates complex relations among the hospitals, radiologists, referring physicians, and patients ("Meeting the Challenge, 1985"). Ethical, legal, and financial problems emerge when some of the referring physicians have financial interests in the success of the freestanding center. A variant is the hospital radiology department that offers mobile mammography services to the community (Krajewski & Gunn, 1987).

Patient convenience and cost-saving incentives stimulated the development of an outpatient intravenous antibiotic program in Minneapolis (Kind, Williams, & Gibson, 1985). Patients of all ages with bone, joint, skin, soft-tissue, and other infectious diseases, such as meningitis, received successful treatment. No significant morbidity and no mortality occurred, patient compliance was high, and cost savings were large. The necessary elements were an enthusiastic medical staff, a central admixture service in the hospital pharmacy, and a team of nurses for IV cannula care. The AIDS epidemic has prompted similar approaches to comprehensive ambulatory treatment of opportunistic infections and other complications of HIV infection (Pascarelli & Holtzworth, 1987). To support these ambulatory services many hospital pharmacies offer durable medical equipment (Smith & Popielarski, 1986), realizing net income while improving the continuity of patient care offered by the institution.

In 1983 the Health Care Financing Administration (HCFA), the governmental agency responsible for the Medicare system, introduced a prospective payment system (PPS) for inpatient hospitalizations. Prior to that time, hospitals received payment for patients on a cost-plus, per diem basis. The longer the patient stayed in the hospital the more money the hospital received. Under the Medicare PPS system, hospitals now receive a set payment based on a diagnostic-related group category (DRG). The longer the patient stays, the more hospitals incur charges that are not reimbursed. This, plus other factors, has led to decreased lengths of hospital stay, with patients being discharged "quicker and sicker." In addition, in 1989 following a law suit, Medicare rules for home care services were clarified, making it easier for Medicare recipients to receive home health services. This, in turn, has led to a marked increase in Medicare home health care, with expenditures increasing at an average annual rate of 40% between 1988 and 1991, reaching $5.4 billion (Bishop, 1993).

Patients are eligible to receive home health services from a qualified Medicare provider if they are homebound, if they are under the care of a specified physician who will establish a home health plan, and if they need physical or occupational therapy, speech therapy, or intermittent skilled nursing care. Skilled nursing care is defined both as technical procedures, such as tube feedings or catheter care, and as skilled nursing observations. Intermittent is defined as up to 28 hours per week for nursing care, and 35 hours per week for home health aide care. Many hospitals have formed their own home health care agencies, finding this a useful way to increase revenues while enabling them to discharge patients from the hospital earlier. In most communities, however, the bulk of home health services are still provided by not-for-profit agencies, such as the Visiting Nurse Service.

More recently, there has been an effort to integrate home health care with community-based services. There are at least four areas in which integration efforts can be focused: acute and long-term care services; the administration and funding of home and community-based care; formal and informal services; and the integration of categorical (mentally disabled, physically disabled, elderly, developmentally disabled) long-term care programs to become long-term care programs for diverse populations (Stone, 1993). In 1985, HCFA began funding an integrated care model, the Social Health Maintenance Organization (SHMO) in four sites-the Kaiser Permanente HMO in Portland, Oregon; the Seniors Plus HMO in Minneapolis, Minnesota; Elderplan, a community-based organization in Brooklyn, New York; and another community-based organization, SCAN in Long Beach,

California. These SHMOS were organized to utilize Medicare HMO funding and to deliver acute and chronic care services, and to provide prescription medicine and eyeglass benefits, all at no increase in total per member cost. All four sites are now, at a minimum, breaking even (Leutz, 1988). These programs, however, have failed to achieve the goal of a truly integrated health care delivery model. They have not been able to coordinate primary care services with community-based long-term care services. A number of integrated demonstration projects are now going on, including the Program of All-Inclusive Care for the Elderly (PACE), the Medicaid Working Group Project, the Minnesota Long Term-Care Option, and the National Chronic Care Consortium (Stone, 1993).

The number of hospitals that have developed health promotion/disease prevention (HP/DP) programs reflects the national interest in these areas. Growing professional awareness of the importance of preventive services and the positive image such services convey for the hospital account for the popularity of these programs. The American Hospital Association's Center for Health Promotion has been a major stimulus and guide for hospitals in developing HP/DP programs. The center has published several books on program development (Bader et al., 1979; Kernaghan & Giloth, 1983; Longe & Wolfe, 1984), many pamphlets and patient-education materials, and audiovisual programs and audiocassettes. Several commercial companies provide HP/DP services, including some specifically designed for hospital employees.

Hospital-sponsored HP/DP programs have potential for improving the health of the American people. In 1990 those who died before the age of 65 suffered a loss of more than 12.3 million years of life (CDO, 1992). More than 60% of all Americans who die each year do so prematurely (McGinnis, 1988–1989) at a cost in medical care and lost productivity in the hundreds of billions of dollars. Successful application of primary prevention measures (immunizations, proper nutrition, exercise, avoidance of smoking and other substance abuse, use of seat belts and other accident prevention strategies, and moderate use of alcohol) and secondary prevention (screening for early detection and treatment of conditions before they become symptomatic) could postpone an estimated 45% of cardiovascular disease deaths, 23% of cancer deaths, and more than 50% of the disabling complications of diabetes.

The programs described above reflect the range of new ambulatory services developed by hospitals to broaden their patient base and strengthen their financial structure. New or expanded ambulatory services have emerged as dominant factors in marketing strategies (Anwar, 1987; Hellstern, 1987; Mashaw, 1987; Maurer, 1987; Phillips & Reeder, 1987; Stafstrom, 1987). This promises to change fundamentally the role of the hospital in U.S. health care.

Health Department Services

Nowhere in the diversity is the scope and variety of health care services provided in the United States more clear than at the level of the local health department. In most parts of the country the health department is responsible for some ambulatory services. These may range from immunization services only to comprehensive departments of health and hospitals offering the full range of acute and chronic health care services to inpatients, outpatients, schoolchildren, and the homebound. No consistent pattern exists for the allocation of responsibility for ambulatory services to municipal, county, or state governments; to health departments or voluntary agencies; or to private physicians under contract for part of their time versus full-time health department employees.

Typically, the local health departments avoid direct competition with private practitioners by restricting personal health services to those areas in which private physicians have little interest (routine well-baby examinations) or lack expertise (case finding, treatment, and contact investigation for venereal disease and tuberculosis). Where financial circumstances make an area unappealing to private practitioners, local health departments may expand the scope of their services to include ambulatory care of acute and chronic illnesses.

Roemer (1975) estimated that local health departments provided less than 3% of áll ambulatory personal health services in 1975, excluding school health services. About half of local health departments provide school health services in their jurisdictions, and the remainder are about evenly divided between cooperative efforts of the school board and the local health department and the school board alone. School health programs focus on screening for vision and hearing problems, assuring that immunization levels are adequate, and case finding for contagious diseases. Students are referred for diagnosis and treatment. A few jurisdictions have integrated the school health program into the community or neighborhood health centers to provide comprehensive ambulatory services for preschool and school-age children.

The most frequently offered personal health services are well-baby care, tuberculosis and venereal disease control, prenatal and family planning services, adult chronic disease screening programs, mental health services, and home public health nursing and homemaker services. All are *categorical programs*, which care for categories of disease or persons. State or federal matching funds frequently stimulate the creation of these programs.

Efforts over the past 70 years to involve health departments in the delivery of comprehensive health services have usually been unsuccessful (Myers et al., 1968; Rosen, 1971). Some have expressed optimism that this can change to improve services to the poor (Cashman, 1967; Miller & Moos, 1981; Miller et al., 1977; Roemer, 1975). Miller (1985) envisioned local health departments as having major responsibility for the delivery of direct social *and* medical services to the poor. The history of local health departments, with their bureaucratic, categorically oriented administrative structure—plus close involvement with politically sensitive, financially pressed local governments—limits the chances for much progress in this direction (Jonas, 1977, Chapters 5, 7).

For example, in 1993, the *financially* strapped New York City Department of

Health agrced to turn over the administration of its child health clinics to the New York City Health and Hospitals Corporation. HHC has the capacity to bill and collect for services provided and is efficient at doing so. Historically, care in the health departments clinics was free, even for patients with health insurance.

Because of the increasing concerns about environmental pollution—the safety of local water supplies, solid waste disposal—and the challenges of containing the AIDS epidemic, it is not surprising that most local health departments feel no desire to expand their role in providing personal health services.

Neighborhood and Community Health Centers

The contemporary community health center (CHC) represents the surviving heir of the Neighborhood Health Center (NHC) movement of the 1960s and early 1970s. Stimulated by funding from the federal Office of Economic Opportunity (OEO), part of the Johnson administration's "war on poverty," NHCs were set up to provide comprehensive ambulatory and social services to the poor living in inner cities and rural areas of the United States. They represented a new form of disciplinary team health care practice, and community involvement in both policy-making and facility operations (Davis & Schoen, 1978; Zwick, 1974). Although the NHCs never served more than 2 or 3% of the American people, they achieved symbolic importance. They demonstrated health services organized to meet community needs with a combination of clinical, preventive, and social services delivered by teams of professionals and community workers dedicated to the ideals of interdisciplinary practice.

Voluntary hospitals, local health departments, and other nonfederal entities sponsored similar NHCs (Schachter & Elliston, 1977; Stoeckle, Anderson, Page, & Brenner, 1972; Tennant & Day, 1974), although their numbers never matched those funded by OEO. All were influenced by the pioneering programs of the Gouverneur and Montefiore Hospitals (Lloyd & Wise, 1968) in New York City and the Tufts-Columbia Point NHC in Boston. The first medical director at Gouverneur, the late Dr. Howard Brown, brought with him the organizational experience of the Health Insurance Plan of Greater New York (HIP), one of the early prepaid group practices (Light & Brown, 1967), to build a comprehensive ambulatory care program that came to serve as a model for many later NHCs.

Although NHCs varied in size, program content, and methods of funding, they shared certain common features. Those established early usually cared for medically underserved inner-city minority groups. Later efforts by OEO stimulated the formation of rural NHCs, which more often served poor populations of mixed racial composition. The NHCs tried to use physicians, nurses, social workers, and community health workers in multidisciplinary team practice—with varying degrees of enthusiasm and success. The community health workers, hired from the service area, provided basic nursing and social service skills. NHCs pioneered in the training and employment of nurse practitioners and physician assistants. The professional staff members were salaried or paid on a sessional basis. The aim of the NHC was to provide comprehensive ambulatory services—preventive and rehabiltative as well as curative services—that were delivered sensitively and were affordable and of high quality, and to intervene in the cycle of poverty.

The typical NHC budget was large. Start-up costs for facilities and equipment were high, and most of the patients had no insurance. The NHCs usually related to a teaching hospital for inpatient services, specialty consultations, sophisticated laboratory and x-ray services, and supervision—if not the direct employment—of the medical staff.

The authorizing OEO legislation mandated "maximum feasible participation" in the operation and administration of the NHCs and the formation of Community Advisory Boards. The board members usually came from the area served by the NHC and previously served by the teaching hospital that now controlled the OEO grant. These hospitals were regarded with suspicion based on prior responsiveness to community needs. The boards frequently demanded the final word on major policy decisions. Eventually, the federal grants went directly to nonprofit corporations representing the served communities. These bodies, frequently called Community Boards, then contracted with the hospital for needed services. They often hired the professional staff directly.

The OEO view that the provision of job opportunities to service-area residents was at least as important as providing health care created additional tensions. The NHCs usually served minority groups living in extreme poverty who had few of the necessary health care skills and training, particularly in the professional and semiprofessional job categories. Control of the jobs for which the local residents might be eligible became a plum, for both positive and negative reasons.

Evaluation of the NHCs included general program evaluations (Orso, 1979; Resource Management Corporation, 1969), evaluations of quality of care (Morehead, 1970; Morehead & Donaldson, 1974), and cost analyses (Sparer & Anderson, 1975). By most accounts, in the mid-1970s NHCs were providing reasonable-quality care. A General Accounting Office report in 1978 noted that some programs were medically underserved areas with no programs at all, and there were some failures to collect third-party reimbursement (Comptroller General, 1978). The tendency toward expansion of service for the nonpoor may have represented an effort to resolve one of the basic contradictions of the original OEO NHC program. The NHCs' emphasis on the poverty population created a curious dilemma. In trying to develop an organization to enhance the health of the poor, the NHC was perpetuating a separate and distinct system of health care for the poor rather than integrating them into the mainstream of medical care.

At the peak of the original OEO NHC program in the early 1970s, an estimated 200 NHCs existed nationwide ("NENA"). By 1974, under the Nixon effort to dismantle OEO, the number had fallen to about 150 (Roemer, 1981). In the mid-1970s the program was renamed the Community Health Center program, and its scope was narrowed to concentrate on the delivery of medical care with less emphasis on the social roles of the NHC. The CHCs were encouraged to expand their services to the nonpoor (Davis & Schoen, 1978, p. 171). By the early 1980s more than 800 CHCs served more than 4.5 million people (Bureau of Community Health Services, 1979; Freeman et al., 1982; Goldman & Grossman, 1982; Sardell, 1983). The program focused on urban and rural medically underserved populations. Support for the CHCs comes primarily from federal grant funds, third-party reimbursements, and fee-for-service on a sliding scale.

By the end of the Reagan presidency the number of CHCs had declined to 561, although 4.7 million people were still receiving care (D. Smith, personal communication, 1989). The strategy for the CHC program includes the following:

1. Work closely with state governments and medical societies.
2. Serve only high-need areas.
3. Support only well-managed projects.
4. Promote self-sufficiency in projects.
5. Help projects to adapt to changing conditions.

With the severe restrictions on federal funds available for discretionary programs imposed by pressures to reduce the deficit, the future of CHCs is uncertain. If, however, legislation is enacted providing health insurance for the 35 million Americans now lacking coverage (Himmelstein & Woolhandler, 1989), the CHCs have appropriate organization and staff to provide comprehensive ambulatory services.

Physician Supply and Specialty Distribution for Ambulatory Services

Physician supply in the United States continues to grow. In 1950 there were 219,900 active physicians (14.1 per 10,000 population), by 1985 there were 534,400 (22.0 per 10,000 population), and by 1989 there were 577,200 (23.3 per 10,000 population) active physicians. By the year 2000, a projected 721,600 physicians will be in active practice (26.9 per 10,000 population) (USDHHS, 1991 Table 97). Despite the dramatic increase in the number of physicians, geographic maldistribution persists. New England continues to have the highest concentration, with 28.6 physicians per 10,000 population in 1989, followed by the Middle Atlantic states with 27.9 and the Pacific states with 23.3. The East South Central states lag far behind at 16.4 and the rest of the central areas of the country range from 17.5 to 20.3 (USDHHS, 1991, Table 96).

Specialty maldistribution also persists in ambulatory care in the United States. The dramatic post-World War II growth in specialization and biomedical research is responsible for the remarkable gains in understanding basic disease processes and in developing effective treatments for many of them. The price of this progress has been the failure to replenish the nation's supply of primary care practitioners. Recognizing the gravity of this problem, the American Medical Association (AMA) in 1966 appointed the Citizens Commission on Graduate Medical Education, usually referred to as the Millis Commission, to review the graduate education of physicians (Millis, 1966). The commission noted that since the Flexner Report a "process of specialization and consequent fragmentation has occurred so that responsibility is diffused and authority divided" [p. vi]. The AMA took the position that the profession should discipline itself in establishing standards of practice and education to improve the balance between general and specialized postgraduate education. Citing the needs of the American people for ambulatory services that offer a balanced array of general and specialty services, the report stated that "medical schools and teaching hospitals should prepare many more physicians than now exist who will have the desire and the qualifications to render comprehensive, continuing health services, including preventive measures, early diagnosis, rehabilitation, and supportive therapy, as well as the diagnosis and treatment of acute and episodic disease states" [p. 30]. The revolutionary changes in medical education needed to produce many more generalists did not, of course, take place.

Two decades later the Association of American Medical Colleges panel on the General Professional Education of the Physician presented its report, "Physicians for the Twenty-First Century," better known as the GPEP Report, describing the same problems of specialty maldistribution that had troubled the Millis Commission (Muller, 1984). The GPEP Report noted that any reform effort must accommodate the following pressures acting on the medical profession in the 1980s:

1. Rapid advances in biomedical knowledge and technology will continue.
2. Chemical, mechanical, and electronic technologies available for prevention and treatment of disease will become ever more complex, powerful, effective, and potentially dangerous.
3. Medical practice using these technologies will require an even higher degree of specialization.
4. There will be an increasing recognition that many factors that determine health and illness are not directly influenced by interventions of the health-care system but are the consequences of life-style, environmental factors, and poverty.
5. Patients will increasingly need and demand advice and counsel from physicians and other health care professionals about how to use special medicinal services to improve personal health.
6. The principal providers of medical service in the near future are likely to be physicians employed by large corporations or by health service organizations covering specific population groups.
7. The environment of medical education will be heavily influenced by the agencies that pay for medical services and that will shape the nature of these

services. In a time of concern for containing medical costs, medical and financial incentives will be less and less congruent, complicating and intensifying ethical dilemmas in medicine (Muller, 1984).

How the profession responds to these pressures will profoundly influence the organization and delivery of ambulatory care. This is especially true in the private sector, where the laws of supply and demand for specific services are less modulated by administrative planning than they are in organized settings. The past inertia of the medical education establishment and the nurturing and conservation of professional values conspire to resist the kind of changes called for by the Millis Commission and the GPEP Report (Jonas, 1978). Modern treatment successes have built on the growth of biomedical research and the training of specialists, clinical investigators, and basic researchers since World War II. During this same period the ranks of the primary care physicians in private practice thinned drastically. They reached a nadir about 1975, when only 16% of nonfederal physicians providing patient care in the United States described themselves as general or family practitioners (USDHHS, 1986, Table 73).

In 1975 there were 28,070 internists (9.8% of clinically active physicians) and 12,559 pediatricians (4.4% of active physicians). Even if all were functioning as primary care physicians—in fact, most of the internists practiced as consultants in 1975—only 30% of U.S. physicians were in primary care specialties. Experience with the National Health Service in the United Kingdom and with the Kaiser-Permanente Health Plan had already shown that a proper mix for an industrialized country was 50 to 60% primary care and 40 to 50% specialty and subspecialty practitioners.

Policymakers in the 1960s interpreted the growing shortage of primary care physicians as a shortage of all physicians. New medical schools were built and existing ones expanded in response to capitation payments from the federal government (Hatch, 1986). The total number of professionally active physicians increased from 340,280 in 1975 to 536,755 in 1989. In 1989, however, the proportion of primary care specialists (general and family practice physicians) remained just under 12%. The overall growth in physician supply produced an actual decline in the proportion of family and general practitioners from 14% to 11% as newly trained generalists did not keep pace with losses from death and retirement. Rural areas were particularly hard hit as aging generalists died or retired and no primary care practitioners replaced them. With recent improvements in physician supply, rural residents are making more use of health services (Krishan et al., 1985).

Despite the dramatic increase in the number of residency programs in family medicine that occurred after establishing this new specialty in 1969, the ranks of general and family practitioners increased only modestly from 46,347 in 1975 to 56,318 in 1989. Much faster growth rates for internal medicine and pediatrics almost doubled the total numbers in these disciplines while producing proportional gains of 8% to 11% and 4% to 5%, respectively (USDHHS, 1991, Table 97). Nonetheless, the Graduate Medical Education National Advisory Committee (GMENAC) projected continued specialty maldistribution into the 1990s, with excessive numbers of subspecialists and barely adequate numbers of primary care physicians (Report of GMENAC). The GMENAC used a needs-based requirement approach rather than an economic demand-based model. Weiner et al. (1987), using data from more than 10,000 children in three large HMOs, tested the validity of GMENAC for pediatrics. Delphi panels of pediatricians in the same sites provided normative data. If the HMO data rather than GMENAC's ideal projections were used, fewer pediatricians would be needed. Increased rates of delegation of pediatric care to nonphysicians (nurse-clinicians and physician assistants) in the HMOs made the Delphi panel projections still lower. There are some signs that the United States may have already moved from a position of physician shortage to one of patient shortage (Iglehart, 1988).

In 1974 the Robert Wood Johnson Foundation started a program to encourage academic medical centers to develop primary care training programs in internal medicine and pediatrics (Lawrence et al., 1977). The Department of Health and Human Services funded a few pilot programs at the same time. In 1976 Congress passed Pulbic Law 94-484, authorizing funding for postgraduate training in the three primary care disciplines: family medicine, internal medicine, and pediatrics. Guidelines for the new programs funded by the federal government required a minimum of 25% of training in ambulatory settings providing continuity of care.

For the first time educators made a concerted effort to plan the curriculum for the knowledge base of ambulatory care on the descriptive epidemiology of presenting problems. The planners hoped to avoid the problem described by Hodgkin (1966) in England: "A study of general practitioners . . . shows an inverse correlation between the frequency of disease and the emphasis given to instruction about diseases during medical training." The new training programs tried to capture the reality of the world of practice and prepare their trainees for satisfying and effective roles in ambulatory care. The emphasis was on learning how to manage "common problems uncommonly well" (Hatem, Lawrence, & Arky, 1978).

Rosenblatt et al. (1983), in their study of the content of ambulatory care, found that 50% of office visits to private doctors in the United States involved only 15 diagnostic clusters. For primary care internists and family practitioners only 11 diagnostic clusters accounted for 50% of visits. Some of these diagnostic clusters include conditions infrequently seen on the inpatient service of the typical teaching hospital. With family practice programs having pioneered a new and more balanced approach to ambulatory training, internal medicine and pediatrics programs incorporated more orthopedics, dermatology, office gynecology, and psychiatry in their curricula. The mismatch between training and practice finally began to disappear. The more rigorous 3-year residency training in family medicine that had replaced the 1-year rotating internship addressed lingering concerns about the competence of the general practitioner.

The changes taking place in hospital care reinforced the new interest in teaching students and house officers in ambulatory settings. Shorter lengths of stay under the DRG (diagnostic related groups) system of reimbursement and changes in case mix among hospitalized patients brought about by new technologies and day surgery programs have worked to reinforce the value of training in ambulatory settings (Perkoff, 1986). Other reasons for renewed interest in ambulatory training are the growing need for well-trained primary care physicians by organized medical groups and the increasing expectation among patients that their care will be more personal than it has been in the past. Paradoxically, some of the very organizations that need more primary care physicians are having a profound effect on the academic medical centers that train such physicians. Driven by strategies of cost containment, HMOs and similar provider systems both limit lengths of stay in hospital and restrict referrals to their own specialists, often at the expense of medical center faculty and specialty clinics (Vanselow & Kralewski, 1986).

A survey of all HMOs in the United States in 1986 (with a 44% response rate) showed a desire for the curricula of medical schools and residency programs to emphasize four topics:

1. Cost-effective use of diagnostic and treatment services.
2. Utilization review and quality assurance.
3. The role of the primary care "gate-keeper."
4. The financing of health services (Jacobs & Mott, 1987).

The HMOs identified the most important criteria for selecting physicians as board eligibility, motivation, bedside manner, ability to function as part of a team, adaptability to a changing health care environment, training in a U.S. medical school, ability to relate to nonphysician staff members, and the reputation of the residency program in which the physician trained.

Including cost-effective use of diagnostic services in the curriculum addresses but one determinant of physician behavior. Epstein and McNeil (1985) reviewed physician characteristics and organizational factors that influenced the use of ambulatory tests. They found that specialty training, more recent physician graduation, and large group practice settings correlate with significantly higher test use. Data about other physician characteristics and organizational factors remain equivocal.

The United States is unique among industrialized countries in having no one dominant form of primary care practitioner. Excluded by the definitions used in P.L. 94-484, obstetrician-gynecologists continue to provide large amounts of primary care to their female patients. The AMA includes obstetricians in its definition of primary care physicians.

Despite the claims of organized internal medicine as addressing the primary care manpower needs of the country, most internists continue to function as subspecialists (Steinberg & Lawrence, 1980). The landmark studies by Mendenhall et al. (1978, Mendenhall, 1979) documented the phenomenon of "principal care." Subspecialists, such as those in nephrology or oncology, restrict their practices to patients having diseases in their subspecialty domain while accepting responsibility for management of most of the primary care needs of those patients (Mendenhall). Similarly, many surgeons function as part-time generalists when there is not enough demand for their surgical skills. They have neither the proper training nor, in many cases, the temperament to function effectively in this role.

Debate continues among those who favor the family practitioner model, those who favor separate care for adults and children by internists and pedicians, and those who favor family-oriented care provided by internist-pediatrician teams (Hudson & Nourse, 1975; McWhinney, 1975; Perkoff, 1978; Petersdorf, 1975). Academic units in family medicine have prospered in state-supported medical schools, but private universities have been inhospitable to the new specialty, preferring instead to develop primary care internal medicine and general pediatrics programs. Patients have accepted family practitioners well, especially in rural areas and physician-shortage areas.

Efforts to create a common primary care discipline have been sporadic and thus far unsuccessful. This is so despite the logic of shared goals, scarce resources for medical education, and a common desire for reform of reimbursement policies to establish parity between "cognitive" services provided by primary care physicians and "procedural" services delivered by specialists. The Primary Care Initiative at Brown University has established a pilot program of a common first year of postgraduate training for family practitioners, internists, and pediatricians, followed by disciplinary training in a shared ambulatory setting (D. S. Greer, personal communication, 1989). With growing signs of a physician surplus in the United States, it is hard to predict whether increasing competition for patients will encourage or discourage efforts to train a prototypical primary care physician.

Bertakis and Robbins (1987) studied patients randomly assigned to the care of family practice residents or primary care internal medicine residents in a teaching hospital ambulatory care setting. After 2 years, patients randomized to the internal medicine practice had a significantly higher frequency of visits to the primary care clinic, emergency room, and acute-care clinic and broken appointments. Internal medicine patients also had a significantly higher number of visits to all non-primary care clinics, especially dermatology, obstetrics-gynecology, and general surgery. Whether these differences in practice styles reflect basic characteristics of those trainees attracted to one form of primary care over another or the attitudes and behaviors of the supervising faculty was indeterminate.

Brook et al. (1987) evaluated 15 group practices in general internal medicine located in university hospitals and used data on the quality of residency education provided, access to and quality of care, and patients' satisfaction with that care to predict changes in ambulatory care programs. One-third of the patient population had no health insurance, the patients had twice the chronic illness rate of the general population, and 40% of the patients remained with the practice at least 2 years. Residents worked in the practice an average of 4 hours per week; few faculty members practiced more than 14 hours per week in the setting. Patient satisfaction was greater than in the general population despite waiting times that were regarded as excessive. Only 10% of eligible patients received an annual influenza vaccination. Most distressing was the finding that the residents did not value their educational experience in the practice.

There is a growing consensus that in order to hold down costs of medical care and to provide more coordinated and comprehensive care, the ratio of practicing generalist physicians to specialist physicians must increase markedly, from 30:70 to 50:50. Among the groups supporting this are the American Medical Association, the Accreditation Council on Graduate Medical Education, the National Governors Council, and the National Council of State Legislatures. The number of physicians in the United States, about 255 nonfederal physicians per 100,000 population, is about what it is in other economically developed countries. The difference is in what they do; in other developed countries generalists make up 50 to 70% of practicing physicians while in the United States they number 29%. That percentage is unlikely to change easily: only 15% of the medical school graduating classes in 1991 and 1992 planned generalist careers (Schroeder, 1993). As this chapter is being written, the Clinton administration has sent to the Congress a blueprint for a major change in the delivery of health care in the United States. This blueprint calls for, among many other things, a change in the distribution and number of graduate medical training positions. In the end the total number of entry level residency positions will likely decrease from about 22,000 to 17,000–18,000, with the percentage of generalists trained rising to 50–55%.

How the percentage of practicing generalists will increase is unknown. Changing the generalist to specialist ratio to 50% of newly trained physicians by 1995 would still not produce the required number of generalists until the year 2040. Market forces may play a significant role as the number of individuals participating in managed care plans increases. The percentage of generalists in those plans is 50 to 60%. Simple arithmetic shows that, in many parts of the country, this will cause an oversupply of specialists. One of the side benefits may be the movement of specialists to areas of the country where shortages of specialists exist. Some specialists may have to restrain, and become generalists, or worse, will start practicing primary care without appropriate retraining.

Another unknown is the future magnitude of the role nurse practitioners (NPs) and physician assistants (PAs) will have in the delivery of primary care ambulatory services. There are an estimated 24,000 PAs and 56,000 NPs, with about 55 to 60% practicing primary care (Fowkes, 1993). NPs and PAs can substitute for an estimated 60 to 70% of the primary care functions physicians now provide (Brown et al., 1992; Schaftt, 1987). NPs in primary care roles, when compared to physicians, have a lower average cost per visit, spend 50% more time with patients, see as many total patients, and score better on patient compliance and patient satisfaction measures. Their patients also have fewer hospitalizations (Brown et al.,

1992). A study from the Kaiser Permanente Northwest Region, a large HMO located in Portland, Oregon, had similar findings for their NPs and PAs (Hooker, 1993). When compared to physicians, they saw similar numbers of patients per hour, prescribed less medication, and had similar patient satisfaction and dissatisfaction rates.

As the "brave new world" of health care tries to control costs and maintain or improve quality, and as the federal government changes its policies on graduate medical education, it is likely that NPs and PAs will have an expanding role in providing primary care services. It is impossible to predict at this time the success that market forces, medical schools, residency training programs, and retraining programs for specialist physicians will have in increasing the percentage of practicing generalist physicians. It is clear, however, that the makers of health policy in the United States are demanding that the costs of health care be reduced. It is also clear that they see increasing the ratio of generalist to specialist providers as an important mechanism for controlling those costs. It is even possible that physicians will choose not to remain the major provider of primary care services, and allow that role to be taken over by nurse practitioners and physician assistants.

Conclusions

The health care system in the United States contains several paradoxes. We stand at the forefront of biomedical technology and are admired and emulated the world over for the sophistication of our specialty care, while millions of our citizens are denied access to these services by financial and social barriers. Our medical education institutions are preeminent yet seem unable to respond to the recommendations of the Millis Commission and GPEP for fundamental reform of their curricula. Specialty and geographic maldistribution persist despite two decades of federal and philanthropic efforts to stimulate programs in primary care service and education.

Ambulatory care is central to the resolution of these paradoxes. We need to pay more attention to the content of ambulatory services, to the potential for integration of preventive services with clinical care, and to the numbers and types of personnel needed to deliver these services to a population that is experiencing an unprecedented demographic shift. Failure to develop more effective, comprehensive ambulatory services by the end of this century will exact a heavy price in overburdened inpatient services filled with sick, elderly patients while younger adults die prematurely of preventable conditions.

References

Abramowitz, K. "Hospital Role on Decline." *Physician Executive 12*(1), 2, 1986.
Adams, G. "Urban Hospital's Innovations Save Money, Win Support." *Health Progress*, 69(1), 56–58, 62, 1988.

American College of Emergency Physicians, "Categorization of Emergency Services" (policy statement). *Annals of Emergency Medicine, 13*, 546, 1984.

American Hospital Association, *Hospital Statistics*. Chicago: AHA 1992–93.

Anwar, R. H., "Marketing the Ambulatory Care Physician." *Ambulatory Care, 7*(7), 29, 1987.

Bader, B., et al., *Planning Hospital Health Promotion Services for Business and Industry*. Chicago: American Hospital Publishing, 1979.

Barnett, G. O., "The Application of Computer based Medical Record Systems in Ambulatory Practice." *New England Journal of Medicine, 310*(25), 1643, 1984.

Berryman, J. M., "Development and Organization of Outpatient Surgery Units: The Hospital's Perspective." *Urologic Clinics of North America, 14*(1), 1, 1987.

Bertakis, K. D., & Robbins, J. A., "Gatekeeping in Primary Care: A Comparison of Internal Medicine and Family Practice." *Journal of Family Practice, 24*, 305, 1987.

Billings, J., & Hasselblad, V., Blueprint, United Hospital Fund, New York, New York, Fall, 1990.

Bishop, C., & Skwara, K. C., Recent Growth of Medicare Home Health, *Health Affairs*, 12:95–107, 1993.

Brook, R. H., Fink, A., Kosecoff, J., Linn, L. S., et al., "Educating Physicians and Treating Patients in the Ambulatory Setting. Where Are We Going and How Will We Know When We Arrive?" *Annals of Internal Medicine, 107*, 392, 1987.

Brooks, E. F., & Johnson, S. L., "Nurse Practitioner and Physician Assistant Satellite Health Centers: The Pending Demise of an Organizational Form?" *Medical Care, 24*(10), 881, 1986.

Brown, S. A., & Grimes, D. E., *Nurse Practitioners and Certified Midwives: A Meta-Analysis of Nurses in Primary Care Roles*, Washington, D. C., American Nurses Association, 1993.

Bureau of Community Health Services. *Community Health Centers*. Rockville, MD: U.S. Department of Health, Education and Welfare, 1979.

Cashman, I., *What Thirteen Local Health Departments Are Doing in Medical Care*. Washington, DC: Public Health Service, 1967.

Centers for Disease Control, *1992 Fact Book*, 1992.

Chesteen, S. A., Warren, S. E., & Woolley, F. R., "A Comparison of Family Practice Clinics and Free-standing Emergency Centers: Organization Characteristics, Process of Care, and Patient Satisfaction." *Journal of Family Practice, 23*(4), 377, 1986.

Chirikos, T. N., & White, S. L., "Competition in Health Care Markets and the Development of Alternative Forms of Service Delivery." *Health Policy, 8*(3), 325, 1987.

Cohen, D. I., Breslau, D., Porter, D. K., Goldberg, H. I., et al., "The Cost Implications of Academic Group Practice. A randomized Controlled Trial." *New England Journal of Medicine, 314*(24), 1553, 1986.

Comptroller General. *Are Neighborhood Health Centers Providing Services Efficiently and to the Most Needy?* (Pub. No. HRD-77-124). Washington, DC: General Accounting Office, 1978.

Daily, M.C., "Women's Primary Care Clinics: Addressing the Women's Market. "*Group Practice Journal, 35*(4), 22, 1986.

Darnell, J. C., Hiner, S. L., Neill, P. J., Mamlin, J. J., et al., "After-hours Telephone Access to Physicians with Access to Computerized Medical Records: Experience an Inner-City General Medicine Clinic." *Medical Care, 23*(1), 20, 1985.

Davis, K., & Schoen, C., *Health and the War on Poverty: A Ten Year Appraisal.* Washington, DC: Brookings Institution, 1978.

Dutton D. B., "Patterns of Ambulatory Health Care in Five Different Delivery Systems." *Medical Care,* 17, 221, 1979.

Epstein, A. M., & McNeil, B. J., "Physician Characteristics and Organizational Factors Influencing Use of Ambulatory Tests." *Medical Decision Making,* 5(4), 401, 1985.

Ermann, D., & Gabel, J., "The Changing Face of American Health Care: Multihospital Systems, Emergency Centers, and Surgery Centers." *Medical Care,* 23, 401, 1985.

Ervin, S. L., Showe, B. L., & Mehta, S., "Social HMOs and Employers: A Budding Relationship for Retiree Health Care." *Health Cost Management,* 4(4), 11, 1987.

Foreman, S., *Social Responsibility and the Academic Medical Center: Building Community-Based Systems for the Nation's Health,* Chairman's Address, Association of American Medical Colleges, Washington, DC, November 8, 1993.

Fowkes, V., Meeting and the Needs of the Underserved: The Roles of Physician Assistants and Nurse Practitioners, in *The Roles of Physician Assistants and Nurse Practitioners in Primary Care,* Eds., Clawson, D. K., Osterweis, M., Association of Academic Health Centers, Washington, DC, 1993.

Freeman, H. E. et al., "Community Health Centers: An Initiative of Enduring Utility." *Health and Society,* 60, 245, 1982.

Freymann, J.G., *The American Health Care System: Its Genesis and Trajectory.* New York: Medcom Press, 1974.

Gersonde, R. J., "Two Approaches to Providing Physicial Coverage in E.R." *Hospital Topics,* 49, 50, 1971.

Gibson, G., "Evaluative Criteria for Emergency Ambulance Services." *Social Sciences and Medicine,* 7, 425, 1973.

Gibson, G., "Emergency Medical Services." *Proceedings of the Academy of Political Sciences,* 32, 121, 1977.

Giglio, R. J., & Papazian, B., "Acceptance and Use of Patient-carried Health Records." *Journal of the American Medical Record Association,* 58(5), 32, 1987.

Goldberg, H. I., Cohen, D. I., Hershey, C. O., Hsiue, I. L., et al. "A Randomized Controlled Trial of Academic Group Practice: Improving the Operation of the Medicine Clinic." *Journal of the American Medical Association,* 257(15), 2051, 1987.

Goldman, F., & Grossman, M., *The Production and Cost of Ambulatory Medical Care in Community Health Centers.* Cambridge, MA: National Bureau of Economic Research, 1982. (Working paper No. 907)

Goodspeed, S. W., & Earnhart, S. W., "Planning, Developing, and Implementing a Freestanding Ambulatory Surgery Center." *Health Care Strategic Management,* 4(2), 18, 1986.

Goulet, C. R., "Blue Cross/Blue Shield Alternate Delivery System." *Health Matrix,* 4(4), 7, 1987.

Greenberg, J. N., Leutz, W. N., & Abrahams, R., "The National Social Health Maintenance Organization Demonstration." *Journal of Ambulatory Care Management,* 8(4), 32, 1985.

Gruber, L. R., Shadle, M., & Polich, C. L., "From Movement to Industry: The Growth of HMOs." *Health Affairs,* Summer 1988, p. 198.

Hannas, R. R., "Emergency Medicine—a Survey." *Southern Medical Bulletin,* December 1971, p. 11

Harrell, G. D., & Fors, M. F., "Marketing Ambulatory Care to Women: A Segmentation Approach." *Journal of Health Care Marketing, 5*(2), 19, 1985.

Harrington, C., & Newcomer, R. J., "Social/Health Maintenance Organizations: New Policy Options for the Aged, Blind, and Disabled." *Journal of Public Health Policy, 6*(2), 204, 1985

Harvey, J. C., "The Emergency Medical Services Systems Act of 1973." *New England Journal of Medicine, 292,* 529, 1975.

Hatch, T. D., "Health Human Resources in the United States of America." *Education Medica y Salad, 20*(3), 388, 1986

Hatem, C. J., Lawrence, R. S., & Arky, R. A., *A Curriculum for the General Education, and Training of Physicians in Primary Care Medicine.* Hartford, CT: National Fund for Medical Education, 1978.

Hellstern, R. A., "The Future of the ACC Industry and NAFAC (National Association for Ambulatory Care)." *Ambulatory Care, 7*(2), 18, 1987.

Heyssel, R. M., *The Academic Medical Center: Old Responsibilities and New Realities,* The Richard and Hilda Rosenthal Lectures at the Institute of Medicine, April, 1990.

Himmelstein, D. U., & Woolhandler, S., "A National Health Program for the United States." *New England Journal of Medicine, 320,* 102, 1989.

Hodgkin, K., *Towards Earlier Diagnosis.* Edinburgh: Livingstone, 1966.

Hoffer, E. P., "Emergency Medical Services, 1979." *New England Journal of Medicine, 301,* 1118, 1979.

Hooker, R. S., The Roles of Physician Assistants and Nurse Practitioners in a Managed Care Organization, in *The Roles of Physician Assistants and Nurse Practitioners in Primary Care,* Eds. Clawson, D. K., Osterweis, M., Association of Academic Health Care Centers, Washington, DC, 1993.

Hudson, J. L., & Nourse, E. S. "Perspectives in Primary Care Education, Part 2." *Journal of Medical Education, 50,* 23, 1975.

Iglehart, J. K., "From Physician Shortage to Patient Shortage: The Uncertain Future of Medical Practice." *Health Affairs (Millwood), 5*(3), 142, 1988.

Jacobs, I. M. et al., "Prehospital Advanced Life Support: Benefits in Trauma," *Journal of Trauma, 24,* 8, 1984.

Jacobs, M. O., & Mott, P. D., "Physician Characteristics and Training Emphasis Considered Desirable by Leaders of HMOs." *Journal of Medical Education, 62,* 725, 1987.

Jonas, S., "Some Thoughts on Primary Care: Problems in Implementation." *International Journal of Health Services, 3,* 177, 1973.

Jonas, S., *Quality Control of Ambulatory Care: A Task for Health Departments.* New York: Springer, 1977.

Jonas, S., *Medical Mystery: The Training of Doctors in the United States.* New York. W. W. Norton, 1978.

Jonas, S. et al., "Monitoring Utilization of a Municipal Hospital Emergency Department." *Hospital Topics, 54,* 43, 1976.

Kernaghan, S., & Giloth, B. E., *Working with Physicians in Health Promotion.* Chicago: American Hospital Publishing, 1983.

Kessler, M. S., & Wilson, K. C., "Emergency Department Key Factor in Hospital Admissions." *Hospitals,* Dec. 16, 1978, p. 87.

Kind, A. C., Williams, D. N., & Gibson, J., "Outpatient Intravenous Antibiotic Therapy: Ten Years' Experience." *Postgraduate Medicine, 77*(2), 105, 1985.

Koster, A., Waterstraat, F. L., Jr., & Sondak, N., "Automated and Ambulatory Record Systems: A Comparative Cost Analysis." *Journal of the American Medical Record Assocation, 58*(11), 26, 1987.

Krajewski, D., & Gunn, S., "Mobile Mammography Project." *Radiography, 53*, 69, 1987.

Krishan, I., Drummond, D. C., Naessens, J. M., Nobrega, F. T., & Smoldt, R. K., "Impact of Increased Physician Supply on Use of Health Services: A Longitudinal Analysis in Rural Minnesota." *Public Health Reports, 100*(4), 379, 1985.

Lawrence, R. S., "Harvard Primary Care Program." Paper presented at the First Conference on Primary Care Delivery, Education and Research in Teaching Hospitals, September 28–30, 1977. *Journal of Ambulatory Care Management, 2*, 55, 1979.

Lawrence, R. S., DeFriese, G. H., Putnam, S. M., Pickard, C. G., Cyr, A. G., & Whiteside, S. W., "Physician Receptivity to Nurse Practitioners: A Study of the Correlates of the Delegation of Clinical Responsibility." *Medical Care, 15*, 289, 1977.

Leutz, W., Abrahams, R., Greenlick, M., Kane, R., & Prottas, J., "Targeting Expanded Care for the Aged: Early SHMO Experience." *Gerontologist, 28*(1), 4, 1988.

Lewis, R. P. et al., "Effectiveness of Advanced Paramedics in a Mobile Coronary Care System." *Journal of the American Medical Association, 241*, 1902, 1979.

Light, H. L., & Brown, H. J., "The Gouveneur Health Services Program: An Historical View." *Milbank Memorial Fund Quarterly, 45*, 375, 1967.

Madison, D. L. "The Case for Community Oriented Primary Care." *Journal of the American Medical Association, 249*, 1279, 1983.

Mak, H. K., "Hospital Outpatient Medical Summary." Medical Records and Health Care *Information Journal 28*(1), 10, 1987.

Mashaw, R., "Marketing, Media and medicine: Competing for ACC Patients." *Ambulatory Care, 7*(7), 31, 1987.

Maurer, M. P., "Marketing Planning for Ambulatory Care: Twelve Key Steps." *Journal of Ambulatory Care Marketing, 1*(1), 3, 1987.

MacLeod, G. K., An Overview of Managed Health Care, *The Managed Health Care Handbook*, Gaithersburg, MD, Aspen Publishers, 1993.

McDonald, H. P., Jr., "Office Ambulatory Surgery in Urology. *Urology Clinics of North America, 14*(1), 27, 1987.

McGinnis, J. M., "National Priorities in Disease Prevention." *Issues in Science and Technology*, Winter 1988–89, p. 48

McManis, G. L., & Hopkins, M., "Managed Care Plans: CFOs weigh the Benefits." *Healthcare Financial Management, 41*(5), 52–54, 58, 1987.

McWhinney, L. R., "Family Medicine in Perspective." *New England Journal of Medicine, 293*, 175, 1975.

Mechanic, D., "Cost Containment and the Quality of Medical Care: Rationing Strategies in an Era of Constrained Resources." *Milbank Memorial Fund Quarterly: Health and Society, 63*(3), 453, 1985.

"Meeting the Challenge of Freestanding Imaging Centers: Options for Hospitals and Hospital-based Radiologists." *Journal of Health Care Technology, 1*(4), 257, 1985.

Mendenhall, R. C., "A National Study of Medical and Surgical Specialties. Part 3. An Empirical Approach to the Classification of Patient Care." *Journal of the American Medical Association, 241*, 2180, 1979.

Mendenhall, R. C., et al., "A National Study of Medical and Surgical Specialties: Part 1.

Background, Purpose and Methodology." *Journal of the American Medical Association, 240,* 848, 1978.

Merz, M., "Preferred Provider Organizations: The New Health Care Partnerships." *Hospital and Health Services Administration 31*(6), 32, 1986.

Miller, C. A., "An Agenda for Public Health Departments." *Journal of Public Health Policy, 6,* 158, 1985.

Miller, C. A., & Moos, M. K., *Local Health Departments: Fifteen Case Studies.* Washington, DC: American Public Health Association, 1981.

Miller, C. A. et al., "A Survey of Local Public Health Departments and Their Directors." *American Journal of Public Health, 67,* 931, 1977.

Millis, J. S., "The Graduate Education of Physicians. Report of the Citizens Commission on Graduate Medical Education." Chicago: American Medical Association, 1966.

Moore, W. B., "CLO's Plan to Expand Home Health Outpatient Services." *Hospitals,* January 1, 1985, p. 74.

Montgomery, B. J., "Emergency Medical Services a New Phase of Development." *Journal of the American Medical Association, 243,* 1017, 1980.

Morbidity and Mortality Weekly Report. 37(20), 319, 1988.

Morehead, M. A., "Evaluating Quality of Care in the Neighborhood Health Center Program of QEO." *Medical Care, 2,* 118, 1970.

Morehead, M. A., & Donaldson, R., "Quality of Clinical Management of Disease in Comprehensive-Neighborhood Health Centers." *Medical Care, 12,* 301, 1074.

Mullan, F., "Community-Oriented Primary Care." *New England Journal of Medicine, 310,* 193, 1984.

Mullan, F., & Conner, E., (Eds.). *Community Oriented Primary Care—Conference Proceedings.* Washington, DC: National Academy Press, 1982.

Muller, S., "Physicians for the Twenty-first Century: Report of the Panel on the General Professional Education of the Physician and College Preparation for Medicine." Washington, DC: Association of American Medical Colleges, 1984.

Myers, B. A. et al., "The Medical Care Activities of Local Health Units." *Public Health Reports, 83,* 757, 1968.

National Conference on Cardio Pulmonary Resuscitation and Emergency Cardiac Care. "Standards for cardio pulmonary resuscitation (CPR) and emergency cardiac care (ECC)." *Journal of the American Medical Association, 227* (Suppl.), 837–868, 1974.

Nelson, S. R., "Hospital Sponsored Group Practice." *Health Matrix, 2*(1), 7, 1984.

Nutting, P. A. et al., "Community-Oriented Primary Care in the United States." *Journal of the American Medical Association, 253,* 1763, 1985.

Office of Disease Prevention and Health Promotion, U.S. Department of Health and Human Services. *Disease Prevention/Health Promotion: The Facts.* Palo Alto, CA: Bull Publishing, 1988.

Olson, L. L., *Establishing Freestanding Ambulatory Surgery Centers: The Planning and Regulatory Process.* Chicago: American Medical Association, 1982.

Orso, C. L., "Delivering Ambulatory Health Care." *Medical Care, 17,* 111, 1979.

Oswald, E. M., & Winer, I. K., "A Simple Approach to Quality Assurance in a Complex Ambulatory Care Setting." *Quality Review Bulletin, 13*(2), 56, 1987.

Parker, M. I., Bell, P. A., Kraas, M., *Interstudy Competetive Usage, 1*(10), 1992.

Pascerelli, E. F., & Holtzworth, A. S., "Developing an Ambulatory Care Program for AIDS Patients." *Journal of Ambulatory Care Management, 10*(1), 44, 1987.

Perkoff, G. T. "General Internal Medicine, Family Practice or Something Better?" *New England Journal of Medicine, 299,* 654, 1978.

Perkoff, G. T., "Teaching Clinical Medicine in the Ambulatory Setting: An Idea Whose Time May Have Finally Come." *New England Journal of Medicine 314*(1), 27, 1986.

Petersdorf, R. B., "Internal Medicine and Family Practice." *New England Journal of Medicine, 293,* 326, 1975.

Phillips, J. H., & Reeder, C. E., "Ambulatory Care Centers: Structure, Services, and Marketing Techniques." *Journal of Health Care Marketing, 7*(4), 27, 1987.

Report of the Graduate Medical Educational National Advisory Committee (GMENAC) to the Secretary (Publ. No. 81-651). Hyattsville, MD: U.S. Government Printing Office.

Resource Management Corporation. *Evaluation of the War on Poverty: Health Programs.* (Contract No. GA-654). Washington, DC: General Accounting Office, 1969.

Robert Wood Johnson Foundation, Special Report: *Access to Health Care in the United States: Results of a 1986 Survey.* Princeton, NJ: Johnson Foundation, 1987.

Roemer, M. I., *Ambulatory Health Services in America.* Gaithersburg, MD: Aspen Systems Corp., 1981.

Rogers, D., "Policy Changes and Their Possible Impact on Hospital-Based Ambulatory Care." *Journal of Community Health, 10*(4), 226, 1985.

Rosen, G., "The First Neighborhood Health Center Movement—Its Rise and Fall." *American Journal of Public Health, 61,* 1620, 1971.

Rosenblatt, R. A., Cherkin, D. C., Sehneeweiss, R., & Hart, L. G., "The Content of Ambulatory Medical Care in the United States: An Inter-Specialty Comparison. *New England Journal of Medicine, 309,* 892, 1983.

Roth, R. et al., "Out-of-Hospital Cardiac Arrest: Factors Associated with Survival." *Annals of Emergency Medicine, 13,* 237, 1984.

Sadowy, H. S., & Wood, S. C., "The Growth of Alternative Delivery Systems and the Implications for Hospitals." *Health Care Strategy Management 4*(7), 14, 1986.

Sardell, A., "Neighborhood Health Centers and Community-based Care: Federal Policy from 1965 to 1982." *Journal of Public Health Policy, 4,* 484, 1983.

Schafft, G. E., Cawley, J. F., *Physician Assistants in a Changing Health Care Environment,* Rockville, MD, Aspen Publishers, 1987.

Schroeder, S. A., Training an Appropriate Mix of Physicians to Meet the Nation's Needs, *Academic Medicine,* 68, 1993.

Selzer, S. R., & Scholl, J. G., "Development of a Campus-based Satellite Medicine Clinic." *Journal of Medical Education, 60*(6), 461, 1985.

Sherman, M. A., "Mobile Intensive Care Units: An Evaluation of Effectiveness." *Journal of the American Medical Association, 241,* 1899, 1979.

Showstack, J., Fein, O., Ford, D., et al., JAMA, 267:2497–2502, 1992.

Smith, D. R., Anderson, R. J., Community Responsive Medicine: A Call for a New Academic Discipline, *Journal of Health Care for the Poor and Underserved,* 1, 219–228, 1990.

Smith, J. E., Popielarski, E., "Hospital Outpatient Pharmacies and Durable Medical Equipment." *American Journal of Hospital Pharmacy, 43*(4), 928, 1986.

Sparer, G., & Anderson, A., *Cost of Services at Neighborhood Health Centers: A Comparative Analysis.* Washington, DC: Office of Economic Opportunity, 1975.

Stafstrom, A., "The Right Staff—The Human Role in Financial Success." *Ambulatory Care,* 7(2), 8, 1987.

Steinberg, E. P., Lawrence, R. S., "Where Have All the Doctors Gone? Physician Choices between Specialty and Primary Care Practice." *Annals of Internal Medicine, 93,* 619, 1980.

Stone, R. I., *Integration of Home and Community-based Services: Issues for the 1990s,* Prepared for the Visiting Nurse Service of New York and the Milbank Memorial Fund Home-based Care for a New Century Project, New York, Sept. 1993.

Tennant, F. S., Jr., & Day, C. M., "Survival Potential and Quality of Care among Free Clinics." *Public Health Reports, 89,* 558, 1974.

Torrens, P., & Yedvab, D., "Variations among Emergency Room Populations: A Comparison of Four Hospitals in New York City." *Medical Care, 8,* 60, 1970.

Tulli, C. G., Jr., "One Key to Practice Growth: Improving Other Practice Encounters." *Group Practice Journal,* 36(6), 58, 1987.

U.S. Department of Health and Human Services, *Health United States, 1986* (DHHS Pub. No. PHS 87-1232). Washington, DC: U.S. Government Printing Office, 1986.

U.S. Department of Health and Human Services, *Health United States, 1991* (DHHS Pub. No. PHS 88-1232). Washington, DC: U.S. Government Printing Office, 1991.

Vanselow, N. A., & Kralewski, J. E., "The Impact of Competitive Health Care Systems on Professional Education." *Journal of Medical Education, 61,* 707, 1986.

Wagner, E. R., "Types of Managed Care Organizations." *The Managed Care Handbook.* Gaithersburg, MD: Aspen Publications.

Weiner, J. P., Steinwachs, D. M., Shapiro, S., Coltin, K. L., et al., "Assessing a Methodology for Physician Requirement Forecasting. Replication of GMENAC's Need-based Model for the Pediatric Specialty." *Medical Care,* 25(5), 426, 1987.

Weinerman, E. R. et al., "Yale Studies in Ambulatory Medical Care: V. Determinants of Use of Hospital Emergency Services." *American Journal of Public Health, 56,* 1037, 1966.

Wilensky, G. R., & Berk, M. L., "The Health Care of the Poor and the Role of Medicaid." *Health Affairs, 1*(4), 50, 1982.

Wolinsky, H., "New Trend in Patient Care: Women's Health Centers." *American College of Physicians Observer, 6*(7), 1, 23, 1986.

Zwick, D. I., "Some Accomplishments and Findings of Neighborhood Health Centers." *Milbank Memorial Fund Quarterly,* October 1972. Reprinted in I. K. Zola and J. B. McKinlay (Eds.), *Organizational Issues in the Delivery of Health Services,* New York: Prodist, 1974.

7

Hospitals

Anthony R. Kovner

Smith and Kaluzny (1986) have characterized the health care system as a white labyrinth "so large, complex and subtle that it defies description." To many Americans, hospitals are just such white labyrinths. People often know little about how their local hospital works, and even those who work in hospitals often know little about departments or occupations other than their own. Yet hospitals, like other, more familiar local organizations, open, grow, merge, and even close.

This chapter surveys the following topics concerning hospitals: (1) historical development, (2) hospital statistics and characteristics, (3) factors affecting costs, (4) hospital structure, and (5) forces propelling and constraining change in hospitals. The primary focus is on the most common type of hospital—that which provides short-term, general, and acute care.

Historical Development

The development of American community hospitals can be divided into five periods:

1. The beginning, before 1870.
2. The first period of rapid growth, 1870–1910.
3. The period of consolidation, 1910–1945.
4. The second period of rapid growth, 1945–1980.
5. The present period of maturation and perhaps the end of growth in terms of the number and size of hospitals, 1980 and onward.

The section on Historical Development in this chapter remains in large part the same as in the first and second editions and was authored by Michael Enright and Steven Jonas.

The first hospitals were primarily of a religious and charitable nature, tending to provide care for the sick rather than providing for medical cure (Freymann, pp. 28–29; Starr, 1982, Chapter 4; Rosenberg).

In the American colonies, the earliest hospitals were actually infirmaries in poorhouses.

Private voluntary hospitals (those provided or supported by community leaders) in the United States go back to the 18th century (Freymann, pp. 22–24). These institutions also cared for the poor: Since hospitals could do little for their patients, there was no reason for the self-supporting sick to use them. By 1873, there were an estimated 178 hospitals in the United States (Stevens, p. 52).

From 1870 to 1910, as biomedical science and technology developed effective means of intervention, hospitals evolved into local physicians' workshops for all types and classes of patients. More effective hospital care was achieved primarily through advances in general hospital hygiene, including the development of trained nurses and techniques for asepsis and surgical anesthesia. Between 1870 and 1910 there was a period of spectacular growth, the number of hospitals increasing from 178 in 1873 to more than 4,300 in 1909 (Stevens, p. 52). Medical care had become too complex for physicians to carry their entire armamentarium in their black bags; special equipment and consultation with other medical specialists became essential.

According to Starr (pp. 169–170), the period from 1750 to 1850 saw the formation of voluntary and public hospitals. From 1850 to 1890 there developed religious or ethnic institutions and specialized hospitals for certain diseases or categories of patients, such as children and women. The period from 1890 to 1920 saw the spread of for-profit hospitals owned by physicians. The period between 1910 and 1945 showed less growth than in the periods before and after.

The types of patients in the hospitals changed with each medical discovery. In 1923, the discovery of insulin drastically changed the character of treatment for diabetes. Liver extract reduced the incidence of pernicious anemia in 1929. Sulfonamides began to affect the treatment of pneumonia and some other infectious diseases in 1935, a trend that accelerated with the widespread use of antibiotics beginning in 1943, as well as the continuing development of immunization techniques. The development of rehabilitation services began to bring more disabled patients to the hospital. The 1950s saw chronic illness becoming progressively more important as a hospital problem. As infectious diseases generally have been conquered (with the notable exception of AIDS), hospitals are increasingly focusing on the pathology of trauma and degenerative and neoplastic disease.

The fourth period, 1945 to 1980, was a second major growth era for hospitals. It was marked by a tremendous increase in hospital services, costs, and technology and by a more modest expansion in the number of hospitals. Many small rural hospitals were built during this period, financed by federal monies

under the Hill-Burton Act. A major factor influencing the increased breadth and
intensity of inpatient hospital services was the rapid growth of hospital insurance.
The Blue Cross system originally was developed during the Great Depression in
order to help assure payment to hospitals. Hospital insurance developed rapidly
through World War II as a result of collective bargaining agreements. In that
period the federal government limited wage increases but not benefits. Finally,
in 1965 the Medicare and Medicaid programs were created, the former providing health insurance for the elderly and the latter providing health benefits for
the poor.

Since 1980, hospital occupancy rates have decreased, both with regard to the
mean discharge rate (which is the ratio of total discharges in a year to number of
beds) and average length of stay. Between 1981 and 1991, the average occupancy
rate of community hospitals in the United States declined nearly 15%—from 76%
to 66.1% (AHA, 1992b; 1993). At the same time that hospital occupancy has been
decreasing, there are fewer independent hospitals. There has been an emergence
in the industry of investor-owned and not-for-profit multihospital corporations
(Starr, 1982, pp. 420–450). In 1991 multihospital systems owned, leased, or sponsored 2,368 hospitals and managed under contract 505 hospitals, putting more than
43% of U.S. hospitals under multihospital systems (AHA, 1992a).

Hospital care is big business. In 1990, hospital expenditures amounted to $256.0
billion, representing 38% of the nation's health expenditures and 4.1% of the
nation's gross national product, or $2,566 per American (U.S. Bureau of the Cen-
sus, 1992). This compares with a 1980 expenditure level of $102.4 billion, which
was 9.2% of the nation's health expenditures and 3.8% of the nation's gross national product (U.S. Bureau of the Census, 1992).

Hospital Statistics and Characteristics

There are two major agencies that count and classify hospitals in the United States:
the American Hospital Association (AHA) and the National Center for Health
Statistics (NCHS) of the U.S. Department of Health and Human Services. The
AHA annually publishes the Hospital Guide issue of its journal *Hospitals*, followed by a companion publication, *Hospital Statistics*. These publications list each
AHA-registered hospital, giving its basic characteristic as well as much summary
data. The NCHS publishes the results of its Hospital Discharge Survey periodically in *Monthly Vital Statistics Report* and *Health and Vital Statistics*. The Hospital Discharge Survey gathers and analyzes data from a sample of hospitals on
demographic characteristics of patients, descriptors of hospitals, morbidity and
diagnoses, and surgical operations. Since 1976 a congressionally mandated annual report to the president, titled *Health: United States*, has appeared. It includes
some data on hospitals, as well as health and financial data.

Hospital Statistics

Table 7.1 provides summary statistics on community hospitals. Community hospitals include general short-term hospitals under not-for-profit (voluntary), public (governmental), and investor-owned (proprietary) auspices. Other hospitals include federal hospitals and nonfederal, long-term mental and other hospitals.

Table 7.2 provides some additional key facts on community hospital size, utilization, employment, and expenditures. Community hospitals admitted more than 31 million patients in 1991, with an average stay of 7.2 days. Hospital occupancy, which is determined by dividing available bed days by patient days, was 66.1% in 1991 (AHA, 1993–1994). This is down from 1981 volume: by 5 million patients admitted, .4 days average stay, and 9.9% in hospital occupancy (AHA, 1993–1994).

TABLE 7.1 Community Hospital Facts: 1991

	1981	1991
Total number of hospitals	5,813	5,342
Beds (thousands)	1,003	924
Patient admissions	36,438	31,064
Births (thousands)	3,465	3,965
Surgical operations (thousands)	19,236	22,405
Outpatients (thousands)	202,768	322,048
Hospital size, by number of beds		
6–24	244	222
25–49	977	922
50–99	1,449	1,244
100–199	1,402	1,311
200–299	717	741
300–399	427	398
400–499	276	223
500 or more	330	281
Community hospitals by type		
Nonprofit	3,340	3,175
Investor-owned	729	738
State and local government	1,744	1,429

Note: Community Hospitals are nonfederal, short-term general and special hospitals (excluding psychiatric hospitals, tuberculosis and respiratory disease hospitals, and hospital units of institutions) whose facilities and services are available to the public.

Source: Adapted from the American Hospital Association, *Hospital Statistics, 1992–93* (AHA, 1993–94).

TABLE 7.2   Community Hospital Key Facts: 1991

Average size	173 beds
Average length of stay*	7.2 days
Hospital occupancy	66.1%
FTEs per 100 adjusted census	431
Expenditures (millions)	$225,023

*An aggregate figure including inpatient days plus an estimate of the volume of outpatient days, expressed in units equivalent to an inpatient day in terms of level of effort.

Source: Adapted from *Hospital Statistics, 1992–93* (AHA, 1993–94).

Although the number of community hospitals (see Table 7.1) has remained relatively the same—at about 5,800—since 1972, the average size of these hospitals has increased from 163 beds in 1976 to 173 beds in 1991 (AHA, 1993–1994). Community hospitals employed 3,535,000 full-time equivalent staff in 1991. Community hospitals expenditures totaled $225 billion in 1991, of which labor expenses were $102 billion of 45%.

Hospitals other than community (nonfederal, short-term general, and special hospitals) include federal, nonfederal psychiatric, tuberculosis and other respiratory disease hospitals, long-term general, and other special institutions. In 1991 there were 1,292 of these hospitals, with 278,000 beds, 2.5 million admissions, and an average length of stay ranging from 23 to 93 days, as shown in Table 7.3.

Hospital Characteristics

Hospitals differ from one another with respect to size, mission, ownership, complexity, competitive environment, population served, endowment and financial situation, physical facilities, and costs per day of care or cost by patient diagnostic category.

As of 1991, 1,144 community hospitals had fewer than 50 beds apiece. Many of these hospitals were in areas with sparse populations, the nearest hospital being an hour's drive away from residents in the community. The 281 largest community hospitals of more than 500 beds (5.3% of the total) had about 22% of the nation's total community hospital admissions (AHA, 1992b; 1993).

For example, according to the 1992 AHA Hospital Guide, Nor-Lea General Hospital in Lovington County, New Mexico had 28 beds and provided the following services: ambulatory surgery, health promotion, respiration therapy, physical therapy, ultrasonography, blood bank, rehabilitation outpatient services, organized outpatient department, hospital auxiliary, patient representation, acute

Table 7.3 Trends among Other Than Community Hospitals

	Hospitals		Beds (000's)		Admissions		Avg. LOS	
	'81	'91	'81	'91	'81	'91	'81	'91
Federal hospitals	348	334	116	97	2032	1658	16	15
Nonfederal psych. hospitals	549	800	202	154	558	740	114	61
Nonfederal TB and other respiratory disease hospitals	11	4	2	0	8	2	46	80
Long-term general and other special	146	126	35	25	77	83	144	93
Short-term units of institutions	66	28	3	2	55	19	9	23

Source: Adapted from *Hospital Statistics, 1992–93* (AHA, 1993–94).

pediatric inpatient care, speech therapy, occupational therapy, inpatient care for AIDS/ARC, emergency services, emergency response (geriatric) (AHA, 1992a). New York University Medical Center in New York City had 878 beds and was listed as providing all of the services that Nor-Lea provided, other than emergency response (geriatric) services. In addition, NYU Medical Center provided cardiac catheterization laboratory, open heart surgery, angioplasty, chronic obstructive pulmonary disease services, patient education, community health promotion, worksite health promotion, hemodialysis, intensive care unit (medical, surgical or other), histopathology laboratory, neonatal intensive care unit, obstetrics unit, psychiatric inpatient services and consultation/liaison, megavoltage radiation therapy, radioactive radiation theapy, CT scanning, magnetic resonance imaging, inpatient rehabilitation, reproductive health services, single photon emission computerized tomography (SPECT), organized social work services, outpatient social work services, emergency department social work services, volunteer services department, organ/tissue transplant, orthopedic surgery, recreational therapy services, health sciences library, and noninvasive cardiac assessment services (AHA, 1992a).

Hospitals are similar to one another in that they provide inpatient care by nurses and physicians, the latter having a great deal of autonomy in deciding whom to admit and what services patients should receive. As organizations, hospitals have to be financially solvent. They all seek to survive and grow. Hospitals provide services every day and at every hour of the day. Some hospitals services are difficult to quantify and measure; for example, how can one measure the amount of health education services a patient receives? But all hospitals must be organized so that standby capacity is available to meet medical emergencies and to deal with critical and life-threatening situations. Hospitals are characterized by hierarchy and rules. There is little but increasing standardization of patient care. Nevertheless, there is overall agreement about the principal objectives of hospitals: curing and caring.

Some Important Types of Hospitals

The American Hospital Association classified hospitals in several ways. Those in which the average length of stay is 30 days or less are short-term hospitals. In long-term hospitals the average length of stay is more than 30 days. There are specialty hospitals—for example, ear, nose, and throat hospitals and those for women's diseases—and general hospitals. There are teaching and nonteaching hospitals, hospitals that are independent or are part of multihospital systems, public and private hospitals, and nonprofit or for-profit hospitals.

The following important types of short-term hospitals will be discussed: teaching, those in multihospital systems, public, and rural. These categories are not mutually exclusive. For example, Bellevue Hospital in New York City's Health and Hospital Corporation is a public teaching hospital that is part of a multihospital system.

Teaching Hospitals. In 1991, there were 285 nonfederal hospitals belonging to the Council of Teaching Hospitals (COTH) of the Association of American Medical Colleges. These COTH hospitals represent 6% of all hospitals. Relative to other hospitals, COTH hospitals are larger and are located in large urban areas. They offer more specialized services and provide more uncompensated care than non-COTH hospitals. Although COTH hospitals only represent 6% of the nation's hospitals, in 1991 23% of the nation's total outpatient visits were to COTH hospitals, as well as 19% of the total surgical operations. COTH hospitals employed 26% of the total FTEs for all hospitals in 1991 (AAMC, 1993).

Because of their commitment to the triad of teaching hospital missions—education, research, and patient care—COTH members also offer a large percentage of tertiary or highly complex services. For example, in 1991, 92% of COTH members reported having a cardiac catheterization lab (vs. 26% for non-COTH members); 82% reported a megavoltage radiation facility (only 16% for non-COTH hospitals); and 47% of COTH institutions reported the capability to perform kidney transplants and 45% could perform other organ transplants (only 9% of non-COTH hospitals reported the capability to perform kidney transplants and 15% reported the capability to perform other organ transplants).

In 1990, COTH members comprised 6% of the nation's short-term nonfederal hospitals but claimed 50% of the total deductions for charity care (approximately $2.98 billion) and 28% of the deductions for bad debt (approximately $3.1 billion) (AAMC, 1993).

Multihospital Systems. Hospitals are part of a multihospital system when they are either leased under contract management or are legally incorporated by or under the direction of a board that determines the control of two or more hospitals (Ermann & Gabel, 1984). In 1991, there were 309 multihospital systems, which included 2,873 hospitals and 548,759 beds (AHA, 1992a). In 1991, 43% of the nation's hospitals and beds were in multihospital systems

Once the largest chain, Hospital Corporation of America (HCA), founded in 1968 with one hospital, sold 104 facilities to an employee group in 1987. HCA now owns 90 facilities and approximately 21,000 beds, which produced $5.126 billion in revenues in 1992; 95% of revenues were from medical/surgical operations and the balance was from psychiatric operations (personal communication, 1993). National Medical Enterprises (NME), another investor-owned system, is one of the nation's largest healthcare services companies with operations in 34 states, the District of Columbia, and abroad. In the United States and abroad, National Medical Enterprises owns or operates 161 facilities that provide acute, psychiatric, physical rehabilitation and substance abuse services (NME, 1992).

According to Ermann and Gabel (1984), investor-owned and nonprofit systems have different patterns of growth. Investor-owned systems average 23 hospitals per system and tend to be dispersed among many states. Individual nonprofit systems average 7 hospitals per system and tend to be regional, located in one or two states.

Large, public multihospital systems include those of the federal Veterans Administration with over 160 hospitals, and the Health and Hospitals Corporation of New York City, whose 11 short-term hospitals have 7,899 beds. Large nonprofit hospital systems include 28 Kaiser hospitals, which are part of the Kaiser-Permanente prepaid group practice system, (with revenues of over $9.8 billion in 1991) and the 16 community health systems owned by Sisters of Mercy Health Corporation in three midwestern states which in some cases have multiple hospitals (personal communication, 1993).

Public Hospitals. Public hospitals are owned by agencies of federal, state, and local government. Federal hospitals typically have been designed for special beneficiaries: American Indians, merchant seamen, military personnel, and veterans. State hospitals typically have provided long-term psychiatric and chronic care, in the past especially for patients with tuberculosis. There are also state university or teaching hospitals that provide short-term general acute care.

There are two main types of local, short-term general public hospitals. The first type has similar characteristics to smaller nonprofit hospitals, is located in small towns or cities of moderate size, is used by private attending physicians, and serves paying and indigent patients.

The second type is located in major urban areas. Physician staff is mostly salaried and mostly residents in training. The hospital's deficits are paid for from taxes. As of 1991, there were 1,448 state and local government general and other special hospitals with a total of 170,000 beds (AHA, 1993–94a). These 1,448 hospitals (27% of all community hospitals) provided 18% of the beds, 16% of the inpatient admissions, and 19.8% of the outpatient visits for all community hospitals (AHA, 1992b; 1993).

Rural Hospitals. Rural areas are areas falling outside a metropolitan statistical area, which is defined as containing a city with a population of at least 50,000 or an urban area with a population of at least 50,000 and a total metropolitan population of at least 100,000 (AHA, 1992b). In 1992, 2,285 of the nation's hospitals (43%) were rural. Seventy-one percent had fewer than 100 beds (AHA, 1993).

Between 1982 and 1992, admissions to rural hospitals dropped from 8.3 million to 5.1 million, a 39% decline. Between 1980 and 1990, 280 rural community hospitals stopped providing inpatient acute health services (AHA, 1992b). Key problems of rural hospitals include: threat of closure, thereby depriving local residents of access to care; the questionable financial viability of hospitals with fewer than 50 beds; difficulties in assuring quality of care in such hospitals when operated as independent units; and, difficulties in attracting skilled professionals to work in isolated rural localities. Rural American counties face different kinds of problems depending on economic structure. Although they are often thought to consist only of farm areas, rural counties can be classified as economically dependent on farming; manufacturing; mining; oil and energy; large federal, state, or local government installations; federal lands; and retirement settlement communities or characterized by persistent poverty (AHA, 1988).

To survive in more competitive hospital markets, rural hospitals have undertaken a variety of innovative measures. According to the AHA rural hospital assessment (1988), these include seeking to increase patient volume by introducing or expanding ambulatory or long-term services. Many have sought to expand technological capabilities, increase referrals, or reduce costs through shared service or networking arrangements and consolidation activities. By 1992 nearly 34% of rural hospitals are part of multi-hospital systems (AHA, 1992b).

An Example

Let us use a fictitious example to illustrate how decreasing the supply of beds and also decreasing the length of stay per admission will impact on hospital costs and capacity. Assume in year 1 (as shown in Table 7.4) a hospital per diem rate of $300 (or $2,280 per 7.6-day stay) in a city with a population of 1 million and a ratio of 4.0 beds per 1,000 people. Assume that in year 2 the same number of hospital admissions and the same resources per day are used to provide care. But now decrease hospital bed capacity by 10% and also decrease the average length of patient stay by 10%. Other things being equal, this would result in savings of $32.85 million, or 10%, and the same hospital occupancy rate of 75%. Other things are not equal, however. In reality, the effect on costs of decreasing capacity varies depending upon how many beds are taken out of service in how many hospitals. If hospital costs are similar in each of ten 400-bed hospitals, cost savings will be greater through closure of one hospital than through taking out of service one 40-bed wing in all 10 hospitals. This is because fixed costs eliminated by closure

TABLE 7.4 Hospital Supply, Utilization, and Costs in Years 1 and 2 in City X with Population of 1,000,000

YI		
(1) Bed capacity (4.0 per 1,000)		4,000
(2) Patient days at 75% occupancy (4,000 beds x 365 days x 75%	=	1,095,000
(3) Cost at $300 per day (1,095,000 patient days x $300)	=	$328,500,000
(4) Admissions (1,095,000 patient days ÷ 7.6-day average length of stay)	=	144,079
Y2		
(1) Bed capacity (3.6 per 1,000) (decrease by 10%)		3,600
(2) Patient days (decrease length of stay by 10%) (144,079 admissions x 6.84-day average length of stay)	=	985,000
(3) Cost at $300 per day (985,500 patient days x $300)	=	$295,650,000
(4) Occupancy (985,500 actual patient days ÷ 1,314,000 available patient days)	=	75%
SAVINGS		
$328,500,000 − $295,650,000 = $ 32,850,000 or 10%		

of an entire hospital are greater than fixed costs eliminated by closing 10 nursery units in 10 hospitals. Fixed costs include costs such as a proportion of the administrator's salary or of the salary of the security force or of the heating bill, which continue if one nursing unit is closed but not if one entire hospital is closed.

The purpose of this example is to begin to outline the factors that affect hospital costs and that policymakers and managers attempt therefore to influence. To illustrate the further complexity underlying the same example, costs per hospital day may actually increase in year 2 because of inflation and because more employees or more highly skilled employees and more nonlabor inputs of higher cost are used to provide the same days of service. This effect is called "increased intensity of service." Area hospital costs may rise even if one hospital is actually closed, for example, if it is a low-cost hospital and if other hospitals' costs per day of care do not fall because of higher volume. Even if area costs do not rise, access costs will increase for patients who live near a hospital that is closed.

Hospital Utilization

There are several measures of hospital utilization, including number of admissions; average daily census (average number of patients in the hospital); occupancy rate (percentage of beds occupied); average length of stay; total patient days (average daily census multiplied by number of days in time period considered); and discharges. These data can be modified and compared in various cross-tabulations: by geography (region, state); by hospital characteristics (bed, size, type, category of ownership); and by patient age, sex, and demographic modifiers. Analyses of hospital utilization data are vast; I shall cover only a portion of them.

In 1991, there were 33.6 million admissions to hospitals in the United States (AHA, 1992–93). Of the admissions, 93% were to community hospitals, and 75% of the patient days were in such hospitals (AHA, 1992–93). Although only 2.2% of admissions were to nonfederal short- and long-term psychiatric hospitals, these accounted for 15% of the total average daily census.

There are many determinants of hospital admission. Being separated or divorced, having comprehensive insurance, and having a long traveling time to a regular source of care all increase an individual's chance of being hospitalized (Andersen et al., p. 13). Length of stay in a hospital varies by sex, age, and diagnosis, as well as family structure, degree of anxiety about health, beliefs about health care, and availability of alternatives to hospitalization, such as nursing homes and home health services (Andersen et al., p. 13).

Women are more likely to be hospitalized than are men (NCHS, 1983, p. 144). When obstetrical admissions are elminated, the average length of stay (ALOS) is about the same for males and females. Length of stay in a hospital decreases as the patient's level of education and income rise, and it increases with age (Phelps, p. 112).

The use of community hospitals varies among age groups. In 1991, persons aged 65 years and over were discharged from the hospital at 3.4 times the rate of persons aged 15 to 44 and 7.5 times the rate of those under 15 years of age (NCHS, unpublished data).

Diagnosis-specific length of stay has been declining with medical progress. In the 1950s physicians often recommended hospital stays of 4 to 8 weeks for a myocardial infarction. In the 1960s, for an uncomplicated myocardial infarction, this was shortened to 3 weeks, to 2 weeks in the 1970s, to 7 to 10 days in the 1980s, and then to an average of 8.1 days in 1991.

In 1991, the most common DRGs (diagnosis related groups) accounted for 35.8% of all discharges in the National Center for Health Statistics' (1991) sample of 484 hospitals as shown in Table 7.5 (NCHS, unpublished data, 1991). These 21 DRGs also accounted for 31.8% of total patient days and had an overall average length of stay of 5.69 days. Note that individual case-mix proportions vary from year to year with respect to changing coding practices to enhance hospital reimbursement. Changing practice patterns and medical technology may also be attributable to changes in case-mix. Over the years, for certain medical conditions, patients have moved from inpatient to outpatient settings (Farley).

The ALOS in community hospitals in 1991 was 7.2 days (AHA, 1993–94). This compares with 7.6 days in 1981. There is a wide variation in length of stay by age (AHA, 1985). In 1991, patients aged 65 and over stayed an average of about

8.6 days; those 65 and under stayed about 5.2 days per admission (AHA, 1993–94). There is a variation in the ALOS by region and hospital bed size. For example, the ALOS in community hospitals ranged 5.2 in Utah and 5.6 in Washington to 8.7 in Minnesota and 9.9 in New York (AHA, 1993–94). In 1991 ALOS in community not-for-profit hospitals ranged from 5.5 days in hospitals with fewer than 25 beds to 7.9 days in hospitals with more than 500 beds. Variation in ALOS by hospital size may be explained in part by variation in severity of disease, but regional differences are difficult to explain on medical bases alone. In 1991 ALOS variance by type of short-term hospital was 6.3 days in investor-owned hospitals and 7.2 days in the nonprofits, with local government hospitals averaging 7.8 days (AHA, 1993–94).

What Do Hospital Services Cost?

An article in *Harpers* in March 1984 detailed how high hospital costs can be (Hellerstein, 1984). Costs were presented for 25 days in the life of "Mrs. K.," whose hospitals stay was in a New York City hospital. Costs were probably higher in this hospital, because of its location, age, and other factors, than in most other hospitals, and are certainly higher for this episode of illness because of the special services that Mrs. K. received. Since this example was effective in illustrating hospital costs for 1983, the total costs for 25 days in the hospital for Mrs. K. were adjusted for inflation in Table 7.6 to reflect 1992 hospital costs.

In 1983, total costs for 25 days of care, nearly all of this intensive care, was $47,311 (not including doctor's bills). In 1992, these 25 days in the hospital would have cost $98, 257, representing an increase since 1983 of 108%. Mrs. K. died on the 25th day. Questions can be raised as to whether all of the services she received were necessary, whether they could have been provided more cheaply, and whether Mrs. K.'s admission was necessary. If she were going to die anyway within 25 days, should $98,257 be spent on her care today? How one might answer these questions may differ depending on whether one is Mrs. K.'s daughter, the hospital administrator, or Mrs. K.'s employer.

Economic Impact

The impact of hospitals on local economies can be very important. In small communities, hospital closure can remove a vital source of local employment and revenues to local hospital suppliers. Construction of a hospital means numerous jobs for construction workers and future hospital employees.

Ginzberg and Drennan (1985) estimated the economic impact of hospitals in New York City to include the following: In 1983, the city's 102 hospitals spent $8.2 billion dollars. In 1981, these hospitals employed 127,676 workers. Also in

TABLE 7.5 Casemix (Percentage of Discharges) and ALOS (Days) for the 21 Most Common DRGs, 1991

Diagnosis related group (DRG)	# of patients discharged (000's)	% of total discharges	Patient days per DRG (000's)	DRG-specific ALOS (days)
373 Vaginal delivery without complicating diagnoses	2, 547	8.19	5,517	2.17
127 Heart failure and shock	793	2.55	5,976	7.53
371 Cesarean section without complications or comorbidity	744	2.39	2,981	4.01
430 Psychoses	742	2.38	10,472	14.11
089 Simple pneumonia & pleurisy age > 17 with complications or comorbidity	537	1.73	4,481	8.34
359 Uterine & adnexa procedures for nonmalignancy without complications or comorbidity	522	1.68	1,933	3.70
140 Angina Pectoris	483	1.55	2,017	4.18
014 Specific cerebrovascular disorders except transient ischemic attack	479	1.54	5,006	10.45
182 Esophagitis, gastroent & miscellaneous digestive disorders age > 17 with complication or comorbidity	411	1.32	2,435	5.92
243 Medical back problems	396	1.27	2,059	5.20
209 Major joint & limb reattachment procedures	392	1.26	3,842	9.80
183 Esophagitis, gastroent & miscellaneous digestive disorders age > 17 without complications or comorbidity	388	1.25	1,445	3.72
098 Bronchitis & asthma age 0-17	347	1.12	1,076	3.10

296 Nutritional & miscellaneous metabolic disorders age > 17 without complications or comorbidity	339	1.09	2,890	8.53
088 Chronic obstructive pulmonary disease	329	1.06	2,197	6.68
215 Back & neck procedures without complications or comorbidity	308	0.99	1,525	4.95
112 Percutaneous cardiovascular procedures	303	0.97	1,538	5.08
198 Total cholecystectomy without common duct exploration without complications or comorbidity	290	0.93	1,040	3.59
096 Bronchitis & asthma agge > 17 with complications or comorbidity	276	0.89	1,815	6.58
138 Cardiac arhythmia & conduction disorders with complications or comorbidity	261	0.84	1,458	5.59
174 Gastrointestinal hemorrhage with complications or comorbidity	261	0.84	1,679	6.43
All patients in 21 most common DRGs, combined	11,148	35.8	63,382	5.69

Source: National Center for Health Statistics, unpublished data from the National Hospital Discharge Survey, 1991.

Note: Data were compiled from a survey of 484 short-stay nonfederal hospitals. Calculations were based on 274,000 abstracts of patients records.

TABLE 7.6   Breakdown of Charges Rendered to
"Mrs. K." during 25-day Hospitalization

	Charges for 1983	Charges for 1983 adjusted for inflation— 1992
Intensive care	12,000	25,560
Laboratory	11,201	23,858
Therapy	8,734	18,603
Drugs	6,365	11,966
Supplies	3,698	6,952
X-ray	2,870	6,113
Blood service	1,389	2,959
Operating room	521	1,110
EKG, EEG, etc.	366	780
Miscellaneous	167	356
Total	47,311	98,257

Source: U.S. Department of Labor, Bureau of Labor Statistics, CPI Detailed Report, January 1984. U.S. Department of Labor, Bureau of Labor Statistics, CPI Detailed Report, January 1993.

Note: Inflation calculated using Consumer Price Indexes, 1983 & 1992 Annual Averages .88 for drugs and supplies (medical care commodities) 1.13 for all other charges (hospital and related services)

1981, 120,000 out-of-city patients (11% of discharges) received inpatient services in New York City hospitals. According to Ginzberg and Drennan, revenues from such patients are equal to those spent by 600,000 tourists on 4-day visits. Assuming a per diem inpatient average reimbursement rate of $360 and an average stay of 10.2 days, 120,000 nonlocal patients generated hospital revenues of $440 million in 1 year. Applying an economic multiplier effect of about 2.0, as is done in analyzing tourist spending, the total economic impact of noncity-resident hospital stays is estimated at $888 million. Hospital expenditures, therefore, have an impact on the revenue side for hospital employees and suppliers as well as on the cost side for taxpayers and insurance purchasers.

Hospital Organizational Structure

The principal departments of the acute-care general hospital are the medical and dental, nursing, other diagnostic and therapeutic support, financial, personnel, and hotel services. Most hospitals provide services both to inpatients who are admitted and assigned a bed and to outpatients who come to an emergency department, an outpatient clinic, or for a diagnostic or therapeutic service for a procedure not requiring admission.

Medical and Dental Departmental Organization

Physicians and dentists relate to hospitals in different ways. Attending physicians on the hospital staff who are not salaried often conduct much of their business in private offices that they own or rent. These physicians may admit patients to more than one hospital and may compete with the hospital for patients or customers. Other physicians may be salaried or paid by the hospital, relative to the amount of hospital work they do. These physicians often see patients or perform related activities in offices that are provided for them by the hospital. Some hospitals employ physicians to provide primary care in competition with other physicians who are attendings or local nonhospital-affiliated practitioners. Other hospitals contract with physician groups to provide emergency care or subspecialist services on hospital premises or in satellite centers. Some physicians are attendings who maintain their own practices distinct from the hospital but who also receive a part-time salary from the hospital for administrative work.

When physicians admit patients to the hospital, in most instances they are free to order whatever tests or treatments they deem necessary. Thus the physician basically determines the amount of services used and the consequent costs of patient care. Physicians have every reason to want the best possible hospital setting in which to practice medicine, especially when it is provided at little personal cost to them.

Although the physician is technically a guest in the hospital, the hospital is responsible for the care its staff renders patients on a physician's orders. Until relatively recently, hospitals could not be held liable for the wrongful conduct of a physician, but this principle has been significantly changed by a series of judicial decisions (Southwick, 1978). Changing legal doctrines regarding negligence and the corporate liability of hospitals have established that hospitals are legally responsible and, to the extent that hospital negligence is involved, financially responsible for the care provided by their entire professional staff, including physicians.

Physicians are primarily organized along the lines of the medical specialties. The larger the hospital and the more specialized the medical services, the greater the number of separate medical departments. There is no universal logic to the way in which medical departments are categorized. Some are separated from the others by type of skill involved, some by the age or sex of their main patient group, and some by the organ or organ system that is their primary purview. Departments found in most hospitals include:

1. *Internal medicine*: general diagnosis and therapy of adults for problems involving one or more internal organs or the skin, in which the principal tools do not involve a physical alteration of the patient's body by the physician.
2. *Surgery*: diagnosis and therapy in which the principal tools involve a physical alteration of a part of the patient's body by the physician.
3. *Pediatrics*: general diagnosis and therapy for children, primarily but not entirely with nonsurgical techniques.
4. *Obstetrics/gynecology*: diagnosis and therapy relating to the sexual and reproductive system of women, using both surgical and nonsurgical techniques.
5. *Psychiatry/neurology*: diagnosis and therapy for people of all ages with mental, emotional, and nervous system problems, using primarily nonsurgical techniques.
6. *Radiology/diagnostic imaging*: diagnosis and therapy, primarily through the use of x-ray and other internal imaging techniques.
7. *Pathology*: diagnosis, both before and after treatment.
8. *Anesthesiology*: principally concerned with preparing patients so that they may be surgically operated upon with no pain or discomfort during the procedure.

Other general medical departments include family and emergency medicine. Other, more subspecialized medical departments tend to be organized around organs and organ systems, for example, ophthalmology (eye); otolaryngology (ear, nose, and throat); urology (male sexual/reproductive system and the renal system for both males and females); orthopedics (bones and joints); and so on.

There are 23 medical specializations for which professional certification may be attained by passing a medical specialty board examination. Specialties other than the ones previously mentioned include allergy and immunology, proctology, dermatology, neurosurgery, nuclear medicine, physical medicine and rehabilitation, plastic surgery, preventive medicine, and thoracic surgery. There are clinicians other than physicians who also may be granted admitting privileges to a hospital; these include dentists and podiatrists.

Physicians and dentists practicing in hospitals have their own medical and dental staff organization, with bylaws, rules, and regulations that must be approved by the hospital's governing board. The medical staff bylaws specify procedures for election of medical staff officers by membership. The officers are given authority under the bylaws to enforce rules and regulations. The officers delineate privileges and recommend disciplinary action when necessary, through the committee structure. They enforce the bylaws and must oversee the committee structure and submit reports of medical staff activities to the governing board.

There are numerous medical staff committees in the hospital, some of which may include nonphysicians, particularly nurses, as members. The executive committee, if there is one, coordinates all activity, sets general policies for the medical staff, and accepts and acts upon recommendations from the other medical staff committees. The joint conference committee, if there is one, acts as a liaison between the medical staff and the governing board in deliberations over matters involving medical and nonmedical considerations. The credentials committee reviews applications by physicians to join the medical staff and considers the qualifications of education, experience, and interests before making recommendations to the executive committee, which will then make recommendations for appointment to the governing board. In some hospitals the joint conference committee is also involved in the process.

The infections control committee is responsible for preventing infections in the hospital, through routine preventive surveillance, tracking down of outbreaks of infection, and education of hospital personnel. The pharmacy and therapeutics committee reviews pharmacologic agents for inclusion in the list of drugs approved for use in the hospital. The tissue committee is responsible for ensuring quality control of surgery, principally by examining and evaluating bodily tissues removed during operations.

The medical records committee is responsible for certifying complete and clinically accurate documentation of the care given to patients. This committee also acts as a judge of clinical care, based on the written record. The utilization review committee evaluates the appropriateness of admissions and length of stay in the hospital and may review use of services and facilities for patients whose hospital care is being paid for by Medicare, Medicaid, and in certain cases by private insurers.

The tissue, quality assurance, and utilization review committees provide for review of each physician's professional work by other physicians. As the hospital has become more complicated and more critical of medical practice, the medical staff has been subjected to more scrutiny. In the hospital, the medical chain of authority exists side by side with an administrative chain. There are many areas of confused jurisdiction and overlapping or conflicting powers. Managers and physicians working together can attempt to integrate these hierarchies. Physicians are becoming more involved in hospital governing boards; boards of trustees are reviewing more closely the methods used to appoint physicians to hospital staff; and more full-time salaried physicians have been hired by hospitals, resulting in more direct physician-hospital reporting lines.

Because of the vested interests of various medical departments in a hospital, the addition of a full-time or part-time salaried chief of the medical staff and of medical departments can create latent or open conflict with trustees or management. To lessen controversy, in some hospitals appointments of chiefs are made for a specified period of time rather than for indefinite or lifetime tenure. As full-time chiefs of service become more common, many functions formerly handled by volunteer committees—such as quality-of-care review, medical records, and continuing medical education—have been taken over by full-time paid employees.

Many hospitals are now hiring salaried medical directors and quality-of-care review teams. As hospitals are made more accountable for alleged misconduct of attending physicians, much attention has been focused on the concept of due process. If a physician is to be deprived of his medical staff privileges, the process by which the decision is made must be capable of standing up to the scrutiny of the courts (Southwick, 1978). Further, many hospitals now require physicians to have malpractice insurance as a condition of staff membership (Hollowell).

There were 83,389 resident physicians in training in American hospitals in 1990 (AMA, 1992). The number of hospital-salaried physicians other than resident physicians has more than quadrupled, from 10,000 in 1963 to 50,795 in 1990 (AMA, 1992). Salaried physicians are employed in the hospital to supervise medical care in intensive care units, outpatient departments, and medical education. Attending physicians are affected by such hiring, as hospital-employed physicians may compete with them for patients, deny them medical staff privileges (particularly to physicians new to the community), more closely supervise their practices, and change a traditional patient-care orientation to more emphasis on teaching and research.

Models of Medical Services Organization

Shortell (1985) has conceptualized four different models of organization among physicians: traditional (departmental), divisional, independent-corporate, and parallel. Under the traditional model, while each department retains relevant medical specialists, it does not contain the support services required by the physicians to provide care. These include nursing, housekeeping, dietary, and clerical staff. Figure 7.1 illustrates a traditional hospital organizational chart, in which support services are organized separately from medical services. The medical staff's relationship to the hospital is indirect, as shown by the dotted line. Physicians are not a part of the hospital chain of command, as are nurses or assistant administrators. In hospitals, this is referred to as a *dual authority structure* (Smith, 1955). Most physicians are not hospital employees. Many physicians do not see themselves as obeying the hospital administration but rather as independent practitioners who must practice according to medical staff bylaws, rules, and regulations.

Shortell's second model of medical services organization, the divisional model, is characterized by the placement of functional support services within medical divisions, which are organized along departmental lines. Each division, such as medicine or physical medicine, includes many of the support services, such as nursing and clerical (and sometimes dietary and medical records and other services), it needs to do its tasks. Each medical division leader is responsible for management, including financial management, of both medical and support services. The Johns Hopkins Hospital in Baltimore, Maryland, is organized along these lines (Heyssel et al., 1984).

FIGURE 7.1   Traditional (Departmental) Organizational Structure for Hospital Medical Services

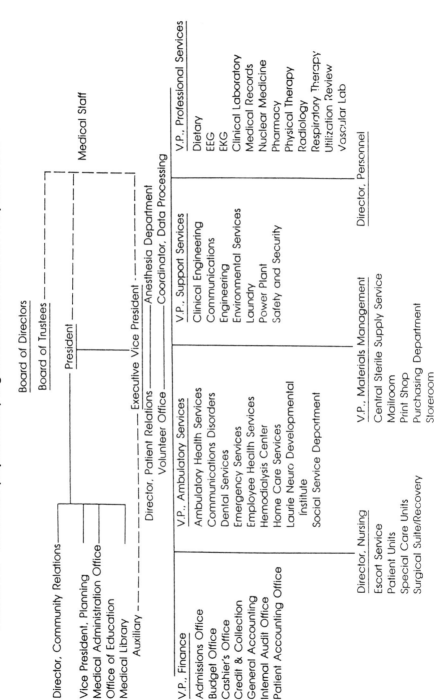

181

Under Shortell's third model, the independent-corporate model, the medical staff becomes a separate legal entity that negotiates with the hospital for its services in return for receiving support services. An independent group of physicians provides medical services to the hospital, under contract. A version of this type of model of organization is carried out by the Permanente medical groups, which have contractual relationships with the Kaiser Health Plan to form the Kaiser-Permanente medical care program, the nation's largest health maintenance organization.

Shortell's fourth model, the parallel model, involves the creation of a separate organization in order to conduct certain activities that are not handled well by the formal hospital organization. Certain physicians are selected to participate in a parallel organization for some percentage of their time, to work on important problems and report back to the formal structure. Some of these physicians would have positions in the formal structure as well. Shortell reports that parallel structures have been implemented at Saint Johns Hospital in Santa Monica, California, and at Fairfax Hospital in Virginia.

Other Patient Care Services

The functional divisions of the nursing service follow the patterns discussed in Chapter 5. Hospital diagnostic and therapeutic services, which may or may not be attached to one of the medical departments, include laboratory, usually under the direction of the department of pathology; electrocardiography, usually a part of internal medicine; electroencephalography, part of neurology; radiography, part of radiology; pharmacy; clinical psychology; social service; inhalation therapy, often part of anesthesiology or pulmonary medicine; nutrition as therapy; physical, occupational, and speech therapy, often attached to the department of rehabilitation medicine if there is one; home care; and medical records, among others.

Hospital Administrative Structure

The nonclinical services that the hospital provides can be categorized into four subsystems; finance, facilities and equipment, human resources, and management.

The financial subsystem includes capital, operating costs, and cash budgeting; pricing and cost allocation; long-range financial planning; and collection policies. In addition, some hospitals also have endowments to invest and grants to prepare and administer.

The facilities and equipment subsystem includes dietary, engineering, and environmental services; clinical engineering; power plant; grounds; housekeeping, communications, and purchasing services; and storeroom, among others.

The human resources system includes job analysis and description, job evaluation, wage and salary administration, recruitment, screening and selection, communication to employees, training and development, organizational development, collective bargaining, and labor contract administration.

The management subsystem includes planning and marketing; community, patient, and public relations; data processing and management information systems; legal services; and compliance with regulations, among others.

The organizational structure for a multihospital system is more complex and comprises a central headquarters, sometimes an intermediate divisional organization as well as the hospitals and other health care organizations, as shown in Figure 7.2.

New Developments in Hospital Organization

Over the last 5 years, there has been continued pressure on hospitals to contain costs, improve quality, and to justify resources used relative to contribution to community health. Hospitals have adapted to these pressures in many ways. In the 1980s, this included mergers, corporate restructuring, and the development of new information and quality assurance systems. Three new developments in hospital adaptation which may be widely implemented in the 1990s include continuous quality improvement, patient-focused care and community health benefit.

Continuous Quality Improvement

Continuous quality improvement (CQI), also called total quality management, is a concept which has been applied for many years in American business, particularly in response to widespread Japanese implementation of CQI ideas developed by Americans such as Deming (1986), Juran (1964), and Crosby (1979). The basic approach is to measure variation in a work process in relation to a standard, and then to implement programs to decrease process variation and improve performance results.

CQI begins with a definition of what quality is for a particular process, such as a hospital infection rate. Focus is on the consumer of the product or service, whether this is a doctor who wishes quick turnaround in x-ray reports, or a patient or a potential patient seeking a diagnosis or a cure. Everyone involved in providing the product or service becomes involved in understanding how quality is measured and in discussing how to improve quality. Rather than focusing on poor quality outcomes and how to avoid them, the work team becomes involved in setting continuously improving standards for better performance and in finding ways to meet those standards.

FIGURE 7.2 Multihospital System Organizational Chart

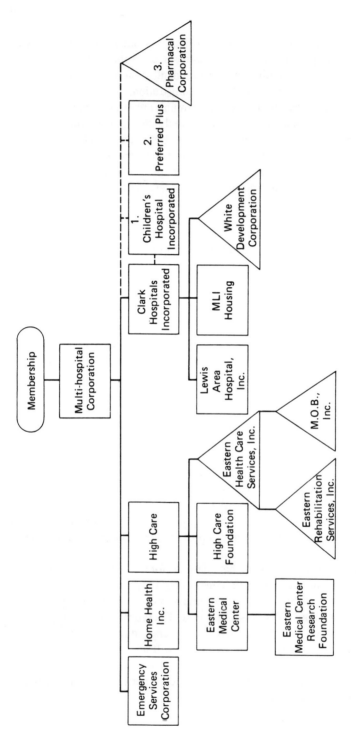

Key: △ for-profit corporation
     ☐ not-for-profit corporation

1. Participation Agreement with Multi-hospital; shared services with Clark Hospitals Incorporated

2. Management Contract

3. Joint Venture with Bliss Corporation (Multi-hospital owns ½ of the stock).

The benefits of CQI can perhaps best be understood by comparing CQI with traditional ways of doing work in which managers are in charge, focus is on production and slogans, and emphasis is placed on getting the work done in the cheapest way assuming given levels of quality rather than on meeting or exceeding consumer or user expectations.

The steps of the CQI process are as follows: find a process to improve; organize a team that knows the process; clarify current knowledge of the process; understand the causes of variation in the process; select the process improvement and continue data collection; do the improvement, data collection and analysis; check the results and lessons learned from the team effort; and, act to hold the gain and to continue to improve the process.

Examples of hospital processes which can be improved are: increasing the preadmission rate to reduce turnaround time in the operating room (in this way there are less hold ups on patients scheduled for surgery due to tests not being done or redone); to make maximum use of registered nurse skills and employ fewer agency nurses and improve the recruitment and retention of staff nurses; and, lowering the hospital Cesarian rate.

Highlights for this last process, implemented at the West Paces Ferry Hospital, a Hospital Corporation of America hospital in Florida (McEachern & Neuhauser, 1987) were as follows. Twelve physicians were taught how CQI works on two evenings and a Saturday from 8:00 A.M. to 2:00 P.M. The C-section rate nationally was 25%, at West Paces Ferry hospital the rate was 21%; at competitor hospitals the rate was 17%. An eleven-person cross-functional team was organized. They saw an opportunity to improve clinical outcomes and patient satisfaction by having fewer Cesarian deliveries. A variation was noted of C-section rates from 15 to 26% of all births, and among physicians with over 44 patients per year from 16 to 44%. Forty percent of the C-sections were caused by the baby's failure to progress in the birth canal. A mother's previous C-section accounted for 13% of the cases (27% of these were at the patient's request). The cross-functional group then changed their CQI opportunity statement to focusing on education to avoid the repeat C-sections, which was subsequently accomplished.

According to Deming (1986), there are 14 points which must be followed to successfully implement CQI. These are as follows: create constancy of purpose for improvement of product and service; adopt the new philosophy; cease dependence on inspection to achieve quality; don't award business on the basis of price tag alone, improve constantly every process for planning, production and service; institute training on the job; institute leadership; drive out fear; break down the barriers between staff areas; eliminate slogans, exhortation, and targets for the workforce; eliminate numerical quotas for the work force and numerical goals for management; remove barriers that rob people of pride of workmanship; institute a vigorous program of education and self-improvement for everyone; and put everyone in the organization to work to accomplish the transformation.

The Patient-Focused Hospital

"The Patient-Focused Hospital" is an attempt to contain hospital in-patient costs and improve quality by restructuring services so that more of them take place on nursing units rather than in specialized units in other hospital locations, and by cross-training staff on the nursing units so that they can do several "jobs" for the same small group of patients rather than one "job" for a large number of patients. Thus, for example, x-ray, pharmacy, and admitting services can all be done in the nursing unit by staff who can do more than one function. The same staff can, for example, serve the patient food, clean the patient's room, and assist in the patient's nursing care.

As services have been customarily organized in hospitals, to get a routine x-ray for an inpatient can require 40 separate steps and consume 140 minutes of personnel time. Up to 24 hours of time may elapse from the doctor's initial request to receipt of the report, and it can involve 15 to 20 employees. Moreover, most of the steps are not medical or clinical activities.

According to Smith (1990), hospital staff spend most of their time on nine activity categories: medical technical and clinical; hotel and patient services; medical documentation; institutional documentation; scheduling and coordination, patient transportation, staff transportation; management and supervision; and being "ready for action" (i.e., standing by in the emergency department whether or not patients are there requiring services). In a study at Lakeland Regional Medical Center, a 750-bed hospital in central Florida, Smith and his colleagues found that only one-sixth of personnel-related costs were consumed by medical, technical, and clinical activity, and that almost twice that amount of time was spent on writing things down. Scheduling and coordination took as much time as medical activity, and ready-for action time consumed more.

Smith (1990) suggests that restructuring services can result in reducing the number of staff required for patient care activities from 2,200 to from 1,200–1,300, and that this can actually improve the quality of care and service levels. Lakeland Hospital would be divided into five, 125-bed, operating units. The area allotted to each unit would be sufficient to contain: a mini-lab, diagnostic radiology rooms, linen and general supply, stock rooms, and so on. Medical documentation could be reduced by almost two-thirds, scheduling and coordination by more than two-thirds, and ready-for action time by two-thirds.

If the patient-focused hospital is such a good idea, why haven't more hospitals already implemented it? We can only speculate on the reasons: (1) because hospitals have, traditionally, never had to control costs in order to receive adequate reimbursement; (2) because hospital interest groups such as doctors and nurses may oppose changing the status quo with a lack of champions who will benefit from implementing what are costly and expensive processes; and, (3) because in many hospitals such changes will require extensive physical plant renovations. This situation is becoming more favorable for such change, perhaps as a result of governmental actions to contain costs and because of competitive pressures facing hospitals which are related to considerable overcapacity.

Hospital Community Benefit Programs

Rising public concern about the high cost and inaccessability of quality health services has focused on the community hospital as one of the major causes of the problem, rather than as a catalyst for reform. Increasingly, the hospital is viewed as more concerned with: generating income for survival than with the health of the community; competing to offer the latest application of high technology than with meeting community need and avoiding unnecessary duplication of facilities; meeting the needs of professionals than with serving the poor and disadvantaged; and, filling beds with inpatients than with responding to community problems affecting the health status and pocketbooks of people.

The Hospital Community Benefit Standards Program (Hospitals, 1992) was funded by the W. K. Kellogg Foundation to demonstrate that: new credible standards could assist and encourage leading hospitals to manage highly effective community benefit programs; and, that community benefit programs based on these standards can put hospitals in the forefront of efforts to reform the health care system and help to resolve the perception of a national health care crisis.

This Program adopted four standards (Kovner & Hattis, 1990): (1) there is evidence of the hospital's formal commitment to a community benefit program for a designated community; (2) the scope of the program includes hospital-sponsored projects for the designated community to improve health status, access to care, and contain the growth of community health care costs; (3) the hospital's program includes activities designed to stimulate other organizations and individuals to join in carrying out a broad health agenda in the designated community; and, (4) the hospital fosters an internal environment that encourages hospitalwide involvement in the program.

Forty-nine hospitals participated in the national demonstration, many of which made substantial movement toward local reform of health services. Community benefit can be viewed as an extension of continuous quality improvement and of the patient-focused hospital beyond the hospital walls and into the community. Focus is on problems of health status, access to care and containment of community health care costs about which the hospital, other health care providers and community leaders can do something meaningful, based on national standards that can be adapted locally which will alter current resource distribution patterns.

Examples of such demonstration site programs include: providing more prenatal care, especially to at-risk mothers, thereby improving the health status of mother and child, improving access to care and reducing health care costs such as low-weight babies resulting in part by the absence of prenatal care; closing duplicative facilities and services, and establishing special programs to reach groups lacking access to health care, for economic, social, linguistic, and cultural reasons.

Why would hospitals want to spend time or money on community benefit programs when they neither receive any money for participating nor are required to do so by government? This is because these and other hospitals are so committed to serving their communities that they believe that they can serve their communities better by learning from others and by being recognized for the success of their efforts.

Why don't more hospitals become actively involved in community benefit programs? Again, we can only speculate on the reasons: (1) because the hospital leadership sees other priorities such as acquiring new technology as more important; (2) because of a lack of support for community health priorities by specialist physicians and among other hospitals and health care providers serving the same community who may see their vital interests threatened by such an initiative; and (3) because they lack the skills and experience in working with community leaders, getting the data that they need to develop programs to improve health status, access to care and containment of community health care costs, and the experience and know-how to integrate community benefit and other hospital activities in decisions to allocate money and staff time.

Forces Propelling and Constraining Change in Hospitals

As the 20-year period of expansion following passage of Medicare and Medicaid comes to an end, hospitals are changing rapidly. The forces that are constraining hospitals as they attempt to survive and grow include purchaser pressure for cost containment, competition from vertically integrated multihospital systems and local physicians, the conservatism of some traditionally oriented practicing physicians, the cost of rapidly changing new technology, slower growth of the national economy, and a changing philosophy of government toward hospital and health care expenditures.

The forces that are propelling hospitals to continued survival and growth include increased power of hospital managers, weakening power of physicians, new forms of hospital organizational structure, new markets for hospitals, the aging of the population, and changing customer expectations for service. These constraining and propelling forces are shown in Table 7.7.

Constraining Forces

Increasingly, limits are being placed on hospital reimbursement, at least for inpatient services. Revenues are being constrained in ways that they never have been previously. When costs run over the prospective reimbursable limits, this constrains

TABLE 7.7 **Constraining and Propelling Forces Affecting Hospitals**

Constraining	Propelling
1. Governmental and third party purchaser pressure for cost containment	1. New health markets other than inpatient care
2. Competition from multihospital systems and local physicians	2. Weakening power of physicians in the hospital
3. Conservatism of some traditionally oriented practicing physicians	3. New organizational structures
4. Cost of continuing technological advances	4. Increasing power of a more business-oriented management team
4. Slower growth of the economy	5. Aging of the population
6. Changing governmental philosophy toward health care	6. Changing customer expectations for service

future hospital investment and forces decision makers to make changes in the services they provide or in how they provide them. Furthermore, it is expected that the annual percentage increases allowed under the new reimbursement ceilings will increase more slowly than before, in relation to the historical ratio of medical to nonmedical price increases.

Large purchasers other than government, such as industrial corporations or coalitions of such corporations and their insurance carriers, are also pressing for cost containment. In exchange for "preferred provider" status and presumably increased or at least a guaranteed volume of business, hospitals are being required increasingly to offer discounted or guaranteed rates to large purchasers.

Hospitals in financial difficulty and lacking sophisticated managerial controls are increasingly merging with or being managed contractually by large multihospital systems, creating competition, a second external force constraining local hospitals. These systems, particularly those that are investor-owned, have greater access to capital markets as sources of money for expansion and renovation. As these systems lack local community ties, it is easier for them to close or sell local hospitals or particular services in geographical areas that are losing population or have increasing unemployment. There also is increased competition from local physicians. Hospitals are losing their monopoly in providing surgery, emergency care, diagnostic services, routine obstetrics, and rehabilitation. Such services are increasingly being provided locally by physicians and by new freestanding organizations, which are employing physicians who may be on a hospital's own attending staff.

A third constraining force is the continuing conservatism of older, more traditional attending physicians, who continue to view the hospital primarily as a doctors' workshop. From the perspective of these physicians, hospitals should be organized primarily to provide services to help physicians take care of their own patients. Physicians with these views lack interest in hospitals providing new services, which they may see as competitive with their own practices or as diluting allocation of resources away from the inpatient support services with which they are familiar and which they see as critical to their private practices.

The Medicare/Medicaid years have been marked by tremendous and costly technological changes in hospitals, the fourth constraining force. These include development and widespread implementation of computerized axial tomography (CAT) scanners, nuclear magnetic resonance (NMR) machines, radiation therapy, ultrasound, cardiac and intensive care, burn units, kidney dialysis, and organ transplants. It is difficult to forecast now what will be the high-technology innovations of the early 1990s, but they probably will be expensive. Fewer hospitals will be able to afford them or will wish to provide them because of the increased financial risks.

The same point applies to new technological advances in computers and information systems. Only certain hospitals, particularly those in multihospital systems, will be able to make the necessary investments and risk higher short-run costs now, in return for expected quicker response time, fewer recording errors, and eventual possible lower unit costs for greater volumes of information in the future.

The final two constraining forces on hospitals are the health of the economy and the philosophy of government officials toward hospital services. During the late 1970s and early 1980s, in contrast to the 40 years following World War II and including the last 20 years of Medicare and Medicaid expansion, the U.S. economy has been growing at a much slower rate than it did previously. There is considerable feeling among federal and state government officials that not only must the rate of increase in hospital and health care expenditures be lowered but also that some competing areas of the economy require increased levels of investment relative to those required in health care. Such areas include defense; infrastructure, such as roads and bridges; criminal justice; and education.

Propelling Forces

Propelling forces are driving hospitals to respond to factors that threaten or constrain them and to take advantage of opportunities for enhanced survival and continuing growth. Our first propelling force is the identification and availability of new health care markets. Being constrained with regard to inpatient revenues, short-term hospitals are considering and implementing new services, such as home care and chronic care, which have been provided previously primarily by visiting nursing agencies, state mental hospitals, for-profit nursing homes, and other providers. Other newly organized services focus on ambulatory care. These include ambulatory surgery, freestanding emergency departments or urgent care centers, rehabilitation, day care, and health promotion/disease prevention programs. Some hospitals also are providing new support services in areas related to inpatient care, such as pharmacies, nurse registries, and parking lots, and even in areas not directly related to health care, such as motels and restaurants.

A second force propelling hospitals to move in new directions is the weakening organizational power of physicians in some hospitals, particularly those in multihospital systems. The accelerating development of a surplus supply of physicians diminishes physician leverage in opposing hospital responses to new market opportunities and enhances hospitals' negotiating positions with physicians for contractual relationships and joint ventures. It is becoming more difficult for physicians to gain hospital privileges or to admit patients to more than one primary hospital. Since multihospital systems operate in numerous markets rather than in a single geographical market, they tend to be less susceptible to local physician pressure than independent community hospitals.

Related to the weakening power of physicians in some hospitals are new organizational structures, a third propelling force and one that drives hospitals to focus effort in a few key directions. There may be separate organizations for different businesses, such as fundraising, research, or satellite health centers. Even within their main line of business—inpatient care—more hospitals are appointing medical directors and salaried chiefs of services to "administer" physician services. As physician leaders become more integrated into the hospital organizational structure, this streamlines the hospital decision-making process, thus enabling more options to be considered and implemented in a more timely way by hospital management.

A related, fourth propelling force is the increasing power, relative to that of the trustees and physicians, of a more business-oriented hospital management team. Medical services are being administered increasingly by salaried physician leaders who are being selected and rewarded for their management competence. Lay hospital managers are better trained and are being rewarded for taking more risks.

Partly as a result of improved medical care, life expectancy of Americans is increasing; hence, a fifth propelling force is the aging of the population. Those over 65 and those over 75 are making up an increasing proportion of the total population. The aged use more hospital services per capita than the rest of the population. They also use more of other types of health services, which hospitals also can provide and increasingly are providing. Such services range from retirement villages and congregate housing to nursing homes and include day-care, home care, and hospice care.

In a time of increasing competition among providers and of oversupply of providers, we can expect increased competition for hospitals in terms of quality of service as well as price. This is our sixth propelling force. In response to purchaser pressure, certain hospitals will compete primarily on price, while other hospitals will seek a niche in the marketplace by responding to the needs of those who are willing to pay more for customized services. For example, certain obstetrical hospitals can be marketed directly to women, more as a combination luxury hotel and beauty salon than as a workshop for physicians delivering babies for mothers. General hospitals may be preferred because, even though costs are higher, their food and nursing services are perceived to be better.

Summary

In this chapter we have reviewed the historical development of hospitals, key hospital characteristics, how hospitals differ from and are similar to each other, some of the key aspects of hospital costs, hospital organization, and some propelling and constraining forces for change in hospitals. Undaunted by the risks inherent in forecasting the future, I predict continuation of the following trends for hospitals in the 1990s:

- Growth of larger multihospital systems that will become increasingly vertically integrated.
- Continuing high costs of hospital care.
- Increasingly differentiated hospitals or larger units within hospitals for patients of similar demographic characteristics and medical problems.
- Increasing standardization of treatment for patients of similar demographic characteristics and medical problems.

The reasons for these changes have to do with the increasing rationalization of the hospital industry. Larger hospital multiunit systems are formed for better response to competitive demands of large purchasers for adequate quality and lower cost. Such large systems can afford functional specialists in areas such as quality assurance and cost accounting and information systems so that treatment can be standardized and costs allocated for patients of similar age and sex and medical problems. New technology, information systems, and professional manpower is increasingly expensive, reimbursement is limited, and all hospitals cannot generate sufficient volume to provide a full range of services. So hospitals will increasingly specialize in the types of patients they can best take care of. This is less true in large areas of the country with dispersed populations, but even in those areas, hospitals will increasingly share services with other hospitals and partition services between periphery and central hospitals.

References

American Hospital Association. *Hospital Statistics*, Chicago: AHA, 1993–94.
American Hospital Association. *Guide to the Health Care Field*, Chicago: AHA, 1992a.

American Hospital Association. *Environmental Assessment for Rural Hospitals*, Chicago: AHA, 1992b.

American Medical Association. *Physician Characteristics and Distribution in the U.S.*, Chicago: AMA, 1992.

Assocation of American Medical Colleges. *AAMC Data Book: Statistical Information Related to Medical Education*, Washington DC: AAMC, January 1993.

Crosby, P. B., *Quality is Free*, New York: New American Library, 1979.

Deming, W. E., *Out of Crisis*, Cambridge, MA: MIT-CAES, 1986.

Ermann, D., & Gabel, J., "Multi-Hospital Systems: Issues and Empirical Findings." *Health Affairs*, *3*(1), 50, 1984.

Farley, D. E., *Trends in Hospital Average Lengths of Stay, Casemix and Discharge Rates, 1980–1985* (Hospital Studies Program, Research Note 11). Washington DC: U.S. Department of Health and Human Services, 1988.

Freymann, J. G., *The American Health Care System: Its Genesis and Trajectory*. New York: Medcom Press, 1974.

Ginzberg, E., & Drennan, M. P., *The Health Sector: Its Significance for the Economy of New York City*. New York: Commonwealth Fund, 1985.

Hellerstein, D., "The Slow, Costly Death of Mrs. K." *Harpers*, pp. 84–89, March 1984.

Heyssel, R. M., Gaintner, R., Kues, I. W., Jones, A. A., & Lipstein S. H., "Decentralized Management in a Teaching Hospital: Ten Years Later at Johns Hopkins." *New England Journal of Medicine*, 310, 1477, 1984.

Hollowell, E., "No Insurance—No Privileges," *Legal Aspects of Medical Practice*, April 1978.

Hospitals, July 5, 1992, pp. 102–110.

Juran, J. M., Managerial Breakthrough. New York: McGraw-Hill, 1964.

Kovner, A. R., & Hattis, P. A., "Benefitting Communities," HMQ Fourth Quarter 1990, pp. 6–10.

McEachern, J. E., & Neuhauser, D., "The Continuous Improvement of Quality at The Hospital Corporation of America, *Health Matrix*, *7*(3), 5–11, 1987.

National Center for Health Statistics. *Health and Prevention Profile*. Washington, DC: U.S. Government Printing Office.

National Medical Enterprises, Inc., *Fact Book*, California: NME, 1992.

Rosenberg, C. E., *The Care of Strangers*, New York: Basic Books, 1987.

Shortell, S. M., "The Medical Staff of the Future: Replanting the Garden." *Frontiers of Health Services Management, 1*(3) 3, 1985.

Smith, D. B., & Kaluzny, A. D., *The White Labyrinth*, (2nd ed.). Ann Arbor, MI: Health Administration Press, 1986.

Smith, H. L., "Two Lines of Authority Are One Too Many." *Modern Hospital*, pp. 59–64, March 1955.

Smith, J., *"The Patient Focused Hospital*, Hospital Management International, 1990, pp. 185–187.

Southwick, A., *The Law of Hospital and Health Care Administration*. Ann Arbor, MI: Health Administration Press, 1978.

Starr, P., *The Social Transformation of American Medicine*. New York: Basic Books, 1982.

Stevens, R., *American Medicine and the Public Interest*. New Haven, CT: Yale University Press, 1971.

U.S. Bureau of the Census, Washington, DC: U.S. Government Printing Office, 1992.

8

Long-Term Care

Hila Richardson

The rapid growth of the elderly population and the increasing financial burden of long-term care on individuals and government have intensified the focus on access, cost, and quality of long-term care services. This chapter will describe the major institutional and community-based long-term care services, discuss the persistent issues of access, cost, and quality of those services and, finally, review the current and future policy developments that are being suggested to address them.

Definition and Overview of Long-Term Care

Long-term care is a range of health, personal care, social, and housing services provided to people who have lost or have never developed the capacity to care for themselves independently as a result of chronic illness or mental or physical disability. The level of assistance needed is on a continuum beginning with minimal help in performing basic activities in the home such as bathing, dressing, using the toilet, ambulation, help with shopping, meal preparation, transportation, house cleaning, and other activities important for self-sufficiency. On the other end of the continuum is complete dependency on nursing services in a nursing home for all basic activities, plus care for such needs as ventilator-assisted breathing and tube feedings. The assistance provided can be continuous or intermittent, but it is assumed that most people will usually need it with increasing intensity for years, often for the remainder of their lives (Kane & Kane, 1987; Kutza, 1981).

The essential element in defining the need for long-term care, therefore, is functional capacity. The level of mental and physical functioning varies enormously within age groups and chronic conditions such as diabetes, arthritis, or Alzheimer's disease. Therefore age or diagnosis cannot solely predict the amount of long-term care a person needs. Neither can the location of services nor the type of service determine the amount of long-term care services needed because people of all levels of dependency use nursing homes or receive rehabilitation in their homes.

A fact often overlooked is that people of all ages need long-term care services, although the elderly use them most frequently. Young people, including babies, can need long-term care services because of mental and physical limitations at birth, spinal cord or brain injury resulting from traumatic accidents, and chronic debilitating conditions such as multiple sclerosis. Increasingly, persons with AIDS or HIV illness rely on home health or nursing homes as new treatments are extending their lives.

Over 70% of chronically disabled people receive long-term care services in their homes from family members and friends (Soldo, 1984). When circumstances require more assistance than can be provided by this informal system, people can use the formal care system, which includes services such as home health, mental health programs, social services, transportation and, finally, institutional services in nursing homes, rehabilitation facilities, and various residential settings. However, these services can be expensive if purchased privately, and publicly funded programs have eligibility requirements that exclude many elderly.

The uncertainty in predicting the levels and types of long-term care services a person will need leads to uncertainties in planning for, budgeting for, or insuring against the demand for long-term care, making it a major health policy and financing issue. In the last 10 years it has gained even more attention as projected growth in the aging population has raised increasing concern about future demand and expenditures for long-term care.

The Elderly and the Need for Long-Term Care

In evaluating the elderly population's need for long-term care, surveys use measures of functional capacity called activities of daily living (ADLs) and instrumental activities of daily living (IADLs). The ADLs are a measure of a person's dependence on others for assistance with personal care functions (i.e., bathing, dressing, feeding oneself, toileting, and transferring from bed to chair). The IADLs measure a person's ability to perform household and social tasks such as preparing meals, shopping, housework, getting around the community, and managing money. Not all people with ADL or IADL limitations need assistance from another person, but can perform the task independently with aids such as canes, walkers, and adaptive devices for kitchens and bathrooms.

According to the 1987 National Medical Expenditure Survey (NMES) 3.6 million or 12.9% of the total persons living in the community over the age of 65 had difficulty with at least one ADL. Of this group, 17.5% had difficulty with at least one IADL task. The older the person was, the more likely they were to have limitations in one or more of both measures (Leon & Lair, 1990).

Accompanying the increase in dependency, there is strong evidence that use of acute-care services, physician services, and nursing home services increases steadily with age with a marked increase for hospital and nursing home services after 75 years. Those 85 and older have a threefold greater risk of losing their independence, seven times the chance of entering a nursing home, and two and one-half times the risk of dying, compared to persons 65 to 75 years of age (Soldo & Manton, 1985). Yet it should be noted that dependency increases gradually over a period of 15 to 20 years. Further, these studies show that even in the oldest age group, about 50% of the elderly still do not have difficulty performing these daily activities. Other studies have shown that a small group of elderly persons account for most of the use of health services among the elderly (Kane & Kane, 1987).

As the number of elderly people is expected to increase, so the number requiring high levels of assistance and health services is also expected to increase. This has been referred to as the demographic imperative for long-term care. It is based on the fact that for most of the twentieth century the elderly have increased far more rapidly than the rest of the population. At the beginning of the century, fewer than 1 in 10 Americans was 55 or over, and 1 in 25 was age 65 or over. By 1986 one in five Americans was at least 55 years old, and one in eight was at least 65 (U.S. Senate Special Committee on Aging, 1988).

The most important projection in terms of estimating the need for long-term care is the number of people surviving into the oldest age ranges. As Figure 8.1 shows, the percentage of persons over 75 years of age is expected to represent nearly 50% of all persons 65 years or older by the year 2000. By 2050, 55% of persons over 65 years of age will be 75 years or older. The percentage of the oldest elderly, those over 85 years, is projected to increase from 10% of those over 65 years in 1990 to 24% in 2050.

Although these numbers are striking, there is no agreement on how to translate them into increased need for long-term care services. There are many unknowns in predicting the influence of different life-styles and better medical management of chronic conditions such as arthritis, dementia, heart conditions, osteoporosis, and incontinence, all major contributors to dependency in the elderly. Nevertheless, there is agreement that the increase will occur and will have a major impact on the delivery of health services in this country.

Long-Term Care Services: Delivery and Financing

Informal Care System

Informal caregiving refers to unpaid care provided to an elderly person who has some degree of physical, mental, emotional, or economic impairment which limits independence and requires ongoing assistance. As stated earlier, Soldo (1984) estimated that over 70% of the care provided to elderly dependent persons in the

FIGURE 8.1   Persons Age 75 and Over and a Percentage of Persons Aged
65+, Actual and Projected, 1980–2050

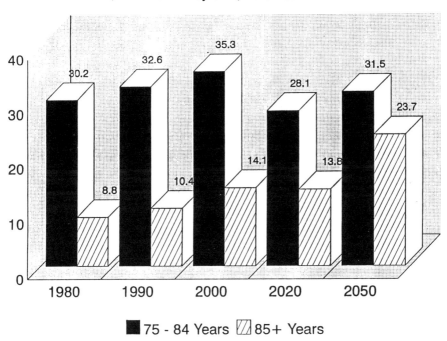

■ 75 - 84 Years ▨ 85+ Years

Source: U.S.Senate Special Committee on *Aging, Aging America: Trends and Projections*
1987–1988.

community comes from relatives, friends or neighbors, many of whom are elderly
themselves. According to a 1982 Informal Caregivers Survey of two million
caregivers providing unpaid assistance to 1.5 million impaired elderly, approximately 72% of the caregivers were female. Daughters were 29% and wives were
23% of the caregiving population. The average age of caregivers was 57 years
with one-quarter aged 65 to 74 and another 10% aged 75 or older (U.S. House of
Representatives Select Committee on Aging, 1987a).

Research has shown that when possible, elderly people turn to the informal
network for support first and most frequently. Only when the informal arrangements are not available or are inadequate do they seek help from formal organizations (Cantor, 1984). Moreover, when formal assistance is necessary, it does
not substitute for informal care but provides additional services, particularly those
requiring more technical and medical services beyond the ability of the informal
caregivers (Soldo, 1984).

The dependent elderly living in the community is estimated to be 4.9 to 5.2
million people, two-thirds of whom are women (General Accounting Office, 1988).

Therefore, informal caregivers play an important role in controlling the amount of long-term care services that would have to be purchased publicly or privately. As a result, programs to maintain the support from existing, informal caregiver arrangements have been gaining interest. These will be discussed later in the chapter.

Formal Care System

Nursing Homes. There were 19,100 nursing homes and related care homes and 1,624,200 nursing homes beds in the United States in 1985, the year of the last national survey. This number represents more than three times the number of community hospitals and double the number of community hospital beds. There has been a 22% increase in the number of nursing homes and a 38% increase in the number of beds since 1974 (Strahan, 1987). However, there is a recognized shortage of nursing home beds because the growth of the elderly population has outpaced the growth of beds. Projected nursing home demand indicates that based on current utilization rates of nursing home beds and population projections, there will be a need for 600,000 more beds in 2010 (Porter & Witek, 1991).

Over 75% of nursing homes are owned by proprietary organizations. Only 20% are owned by voluntary groups or hospitals, and 5% are government owned. Nursing homes have remained mostly small, with an average of 85 beds. Those owned by voluntary groups average 98 beds per facility, whereas the 1,000 public nursing homes had the largest average number of beds: 132 (Strahan, 1987).

Just over 50% of nursing homes are operated independently. There has been a significant increase in the number of nursing homes operated by what is referred to as a chain, usually a for-profit organization that operates a group of facilities. In 1977 nursing homes with chain affiliations were 28% of total homes, whereas in 1985 they were 41%.

Examples of the consolidation of chain ownership of nursing homes and beds are Beverly Enterprises, ARA, and Hillhaven, three of the largest chains. In 1973 they accounted for 2.2% of nursing home beds. Ten years later, they owned, managed, or leased 10% of the beds. Beverly alone controlled 40,000 beds in that year (Hawes & Phillips, 1986). This consolidation was largely accomplished by acquisition of existing homes. Since 1986, however, these major chains began to decrease their share of the nursing home market. For example, Beverly Enterprises announced plans to sell 170 facilities, or 15,000 to 20,000 beds, in 1988. Hillhaven also planned to sell about 30 homes (Mayer, 1988).

Until 1989 nursing homes were classified as either skilled nursing facilities (SNFs) for Medicare or Medicaid residents or intermediate care facilities (ICFs) for those covered by Medicaid. Each type of facility met distinct but overlapping conditions of participation to be certified to admit patients under the Medicare and Medicaid programs.

The SNFs were designated to provide a higher level of care to sicker patients and therefore required a licensed nurse on duty 24 hours a day and a registered nurse on day shifts. ICFs were considered to provide a lower level of care, more custodial than clinical, and were required to have a licensed nurse on duty only during the day. In practice, the distinctions between SNFs and ICFs always have been artificial because both types of facilities have served persons with a wide range of needs that often fluctuated between the definition of the two levels of care. The Nursing Home Reform Act, passed in 1987, ended the difference in staffing levels and mandated that ICFs provide the same range of services as SNFs. Since the statute has been fully implemented, nursing homes are often referred to as nursing facilities (NFs).

Although nursing home care is the service most closely associated with long-term care, only a small minority of the elderly are in nursing homes on any day. In 1985, of the 28.5 million persons over 65 years of age, 5%, or 1.3 million, lived in nursing homes (Hing, 1987). This proportion of the total elderly population residing in nursing homes has remained stable since 1973–1974, when the first National Nursing Home Survey (NNHS) was conducted (Hing, 1987).

However, 20% of the functionally dependent elderly people were in nursing homes in 1985. In fact dependency in ADLs is one of the major predictors of nursing home admission. Other predictors include age, diagnostic condition, living alone, marital status, race, income, and lack of social support (Kane & Kane, 1987).

Those in nursing homes were typically the older elderly with the larger group being 85 years and over (45%), followed by those aged 74 to 85 years (39%) and 65 to 74 years (16%). The rate of nursing home use increases with age with only 1% of persons between 65 to 74 years in nursing homes compared to 22% of those 85 years and older. It is also twice as likely for elderly females to be in nursing homes than it is for elderly males. Six percent of elderly females compared to 3% of elderly males were in nursing homes in 1985 (Hing, 1987). It has been projected that if past utilization patterns continue, over half of the women and almost one-third of the men who turned 65 in 1990 can be expected to use a nursing home sometime before they die (Murtaugh, Kemper & Spillman, 1990).

Elderly white people are more likely to use nursing homes than elderly who are black or of other races. This is particularly true if they are over 85 years of age. This can be the result of more substitution of informal care or from discriminating admission practices by nursing homes (Hing, 1987).

Given the age of nursing home residents, it is not surprising that they have high levels of functional dependency. Thirty percent of the residents required assistance in six ADLs and only 8% were independent in all six activities. The level of dependence increased with age and females were more dependent in ADLs than males. The functional dependency has been increasing in nursing residents and may be one of the major reasons why people enter a nursing home (Hing, 1987).

Another indication of the level of dependence is urinary and bowel incontinence and mental disorders of nursing home residents. Residents with one or more of these impairments, require high levels of assistance with ADLs and frequent supervision for problem behaviors. Over half of nursing home residents had difficulty controlling their bladder while for 43% bowel incontinence was a problem.

Nearly 60% of nursing home residents had some type of mental disorder, including dementia (28.7%), dementia combined with other mental disorder (13.7%) or only a mental disorder not accompanied by dementia (15.5%). In addition, slightly less than half of nursing home residents exhibited problem behavior such as wandering, yelling, and hurting themselves and others. More than two-thirds of residents had one or more psychiatric symptoms including depression, delusions, and hallucinations (Lair & Lefkowitz, 1990).

Overall, these data present a profile of the nursing home population of mentally and physically frail elderly with high levels of functional dependency. This reflects a population who requires intensive resources, particularly staffing to care for and supervise them. Given that 20% of nursing home residents could stay 5 years or more, the implication for cost and quality are enormous and require careful exploration to determine the appropriate role of nursing home care in the long-term care continuum of services (Lair & Lefkowitz, 1990).

Although 90% of nursing home residents fit the profile of frail elderly, the remaining 10% are under 65 years of age and have physical and mental disabilities that prevent them from living in the community due to limited resources or financing for their care. Within this age group, 4.7% are between the ages of 18 to 54 years and 5.6% are 55 to 64 years. In contrast to the typical nursing home resident, the number of men and women is about evenly distributed. Also, roughly 20% between the ages of 18 and 54 were black compared to 10.8% in ages 55 to 64 and 6.4% over 65 years. This may reflect the higher risk of both men and blacks for serious accidents resulting in spinal cord injury or head trauma. Also, this group may be institutionalized because Medicaid will not pay for their care in the community. More than 36% of nursing home residents between 18 and 54 years had disorders of the central nervous system such as multiple sclerosis, cerebral palsy, paralysis, and epilepsy. Although these disorders were common among the 55 to 64 age groups, the most prevalent conditions in this age group were psychoses and nonpsychotic mental disorders. This older group was also more likely than young ages to have diseases of aging such as ischemic heart disease and hypertension (Lair, 1992).

The number but not necessarily the proportion of younger nursing home residents is expected to grow because: (1) the disabled born during the baby boom of the 1940s and 1950s have aging parents who are dying or becoming too old to care for them; (2) medical technology can now keep people alive who are severely disabled at birth or experience traumatic injuries and who can require institutional long-term care for decades; (3) the individuals with HIV illness and AIDS will increasingly need long-term care as their life expectancy increases (Lair, 1992). This younger institutionalized population often requires very different activities and support services than the typical frail elderly resident of nursing homes. Age appropriate therapeutic recreation, flexibility in institutional routines such as getting up and going to bed, and more private space are among a few of the considerations that nursing home programs must adopt (Blustein, Schultz, Knickman, Kator, Richardson & McBride, 1992).

The financial burden of nursing home care is shared almost equally between Medicaid (47.4%) and individuals (43.1%) (see Figure 8.2). Private insurers and Medicare paid only a small percentage of nursing home care in 1991.

Hospital-Based Services. Because of the national decline in hospital occupancy, hospitals are looking for new services or conversions of existing facility space to more profitable uses than general acute care. The growing numbers of elderly in need of long-term care have become a primary target of hospital expansion. A 1985 survey found that 24% of hospitals owned SNFs, 12% owned intermediate care facilities, 33% provided home health services, and 14% provided homemaker services (Capitman et al., 1988). A survey by the American Hospital Association of more than 3,000 hospitals found that 15% planned to add long-term care beds in the future. Of this 15%, 61% planned to convert acute-care beds to skilled-nursing-care beds, and 29% planned to build new facilities (Pierce, 1987).

FIGURE 8.2 Distribution of Nursing Home Expenditures by Payer, 1991 (Total Expenditures = $59.9 Billion)

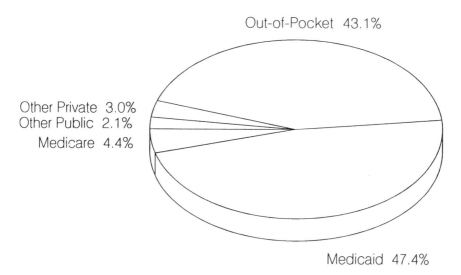

Source: Letsch, S. W., Lazenby, H. C., Levit, K. R., & Cowan, C. A., National Health Care Expenditures, 1991, *Health Care Financing Review*, 14(2), Winter 1992.

Another example of how hospitals provide long-term care is the swing-bed, a hospital bed that can be used interchangeably to provide acute, skilled, or intermediate care to patients. However, participation in swing-bed programs is currently limited to rural hospitals with fewer than 100 beds. To provide services, the hospitals must comply with most of the Medicare conditions of participation for nursing homes (Richardson & Kovner, 1987). In July 1986 there were 900 rural hospitals certified to provide swing-bed services (Shaughnessey, Schlenker & Hittle, 1987).

Home Care. Home care encompasses a broad array of health care and social services provided to individuals and their families in their home or other residential settings. Generally, home care is classified as services related to medical needs or personal care and social needs. The medically related services are often referred to as "home health care" and consists of home visits by health professionals only, i.e., nurses, physical therapists, occupational therapist, or professional plus a paraprofessional "home health aide" to provide assistance with ADLs. For medically related home health care, there must be a plan of care prescribed by a physician and the care provided in the home must be supervised by a professional, usually a nurse. Medically related services provided in the home include giving oral medications, injections, dressing changes and other nursing treatments, teaching the patient and family, and assistance with ADLs.

The personal care and social services are usually referred to broadly as "home care." These services include assistance with direct personal needs such as bathing, dressing, and grooming. These services are performed by a "personal care aide" or a "home health aide." In addition, this classification of services includes help with IADLs such as shopping, cooking, and cleaning, which are performed by "homemakers," "housekeepers," or personal care aides.

The National Association for Home Care (NAHC) has identified a total of 12,497 home care agencies in the US. These agencies include 6,129 Medicare-certified home health agencies, 1,110 certified hospices, and 5,258 noncertified home health agencies, home care aide organizations, and hospices that do not participate in Medicare. When Medicare included home health services, primarily short-term skilled-nursing and restorative therapy, as one of its covered services, the Medicare-certified home health agency grew very rapidly and became the major type of home care agency. In 1967, there were 1,753 Medicare-certified Home Health Agencies (CHHAs), in 1987 there were 5,785 CHHAs and in 1992 the number had risen to the high of 6,129. To become certified by Medicare, an agency has to meet the conditions of participation established by Medicare. This includes having certain policies, record-keeping practices, training requirements, utilization review, and quality assurance committees and maintaining Medicare eligibility requirements for serving patients.

As the numbers indicate, many home care agencies do not become Medicare-certified because they only target private pay clients, do not provide the services Medicare requires, or do not want to meet all the conditions of participation. The noncertified agencies can be licensed by the state, if the state has licensure requirements, or the agency can operate as a nonlicensed agency. As an example of the complexity and fragmentation of the home care system, a comparative study of formal home care providers in California showed that at least seven types of formal providers were found to deliver home care and related services: licensed-only, noncertified home health agencies, licensed and certified home health agencies, nurse' registries, employment agencies, unlicensed temporary personnel agencies, other unlicensed agencies, and unlicensed individual providers. These providers varied in services provided, sources of payment, payment arrangements, regulatory agencies and requirements, duration of care, supervision of care and utilization of services (Harrington & Grant, 1990).

The growth in the number of CHHAs has been accompanied by changes in the mix of organizations that own or sponsor them. As Table 8.1 shows, the Visiting Nurse Associations (VNAs) and the public agencies represented 90% of the CHHAs in 1967. There were no proprietary or private not-for-profit (PNP) agencies that year because an initial Medicare legislation prohibited the certification of agencies with that ownership. However, the prohibition was lifted in 1980 and the dramatic growth in the proprietary CHHAs can be seen. By 1987, proprietary CHHAs were 32% of all CHHAs. Also, the hospital-based CHHA experienced a rapid growth going from 7.6% in 1967 to 25% in 1987. This growth reflects both the influence of the implementation of the Diagnostic Related Group hospital reimbursement and the broadening of the home care benefit in the 1980s to encourage home health as an alternate to costly recuperative days in the hospital. In 1992, the proprietary and PNP agencies represented over 40% of the CHHAs with the hospital-based agencies, many of who also have proprietary and PNP ownership, representing slightly less than 30%. The VNAs and the public agencies stabilized at 10% and 19%, respectively after experiencing a dramatic decrease between 1967 and 1987.

TABLE 8.1 Medicare-Certified Home Health Agencies, by Ownership, 1967, 1987, & 1992

Auspice	1967 No.	1967 %	1987 No.	1987 %	1992 No.	1992 %
VNA	642	36.6%	551	9.5%	604	9.9%
Public	939	53.6	1,073	18.5	1,149	18.7
Proprietary	0	0.0	1,846	31.9	1,953	31.9
PNP	0	0.0	766	13.2	594	9.7
Hospital-based	133	7.6	1,439	24.9	1,688	27.5
Other	39	2.2	110	1.9	141	2.3
Totals	1,753	100.0%	5,785	100.0%	6,129	100.0%

Source: National Association for Home Care, *Basic Statistics About Home Care*, 1992.

In addition to the array of formal direct providers of home care services, the home care sector now includes the home medical equipment and home infusion therapy industries. Advancements in technology for the home have made it possible to provide in-home therapies that previously could be provided only in the hospital (e.g., intravenous therapy, respirators, and parenteral nutrition). This sector has experienced a high growth rate with estimated expenditures for infusion therapies, as an example, growing from $684 million in 1986 to almost $3 billion in 1992 (National Association for Home Care, 1993).

Nearly 6 million people or 2.5% of the civilian noninstitutionalized population received some type of home health services in 1987 (Altman & Walden, 1993). As Table 8.2 shows, just over 50% of those receiving services were ages 65 and older with an increasing use of services with age. For example, 31% of those 85 and older received home health services while only 7% of those between the ages of 65 to 74 received services. What is most striking about the data is that persons under 40 years of age received almost 30% of the home health visits received in 1987. Those over 65 years of age received 40% of the visits. This clearly shows that home health is not only a service for the elderly but is used by all age groups.

Women used services slightly more than men, but there was no difference in use between whites, blacks, or Hispanics according to the 1987 National Medical Expenditure Survey (NMES). However, different levels of limitations in function were associated with increases in the percentage of the population using home health services (Table 8.2). Only 1.2% of those without ADL/IADL limitations used home health services. In contrast to this small use rate is the 23% with 1 to 2 ADL limitations and 41% with 3 or more ADL limitations. It should be noted, that nearly 50% of those receiving home health services were not limited in their ADL/IADL limitation. Any restrictions of benefits based on ADL/IADL need would exclude this group from services.

A total of $11.6 billion was spent on all formal home health services in 1987 (Altman & Walden, 1993). The mean annual expense per person in that year was $1,967 with the annual expenditures increasing with age. For those 85 years and older the average spent was $3,292 per person while 65 to 74 years of age spent an average of $2,014. Of the total expenditure of more than $11 billion, 43% was paid out of pocket by individuals (Figure 8.3). Medicaid paid 24.5%, Medicare 19.2 % for a total of public payments of 43.7%. Private insurance paid only 10.7% of annual home health expenditures. The other programs that pay for some home health services are the Older Americans Act, Title XX of the Social Services Block Grants, the Veterans Administration, and CHAMPUS.

Medicare is the major public payer for home care, but as previously stated, it pays for only short-term, post-acute care. In 1991, Medicare home health expenditures were $5.5 billion, accounting for just over half of a total of $9.6 billion of publicly funded home health care. Although still only 4.8% of total spending for home health, Medicare's share has been steadily increasing (National Association for Home Care, 1993)

TABLE 8.2 Use of Home Health Services: Percentage of Persons Receiving Home Health Visits and the Percentage of Home Health Visits Received by Age and Functional Limitation

Population characteristic	Total U.S. population (in thousands)	Percent receiving at least 1 home visit	Number receiving at least 1 home visit	Percent of home health visits received
Total	239,393	2.5	5,985	
Age in years				
Under 40	153,128	1.1	1,684	28
Under 6	24,838	2.5	621	10
6–17	41,950	0.6	252	4
18–39	84,340	1.0	863	14
40–64	59,744	2.0	1,195	20
65–74	16,378	7.1	1,163	20
75–84	8,111	14.5	1,176	20
85 and over	2,032	30.9	628	11
ADL/IADL difficulties				
None	227,004	1.2	2,724	46
IADL difficulties only	4,910	17.7	869	15
1–2 ADL"	4,625	22.9	1,059	18
3 or more ADL difficulties	2,854	41.4	1,182	20

Source: Altman, B. M. and Walden, D. C. *Home Health Care: Use Expenditures, and Sources of Payment,* (AHCPR Pub. No. 93-0040) National Medical Expenditure Survey Research Finding 15, Agency on Health Policy and Research, Rockville, MD, Public Health Service, 1993.

FIGURE 8.3   Sources of Payment for Home Health Care, 1987

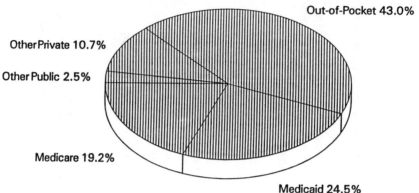

Out-of-Pocket 43.0%

OtherPrivate 10.7%

Other Public 2.5%

Medicare 19.2%

Medicaid 24.5%

Source: Altman, B., and Walden, D., *Home Health Care: Use Expenditures and Sources of Payment*, Agency for Health Care Policy Research (AHCPR Pub. No 93-0040) Public Health Service, Rockville, MD, 1993.

In contrast to Medicare policies, Medicaid benefits for home health services can be extensive, depending on the state. They can include services by nurses, home health aides, social workers, housekeepers, and various therapists. Most states expanded their home health and community-based services under Section 2176 waivers (Home and Community Based Waiver Program) in the 1981 Omnibus Reconciliation Act. In 1991, $4.1 billion of the $9.6 billion in public funds expended for home health were from the Medicaid program. Although home health programs have increased as a proportion of total Medicaid spending, they remain a small percentage (4.3%) of total Medicaid spending in 1991 (National Association for Home Care, 1993).

Community-Based Services.   Services based in the community are provided through voluntary, public, or proprietary organizations and include adult day care, hospice, respite, congregate meals, transportation, and case management programs. These services are supported by a combination of funds from Medicare, Medicaid, Title III of the Older Americans Act, and other federal, state, and local social services programs. The extent of the services provided and the eligibility requirements vary by funding source and by state and locality.

Through the social services block grant program, states may provide homemaker, home health aide, chore, adult day care, and adult foster care services. Under Title III of the Older Americans Act, established in 1965, available services include transportation, homemakers, and chore and home health aide services. In 1987 the Administration on Aging estimated that the number of client contacts for these services ranged from 6.3 million for transportation to almost 1 million for homemaker and home health aide services. Amendments to the Older Americans Act in 1987 authorized funds for nonmedical in-home services that included visiting and telephone reassurance, chore maintenance, and in-home respite and adult day care respite for families (General Accounting Office, 1988).

Adult Day Care Services. Adult day care is a program that offers a wide range of health and social services to the elderly during the day and out of the home. Adult day care services are usually targeted to elderly in families where the caregivers work or to elderly living alone. Their goal is to delay or prevent institutionalization and provide respite for the caregiver. The services offered follow a medical or social model. The social model emphasizes social and recreational activities, crafts, discussion groups, and exercise. The medical model incorporates more rehabilitation, physical and mental assessment, nursing and medical care.

Data on adult day care programs are still limited, but a survey done by the National Council on Aging found that there were about 1,200 adult day care centers in 1983. Programs were most commonly sponsored by nonprofit human services organizations, including government. Programs served an average of 19 clients per day, the typical participant being a 73-year-old female who lives with a spouse, relative, or friends (Von Behren, 1986).

Most adult day care programs surveyed offered social services, crafts, current events discussions, family counseling, reminiscence therapy, nursing assessment, physical exercise, ADL rehabilitation, psychiatric assessment, and medical care. The average daily fees charged were just over $20. Forty-three percent of the participants were Medicaid-eligible.

States finance adult day services with Medicaid funds and Social Security block grants. Medicare does not cover adult day care. Most elderly people and their families pay for adult day care out of pocket.

There is conflicting evidence about the benefits of adult day care programs for clients. Some studies have shown improvement in mental and physical functioning of adult day care clients that delays nursing home admission, whereas others have concluded it does not have that effect (Kane & Kane, 1987). The conflicting evidence may be a result of the programs themselves, which tend not to be targeted to the highest-risk population groups or are not well integrated with rehabilitation services and medical supervision that might improve or maintain functioning. Adult day care programs may not appeal to the elderly unless they or their caregivers feel they are close to institutionalization. In such cases it may be a last attempt to forestall admission to a nursing home. Otherwise, the elderly may prefer other, less institutional sources of social and recreational activities, like senior centers and social clubs.

Respite Services. Respite services provide a temporary respite, or break, for the caregivers of the frail elderly or disabled chronically ill. There is no uniform definition of respite care. The services can be provided in or out of the person's home. In-home respite provides temporary homemaker, chore, or home health services. Out-of-home care includes adult day care and temporary stays in nursing homes, hospitals, group homes, or foster care homes. The type and scope of services and eligibility for services vary considerably among states (Kane & Kane, 1987; Meltzer, 1982). States started using respite services for developmentally disabled and mentally retarded children in the 1960s. Research had shown that the ability to free the parents to care for nondisabled family members, including themselves, reduced their level of stress, anxiety, and isolation (Meltzer, 1982). The application of the concept to the elderly grew out of a combination of increasing interest in the role of the informal caregiver and the cost-containment effort to reduce expenditures of institutionalization.

Respite care may be paid for by Medicaid, a social services block grant, Older Americans Act funds, state general revenues, or privately. Medicaid rules require that respite care be provided only to elderly at risk of institutionalization. Some states require an assessment of functional limitations for admission to respite services (Pierce, 1987). With the passage of the Medicare Catastrophic Coverage Act in 1988, Medicare coverage was extended to respite services. The new benefit paid for the temporary services of a home health aide to provide respite for a spouse, relative, or friend caring for a Medicare beneficiary who cannot be left alone. This benefit was lost when the Act was repealed in 1989.

Few studies have been done to evaluate how respite care benefits the patient. One study of a group of Alzheimer's disease patients found that a 2-week in-hospital respite program had little effect on the patient's cognitive status and level of functioning. The changes, both positive and negative, that did occur depended on the patient's level of functioning on admission (Seltzer et al., 1988)

An earlier study of a short-term respite program in nursing homes showed an unexpectedly high rate of institutionalization (12%) of the respite population within 1 month of use of respite services. Meltzer (1982) identified two possible explanations: (1) the use of respite might have been one last attempt to keep the patient with the family, suggesting that the institutionalization rate might have been even higher without respite; and (2) the respite experience reduced the family's resistance to institutional placement.

All in all, little is known about the respite concept. Research has not supported or refuted the hypothesis that respite care avoids institutionalization and reduces costs, nor has it demonstrated how services should be organized and provided to ensure a positive outcome for the patient and the caregiver.

Hospice Services. Hospice services are provided to the terminally ill and their families. Hospice is based on a philosophy of care imported from England and Canada, that during the course of terminal illness the patient should be able to live life as fully and comfortably as possible. In the hospice approach, the family is the unit of treatment. An interdisciplinary team provides medical, nursing, psychological, therapeutic, pharmacological, and spiritual support during the final stages of illness, at the time of death, and during bereavement. The main goals are to control pain, maintain independence, and minimize the stress and trauma of death.

Most patients who need hospice care are elderly persons with cancer. More than 75% of hospice patients are over 65 years of age. The pool of younger patients, however, is growing due to the needs of persons with acquired immune deficiency syndrome (AIDS). The palliative care and emotional support in a hospice, as well as less expensive care, have been accepted as a humane way to treat AIDS patients (Strahan, 1987).

Increased federal and private insurance have spurred a boom in hospice care. In 1983, Medicare added hospice benefits and the number of programs increased from 516 in 1983 to 1,000 in 1992. The majority of hospices (65%) participate in the Medicare program (Strahan, 1987). The nonparticipating hospices either cannot meet Medicare standards or do not apply for certification because of regulatory or financial provisions that discourage participation in Medicare (General Accounting Office, 1989).

The funding for hospice under Medicare strongly reinforces the intent to use hospice as a cost-saving measure. For example, it is required that for at least 80% of the days in a hospice program, the patient is not in an inpatient setting like a hospital or nursing home. Also, the patient must waive other types of acute care, the patient's doctor must certify that life expectancy is 6 months or less, and 5% of services have to be furnished by volunteers in the patient's home with documentation of the cost savings from volunteers' services.

Despite these restrictions, the Medicare hospice benefits cover a comprehensive array of medical, nursing, and rehabilitation services in addition to medical appliances and supplies. There is a small coinsurance required for drugs. Inpatient respite care is provided for up to 5 consecutive days, and bereavement counseling is required but not reimbursed. To encourage the patient to remain in the home during crisis, Medicare will cover nurses, nurse's aides, and homemakers 24 hours per day. Reimbursement for hospice care was limited to a lifetime benefit of 210 days until 1989 coverage was allowed to continue if the beneficiary is recertified as terminally ill by an attending physician or hospice director (General Accounting Office, 1989).

Hospice services have gained acceptance as an alternative to hospital care for the terminally ill. It is likely that hospices will continue to grow because of their philosophy toward caring for those at end of life and because services have been determined to be less expensive than those provided to patients in hospitals.

Case-Management Programs

Generically, case management refers to a method of linking, managing, or coordinating services to meet client needs and typically includes client assessment, service provision and follow-up (Zawadski & Eng, 1988). Case management demonstrations grew out of a concern about the cost of long-term care services, particularly nursing home care. Their goal was to reduce public costs through substitution of community care for nursing home and hospital services.

Case management of community-based services was authorized for Medicaid reimbursement under Section 2176 of the Home and Community Based Waiver Program of 1981. Today many states have assigned case management activities to agencies like the Department of Social Services, Area Agencies on Aging, or Health Department special units. Also, case management for high-cost patients is offered by virtually all private insurers and many health management firms (Henderson, Sonder, Bergman & Collard, 1988).

Zawadski and Eng (1988), in their review of eight demonstrations, differentiated the following three models of case management:

1. The prior authorization screening model, in which a health professional assesses the individuals considering institutional placement, determines whether alternative community services could be provided, and arranges for those services. Wisconsin has reported one of the most successful preadmission screening programs by assessing only those who were actually nursing home applicants, rather than all elderly at a high functional impairment level (Lindberg & Monson, 1989).
2. The brokerage model, wherein a health professional independently assesses an impaired individual, arranges services through other providers, and regularly reassesses and follows the client. This is the model used by most private insurers.
3. The consolidated model, in which a multidisciplinary team assesses needs and provides the services directly or under contract with other providers (e.g., hospitals, lab, home health agencies). The two most famous examples of this model are the Social Health Maintenance Organizations (SHMOs) and the On Lok Senior Health Services in San Francisco.

SHMOs are community-based programs that arrange for the provision of all primary, acute, and long-term care services, including personal care and social services, for a fixed monthly prepaid fee. The sponsoring agency is therefore financially "at risk" and uses case-management services to control the use of hospital and nursing home care while providing expanded home and support services. A federal demonstration of this concept is underway in four cities, serving about 15,000 elderly persons (Leutz et al., 1988).

On Lok Senior Health Services is an extremely integrated model of acute and long-term care case management; the primary medical care, hospital care, nursing home care, home health and respite services are provided by On Lok multidisciplinary staff teams, which therefore maintain complete control over all of the services used. On Lok receives prospective monthly payments from Medicare, Medicaid, and individuals for whom it assumes full financial responsibility for the total health care of 300 physically and mentally frail elderly. A per diem fee is negotiated for hospital and nursing home services. A central feature of the program is a day health center linked to home health and in-home supports. Data from the program show a significant reduction in high-cost hospital and nursing home services and an increase in community services, particularly in-home personal care and support services (Zawadski & Eng, 1988).

Housing Services for Elderly People

Assisted Living

Housing is increasingly recognized as playing a significant role in the continuum of long-term care services. For example, the availability of affordable and appropriate housing for elderly people, particularly for those who are physically and mentally impaired, determines the need for institutional long-term care services in the community. Increasing numbers of disabled older people now live in assisted living settings where they receive individualized personal care in homelike accommodations that offer privacy, space, and dignity.

Assisted living is generally defined as any group or residential setting (licensed or unlicensed) providing personal care and meeting unscheduled needs for older, disabled persons. Assisted living may be board and care homes with additional services, residential units owned by and adjacent to nursing homes, congregate housing settings that have added services, housing built for the purpose of assisted living or Continuing Care Retirement Communities (CCRCs). Ownership may be either nonprofit or for-profit with the latter including chains of varying sizes.

Assisted living varies across the states in sponsorship, size, physical environments, target populations, admission and retention practices and service and staffing requirements. The variation is in part a response to state regulations with some states having stricter limits on admission and retention than others, and states using a variety of indirect funding mechanisms that can hinder the development of assisted living. Oregon is the one state that has deliberately encouraged the expansion of assisted living as an alternative to nursing homes. Regulations for licensing assisted living were developed in 1989 and a Medicaid waiver was obtained to cover assisted living for Medicaid recipients who are nursing home certifiable. The Oregon model requires high environmental standards for private rooms, kitchenettes, and showers but permits flexible staffing. This allows programs to keep their costs at 80% of nursing homes costs (Kane & Wilson, 1993).

The most common assisted living options are as follows.

Congregate Living. This includes a variety of group-living and supportive service arrangements. Congregate housing generally occurs in multi-unit apartment complexes. Residents usually can walk and eat independently. They may need assistance with housekeeping and personal care, and they have the option to have meal services. Congregate housing programs are operated by communities and public service agencies. Various efforts have been made to add services to congregate housing to meet the needs of residents as they "age in place" and delay their placement in nursing homes.

Board-and-Care Homes. This is a broad category of housing that covers adult foster care homes, sheltered care facilities, halfway houses, and adult homes. They provide rooms, meals, help with ADLs, and some degree of protective oversight. Depending on the state, services may include supervising the use of medications by residents and linking residents to community services. A nationwide survey in 1987 reported approximately 41,000 licensed homes with about 563,000 beds (General Accounting Office, 1989b). Data are not available on unlicensed homes. The residents pay for services themselves or receive Supplementary Security Income (SSI) to help pay for the facility (Kane & Kane, 1987). Board-and-care residents are both elderly people who need assistance with dressing and bathing due to physical and mental impairment and younger people who have mental impairment and cannot function without supervision. However, some residential settings do not admit people who use wheelchairs, are incontinent, cannot transfer, or have cognitive impairments. Also, if people develop these disabilities they may have to be transferred to another setting.

Continuing Care Communities (CCRCs). CCRCs have three levels of living: independent, assisted, and nursing home care. As of 1986, 100,000 to 200,000 (less than 1%) of elderly people lived in about 700 CCRCs. There are predictions that by 1999 there will be 1,500 CCRCs with nearly 450,000 elderly residents. However, the high costs of these communities make them accessible to only a small proportion of the elderly. In 1989, only 13% of people over 75 years of age, the typical age for entering a community, had sufficient income and assets to pay the entrance fee and monthly charge (General Accounting Office, 1988). There is a large range in entrance fees and monthly charges, depending on the services contracted. The median entry fee for a one-bedroom apartment was $49,927, and median monthly fees were $756 a person in 1987 dollars. The entry and monthly fees for a two-bedroom unit were $65,000 and $800, respectively, in the same year. Entry fees can range as high as $150,000. Two-thirds of the CCRCs provide some level of long-term care services, including nursing home care. The others charge fees for these services (Cohen, 1988).

Other Housing Options

Following are other housing programs and resources available to the elderly.

Federal Housing. Federal subsidy has stimulated the building of approximately 1.5 million units of housing for elderly residents who meet income and age requirements. Recently, the issue of the elderly "aging in place" in subsidized housing has expanded support services for tenants to maintain them in their homes. These services include meals programs, homemakers, laundry service, on-site medical personnel, and transportation. The Robert Wood Johnson Foundation, for example, has awarded grants to 10 state housing financing agencies to develop programs to serve the needs of their elderly tenants ("Redefining Elderly Housing").

Home Equity Conversion. These programs allow elderly home owners to convert part of their home equity into cash without having to leave their homes and to be able to live in them until they die. The overall purpose is to provide cash for the 75% of the elderly who are homeowners to purchase long-term services, particularly in-home services and long-term care insurance. However, Scholen (1984) has identified the limitations of the concept: (1) the high cost of care relative to life expectancy and home value; (2) the reluctance of elderly people to sell their homes, their most valuable asset and one that represents their lifetime of labor and their independence; and (3) the complexity of the home equity conversion plans. As a result, the market is expected to be small and to develop slowly. By 1987, only 2,000 home equity conversions had been completed throughout the nation (Rivlin & Wiener, 1988).

ECHO Housing. Elder Cottage Housing Opportunity (ECHO), often referred to as "granny flats" are small, freestanding, and removable units that can be located on the property of adult children to ensure accessibility of informal caregivers. There are no national data on the extent of their use. Thus far, their development seems to be hindered by zoning laws and concerns about loss in property values (Kane & Kane, 1987).

Home Maintenance. These programs help poor elderly home owners with repairs (winterization, painting, plumbing, plastering, etc.) that will assist them in living independently in the homes. The programs are financed by both public (Community Development Block Grant, Title III of Older Americans Act, Title XX of Social Security Act) and private community organizations. National data are not available on these programs.

Shared Housing. This is a living arrangement in which two or more unrelated individuals share a house or an apartment. Examples of shared housing range from elderly people renting spare rooms to state agency-sponsored homes with 4 to 10 residents. In 1986, 670,000 elderly people shared housing with nonrelatives, a 35% increase in the last decade (Pierce, 1987).

Issues in Long-Term Care

There is increasing concern that these existing long-term care services will not be available, affordable, or of adequate quality to meet the needs of the growing number of elderly people. This section will discuss the basis for these concerns by describing the access, cost, and quality problems in long-term care.

Access: Problems in Supply and Eligibility

Access to long-term care service depends on the supply of services relative to the need or demand for them and on the ability to reach services by overcoming financial, transportation, or geographic barriers.

Supply. Nationally, the supply of nursing home beds has not kept pace with the growth in the elderly population (Swan, Harrington & Grant, 1988). There is an estimated national shortage as high as 600,000 beds (Porter & Witek, 1991). For every person in a nursing home, there may be as many as two people not in nursing homes who are equally debilitated (USDHHS, 1987). Most states have restricted the supply of nursing home beds, to control Medicaid expenditures, by using the Certificate of Need (CON) regulations. By 1980, all but three states had CON laws for nursing, home expansion (Kane & Kane, 1987).

The availability of nursing home care is not equally distributed across the nation. The number of nursing home beds per 1,000 of the elderly population ranges from 22 in Florida to 96 in Wisconsin (USDHHS, 1987). There is no apparent correlation between the size of the elderly population and the supply of nursing home beds. Neither is there a correlation between the ratio of beds per 1,000 elderly population and the occupancy rate of nursing homes (USDHHS, 1987). For example, nursing home occupancy rates average 91% but can be as low as 70% and the nursing homes with low occupancy rates are not always in areas where there are more beds per elderly population unit. Such variation in supply affects the use of nursing homes even for elderly people with similar needs. A study of very dependent elderly over 75 years of age, unmarried and with low incomes, showed there was a greater likelihood they would be in nursing homes in the states with the largest number of nursing home beds per 1,000 elderly people (Scanlon, 1988). The findings of the study suggest that unmet needs may exist in those states with a low ratio of nursing home beds.

The access barriers created by the shortage of nursing home beds has made admission to nursing homes particularly difficult for the elderly poor who are very sick. Since nursing home administrators try to achieve a resident mix in their facility that optimizes their reimbursement (Institute of Medicine, 1986; Scanlon, 1980), a shortage of nursing home beds allows them to be more selective in their admissions, accepting more profitable patients—those who are private-pay (and pay higher rates) or who are less sick and require less nursing care. Research has shown that patients who have labor-intensive needs such as tube feedings, those who require assistance with most ADLS, and those with mental and behavioral problems are the most likely to wait for nursing home placement (General Accounting Office, 1990).

Medicaid recipients have more trouble getting into nursing homes than those who pay privately according to a study by the General Accounting Office of access to nursing homes by Medicaid recipients in nine states. The types of Medicaid recipients facing the most difficulty in access to nursing homes varies depending on the difference between the State's Medicaid and private payment rates and the extent to which Medicaid rates are adjusted based on care needs (General Accounting Office, 1990).

When states have narrowed or eliminated the difference between the Medicaid and private-pay rates or based the Medicaid rate on the care needs of nursing home residents, Medicaid recipients appear to have improved access. Requiring equal rates for Medicaid recipients and private-payers eliminates the financial incentive for nursing homes to select private pay residents. Increasing the Medicaid rate without adjusting for patient care needs increases the incentive to select Medicaid recipients who are less expensive to care for, those needing lighter care. Basing Medicaid nursing homes rates on care needs improves access for those with heavier care needs, but unless the needs-based rate is high enough, those with the heaviest needs continue to experience access problems.

Although changing nursing home rates can increase or decrease access to Medicaid recipients, it also increases or decreases the amount of money a state spends on nursing home services. Therefore, a state's financial condition may influence its willingness to increase access to nursing home care. Some states have attempted to ease the access problem through regulatory reform by requiring nursing homes to admit patients on a first-come, first-serve basis regardless of payment source for each admission or until a certain Medicaid census is achieved in the nursing home. There is disagreement over the appropriateness and effectiveness of these approaches and little data has been available to prove either side of the arguments (General Accounting Office, 1990).

Unless states are willing to provide sufficient resources to meet all the need for nursing home beds or appropriate community-based services, payment reforms will only shift the incentives from one patient group to another moving different groups to the top or bottom of providers' lists, depending on the incentive. There also is evidence to suggest that there are unmet needs for services in the community, including home health. The 1982 National Long-term Care Survey showed that 40% or 3.2 million elderly with one or more ADL or IADL dependency were not receiving all the help they needed. Some needs may not be met because home health nurses, aides, homemakers, and other personnel may not be available due to geographic location of the person or the regulatory or financial requirements of the state or locality impede the development of services (General Accounting Office, 1988).

Finally, the inadequate supply of long-term care services extends to housing. There is a widely recognized shortage of federally subsidized housing for elderly households. The decline in funding for new units of federal housing during the 1980s has left many elderly who need this housing unable to obtain it. For example, the ratio of elderly on waiting lists for Section 202 housing to the annual vacancies was 8:1 across the country. Of those on a waiting list, one-third had been on less than a year while 37% had been on a waiting list longer than 2 years (General Accounting Office, 1992a). In addition, there are indicators that board-and-care homes are closing because the costs of operations are exceeding the SSI benefits and payments by the state social service agency (General Accounting Office, 1989).

Eligibility Barriers. In addition to access barriers created by shortages of resources, eligibility and service restrictions for Medicare and Medicaid programs, described earlier, prevent many elderly people from obtaining needed services that are available. Also, the social services block grants, Title III of the Older Americans Act, and Title XX of the Social Security Act, which fund community-based services have limited funding and eligibility requirements. These eligibility restrictions not only create many "cracks" for people to fall through in qualifying for services, they also cause confusion about what services are available. For example, an elderly person may know there is a daycare program available but may not know that it provides transportation. Lack of information about programs can also be a barrier to access. Because of these restrictions, available data show that few elderly people receive community-based services compared to the total number of dependent elderly in the community (General Accounting Office, 1988).

Financing Issues: Private and Public Responsibility

The major financing issue in long-term care is what should be the distribution of public versus private responsibility in paying for services. On the public side, federal expenditures for health care and social programs for the elderly as a proportion of all spending on the elderly (retirement income, disability, housing program, etc.) have increased from 6% in 1960, before Medicare and Medicaid, to close to 30% in 1986 (U.S. Senate Special Committee on Aging, 1986). Expenditures for these programs represented about 53% of the $45 billion spent on long-term care services for the elderly in 1985. However, the remaining 47% was paid for privately, leaving the elderly and their families paying out of pocket for almost half (44%) of all long-term care expenditures. The Congressional Budget Office has projected that long-term care expenditures could increase between 50% and 200% from 1985 to 2000 (General Accounting Office, 1988).

The public programs have not assumed a greater proportion of long-term care costs because of limitation in eligibility and benefits. Medicare was designed to finance medical expenses associated with acute and post-acute restorative care for the aged and disabled. It does not cover nursing homes stays beyond 150 days annually, and home health for those who do not require skilled level of nursing care. Medigap, which are private insurance policies purchased by the elderly to fill the gaps in Medicare coverage, cover deductibles, co-payments, outpatient drugs, etc., but do not finance extended long-term care.

Medicaid, a federal/state program of medical assistance, covers long-term care for certain categories of poor people. Medicaid eligibility, however, requires that individuals be impoverished before benefits begin. Through a process called "spend down" the elderly use their income and assets until they meet state income eligibility requirements for Medicaid. Given that nursing homes average more than $2,000 per month or $25,000 to $30,000 a year, many elderly persons can meet the income requirements as soon as they begin to incur nursing homes expenses. For example, a study of nursing home residents in 1987 showed that 12.7% had spent-down from private-pay to Medicaid. Half of the residents spent down within 6 months of admission and about three-quarters within 2 years. Other estimates of spend-down rates have ranged from 14% to 25% of elderly nursing home residents (Short, Kemper, Cornelius & Walden, 1992).

It is not surprising, therefore, that many elderly who need community or home-based services over years or who must enter a nursing home face impoverishment within only weeks. For example, those over 65 who are living alone and have an annual income between $9,700 and $15,000 would be impoverished after only 17 weeks in a nursing home with an annual average cost of $22,000. If their annual income is between $6,000 and $10,000, it would take only 6 weeks on average in a nursing home for an elderly person to become impoverished and dependent on Medicaid. These are elderly people who otherwise would not qualify for any form of public assistance (U.S. House Committee on Aging, 1987b). As Vladeck (1983) has stated, "Medicaid-reimbursed nursing home services have thus become the largest 'welfare' benefit available to formerly middle-class individuals and their families" (p. 360).

A series of proposals to alter public financing of nursing home care received considerable attention in the early 1990s. They offered universal entitlement to either the front-end or back-end of nursing home stays. These proposals would have shifted some nursing home costs both from individuals and state Medicaid programs. However, the budgetary implications kept the proposals from advancing through the legislative process during an era of federal budget constraints.

In order to defray this personal burden without increasing public expenditures, private long-term care insurance has been proposed. Although long-term care insurance has been available since the late 1970s, only a few companies offered long-term care coverage before 1986, when approximately 125,000 policies were in force (General Accounting Office, 1988). By 1990, almost 2 million policies had been sold with over 125 insurance companies marketing the policies. However, only 4% of the elderly population had purchased a policy in that year. If growth continues at 15% to 20% per year, less that 20% (5 to 6 million) of the elderly will have policies by the year 2000 (Cohen, Kumar, & Wallack, 1993).

A recent study of over 6,000 elderly long-term care insurance purchasers shows that the typical policy sold costs $102 per month, covers 5 years of nursing home care, and pays $69 per day in benefits (Cohen, Kumar, & Wallack, 1993). Assuming the premium remains the same for the average policy, a 65-year-old purchasing the policy would pay $1,224 annually or have paid $12,240 by the age of 75 and $24,480 by the age of 85. A study examining the ability of older people to purchase long-term care insurance by Families USA Foundation and the United Seniors Health Cooperative found that 84% of people between the ages of 65 and 79 could not afford to pay the average cost of basic long-term care insurance policies from nine leading companies (General Accounting Office, 1988).

The expense of premiums is leading to a high percentage of policyholders letting their policies lapse before they receive any covered services. Insurers report that about 20% of long-term care insurance policies are expected to lapse during the first year of policy ownership. The coverage projected lapse rate within the 5 years of policy ownership was 50% for 5 large insurance companies. The General Accounting Office, which conducted the study concluded: "By the time policyholders may need nursing home benefits, many will have let their policies lapse and will no longer have their LTC coverage" (General Accounting Office, 1988).

Another major drawback in private long-term care insurance is that most policies pay a fixed benefit—ranging from $25 to $100—that is not adjusted for inflation. In each year after the purchase of the policy, the benefit will pay for a smaller part of the actual cost of care. Furthermore, there are major differences in the definition of covered nursing facilities, length of time benefits are paid, coverage, and eligibility for benefits.

An analysis of long-term care insurance options by Rivlin and Weiner (1988) found the most optimistic projection to be that only one-quarter to one-half of the elderly will be able to purchase or want to purchase policies by 2,018. There will continue to be a need for public financing to pay for most long-term care, particularly for the low- and middle-income elderly despite the increased availability of private policies.

Quality of Long-Term Care Services

Since most long-term care is provided by family and friends in the privacy of homes, studies related to the quality of long-term care services have historically centered on nursing homes. The nursing home sector has continually been plagued by scandals related to physical danger, filthy conditions, patient abuse, and negligence (Vladeck, 1980). Since 1974 the U.S. Senate Special Committee on Aging has issued two reports documenting the continued existence of these conditions. The most recent report in 1986, found that there had been an increase in violations of major conditions of participation, including a 75% increase in failure to provide physician supervision and a 61% increase in failure to provide 24-hour nursing care (U.S. Senate Special Committee on Aging, 1986).

The committee report and others have blamed the federal nursing home survey and certification regulations and enforcement mechanisms. A 2-year, $1.5 million study of the nursing home regulatory system by the Institute of Medicine (IOM) of the National Academy of Sciences (1986) found the major problem with the current survey and certification system was that it relied on a facility's ability to provide care, not whether the care is actually being delivered. A common example is that the survey process is mainly concerned about the facility having a dietitian, not how the food tastes or even if the patient is given the needed assistance to eat the food near the time it is served. The IOM report called for stronger regulations focused on patient outcomes determined through observation and direct contact with patients.

As a result of this study, a number of nursing home reforms were passed in the Omnibus Reconciliation Act of 1987:

1. Upgrade nurse's aides by setting minimum hour and content standards for training programs and requiring testing of knowledge and clinical skills.
2. Admission screening to prevent admission to nursing homes of people whose only need is for services related to mental illness or mental retardation.
3. Minimal nurse staffing requirements for 24-hour licensed nursing services and a full-time registered nurse 7 days a week.

Although these measures are needed, they will require upgrading in staffing and nurse's aides' training, among other reforms related to patient's rights. If the increased costs associated with these improvements are not recognized through increases in reimbursement, the nursing homes will have to find other ways to cut costs. Ironically, these cost reductions might undermine any improvements in quality gained from the implementation of the legislation. Also, since there is no provision for increasing the wages of the nurse's aides, their positions will be upgraded without a commensurate increase in salary. Without better nurse's aide salaries, the nursing homes will still be faced with turnover and burnout in this labor force.

Defining and measuring quality of care in nursing homes is particularly difficult because a nursing home must be evaluated as an appropriate and sometimes final living situation for the residents. Quality of care over an extended period of time requires periodic and careful assessment of medical, functional, social, and psychological needs of the resident. Not all nursing homes have or can afford skilled professional staff able or motivated to do this.

Also, quality of care in a nursing home is closely related to quality of life, the resident's ability to have a sense of self-determination by making decisions about food, activities, and clothing; pursuing personal interests; having privacy; and being treated courteously and kindly by staff. These can be difficult and costly achievements for even the best nursing homes. Nursing home life must be institutional to some extent, particularly in large facilities. Nursing homes are built to look like hospitals, and the routine is geared to that of hospital staff. Although most nursing homes allow personal furniture and belongings, it is difficult to achieve a homelike atmosphere and privacy in an environment built with the main objectives of making it easy to clean and meeting fire and safety codes.

One of the critical elements of quality of life in nursing homes is the quality of the resident–staff relationship. Most of the care in nursing homes is provided by nurse's aides, who usually are low-paid, receive relatively little training in many states, and are inadequately supervised. They are often required to care for a large number of frail, very old residents many of whom have mental impairments as well as physical disabilities. Not surprisingly, the turnover rate of nurse's aides ranges from 70% to over 100% a year (Institute of Medicine, 1986). Also, the nursing shortage has made it more difficult to recruit licensed and registered nurses for nursing homes, where the wages are lower than in acute-care facilities. This has intensified the problems with inadequate supervision and has put nurse's aides into the position of providing care they are untrained to provide.

According to the IOM report (1986), many of the quality problems can be handled by competent management and staff: "In most regions of the country, very good homes can be found—places that are well-managed, where competent, caring staff provide services in a conscientious, sensitive manner: where the dignity, privacy, and human needs of the residents are respected and provided for in thoughtful, and even imaginative ways." However, it is acknowledged that these remedies increase costs. Reimbursement policies must recognize that maintaining the quality of patient care and life means higher costs.

The quality of home health services is particularly difficult to monitor because most of the time it cannot be observed. The patient contact occurs in the patient's home, often with only a paraprofessional home health aide or attendant and the patient present. Observation of the patient by a professional supervisor may occur only every 2 weeks and then may not include an observation of the care being provided.

Often quality problems in home care are also related to the difficulty home health agencies have in attracting and retaining experienced and reliable staff and to the varying state requirements for training and supervision of unskilled home health workers. The wages of home health workers lag behind most unskilled positions available, such as hotel, laundry, and cleaning workers (Kane, 1989).

Wages are so low that incomes of home health aides or attendants are near or below the federal poverty level. In Los Angeles home care workers made $3.72 per hour in 1987 and received no health insurance or fringe benefits. More than half of them depended on public assistance programs (Lutz, 1988). Until a recent contract settlement, home attendants working for the Medicaid program in New York City made $4.15 per hour, which gave them an annual income level of $7,000, less than the federal poverty level of $7,400 for two persons. Under the new contract, the hourly wages will be increased to $5.90 over a 3-year period, plus an enhanced health insurance benefit.

As with nursing homes, improving the quality of home care staff can also increase the costs of providing care. As Medicare and Medicaid develop more stringent limitations on eligibility for home health services and ratchet down rates, agencies will be less likely to undertake efforts that will improve quality of care. Rapid turnover, poor reliability, low morale and emotional and physical abuse of patient and worker are common problems in the industry. The considerable physical and emotional strain of home health work together with geographic difficulty of supervision makes quality assurance not only a challenging, but also an expensive endeavor for management.

Strategies for Change: Federal and State Approaches

Federal Approach

During the 1980s the federal government limited its role in long-term care largely to funding research aimed at demonstrating whether long-term care costs could be reduced by (1) substituting home and community-based services for nursing home care and (2) using a combination of case management and capitated funding as incentives to control the use of services. The largest Medicare demonstration was the National Long-term Care Channeling demonstration at 12 sites throughout the country. Half the sites were using a case management and brokerage model and half a financial control model. The results of the demonstrations, which intended to substitute community services for nursing home care, showed that expanded community services led to only a small reduction in nursing home use and, in fact, actually increased aggregate costs of services. Although the population served was extremely frail, it turned out to be very difficult to predict who would use nursing home services even among this frail population. The costs of the additional home care provided in most cases to people who would not have entered a nursing home were not offset by reduced nursing home costs leading to a total increased costs (Kemper, 1988). However, the demonstrations did show that the increased services benefitted patients and their families and were most successful in improving their quality of life (Kemper, 1988; Weissert, Cready, & Parvelak, 1988). One additional but unexpected finding, from the evaluation of these demonstrations was that informal caregivers did not stop giving care when formal care was added—an argument often used against expanding community-based services (Christianson, 1988; Kemper, 1988).

The other major federally supported demonstrations on capitation and case management were the SHMOs. The SHMO demonstrations have placed limits on long-term care benefits ranging from $6,500 to $12,000 (Pierce, 1987). This has raised concern about unrealistic restrictions on access to these services because this amount would cover only about 6 months in a nursing home. The four demonstration sites are expected to save $3 million to $6 million over 3 years in decreased use of hospitals and nursing homes (Pierce, 1987).

More recent demonstrations that began in 1991 have been attempts to replicate the On-Lok model of a capitated, comprehensive, risk-based acute and long-term care program. The Program of All-Inclusive Care for the Elderly (PACE) has been developed in eight sites: Boston, Bronx, Chicago, Columbia, South Carolina, Denver, El Paso, Milwaukee, and Portland. The PACE program represents a combination of private and public funding. The Health Care Financing Administration has provided waivers that allow capitated contracts using Medicare and Medicaid funds. The start-up costs of the demonstration have been supported largely by private foundations and sponsoring organizations. The PACE sites are targeting the care of elderly Medicaid clients at risk for admission to nursing homes. The sites will offer a full array of services including supportive housing, an important part of the On-Lok's model success. The sites will also focus on the day health program, the centerpiece of the On-Lok model by trading off some of the inefficiency of some in-home services to a day care setting (Kane, Illston, & Miller, 1992).

Although more systemwide federal reforms have been suggested, they have not been enacted largely due to budgetary constraints. For example, adding a Medicare Part C for long-term care has been advocated to get long-term care disentangled from Medicaid and the state welfare system and make it an entitlement program like the other services under Medicare. Also, establishing federal and minimum standards for Medicaid coverage of long-term care services has been discussed.

In October 1993, the most radical restructuring of the long-term care system since Medicaid and Medicare was proposed by President Clinton in his Health Security Plan. As proposed, the plan guaranteed universal coverage for a basic benefit package of hospital, physician, preventive, and long-term care services. The benefits that address the needs of the elderly and disabled were coverage for home health care and infusion therapy, extended care (up to 100 days per year) in a skilled nursing or rehabilitation facility, annual medical exams for those over 65 years, outpatient prescription drugs and biologicals and durable medical equipment and orthotic devices. In addition, the plan proposed to establish a significant home and community-based (HCBC) program for all people with severe disabilities without regard to income.

The legislation was not enacted and was withdrawn from congressional debate in September 1994. However, the proposal itself raised public consciousness about serious reform of the health system, including the need to restructure long-term care services not only for the elderly but for the one-third who need these services but are younger than 65 years of age. Although it is not clear what changes, if any, will emerge from a second health reform proposal there continues to be longstanding strong public support for the federal government to expand long-term care coverage. A 1987 poll by the American Association of Retired Persons and the Villers Foundation found that 86% of the sample supported government action for a universal long-term care program that would finance care for all income groups and not just the poor. Overall, 75% would agree to increased taxes for this program, although the sample did not identify the amount of increased taxes that would be acceptable (R.L. Associates, 1987).

State Approaches

With the growing pressure on their Medicaid budgets, states have been undertaking their own programs to reduce Medicaid spending on long-term care. The approaches have focused on reducing Medicaid spending in three general areas: (1) targeting access, (2) limiting payment, and (3) encouraging private responsibility through private health insurance and support to caregivers.

Targeting Access. The most widely used method for targeting access is case management, particularly preadmission screening. Preadmission screening is currently used by 45 states (Pierce, 1987). The programs range from a broad screening of applicants who are likely to become Medicaid-eligible within a certain time to screening only those who have decided to enter a nursing home. Wisconsin and South Carolina have been so successful in the latter approach that it is likely to become more widespread. However, savings from keeping less-sick patients in the community ultimately may be offset by limiting nursing homes to heavier-care patients whose care is more costly.

Case management as a targeting function ranges from coordination and monitoring of service delivery to state organizational structure that has a total gatekeeping function. A General Accounting Office study of California, Massachusetts, Connecticut, Maryland, Oregon, and Washington found a wide variation in approaches to case management including differences in responsible agencies, qualifications, and salaries of case-managers and the scope of case-managing activities. Oregon, provides an example of a state that has consolidated all long-term care responsibilities, including both institutional, community-based care, and assisted living under a single agency, the Department of Human Services. Most other states have less integrated case-management approaches but are attempting to move toward the Oregon model.

Major components of the Oregon system include relocation planning, risk intervention, and preadmission screening. All functions are performed by case managers, who assess client needs and develop a care plan authorizing the provision of Medicaid services. They also identify services available through other resources for those not eligible for Medicaid. Other case managers assigned to relocation planning help institutionalized older people return to the community. Since 1982, more than 5,000 nursing home patients have been relocated to community settings (Justice, 1988). This case management function is part of the Senior Services Division (SSD), which has centralized control over all major state funds for the elderly, including Medicaid, social services block grants, Older Americans Act funds, and SSI. The state estimated that in 1986 the combined nursing home and community-based services cost the state $13 million less than if the reorganization had not occurred. This represented an 11% reduction in state expenditures for these services (Justice, 1988). Also, the Oregon model that relocates and arranges for other services can indirectly improve access. Case management without these features is more likely to result in limiting access only.

Limiting Payment. States have been experimenting with ways to avoid the open-ended health insurance reimbursement model that pays retrospectively for services that are prescribed and provided by providers of nursing home care, home health, and other community-based services. The approaches range from tinkering with the nursing home reimbursement system to placing a cap on the total value of services that can be provided. States may be experimenting with more than one approach.

Prospective payment is the most popular reimbursement reform (Pierce, 1987). A specific form of prospective payment, case-mix payment, is gaining in use. Seven states (Illinois, Maryland, Minnesota, Montana, New York, Ohio, and West Virginia) have adopted a case-mix approach to establishing nursing home reimbursement rates (Swan, Harrington & Grant, 1988). Case-mix reimbursement is based on an assessment of each resident's condition and an estimate of the actual amount of nursing time and other resources that patient will need (Schlenker, 1986). The assessment usually measures ADLs, mental status, medical conditions, and behavioral problems. After the assessment, residents can be grouped according to the level of resources they require. Although case-mix systems help prevent facilities from losing money when accepting Medicaid residents with heavier care needs, they are mainly intended to restrict cost by setting ceilings for average costs of different case-mix groups.

There are two concerns about case-mix reimbursement. One is that paying nursing homes less money as residents improve creates the potential for nursing homes to increase the residents' dependency and care requirements to maximize reimbursement (Kane & Kane, 1987; Swan et al., 1988). The second concern is that the increase in reimbursement will not necessarily mean an increase in services. Patient case-mix reimbursement formulas can be targets for "gaming" to increase reimbursement. To control this potential, New York State has implemented a new, more stringent quality assurance system that will be looking more closely at how care is provided and the outcome of the care to determine if the patient has received the needed services. Also, the New York State program has a quality-of-life component that will assess such areas as resident participation in activities as an indicator of their process.

Half of the state Medicaid programs still use retrospective cost-based reimbursement for home care, but it is expected most states will change to prospective payment (Pierce, 1987). Of those who have already changed, 29 states have established prospective maximum payment rates for home health care services adjusted by type of provider (nurse, nurses aide, physical therapist, etc.). Development of case-mix reimbursement for home health services is difficult because there is not a sufficient data base on home health recipients. Also, it is difficult to assess the population with multiple and changing health problems, differing home and family situations, variation in travel time and the time required to perform the same unit of service.

In setting maximum payable amounts for home and community services under the Section 2176 waiver programs, most states have used a percentage of the average cost of nursing home care as the limit above which services may not be authorized. The range is usually between 75% and 90% (Pierce, 1987). Maine has a per-client cap equal to the state's potential expense of providing ICF care for that person. This maximum amount is programmed into the state's Medicaid computer so that spending cannot exceed the limit (Justice, 1988). Arkansas currently limits its personal care services to a maximum of 72 hours per client per month ($442/month). Although Wisconsin does not set maximums for individuals, it sets an average payment level for counties, and the counties are not reimbursed if the average cost for all recipients exceeds the contract level (Justice, 1988).

As states become more restrictive in payment for long-term care, providers are forced to reduce their costs in order to keep operating. To balance the negative effect these reductions might have on quality, Illinois has been using an outcome base reimbursement, a concept originated by Robert Kane at the University of Minnesota. The Illinois scheme uses incentive payments for reaching goals in the resident's condition and in the environment. Despite the potential of this scheme to protect quality of care, it is naive to assume that continually reducing nursing home or home health payments to make them more efficient will not affect quality and access. As Scanlon (1988) has pointed out with respect to nursing homes, "Because of virtually guaranteed high occupancy, nursing homes have little need to compete. A likely response to lower Medicaid reimbursement is therefore a reduction in staff and other resources devoted to providing care."

Encouraging Private Responsibility. Because the insurance industry is regulated by states, they must strike a balance between removing legal and regulatory barriers that discourage the industry's developing private long-term care insurance and protecting the consumer from unscrupulous practices by the industry. States also can take steps to encourage the sale of policies. One of these steps is sponsoring educational campaigns to inform elderly citizens of the limitations of Medicare in covering long-term care services. The Washington State insurance commissioner, for example, runs a program that uses trained senior volunteers to conduct public meetings and assist individuals in assessing insurance policies (Pierce, 1987). Colorado has enacted a tax reduction for purchasing long-term care policies. Other state proposals include waiving Medicaid asset eligibility requirements for those who have used up benefits through long-term care insurance policies and making long-term care insurance available to state employees (Pierce, 1987). The Robert Wood Johnson Foundation funded a national demonstration in four states: New York, Connecticut, California, and Indiana to support state/private initiatives in developing long-term care insurance. These initiatives are still in experimental stages and the ability of long-term care insurance to lead to Medicaid savings will not be known for at least 10 to 15 years, when those purchasing policies now will actually need to use the services covered.

The other major area in which states are able to encourage private responsibility is the use of tax incentives to support family and informal caregiving. States provide tax incentives through use of exemptions, deductions, and tax credits. Only five states (Arizona, Idaho, Iowa, North Carolina, and Oregon) have tax incentive programs. Iowa's program allows informal caregivers to claim a deduction of up to $5,000 for eligible expenses. The disabled relative must be eligible for Medicaid and have a statement from a physician stating the person cannot live independently. The combination of these two requirements means the program is targeting those at higher risks for institutionalization (U.S. House of Representatives Select Committee on Aging, 1987a).

In contrast, Oregon has a very limited program that allows a credit of up to 8% of eligible expenses, to a maximum of $250. Oregon also is the only state of the five to limit income eligibility of the caregivers to $17,500 (Pierce, 1987).

Thirty-five states permit some form of payment to relatives for the provision of home care to elderly clients. This financial incentive is usually restricted to clients at high risk for institutionalization. States also have various guidelines for payments, including requirements that the caregivers demonstrate financial hardship and that the dependent person live in the same household (U.S. House of Representatives Select Committee on Aging, 1987a).

Tax incentive programs have the advantage of keeping the dependent elderly person in the family home, where it is assumed that he or she will get the best care. However, the few programs that exist have been so small, it is unlikely that they will be sufficient incentive for daughters and daughters-in-law to leave the labor force for caregiving responsibilities. As a result, they have limited ability to create more direct care.

Conclusion and Future Direction

In summary, existing problems in access, financing, and quality of long-term care make obtaining appropriate, high-quality long-term care too often a matter of chance. The availability of services depends on the state and locality in which one lives. It also depends on whether one has just the right amount of income and assets to qualify for Medicare, Medicaid, or other public programs or so much income that any amount of services can be purchased. Those who are unlucky enough to fall between those two extremes will be forced to use most of what income and assets they have until they are poor enough to obtain Medicaid. Once services have been obtained, their quality will largely depend on luck in getting personnel who, despite poor wages and little status, will be competent, considerate, and remain on the job. Although these problems and inequities have existed for decades, the policies and programs to address them have been slow in developing because of resistance at both state and federal levels to increased spending. As the elderly population increases, mortality rates decrease and the number of "baby-boom" informal caregivers are unable to manage the time or cost of long-term care to their parents, the development of a national long-term care policy will become increasingly urgent. The goals of a national long-term care system should include:

- Achieving equity in the distribution of resources and the distribution of financial responsibility.
- Ensuring access for functionally impaired persons of all ages based on their need for services including personal care services, homemaker assistance, and housing.
- Expanding support for informal caregivers.
- Funding education, training, and decent salaries to attract health personnel into long-term care.

These goals can most efficiently and appropriately be achieved through a model that integrates acute and long-term care services providing a full range of medical, social, and housing services. Since it is apparent that neither the public nor private sector can cover the cost of such an approach, major new efforts are needed in both sectors. In the public sector, this should include a social insurance model that would provide near universal coverage and would recognize long-term care services as a normal, insurable risk of growing old. As such, it would eliminate the need for anyone, particularly the elderly, becoming impoverished in order to be covered for services. In addition, private insurance companies could increase their role in supplemental coverage for those who can and should participate in cost-sharing for services. This approach acknowledges the reality that private long-term care can never provide comprehensive long-term care coverage for the majority of elderly.

Variations in level of need and demand for long-term care among individuals, localities, and states added to the fact that needed services often cross the boundaries between health, social services, and housing make a strong federal role necessary to address the issues of equity and quality. The health reform under the Clinton Administration may be a first step, but the ultimate goal must go farther to achieve comprehensive reform rather than incremental changes in existing programs.

References

Altman, B. M., & Walden, D. C., *Home Health Care: Use, Expenditures, and Sources of Payment,* (AHCPR Pub. No. 93-0040), National Medical Expenditure Research Findings 15, Agency for Health Care Policy and Research. Rockville, MD: April 1993.

Blustein, J., Schultz, B. M., Knickman, J. R., Kator, M. J., Richardson, H., & McBride, L. C., "AIDS and Long-Term Care: The Use of Services in an Institutional Setting." *AIDS & Public Policy Journal,* 7(1), 32-41, Spring 1992.

Cantor, M., "The Family: The Basic Source of Long-term Care for the Elderly." In P. H. Feinstein, M. Gomick, & J. N. Greenberg (Eds.), *Long-term Care Financing and Delivery Systems: Exploring Some Alternatives.* Washington, DC: Health Care Financing Administration, 1984.

Capitman, J. A., Prottas, J., MacAdam, M., Leutz, W., Westwater, D., & Yee, D. L., "A Descriptive Framework for New Hospital Roles in Geriatric Care." *Health Care Financing Review,* (Annual Supplement), 17-25, December 1988.

Christianson, J. B., "The Effect of Channeling on Informal Caregiving." *Health Services Research,* 23(1), 99, 1988.

Cohen, M. A., "Life Care: New Options for Financing and Delivering Long-term care." *Health Care Financing Review,* (Annual Supplement), 139, December 1988.

Cohen, M. A., Kumar, N., & Wallack, S. S., "New Perspectives on the Affordability of Long-Term Care Insurance and Potential Market Size." *The Gerentologist,* 33(1), 105-113, 1993.

General Accounting Office, *Long-term care for the Elderly.* (HRD-89-4). Washington, DC: Author, 1988.

General Accounting Office, *Medicare Program Provisions and Payments Discourage Hospice Participation.* (GAO/HRD-89-111). Gaithersburg, MD: September 1989.

General Accounting Office, *Nursing Homes: Admission Problems for Medicaid Recipients and Attempts to Solve Them.* (GAO/HRD-90-135). Washington, DC: September 1990.

General Accounting Office, *Elderly Americans: Health, Housing and Nutritional Gaps Between the Poor and Nonpoor.* (GAO/PEMD-92-29). Washington, DC: June 1992a.

General Accounting Office, *Long-term Care Insurance: Better Control Needed in Sales to People with Limited Financial Resources.* (GAO/HRD-92-66). Washington, DC: March 1992b.

General Accounting Office, *Long-term Care Case Management: State Experiences and Implications for Federal Policy.* (GAO/HRD-93-52). Washington, DC: April 1993a.

General Accounting Office, *Long-term Care Insurance: Hiah Percentage of Policyholders Drop Policies.* (GAO/HRD-93-129). Washington, DC: August 1993b.

Harrington, C., & Grant, L. A., "The Delivery, Regulation, and Politics of Home Care: A California Case Study." *The Gerontologist,* 30(4), 451-461, 1990.

Hawes, C. & Phillips, C. D., "The Changing Structure of the Nursing Home Industry and the Impact of Ownership on Quality, Cost, and Access." In B. H. Gray (Ed.), *For-Profit Enterprise in Health Care.* Washington, DC: National Academy Press, 1986.

Henderson, M. G., Sonder, B. A., Bergman, A., & Collard, A. F., "Private Sector Initiatives in Case Management." *Health Care Financing Review,* (Annual Supplement), 89-95, December 1988.

Hing, E., "Use of Nursing Homes by the Elderly: Preliminary Data from the 1985 National Nursing Home Survey." (DHHS Pub. No. PHS 87-1250). Hyattsville, MD: National Center for Health Statistics, 1987.

Institute of Medicine, *Improving the Quality of Care in Nursing Homes.* Washington, DC: National Academy Press, 1986.

Justice, D., *State Long-term Care Reform.* Washington, DC: Center for Policy Research, National Governor's Association, 1988.

Kane, N. M., "The Home Care Crisis of the Nineties." *The Gerontologist,* 29(1), 24-31, 1989.

Kane, R. A., & Kane, R. L., *Long-Term Care: Principles, Programs and Policies.* New York: Springer Publishing Co., 1987.

Kane, R. A., & Wilson, K. B., *Assisted Living in the United States: A New Paradigm for Residential Care for Frail Older Persons.* American Association of Retired Persons. Washington, DC: 1993.

Kane, R. L., Illston, L. H., & Miller, N. A., "Qualitative Analysis of the Program of All-Inclusive Care for the Elderly (PACE)." *The Gerontologist,* 32(6), 771-780, 1992.

Kemper, P., "Overview of the Findings." *Health Services Research,* 23(1), 161, 1988.

Kutza, E. A., "Allocating Long-Term Care Services." In J. Meltzer, F. Farrow, & H. Richmond (Eds.), *Policy Options in Long-Term Care.* Chicago: University of Chicago Press, 1981.

Lair, T. J., "A Profile of Nursing Home Users Under Age 65." Research Findings 13, National Medical Expenditure Survey Research Findings (AHCPR Pub. No. 92-0060), Agency for Health Policy and Research. Rockville, MD: August 1992.

Lair, T. J., & Lefkowitz, D. C., "Mental Health and Functional Status of Residents of Nursing and Personal Care Homes." Research Findings 7, National Medical Expenditure Survey Findings (DHHS Pub. No. PHS 90-3470), Agency for Health Care Policy and Research. Rockville, MD: September 1990.

Leon, J., & Lair, T., "Functional Status of the Noninstitutionalized Elderly: Estimates of ADL and IADL Difficulties." Research Findings 4, National Medical Expenditure Survey Findings (DDHS Pub. No. PHS 90-3462), Agency for Health Care Policy and Research. Rockville, MD: 1990.

Lutz, W., Abrahams, R., Greenlick, M., Kane, R., & Prottas, J., "Targeting Expanded Care to the Aged: Early SHMO Experience." *The Gerontologist,* 28(1), 4, 1988.

Lindberg, G., & Monson, T., "Long-term Care Initiatives in Hennepin County, Minnesota." Notes from the Field. *American Journal of Public Health,* 79(4), 519, 1989.

Lutz, S., "Despite Pitfalls, Home Care Keeps Growing." *Modern Health Care,* 24-37, June 24, 1988.

Mayer, D., "Nursing Home Market Reaches All-Time High." *Health Week,* August 8, 1988.

Meltzer, W., *Respite Care: An Emerging Family Support Service.* Washington, DC: The Center for the Study of Social Policy, 1982.

Murtaugh, C. M., Kemper, P., & Spillman, B. C., "The Risk of Nursing Home Use in Later Life." *Medical Care,* 28(10), 952-962, October 1990.

National Association for Home Care, *Basic Statistics About Home Care 1992.* Washington, DC: 1993.

Pierce, R. M., *Long-term care for the Elderly: A Legislator's Guide.* Washington, DC: National Conference of State Legislatures and the American Association of Retired Persons, 1987.

Porter, M., & Witek, J. E., "The Nursing Home Industry: Past, Present and Future." *Topics in Health Care Financing: Financing Long-Term Care,* (7)4, 42-48, Aspen Publishing, Inc., Summer 1991.

Richardson, H., & Kovner, A. R., "Swing-Beds: Experience and Future Directions." *Health Affairs,* 6(3), 61, 1987.

Rivlin, A. M., & Wiener, J. M., *Caring for the Disabled Elderly: Who Will Pay?* Washington, DC: The Brookings Institution, 1988.

R. L. Associates, "The American Public Views Long-Term Care: A Survey Conducted for the American Association of Retired Persons and the Villers Foundation." Princeton, NJ: October 1987.

Scanlon, W. J., "A Theory of Nursing Home Market. " *Inquiry,* 17(1), 25, 1980.

Scanlon, W. J., "A Perspective on Long-term care for the Elderly." *Health Care Financing Review,* Annual Supplement, 7-15, December 1988.

Schlenker, R. E., "Case Mix Reimbursement for Nursing Homes." *Journal of Health Politics, Policy and Law,* 11(3), 445, 1986.

Scholen, K., "An Overview of Home Equity Conversion." In P. H. Feinstein, M. Gornick, & J. N. Greenberg (Eds.), *Long-term Care Financing and Delivery Systems: Exploring Some Alternatives.* Washington, DC: Health Care Financing Administration, 1984.

Seltzer, B., Rheaume, Y., Volicer, L., Fabiszewski, K. J., Lyon, P., Brown, J. E., & Volicer, B., "The Short-Term Effects of In-Hospital Respite on the Patient with Alzheimer's Disease." *The Gerontologist,* 28(1), 121, 1988.

Shaughnessy, P. W., Schlenker, R. E., & Hittle, D. F., *An Evaluation Study of the National Swing-Bed Program in the 1980s.* Denver: Center for Health Services Research, University of Colorado Health Sciences Center, 1987.

Short, P. F., Kemper, P., Cornelius, L. J., & Walden, D. C., "Public and Private Responsibility for Financing Nursing Home Care: The Effect of Medicaid Asset Spend-Down." *The Milbank Quarterly,* 70(2), 277-298, 1992.

Soldo, B., "Supply of Informal Care Services: Variations and Effects on Service Utilization Patterns." In W. Scanlon (Ed.), *Project to Analyze Long-Term Care Data,* 3, Washington, D.C.: The Urban Institute, 1984.

Soldo, B., & Manton, B., "Dynamics of Health Changes in the Oldest Old: New Perspectives and Evidence." *Milbank Memorial Fund Quarterly,* 63(2), 286, 1985.

Strahan, G., "Nursing Home Characteristics: Preliminary Data for the 1985 National Nursing Home Survey." *Advance Data from Vital and Health Statistics*, No. 131, (DHHS Pub. No. PHS 87-1250). Hyattsville, MD: Public Health Service, 1987.

Swan, J. H., Harrington, C., & Grant, L. A., "State Medicaid Reimbursement for Nursing Homes, 1978-86." *Health Care Financing Review*, 9(1), 33, 1988.

U.S. Department of Health and Human Services, Health Care Financing Administration. *Long-Term Health Care Policies* (HCFA Pub. No. 87-02170). Washington, DC: U.S. Government Printing Office, 1987.

U.S. House of Representatives, Select Committee on Aging, *Exploding the Myths: Caregiving in America*, (Comm. Pub. No. 99-611). Washington, DC: U.S. Government Printing Office, January 1987a.

U.S. House of Representatives, Select Committee on Aging, *Long-Term Care and Personal Impoverishment: Seven in Ten Elderly Living Alone Are at Risk* (Comm. Pub. No. 100-631). Washington, DC: U.S. Government Printing Office, 1987b.

U.S. Senate Special Committee on Aging, *Aging in America*. Washington, DC: U.S. Department of Health and Human Services, 1988.

U.S. Senate Special Committee on Aging, *Nursing Home Care: The Unfinished Agenda*, Staff Report, May 21, 1986.

Vladeck, B., *Unloving Care: The Nursing Home Tragedy*. New York: Basic Books, 1980.

Vladeck, B., "Nursing Homes." In D. Mechanic (Ed.), *Handbook of Health, Health Care and Health Professions*. New York: The Free Press, 1983.

Von Behren, R., *Adult Day Care in America: Summary of a National Survey*. Washington, DC: National Council on the Aging, 1986.

Weissert, W. G., Cready, M. C., & Parvelak, J. E., "The Past and Future of Home and Community-Based Long-term care." *Milbank Memorial Fund Quarterly*, 66(2), 1988.

Zawadski, R. T., & Eng, C., "Case Management in Capitated Long-term care." *Health Care Financing Review*, (Annual Supplement), 75-81, December 1988.

9

Mental Health Services

Steven S. Sharfstein, Anne M. Stoline, and Lorrin Koran

Who is mentally ill? The precise boundaries for the concept of "mental disorder" are not clear and are influenced by philosophic, social, and cultural considerations. This is also true for the concepts of physical disorder and notions of health and disease. Every society includes individuals who present behavioral or psychological deviancy significant enough to qualify for a definition of mental illness. These syndromes are associated with painful emotional symptoms or present as an inability to think, remember, or concentrate. Such syndromes also significantly increase the potential for general medical illness, pain, disability, and even death. The causes of mental disorders may be biological, developmental, psychological, environmental, or combinations of these. The important boundary line is the person's level of distress and dysfunction that is expressed primarily through a behavioral syndrome.

Expenditures for mental health services were estimated at $71 billion in 1991, including $58.7 billion for mental disorders, $9.3 billion for alcohol abuse, and $2.9 billion for drug abuse. Services for psychiatric disease alone accounted for about 8% of the nation's expenditures for health care. At nearly $161.1 billion, indirect costs of mental disorders (including drug and alcohol abuse) in 1991 totaled more than twice the direct treatment costs. Indirect costs of mental disorders ($71.7 billion) resulted from lost wages due to illness or premature death, productivity losses for individuals incarcerated due to conviction related to a psychiatric disorder, and value of time spent by family members of those with psychiatric conditions. Indirect costs of alcohol abuse ($65 billion) and drug abuse ($24.4 billion) result from adverse health effects, accident-related injuries and fatalities, homicides, suicides, fetal alcohol syndrome, productivity lost by addicts, their incarceration due to drug-related crimes, costs incurred by the victims of those crimes, and costs associated with AIDS contracted through intravenous or prenatal exposures (National Foundation for Brain Research, 1992). These dollar estimates can only begin to suggest the magnitude of human suffering caused by mental disorders and substance abuse.

Like the general health care sector, the mental health care sector is experiencing pressures for cost containment. Insurance companies are encouraging psychiatrists to offer their services for lower fees through preferred provider organizations. The federal government, while maintaining its exemption of psychiatric hospitals and inpatient units from Medicare's Prospective Payment System using diagnosis-related groups, continues to research prospective payment methods for psychiatric inpatient care as well. Partly in hopes of lowering fees for psychotherapy, state legislatures are acceding to lobbying by psychologists and other nonmedical psychotherapists to allow them direct access to third-party reimbursement without physician supervision. As policy makers encourage competition to stimulate efficiency, safeguarding the quality of care must not be forgotten.

Despite great progress in the past quarter century, the delivery of mental health care, like the delivery of general health care, is beset by many difficulties. The pluralistic nature of the service delivery system leads to inequitable access based on geography, class, and diagnosis. Different phases of care and interrelations with other human services (general medicine, legal, education, and welfare) are inadequately coordinated. Planning, evaluation, and regulation are fragmented. Many mental disorders can only be ameliorated, not cured. Mental health personnel and community-based treatment programs are in short supply, further threatened by a recent decline in the number of applicants to psychiatric residency programs. The social stigma attached to mental patients (Rabkin, 1974) and public apathy toward their suffering also hamper care. Finally, when mentally ill people are also affected by poverty and racism, delivering adequate services becomes a most formidable task.

Further, the pluralistic delivery system contributes to the major public health problem in the delivery of continuous care for the chronically ill, many of whom have been deinstitutionalized from psychiatric institutions over the past two decades. The public health problem of homeless people, especially wandering individuals with schizophrenia and substance abuse, rivals other major medical crises today, such as the AIDS epidemic. This is partly because of a fragmentation of services, including general medical and social welfare services, and an uneven approach by state government toward the direct care needs of these individuals.

The challenge for the brief remainder of the twentieth century is to find ways to diminish these difficulties. To help the reader respond to this challenge, this chapter will discuss the forms of mental disorder, the kinds of mental health care, the history of that care in the United States, the prevalence of mental disorders, the mental health labor force, the delivery of services, insurance coverage, and legal issues. Although generally included in the category of mental conditions, data for services for substance abuse diagnoses will not be included in the following sections.

Forms of Mental Disorders

The American Psychiatric Association published its first edition of the *Diagnostic and Statistical Manual of Mental Disorders* in 1952. In late 1993, the fifth edition of the *Diagnostic and Statistical Manual of Mental Disorders (DSM-IV)* was released (American Psychiatric Association, 1993). The manual currently includes more than 450 conditions and their subtypes, grouped in 17 categories. The culmination of more than 4 years of effort, *DSM-IV* includes newly recognized diagnostic entities and reorganizes former diagnostic categories to take account of discoveries in recent years regarding the causes, natural history, and treatment responsiveness of many forms of mental disorder. This diagnostic manual undoubtedly will change as the research informing practice and the validity of the diagnostic categories improve. The 17 major diagnostic classes in *DSM-IV* are as follows:

1. Disorders usually first diagnosed in infancy, childhood, or adolescence (including intellectual, behavioral, emotional, physical, and developmental disorders).
2. Delirium, dementia, amnestic, and other cognitive disorders.
3. Mental disorders due to a general medical condition not elsewhere classified (including catatonic disorder personality change, when due to a general medical condition).
4. Substance-related disorders (including alcohol, drugs, and tobacco).
5. Schizophrenia and other psychotic disorders.
6. Mood disorders (conditions with manic, depressive, or mixed symptomatology).
7. Anxiety disorders (including phobias, post-traumatic stress disorder, and obsessive-compulsive disorder).
8. Somatoform disorders (physical symptoms suggesting physical disorders but without organic findings).
9. Factitious disorders (disorders deliberately simulated by the individual for psychological gain, excluding malingering because it aims at environmental gains).
10. Dissociative disorders (including multiple personality and psychogenic amnesia).
11. Sexual and gender identity disorders (including desire, arousal, and paraphiliac disorders).
12. Eating disorders.
13. Sleep disorders (including insomnia and nightmare disorders).
14. Impulse control disorders not elsewhere classified (including pathological gambling and kleptomania).
15. Adjustment disorders (maladaptive reactions to psychosocial stress).

16. Personality disorders (enduring, maladaptive patterns of relating to, perceiving, and thinking about the environment and oneself that cause significant impairment of social or occupational functioning or subjective distress).
17. Other conditions that may be a focus of clinical attention (including malingering, bereavement, and adult antisocial behavior).

The placement of adult antisocial behavior and bereavement in the category "Other conditions that may be a focus of clinical attention represents the attempt to avoid labeling all socially deviant or normal human responses as being "mental disorders." Although a few mental health professionals believe all mental disorders are social myths (Szasz, 1961), the reasoning and evidence to the contrary are powerfully convincing (Kendall, 1975; Moore, 1976; Murphy, 1976), thus making it all the more important to accurately differentiate the constellations of thoughts, feelings, and behaviors that constitute clinical conditions from those that do not.

Prevalence of Mental Disorders

Epidemiological studies of the prevalence of mental disorders have encountered the same problems as have analogous studies of physical diseases: deciding what constitutes a "case," establishing operational diagnostic criteria, and choosing a method of case finding.

The largest, most carefully conceived and executed study of the epidemiology of mental disorders was carried out from 1980 to 1982 by the NIMH Epidemiological Catchment Area (ECA) program. The ECA program was one of the recommendations of the 1978 President's Commission on Mental Health. A reliable structured interview, the Diagnostic Interview Schedule (DIS), incorporating *DSM-III* diagnostic criteria for 32 mental disorders, was administered by trained interviewers to a random sample of nearly 20,000 people in five U.S. cities. After the initial interview (Wave 1), when possible the subjects were interviewed again 1 year later (Wave 2). Recently available results of extensive analysis of this data suggest that the 1-year total prevalence rate of the mental and addictive disorders included in the DIS is 28.1% for the adult U.S. population (Regier et al., 1978). The 1-year prevalence of the most common disorders recorded were phobias (10.9%), any alcohol disorder (7.4%), and dysthymia (5.4%). (*Dysthymia* is one form of depressive disorder.)

The ECA Program also reported the number of individuals who reported the use of services for mental and addictive disorders in a 1-year period. Of the adult U.S. population, 14.7% received some service for a mental or addictive disorder in a 1-year period, but often the service was limited to consulting a voluntary support network or self-help group; only 5.9% of the population received services from specialty providers of mental/addictive services, and 6.4% from general medical physicians (some persons received services from both). Because the results do not include those who may have seen a health care provider for other reasons but received medication or psychosocial treatment for a mental or addictive condition, or those providers who did not report these services, these numbers should be considered conservative, underestimating the number of people receiving services (Regier et al., 1978). Of the 28.1% of the population afflicted by a mental disorder, only about one in five receive any treatment from a mental health professional. Of the 23 million people receiving services in a 1-year period, 54% had a current mental or addictive disorder diagnosis, and 37% met criteria for such a diagnosis in the past. The specialty mental health sector saw 40 to 70% of people treated who had a current diagnosis, while 40 to 50% of persons with diagnosed disorders saw providers in the general health care sector (Narrow et al., 1993). Approximately two-thirds of persons with a diagnosed mental disorder did not receive any mental health or addictive services during the one-year period, although they have been seen by other human service providers such as clergy or social welfare agencies (Regier et al., 1978; Narrow, 1993).

The data that follow focus on the mental health sector of the U.S. health care delivery system. One must remember, however, that only about one in five people who are afflicted with a mental disorder receive care in this sector. Training primary care physicians to recognize and treat mental disorders, and establishing better linkages between the general health sector and the mental health sector are vital to improving the major portion of mental health care (Browskowski et al., 1978; NIMH, 1983a, Series DN, No. 2).

Treatments and Services for the Mentally Ill

The term *mental health care* encompasses diverse preventive, therapeutic, and rehabilitative activities. Preventive mental health care aims at promoting mental health and preventing specific mental disorders. The first objective is difficult to attain because it is vague: few people agree on exactly what *mental health* is. The second preventive aim has met with some success: such disorders as syphilitic dementia and pellagrinous psychoses, for example, now rarely occur. Efforts to prevent childhood mental disorders through prenatal care, neonatal screening, childhood immunizations, adequate nutrition, and preschool education are receiving increased study. But primary prevention of schizophrenia, mania, depression, and other mental disorders of adult life remains beyond our ability (Langsley, 1985).

Therapeutic mental health services include individual, family, and group psychotherapies; hypnosis; psychodrama; expressive therapies such as art therapy; milieu therapy; medications; electroconvulsive therapy; and psychosurgery. Psychotherapies rely primarily on structured conversation aimed at changing a patient's attitudes, feelings, beliefs, defenses, personality, and behavior. The therapist's procedures vary across schools of psychotherapy and with the nature of the patient's problem. Psychoanalysis, for example, employs techniques such as free association and interpretations based on psychoanalytic theory to bring about personality restructuring. Most forms of psychotherapy, however, have much in common (Frank & Frank, 1991). Psychotherapy, hypnosis, and psychodrama are generally used to treat mental disorders other than psychoses and organic brain syndromes. Milieu therapy involves arranging the physical setting and social organization of an inpatient treatment setting to encourage socially acceptable and responsible behavior.

Most drugs effective in treating mental disorders have been available for less than 40 years. These include phenothiazines and other drugs for treating schizophrenia; tricyclic and other antidepressants for depression, panic attacks, and obsessive-compulsive disorders; lithium and carbamazepine for manic-depressive disorders; and benzodiazapines for anxiety states (Schatzberg, 1991). Amphetamines have been used to treat hyperactive children since the 1930s. Electroconvulsive therapy, which is effective for certain forms of depression, schizophrenia, and mania, was introduced in 1938 (Fink, 1979). Psychosurgery (neurosurgery used to treat a mental disorder) was widely used to treat schizophrenia in the late 1940s and early 1950s, but is rarely used today for any mental disorder, and then usually as a treatment of last resort (Bernstein et al., 1975; National Commission, 1977).

A new class of antidepressants that selectively affects the serotonin system has been developed in recent years. These drugs, such as fluoxetine, have low side effect profiles, are safe and effective not only for severe to moderate depression, but are also helpful for obsessive-compulsive disorder and milder depressions. Advances have also been made in pharmacologic treatments of the addictive disorders, such as agents that selectively affect opiate receptors (Schatzberg, 1991).

Rehabilitative mental health care includes occupational therapy, social skills training, and re-education aimed at helping the patient return to normal living patterns. It may begin in an inpatient setting with patient self-government activities and social activities, and can progress through transitional settings such as halfway houses, group homes, or supervised apartments. Rehabilitative care is employed primarily with patients suffering from psychoses, drug addiction, or alcoholism.

In part due to expansion of the NIMH mission in the area of research and neuroscience, our knowledge of the brain continues to increase rapidly. Private sector research, particularly by pharmaceutical manufacturers, adds to the knowledge base as well. Our growing understanding of the brain and the frequent introduction of new treatments of mental disorders combine to make psychiatry one of the most exciting areas in medicine today.

Brief History of Mental Health Care in the United States

Throughout the Colonial period, most mentally ill people were kept at home or wandered from town to town where they were lodged in jails or almshouses (work-houses). This remained the general pattern until the 1840s (Shryock, 1947).

In the early 1800s, the Quakers and American physicians exposed to European psychiatry encouraged the view that mental illness was treatable, and urged kind and sympathetic methods. Partly as a result, a few mental hospitals were opened where "moral treatment" (combining work, recreation, education, and kind but firm management) was predominant (Bockoven, 1972). Violent patients, however, were segregated in separate wards, and in most of the country mentally disordered pau-pers and blacks were sent to workhouses and jails (Mora, 1975). In 1841 an alli-ance of professionals and reformers began lobbying legislatures for improved care.

Despite the reformers' successes, the quality of care in state mental hospitals rapidly declined. Outright neglect and custodial care were fostered by the over-crowding of hospitals with criminals, alcoholics, vagrants, and state paupers; by a tendency to build larger institutions to keep per capita expenditures down; and by an increasing pessimism regarding the curability of mental disorders. Since mental hospitals were located away from population centers, the dismal condi-tions within them were easily ignored for a time. In the 1870s and 1880s a new wave of reform began, with criticisms of commitment procedures, the use of restraints, and the low level of staff training (Deutsch, 1947). Inspection and ac-creditation of mental hospitals was not undertaken by the Joint Commission on the Accreditation of Hospitals until 1958 (see Chapters 8 and 16).

At the beginning of this century, mental health care was primarily hospital-based, and biological approaches dominated etiological theories and applied treat-ments. During World War I, however, psychological and social contributions to cause and treatment were forcibly brought home to professionals and the public alike. Thousands of men were rejected for military service because of psycho-neuroses. War neuroses ("shell shock") accounted for a large proportion of psy-chiatric casualties.

In the 1920s the mental hygiene movement, nurtured by the National Commit-tee for Mental Hygiene and strengthened by Freud's psychological theories and the experience gained in World War I, captured the popular imagination. In the 1930s the advance of the mental hygiene movement slowed under the weight of the Depression, limited scientific knowledge regarding the prevention of mental disorders, and conflicts among various schools of psychiatric theory.

Between 1910 and World War II, psychoanalysis gradually came to dominate psychiatric training, outpatient care, and popular views of the nature of human-ity. Psychoanalysis did little, however, for severely disturbed individuals who, for the most part, remained in poorly funded, sparsely staffed, biologically ori-ented, custodial state institutions. In the 1930s, new hope for these severely dis-turbed patients was raised by the discovery of new biological treatments: insulin coma, drug-induced convulsive treatments, electroconvulsive therapy, and psycho-surgery. The Federal Public Works Administration added more than 60,000 beds to state and local mental institutions.

World War II again focused public attention on mental disorders: 1.75 million men were rejected for service because of mental or emotional disturbances, and a large number of veterans returned with emotional problems. In 1946 Congress passed the national Mental Health Act, which established the National Institute of Mental Health (NIMH) and gave new federal support for mental health services, training, and research. The Veterans Administration established psychiatric hospitals and outpatient clinics. Most inpatient treatment, however, still took place in state institutions whose deplorable conditions were graphically described by two journalists, Mike Gorman and Albert Deutsch. Partly to compensate for limited professional personnel, institutions and outpatient clinics began to use group psychotherapy, which allowed one professional to treat many patients at once.

By the mid-1950s, the number of persons hospitalized in state and county mental hospitals reached its peak at 558,900. At the same time, however, effective drugs for treating schizophrenia and mania were discovered (reserpine and chlorpromazine). These drugs replaced insulin coma and psychosurgery, and allowed many patients to behave more rationally in institutions, to leave them, or to avoid hospitalization entirely. Effective drug treatment stimulated the introduction of milieu therapy, halfway houses, and aftercare.

In 1955 Congress established the Joint Commission on Mental Illness and Health, representing 36 organizations, to examine the nation's mental health care. The Commission's 1961 report, *Action for Mental Health*, concluded that half of the patients in the state mental hospitals were not receiving active treatment. The Commission's recommendations set the stage for the emphasis on community mental health care that marked the 1960s. They recommended establishing one fully staffed community mental health clinic per 50,000 citizens, limiting the bed complement of large psychiatric hospitals to a maximum of 1,000, and encouraging the use of community-based, short-term inpatient care.

Many of the Commission's recommendations were incorporated in a 1963 Message to Congress by President Kennedy, the first Presidential message Congress had ever received on behalf of the mentally ill and the mentally retarded. Congress responded with the Mental Retardation Facilities and Community Mental Health Centers Construction Act, which, in part, created federal support for community-based mental health services delivered by community mental health centers. The 1960s also saw the introduction of additional effective drug treatments for mental disorders: benzodiazepines for anxiety disorders, tricyclic and mono-amine oxidase-inhibiting drugs for depressions, and lithium for manic-depressive psychosis. Behavior therapy became popular for treating certain neuroses and behavior disorders, and research began to demonstrate the effectiveness of various psychotherapies (Bergin, 1971; Malan, 1973; Smith & Glass, 1977).

Congress continued to expand the NIMH financial support for psychiatric and behavioral science research, psychiatric education in medical schools, residency training of psychiatrists, and community mental health centers. The creation of Medicare and Medicaid (Titles VIII and XIX of the Social Security Act; see Chapter 12) helped transfer some of the costs of caring for the chronically mentally ill to the federal treasury. Federal welfare support (Social Security Disability Income) and food stamps provided a minimal level of economic support for chronically mentally ill patients discharged from state hospitals. Unfortunately, the necessary networks of community medical, mental health, and human service agencies were inadequately organized and underfunded.

The 1970s saw a decline in federal support for mental health research and training and slow growth in funding for community mental health centers. The Carter Administration renewed presidential interest in mental health. In 1977 President Carter appointed a President's Commission on Mental Health, with Mrs. Carter as honorary chairperson. The Commission's 1978 report included an extensive review of the magnitude of the nation's mental health problems and of the resources available to meet them. The problems inherent in transferring the care of chronically mentally ill patients from state hospitals to community agencies began to be recognized. Detailed recommendations were made for increasing community services for chronic mental patients; improving access to care for underserved groups (children, minorities, rural citizens, and the aged); improving insurance coverage for mental health services; encouraging federal support for training personnel for underserved areas and population groups; increasing public understanding of mental disorders; protecting patients' rights; and expanding the knowledge base through increased federal support of research (President's Commission, 1978).

The 1980s were a period of fiscal retrenchment, with increasing numbers of Americans on the poverty rolls, cutbacks in programs for the poor, an increase in the number of homeless, and a new public health menace—the AIDS epidemic. During this time NIMH service programs, along with programs aimed at chemical-dependency treatment, were provided as block grants to states, but the NIMH continued a major leadership role through its community support program and demonstration projects aimed at the homeless mentally ill. Indeed, the major public mental health problem in this country became the homeless with mental illness wandering the streets, often hallucinating, rummaging through garbage, and sleeping on grates. This issue, more than others, has received attention through legislative hearings, the media, and public outcry. It is symptomatic of the release of thousands of patients from state facilities and the imperfect psychiatric technology that can help patients in the acute phase of a psychosis, but does not provide a long-term cure. Patients have found themselves in underfunded community mental health programs, and when they discontinue treatment, they are readmitted to hospitals for short-term stays.

The desire for minimal government involvement prevailed throughout the 1980s and early 1990s, until President Clinton's election campaign. His campaign was based on a number of domestic policy issues, health care prominent among them.

Clinton's election in 1992 reflected another shift in national mood, as many Americans became dissatisfied enough with the health care system to support major reform. Soon after his inauguration, he assembled a task force on national health reform, appointing his wife, Hillary Rodham Clinton, as chair of the task force. Vice-President Gore's wife, Tipper, a strong ally of the mentally ill, rallied behind parity coverage of mental illnesses. Clinton's health care reform proposal was released in September 1993, and generated a stormy Congressional debate. The proposal fell victim to political infighting and strong lobbying by special interest groups, and no reform was ratified.

Because citizens with major mental mental illnesses are not an effective political lobby group, the current coalition of former patients, dedicated professionals, and inspired reformers such as Mrs. Gore came together to maintain the momentum of reform. Although national reform was not implemented, they reinvigorated our society's long-standing moral commitment to care for its disabled and vulnerable citizens.

Mental Health Personnel

Many types of mental health professionals serve patients and clients in the mental health sector, including psychiatrists, nonpsychiatric physicians, psychologists, social workers, and registered nurses. In addition, services are provided by vocational rehabilitation counselors, occupational therapists, teachers, and by other health workers such as licensed practical nurses. In 1988, NIMH surveys identified 531,000 filled staff positions in 4,930 U.S. mental health facilities, of which 381,200 were patient care staff. The distribution of these employees is shown in Table 9.1. Almost one half (47%) were professional patient care staff; one-quarter were other patient care staff with less than a baccalaureate degree; and 28% were administrative, clerical, and maintenance staff. Combining part-time and full-time staff into full-time-equivalent (FTE) staff, just over half of FTE staff were employed in state and county mental hospitals (33%) and community mental health centers (21%) (Center for Mental Health Services, 1992).

Psychiatrists

Psychiatrists are physicians with 4 years of postgraduate training. During the first year after medical school at least 6 months of general medicine and neurology are required, followed by 3 years of psychiatric residency training. Psychoanalysts undergo additional years of education and training, including part-time didactics, a personal psychoanalysis, and supervision of their treatment cases, before being certified by a psychoanalytic institute. About 10% of all psychiatrists are psychoanalysts.

TABLE 9.1   Number of Full-time Equivalent Positions in Mental Health Facilities by Staff Discipline: United States, 1988

Staff discipline	All facilities	%
Professional patient care staff	248,430	46.8
Psychiatrists	18,132	3.4
Other physicians	3,959	0.8
Psychologists	23,131	4.4
Social workers	46,218	8.7
Registered nurses	73,387	13.8
Other mental health professionals: B.A. and above (e.g., vocational rehabilitation counselors, occupational therapists, teachers)	71,148	13.4
Physical health professionals and assistants (e.g., dentists, dental technicians, pharmacists, dieticians)	12,455	2.3
Other patient care staff	132,786	25.0
All other staff (administrative, clerical & maintenance)	149,856	28.2
TOTAL	531,072	

Source: Center for Mental Health Services

Between 1970 and 1988, the number of "active" psychiatrists (those neither in training nor retired) increased from about 19,900 (Koran, 1987) to about 33,000 (Dorwart et al., 1992). Of these, about 6,900 had specialized training in child psychiatry, too few, according to the federal Graduate Medical Education National Advisory Committee to meet the needs of the nation's children (Beresin & Borus, 1989). In addition, 4,496 residents were in psychiatric training in 1988, including 491 in child psychiatry (Rowley et al., 1990). Results of the 1988–1989 survey of members and nonmembers of the American Psychiatric Association (Dorwart et al., 1992) indicate that office-based practice was the primary professional activity of about 45% of active psychiatrists. Smaller proportions worked primarily in private, freestanding psychiatric hospitals (16%), state and county hospitals (11%), or other hospitals (6%). About 7% worked primarily in community mental health centers, 6% in university medical centers or medical schools, 2% in clinics or HMOs, 1% in government administrative agencies, and 5% in other settings. Most psychiatrists worked in more than one setting. About 67% of active psychiatrists' time was devoted to direct patient care, 12% to administration, 6% to teaching, 5% to consultation, 4% to research, and 6% to other activities. Psychiatrists working primarily in private office-based practice or HMOs treated an average of 30 patients per week. Across all outpatient settings, psychiatrists' mean monthly caseload (different patients who were seen at least once) was 47 patients (the median was

35 patients). In inpatient settings, where the intensity of service is greater, the mean monthly caseload was 31 patients.

Almost half of full-time psychiatrist positions in mental health facilities in 1971 were in state and county mental hospitals. By 1988, however, only 25% of the 18,182 full-time-equivalent (FTE) positions for psychiatrists were in state and county hospitals, primarily because of the decline in the number of state hospital beds and the increase in psychiatric positions in multi-service agencies (formerly termed community mental health centers) and private psychiatric hospitals (NIMH, 1983a, 1985; CMHS, 1992).

Like other physicians, psychiatrists are unevenly distributed geographically. In 1993, American Psychiatric Association membership distribution ranged from 25 psychiatrists in Wyoming to 4,255 psychiatrists in New York State. Within states, psychiatrists are more concentrated in urban areas than in the general population (APA, 1993). Unfortunately, the same counties that lack psychiatrists also lack other providers of mental health services (e.g., psychologists and family physicians) (Knesper et al., 1984; Olfson et al., 1994).

The largest proportions of patients treated by psychiatrists suffer from affective disorders (24%), schizophrenia (15%), and anxiety disorders (11%) (Dorwart et al., 1992). In outpatient settings, about 52% of psychiatrists' patients are treated with psychotherapy; 61% of these patients also receive medication. About 18% of patients are seen primarily for medication management, and 15% for evaluation or consultation. Thus, medical evaluation and treatment skills are essential for more than two-thirds of psychiatrists' outpatients. Fewer than 3% of outpatients were engaged in psychoanalysis; about 4% were treated with group psychotherapy, and about 4% with couples therapy (Dorwart et al., 1992).

Psychologists

Psychologists are nonmedical professionals who may have either a master's or a doctoral degree in one of many kinds of psychology, including experimental, social, general, or clinical (Rodnick, 1985). Only psychologists trained in clinical psychology programs must have supervised clinical experience. Because most states license individuals generically as psychologists, any psychologist, regardless of training, can open a private psychotherapy practice (Meltzer, 1975).

About 43,000 psychologists (of whom over 82% held doctoral degrees) were providing mental health services in 1993 in mental health facilities, schools, community agencies, and private practices. About 20,000 psychologists providing mental health services were employed full-time in 1993. Private practice was the primary professional setting of one-third of psychologists employed full-time; about 28% practice primarily in organized care settings (including hospitals and clinics), and 31% in educational and academic settings (Office of Demographic, Employment, and Educational Research, 1993). Psychologists working in mental health facilities carry out psychotherapy, diagnostic testing, research, teaching, and administrative duties, and offer consultation to other human service agencies.

More than one-third of clinically active psychologists whose primary work setting is *not* private practice have a secondary work setting that is. All 50 states plus Washington, D.C. and Puerto Rico regulate licensure and scope of practice of psychologists. Psychology applicants in all states are required to have either a Ph.D., or a master's degree in addition to 3 to 5 years of work experience. States can also pass laws regarding independent reimbursement of psychologists by third-party payors (Council of State Governments, 1986). Psychologists have been extremely successful in lobbying the federal and state government to allow third-party payments without requiring physician referral or supervision (Meltzer, 1975). Some states, such as New York, permit psychologists to have independent provider status, and Medicare extended this privilege to psychologists in 1989.

Psychologists have also been pressing for hospital admitting privileges, and they debate with psychiatrists the qualifications necessary for practicing psychotherapy. On the one hand, a medical education is not needed for one to be a skilled psychotherapist or to counsel or treat physically well individuals whose mental disorders do not require medications. On the other hand, only physicians can prescribe indicated psychotherapeutic drugs, and psychiatrists most knowledgeably treat the large proportion of mentally disordered patients who suffer from both physical disease and mental disorder (Hall et al., 1978; Koranyi, 1979; Tsuang & Simpson, 1985), and can be relied upon to recognize physical diseases masquerading behind mental symptoms (Hoffman & Koran, 1984; Lishman, 1978). Psychologists working in organizational settings are also finding themselves in competition with social workers, nurses, and marriage and family counselors, who claim to offer the same psychotherapeutic services at even lower cost to the organization. Some psychologists have lobbied for extension of prescribing privileges to psychologists. The U.S. Department of Defense instituted a Demonstration Psychologist Prescribing Program in 1991. To date, no enrollees have graduated from this program.

Social Workers

Social workers may have a bachelor's, master's, or doctoral degree in social work, although an advanced degree is encouraged for those doing clinical work . Social work education programs are accredited by the Council on Social Work Education.

Social workers' licensure and scope of practice are regulated in all 50 states. Most states recognize more than one category of social worker, based on education and work experience. Three categories are commonly delineated, corresponding to bachelor's, master's, and advanced master's or doctoral level training (Council of State Governments, 1986). Twenty-seven states license social workers with

B.S.W. degrees, although some require additional clinical experience (generally 2 to 3 years) before granting licensure.

The 145,000 members of the National Association of Social Workers (NASW) represent approximately one-half of the U.S. social work labor force. A recent NASW survey indicated that approximately 30,000 NASW members are clinical social workers. In 1988, 12% of patient care staff in mental health facilities were social workers, most holding a master's or doctoral degree (NASW, 1993; Rubenstone, 1991). Approximately 16% of social workers were in private practice in 1990.

Psychiatric social work received great impetus from the mental hygiene movement and child guidance clinics of the 1920s and 1930s. The social worker obtained diagnostic information from the child's parents concerning the child, the parents, and the environment, pooled this information with that gathered by the psychologist and psychiatrist, and then carried out therapy with the child's parents (Modlin, 1975). Today psychiatric social workers bring resources of community health and welfare agencies to bear on their patients' problems; continue in their diagnostic and therapeutic roles; offer consultation to human service agencies; and, to a lesser degree, engage in research, teaching, and administration. NASW estimates that social workers provide more than half of the mental health counseling in the U.S. There is a large projected need for social workers into the next century, and enrollment in social work master's degree programs has grown an estimated 300% in the last 5 years (Rubenstone, 1991).

Registered Nurses

In 1988, registered nurses (RNs) held 14% of FTE staff positions in mental health organizations. RNs accounted for 35% of FTE staff in nonfederal general hospitals and 20% of FTE staff in private psychiatric hospitals, compared to only 11% of such positions in state and county mental hospitals (CMHS, 1992).

Education in psychiatric nursing is part of all generic nursing education programs. The role of the psychiatric nurse includes assessing patient health status; supervising patient interactions on the inpatient unit; administering medications; planning, administering, and supervising others in somatic treatment; helping patients with activities of daily living; and in some instances providing individual, group, or family therapy. A small percentage of registered nurses pursue specialized training in psychiatric nursing and pursue master's or doctoral degrees. Registered nurses are the largest group providing professional care in mental health facilities. Psychiatric nurses with advanced training participate in research, teaching, and administration and offer consultation to nurses and other workers in medical units and public health agencies (O'Toole, 1975).

Recently nurses, following the lead of social workers and psychologists, have been lobbying state legislatures to permit increased autonomous practice; that is, being able to evaluate and treat patients without a prior referral or without supervision. They have been granted these privileges in a few states, however, the scope of practice for nurses has remained quite circumscribed (Carter, 1985).

Delivery of Mental Health Services

From the mid-nineteenth century to the mid-twentieth century, psychiatric services in this country were primarily based in long-stay institutions supported by state government, and patterns of practice were relatively stable. Over the past 40 years, remarkable changes have occurred. These changes include a reversal of the balances between institutional and community care, inpatient and outpatient services, and individual and group practice. Today, of the approximately 35.1 million Americans with a mental disorder, and the 15 million with a substance use disorder, only 9.4 million Americans receive services in the specialty mental health sector (21% of the total of 44.7 million with mental/addictive disorders; note some individuals have both kinds of disorders), and 20% of those afflicted receive no services.

Deinstitutionalization, or the departure of thousands of individuals from the large state hospital system, has occurred over the last three decades and has had a significant impact on the mental health care delivery system. At the peak of public asylum psychiatry in 1955, 559,000 Americans were hospitalized in state and county mental hospitals. Now, long-stay residents in state mental hospitals number well under 100,000, with total bed capacity of about 107,000 (CMHS, 1992). In 1955, three of four patient care episodes took place in state hospitals, one of four in community settings. Today three of four patient care episodes occur in community settings, only one of four in institutional-type settings (Manderscheid & Witkin, 1985). The shift of care to community-based settings began in the public sector. The private sector's bed capacity increased in the 1970s and 1980s, including psychiatric units in nonfederal general hospitals, private psychiatric hospitals, and residential treatment centers for children. Substance abuse centers and child and adolescent inpatient psychiatric units grew particularly quickly in the 1980s, as investors recognized their profitability. However, growth of the inpatient private mental health sector recently has slowed.

These changes have occurred as a result of a number of forces, not the least of which was a change in the legal environment in the 1960s, when patient rights suits established the principle of treatment in "the least restrictive setting." Further, social psychiatrists had established the deleterious effects of long-term institutional care, that is, the so-called social breakdown syndrome. The development of effective psychiatric medications ameliorated patients' behavioral symptoms and allowed discharge into the community. The increased proportion of the population with private insurance coverage for psychiatric services has also stimulated utilization. Probably the most significant factor in spurring the discharge of patients from state hospitals, however, was financing. With the federal Social Security titles—Medicare, Medicaid, Supplemental Social Security—it became advantageous for states to discharge patients into a variety of nursing homes or board-and-care-type settings and utilize new federal dollars to deal with state fiscal concerns. As long as patients remained in state institutions, they were not eligible for federal funds. With the passage of Medicaid (Title XIX) in 1965, patients who moved into the community or long-term-care institutions that were not institutions for mental diseases could be supported through that program, which provided a 50% federal subsidy. In 1972, with the passage of Supplemental Social Security (Title XVI), patients discharged from hospitals could perceive federal payments for board-and-care homes and other group living arrangements and for their daily support and also Medicaid for their treatment costs. This cost shifting strongly encouraged the emptying of state facilities, and reduce because of the fiscal pressure on state budgets.

Admissions to state mental hospitals and the number of psychiatric beds in general hospitals increased dramatically during this same period. Most admissions, however, were actually readmissions, as hospitals experienced a "revolving door," with patients admitted for multiple acute stays. Further, nursing homes have become a substitute for state mental hospitals and have assumed the long-term-care function. One estimate places three-quarters of a million Americans with chronic mental illness in nursing homes (Goldman & Manderscheid, 1987). Most of these patients suffer from behavioral disturbances or inability to care for themselves due to dementia, head injury, or other physical illness. Nearly 100,000 patients, however, have another psychiatric diagnosis, such as schizophrenia or bipolar disorder, that requires extended stay.

Decline in the use of state hospitals has had negative effects. Many patients— perhaps a million—have been discharged into communities that are ill-prepared to provide the therapeutic and rehabilitative services they need, such as halfway houses, aftercare programs, sheltered workshops, and psychosocial rehabilitation (Borus, 1981; Talbott, 1980). Some have become homeless wanderers, shifted from the back wards to living on the streets. Many patients now reside in unlicensed and uninspected board-and-care homes that do not offer or arrange for active treatment (Lamb, 1979).

Since 1978 the NIMH, through its Community-Support Program, has provided leadership to states and local communities to help them build systems of coordinated and cooperative mental health, health, and human services agencies to meet the needs of those with chronic mental illness. By 1984, most states had developed some community support arrangements, with the help of CSP planning grants (Morrissey & Goldman, 1984). Currently, there is a CSP in every state and program grants totalled $16 million in 1992.

In the past quarter-century, outpatient services have exhibited dramatic growth. The rate of additions to outpatient care more than doubled between 1969 and 1988, from 576 to 1,237 per 100,000 population. Most of this growth occurred in community mental health centers, but nonfederal general hospitals and freestanding psychiatric outpatient clinics also registered large increases in patient volume (CMHS, 1992).

Although over 4.5 times their 1969 number, patient additions to partial hospitalization care in 1988 (276,185) still represented only 5% of patient additions to all mental health service organizations (CMHS, 1992).

The Settings for Mental Health Services

The number of organizations providing specialized mental health services rose 65% between 1970 and 1988, from 3,005 to 4,930. Most of the increase is attributed to the growth in psychiatric units in general hospitals, which grew from 797 in 1970 to 1484 in 1988. The number of organizations providing outpatient psychiatric services also grew substantially during this period, increasing 38%.

The number of private psychiatric hospitals also increased, from 150 in 1970 to 444 in 1988, the great majority being part of investor-owned, for-profit medical chains. Costing less to build and operate per bed than general hospitals, psychiatric hospitals are an attractive source of profits for these corporations. On the positive side, corporate management may bring greater efficiency; stimulate innovation; drive down costs via competition; create psychiatric hospitals where none exist; and, by means of marketing, reduce the stigma associated with mental health care. On the other hand, these hospitals are less tolerant of nonpaying patients than are tax-supported or charity-supported hospitals, and they may be somewhat less responsive to local community needs than locally controlled hospitals. Whereas in 1981, 16 states had no hospital of this kind, by 1988 only North and South Dakota were without private psychiatric hospitals. Between 1970 and 1988, the number of beds in private psychiatric hospitals and in psychiatric units of general hospitals increased by 54,000 (from 36,700 to 90,700, almost 250%), resulting in a net increase in the number of psychiatric beds for all organizations (despite shrinking state hospital bed capacity).

In contrast, the number of VA medical centers stayed relatively constant (115 to 138) and the number of state and county mental hospitals decreased (310 to 285) during the same period. Indeed, nearly all of the decrease in inpatient beds during this period can be attributed to reductions in state and county mental hospitals, which decreased their bed counts from 413,000 in 1970 to 107,000 in 1988, a decrease of 74%. As a result, state and county mental hospitals only accounted for about 40% of all psychiatric beds in 1988, compared to 79% in 1970 (CMHS, 1992).

Reflecting the decline in public sector capacity, nonfederal general hospital psychiatric units have become the most common site of inpatient mental health admissions (44% in 1988), followed by private psychiatric hospitals (19%), and state and county psychiatric hospitals (15%). In addition to the admissions to general hospital psychiatric units recorded by NIMH, many more admissions of patients with psychiatric diagnoses to med/surg units in general hospitals are unrecorded (Kiesler & Sibulkin, 1984).

Patient admission data differ in demographic and diagnostic aspects between public and private sector facilities, reflecting source of payment as well as historic responsibilities. State and county hospitals may be returning to their original role—that of providing asylum for disabled patients who cannot function in their communities. If adequately funded, these hospitals can serve patients with special treatment and rehabilitative needs, such as chronically ill patients with no families or social supports, alcoholic patients (particularly those with associated cognitive impairment), and patients chronically dangerous to themselves or others.

Despite the drop in resident population, state and county mental hospitals face a number of problems. Fiscal restraint leaves budgets inadequate for high-quality clinical programs. State hospitals must deal with high readmission rates because publicly supported aftercare services have not been created in sufficient numbers. This has resulted in the so-called "revolving door syndrome." For-profit hospitals have not designed services, nor do they currently have the appropriate financial incentives, to meet the needs of chronically mentally ill patients. As in the general health care sector, a new social consensus must be reached regarding who will pay for those who cannot themselves pay for care. Neither for-profit nor nonprofit hospitals can shoulder this burden without realistic sources of revenue.

Residential treatment centers (RTCs) for emotionally or mentally disturbed children provide inpatient services to children under 18 years of age. Although their focus ranges from personality and behavioral disorders to severe psychoses, RTCs do not attempt to treat all serious mental disorders of children. The programs and physical facilities of RTCs are designed to meet patients' daily living, schooling, recreational, socialization, and routine medical care needs. Because a large number and variety of staff are required, costs are high. Treatments include milieu therapy, psychotherapy, behavior modification, psychotropic drugs, and special education (Lewis & Solnit, 1975). In 1988, there were 440 RTCs with a resident population of 23,000 (CMHS, 1992). The lack of coordination between the mental and general health care, juvenile justice, education, foster care, and child protective service sectors creates severe discontinuities (and more rarely, redundancies) in service delivery for children and adolescents. Improved service coordination is a major focus of reform efforts in the 1990s.

Day treatment patients spend most of the day at the treatment facility in structured therapeutic activities and then return home in the evenings. Day treatment services—including psychotherapy, pharmacotherapy, and occupational therapy—can provide alternatives to inpatient care, a transition from inpatient to outpatient care or discharge, or a locus for rehabilitating or maintaining chronically ill patients.

The number of day treatment programs has increased in response to pressures to decrease length of hospital stays and the increased number of patients discharged from mental hospitals partially recovered and receiving continuing pharmacotherapy. Between 1963 and 1988, the number of day treatment settings increased from 114 to 12,161. In 1988, partial care services were provided to 157,000 admitted persons, about 12% of whom were younger than 18 years of age.

Despite this impressive growth, expansion of day treatment services was slowed by the widespread failure of insurance policies to cover this treatment modality. Only recently have third-party payors been convinced of the cost-effectiveness of the treatment. Medicare has covered this service since 1987, and other plans have followed suit. In rural areas, long travel times continue to impede the use of day treatment.

Psychiatric halfway houses are nonmedical residential facilities that provide room and board in a homelike atmosphere for mentally disturbed individuals who cannot live independently but who can work or occupy themselves productively during the day if given some support and supervision. Most are 15- to 25-bed facilities with in-house staff who provide supervision and some treatment. Where they exist, halfway houses allow patients a graded transition from the extreme dependency of hospital life to the full responsibility of independent living. Admission to a halfway house is also used to prevent hospitalization.

Psychiatric halfway houses provide an important community service, not only through provision of housing for the mentally ill, but as a critical treatment link for those with severe and persistent illness. Despite these advantages, however, residential neighborhoods usually resist their establishment because most patients in halfway houses are not fully recovered. Because residence in a halfway house is usually not covered by insurance, there are far fewer than are needed.

The passage of Medicare and Medicaid unintentionally led to the shifting of many patients with chronic mental illness to nursing and personal-care homes. Since Medicare and federal Medicaid cover care for psychiatric disorders on the same basis as for general medical disorders in these facilities, but limit coverage of psychiatric care in state mental hospitals, states had a clear financial incentive to transfer patients to nursing and personal-care homes. Most patients with mental disorders receive a custodial level of treatment in nursing homes, although many would likely benefit from more active treatment than this setting provides.

If one adds the growth characteristics enumerated above to the growth of the mental health personnel, one can see that the mental health system, in the words of our modern corporate managers, "has expanded and diversified its portfolio." Indeed, expenditures by mental health organizations rose from $3.29 billion in 1969 to $23 billion in 1988, a 700% increase. Measured in constant (i.e., non-inflated) dollars, the increase was only 230%. State and county mental health agency expenditures accounted for 30% of the total, followed by private psychiatric hospitals with 20% and general hospital psychiatry services with 16% (CMHS, 1992). Funding sources vary considerably by type of organization and location across the country. Data regarding expenditures for professional services provided in private practice settings are not available.

In 1963 the federal government initiated a new type of mental health organization: community mental health centers (CMHCs). The CMHC program was an effort to provide access to an integrated set of services to residents of a specific geographic area (catchment area) containing from 70,000 to 200,000 persons. By 1980 there were 798 federally initiated CMHCs providing services in about half the country. Centers had to provide inpatient, outpatient, 24-hour emergency, partial hospitalization, and consultation/education services directly or through affiliative arrangements and had to treat individuals regardless of ability to pay. Later, centers were required to develop additional services, including rehabilitative aftercare services; specialized services for substance abusers, for children and adolescents, and for the elderly; and research and evaluation programs.

By 1980, 46% of the admissions to outpatient care in mental health facilities occurred in federally funded CMHCs, compared to 31% in freestanding psychiatric clinics. In addition, CMHCs accounted for 14% of all inpatient episodes (NIMH, 1983). Although federal grants to CMHCs totaled $314 million in 1980, this represented less than 5% of public funding for mental health services. In launching this program, the federal government bypassed state mental health agencies, which until that time had been slow to establish community-based programs. An unfortunate result was that CMHCs failed to focus on providing services to chronically mentally ill patients discharged from state mental hospitals (Morrissey & Goldman, 1984). Patients with diagnoses of neuroses and personality disorders were the largest group admitted to care (21%), with substance abusers (13%), and depressed patients (13%) next (President's Commission, 1978).

Between 1963 and 1982, successive administrations held varying views of the appropriate federal role in funding mental health services through the CMHC program. Republican administrations tried to limit it to a demonstration program, whereas Democratic administrations sought to expand the program gradually nationwide (Ochberg, 1976). With Public Law 97-35 (the 1981 Omnibus Budget Reconciliation Act), the Reagan administration repealed the legislation authorizing the CMHC program and consolidated all federal funds for mental health and alcohol and drug abuse services into a block grant program for the states, funded at 21% less (30% with inflation) than the previous year's appropriation (Estes & Wood, 1984). In addition, many states took steps to decrease their Medicaid expenditures, which had been an important source of funds for CMHCs. CMHCs ceased to be a federally recognized reporting category for mental health statistics. Depending on the services they operated and controlled directly, they were reclassified as multiservice mental health organizations, freestanding psychiatric outpatient clinics, or psychiatric units of nonfederal general hospitals. A 1983 survey of a sample of former CMHCs revealed that the cutbacks in federal and state funding had caused more than one-third of the centers to reduce staffing and services (Estes & Wood, 1984).

CMHCs were designed to remedy some of the deficiencies long recognized in the U.S. mental health care delivery system; however, the achievement of this laudable aim was blocked by various obstacles. Growth of nonfederal sources of funding was slower than expected. Insurance coverage for some services (day treatment, consultation and education, and home visits) was quite limited. Some CMHCs had difficulty in obtaining provider status under state Medicaid plans, and some states limited CMHC participation in Medicaid. Local governments often allocated very little money to CMHCs, particularly in poverty areas. Nonetheless, older CMHCs depended less on federal funds than younger ones did (NIMH, 1974). The declining participation of psychiatrists in providing services and in administering CMHCs, together with the small percentage of CMHC caseloads represented by patients with severe mental disorders, led some to ask whether CMHCs were evolving into social agencies rather than providers of mental health care (Fink & Weinstein, 1979). Some CMHCs aroused local opposition when, because of their attempts at preventing mental disorders, they plunged into local political conflicts about resource allocation. CMHCs were not able to cure social inequities and injustices rooted in economics, politics, and racism (Musto, 1975).

The long-term effect of the CMHC experiment on the pattern of mental service delivery is yet to be determined. Nonetheless, the experiences of CMHCs with catchment area responsibility; multi-agency agreements the integration of different levels of care; consumer participation; and local, state, and federal politics provide a rich record to be consulted by those interested in planning improvements in general health care service delivery.

Insurance Coverage for Mental Disorders

Insurance coverage for mental health care has always lagged behind coverage for other medical care. Only 13% of the payment for mental illness treatment comes from private insurance dollars, compared with 28% for general medical care. States pay almost 50% of the cost of mental health care, while paying less than 15% of the cost of other medical treatments (Sharfstein et al., 1984).

An analysis of data from the Bureau of Labor Statistics from 1979 to 1984 revealed changes in the level of insurance benefits for mental and nervous disorders in the private sector. Virtually all individuals with private health coverage have some inpatient psychiatric treatment included in the benefit package. Fewer than half of all individuals, however, have coverage for inpatient psychiatric treatment that is equal to the coverage for other illnesses, and this proportion is falling. In 1984, 48% had equal mental and general health coverages, compared to 58% in 1981. The limitations on psychiatric benefits include limitations on days of care and separate dollar limits, including fixed dollar caps on an annual or lifetime basis.

For outpatient care, although the vast majority of those with insurance (96%) has some coverage, this coverage is often quite restricted. In 1984 a total of 89% of all participants—up from 82% in 1981—had some outpatient coverage, subject to limitations such as additional copayment charges, higher deductibles, and specific dollar limitations. In this survey, the percentage of participants with any coverage for the treatment of alcohol abuse increased from 38 to 61% between 1981 and 1984 (Brady, Sharfstein, & Muszynski, 1986).

Differences in insurance for psychiatric versus other conditions arose in the 1920s and 1930s when hospital insurance was first written. Inpatient treatment for mental disorders then occurred largely in state-funded mental hospitals or in private mental hospitals used primarily by the wealthy. Although treatments and treatment settings have changed, rising health care costs, the absence of strong consumer demand for mental health coverage, and insurers' continuing fear of the potential cost of this coverage have kept these restrictions in place.

Today psychiatrists treat approximately twice the proportion of patients with no health insurance as do other physicians. Mental health coverage has been curtailed in a number of plans, including those under the Federal Employees Health Benefits Program (FEHBP). The Blue Cross/Blue Shield FEHBP, for example, in 1982 imposed a 50-visit limit on outpatient mental health treatment and a 60-day annual limit on inpatient care, whereas in the past treatment was limited only by medical necessity (Sharfstein & Taube, 1982).

Psychiatric care will not be adequately covered by insurance until the surrounding economic myths are addressed. The first myth is that costs of psychiatric treatment are uncontrollable and unpredictable, but experience contradicts this. For example, The Blue Cross/Blue Shield FEHBP had no limits on mental health coverage from 1967 to 1981, aside from the same deductibles and copayments as for general medical care. After the initial jump in costs immediately following the introduction of broader psychiatric benefits between 1967 and 1969, mental health care accounted for 7.2 to 7.7% of the total benefits paid from 1970 to 1981 (Sharfstein et al., 1984), suggesting that mental health costs were stable over time.

In 1971 the Rand Corporation began a health insurance study that enrolled 7,500 persons at six sites across the country in 14 different insurance plans. Patient copayments ranged up to 95%, with a maximum dollar expenditure of $1,000 per family (Brook et al., 1983). The study found that expenditures for mental health care constituted only about 5% of the total health care costs for all insurance plan enrollees. Depending on copayment levels, between 7.1 and 9.6% of the population studied used mental health benefits, including visits to general practitioners and internists. Recall that the NIMH Epidemiological Catchment Area study reported mental illness prevalence rates of 28.1% of the population (and included only a portion of all mental disorders) (Myers et al., 1984). Only a small percentage of the Rand study population (0.4%) saw clinicians more than 40 times a year (Brook et al., 1983). This study and others underscore the stability over time of costs for mental health care under insurance (Krizay, 1982; Wells et al., 1982).

Many of the restrictions on insurance coverage for psychiatric care appear to stem largely from concern about the costs of long-term custodial care or intensive psychotherapy. The standard treatment regimen for intensive psychotherapies involves a minimum of three therapy sessions a week. Within the FEHBP, which placed no restriction on the annual number of outpatient visits for more than a decade, the number of persons receiving intensive psychotherapeutic treatment ranged from 0.9% of all psychiatric outpatients treated in 1971 to 1.1% of those treated in 1973. The cost for treatment for this population during the same period ranged from 8.7% to 10.3% of the total cost of physicians' treatment of mental disorders (Sharfstein & Magnas, 1975).

Another myth is that mental health care costs are unstable because liberal coverage encourages unnecessary and excessive use. Supporters of this view cite data such as these: 9% of outpatient users of mental health care in the Blue Cross/Blue Shield FEHBP accounted for 45% of the total cost (Sharfstein & Taube, 1982). That someone with insurance may be more likely to initiate medical care and, once under care, be more likely to opt for more extensive treatment is not a phenomenon limited to mental health care. Insurance encourages utilization of all physician services. The Rand study, for example, reported that 1% of utilizers of medical care in their 7,500-person sample accounted for 28% of the total expenditures (Wells et al., 1982).

A third myth is that mental health care is not cost-effective. This myth is a carryover from the years preceding development of effective psychiatric treatments, when most treatment was custodial instead of curative. Considering costs and benefits from a broad societal perspective, the introduction of lithium for the treatment of manic-depressive psychoses produced a conservatively estimated 10-year savings of $4.2 billion ($2.9 billion in unexpended treatment costs plus $1.3 billion in productivity gains) (Reifman & Wyatt, 1980). In addition to the evident analogies between medical management of psychiatric and nonpsychiatric conditions, a body of evidence suggests that expenditures for psychotherapy produce savings elsewhere in the economy through increased employee productivity, reduced absenteeism, and lower costs for other medical care (Jones & Vischi, 1979; Mumford et al., 1984). For example, beneficiaries covered by the Blue Cross/Blue Shield FEHBP who began outpatient psychotherapy following diagnosis of chronic medical disease used 56% fewer medical services during the third year after diagnosis than did beneficiaries with the same diseases who received no outpatient psychotherapy (Schlesinger et al., 1983).

A final myth is that psychiatric treatment is not accountable to insurance carriers. Utilization review in the form of peer review has become the cornerstone of organized psychiatry's accountability to payers and consumers. Many insurance carriers have chosen to put strict limits on psychiatric care rather than implement peer review procedures. The APA developed peer review services in the early 1970s to give insurers the option of providing psychiatric care limited only by medical necessity, thereby enhancing their opportunity to achieve savings through cost avoidance in other areas of medical care. In 1982 the APA conducted 5,000 reviews for the Civilian Health Medical Program of the Uniformed Services (CHAMPUS) and 965 reviews for other third-party payers.

The cost savings reported from the APA program are impressive. Aetna Life and Casualty's peer review costs in 1981 were about $20,000; its estimated savings were $2.4 million. Mutual of Omaha Insurance Company estimated a savings of about $300,000 during its first year of participation in the program. CHAMPUS reports that peer review has led to "outright savings" of $5 million per year since it began participating 3 years ago. Additional savings in costs of medical care avoided as a result of peer review may be three to four times greater than the direct savings. Peer review in the APA program has been effective in assuring that necessary and appropriate care is delivered (Sharfstein et al., 1984). Although the financial savings in some UR programs are negligible, and opponents of these strategies point to their potential negative impact on patient care, fiscal realities in the 1990s have necessitated that payors implement measures of this type. Managed care strategies are likely to remain an integral component of third-party payors' ongoing search for ways to reduce their outlays.

Medicare

The general benefits and costs of Medicare, a federal program that insures through the Social Security system some health care costs of individuals aged 65 and over and disabled individuals regardless of age, are described in Chapter 12. Under Part A (hospital insurance), benefits for inpatient treatment in a psychiatric hospital are limited to 190 days in a lifetime. Only 150 of these days (90 benefit-period days plus 60 lifetime-reserve days) can be used in any one benefit period. Benefits for psychiatric care in a certified general hospital or extended-care facility are the same as for any other form of medical care. This provision has increased the use of general hospitals to provide psychiatric care for the elderly.

Under Part B (supplementary medical insurance), benefits for physicians' outpatient care for mental illness initially was limited to 50% of the charges or $250, whichever was less. Benefits for physicians' inpatient care for mental illness are the same as for other illnesses; that is, they are not limited. One hundred home visits are also covered and may be provided by mental health agencies.

In 1993, Medicare implemented a reformed reimbursement method for Part B, known as the Resource-Based Relative Value System (RBRVS). Payment is based on skill, risk, resources, and time required for the type of service provided. Although psychiatrists and other providers of cognitive and primary care services were assured that RBRVS would compensate these services adequately, to date hard-fought battles within Congress have been necessary to win fair reimbursement levels.

A relatively small part of Medicare payments are for psychiatric services. In FY 1987, less than 3% of total Medicare funds ($79,750 billion) was spent for alcohol/drug/mental health services. About $1,915 billion was paid for hospital services under Part A, and about $253 million for professional services under Part B

(Lave & Goldman, 1990). This low percentage may reflect both the reluctance of older Americans to seek mental health services in the face of stigma, and the more limited coverage of these services under Medicare than under many private insurance plans. In fiscal year 1988, about 3% of Medicare's expenditures paid for psychiatric services (Lave & Goldman, 1990). Reed and his associates have pointed out that "a comprehensive program of services for the mentally ill, with emphasis on ambulatory care, is not at present a Medicaid requirement and is not included in the Medicaid plans of a number of states" (Reed et al., 1972, p. 144). This deficiency reflects the priority given by both the federal and state governments to the mental health care needs of the poor and near poor. Considered alongside the prevalence of mental disorders among the elderly, these percentages are strikingly low. After reviewing these and other data, the President's Commission on Mental Health recommended increased mental health benefits under Medicare as well as national standards for minimum mental health benefits and other service expansions and improvements under Medicaid (President's Commission, 1978).

In December 1987 Congress expanded the outpatient psychiatric benefit in Medicare as part of the Budget Deficit Reduction Act of 1987. Outpatient benefits were increased in two stages over a 2-year period to $2,200 annually, with a 50% co-payment. This quadrupling in benefits basically keeps the outpatient psychiatric benefit on par with inflation since 1965. Benefits were expanded for partial hospitalization, which was established as a reimbursable service. Perhaps most significantly, all limits and special copayments were removed for "the medical management of psychopharmacologic agents" for Medicare beneficiaries. This type of "medical management" is now covered on a par with outpatient treatment for other medical illnesses, that is, with a 20% co-payment and no visit or dollar limits.

Medicaid

Medicaid is a combined federal and state program that covers certain health care costs for eligible persons with incomes falling below stated levels. Eligibility standards and covered health care services vary from state to state; however, in no state is care of patients under age 65 in mental institutions included. The federal government views this as a responsibility long borne by the states through their own mental hospitals. Although no other restrictions by diagnosis are permitted, states can and have limited the amounts of covered mental health care. An APA survey revealed a typical set of limits in most states:

> For inpatient hospital care most states limit the number of days allowable to 30 or less per year. Inpatient physician visits are generally provided for but allowed charges are usually set unrealistically low. Outpatient physician visits for psychiatric care are typically limited to 20 to 30 visits per year with maximum fees per visit usually set well below prevailing charges. (Muszynski et al., 1984, p. 865).

Few utilization data are available because states are not required to keep records by diagnosis. In 1984 Medicaid spending ranged from $52 per capita in Wyoming to $382 in New York (National Advisory Mental Health Council, 1993). Very approximate estimates suggest that mental health services, primarily in skilled nursing and intermediate care facilities (over $2 billion), and state hospitals (approximately $2 billion) accounted for about 15% of Medicaid expenditures (Taube, et al., 1990).

Legal Issues

Laws and their interpretations change with the times, and laws regulating the delivery of mental health services are no exception. Legal issues receiving substantial judicial attention in the past two decades have included commitment procedures, the right to treatment, the right to refuse treatment, and the insanity defense in criminal proceedings (Stone, 1975). Patient-therapist relationships have also been subjected to judicial and legislative scrutiny (Mills et al., 1987).

Civil commitment to a mental institution deprives a mentally disordered person of liberty, in exchange for treatment. The grounds for civil commitment vary in different states, but include judgments that the person is dangerous to self or others, is unable to care for physical needs, or needs care or treatment. Recent rulings show a movement toward restricting the grounds for civil commitment, reducing the length of time a person can be committed by physicians without judicial review, abolishing indeterminate stays during which the patient cannot initiate discharge or release, and requiring commitment through the courts, with due process guarantees for longer-term commitments (Appelbaum, 1984a). In a 1978 case, *Addington v. Texas*, the U.S. Supreme Court determined that the standard of evidence for civil commitment should be "clear and convincing evidence," rather than the standard of "beyond a reasonable doubt" that applies in criminal proceedings. Appelbaum has argued that the general principle behind these and other decisions of the Burger Court in the mental health arena was the desire to limit judicial intrusiveness into the operation of state-level institutions, such as hospitals, prisons, and schools (Appelbaum, 1984b).

The civil and personal rights of committed and voluntary mental patients have been given increasing statutory recognition. These rights include the right to communicate with persons outside the institution; to keep clothing and personal effects; to practice religion freely; to receive independent psychiatric examination; to manage or dispose of property; to retain licenses, permits, or privileges established by law; to enter into contracts; to marry; and to sue and be sued (McGarry & Kaplan, 1973).

The Mental Health Law Project, sponsored by the American Civil Liberties Union Foundation, the American Orthopsychiatric Association, and the Center for Law and Social Policy, engages in litigation and consults with legislatures and mental health organizations to help secure these and other patient rights. Because of this attention to procedures and rights, seriously disturbed individuals are being given more humane care. But the conflicts, involving patients' rights to liberty, their need for care or treatment, and the state's interests in protecting their welfare and in preventing harm to others, remain (Roth, 1979).

A constitutional right to treatment for involuntarily committed patients was first recognized by a court in *Wyatt v. Stickney* in 1972. Guardians of involuntarily committed patients sued the Alabama mental health commissioner, charging that inadequate care was rendered in a state mental hospital. A federal district court judge agreed that patients had a right to treatment that included the right to certain standards of care. With the aid of medical and psychiatric consultants, he defined these standards to include individual evaluation, active treatment, minimum staffing ratios, detailed nutritional and physical standards, and compensation for work performed. But the judgment had certain limitations. It did not apply to voluntary patients, and it set no penalty for noncompliance. The mental health commissioner, a psychiatrist, did not contest the inadequacy of care at the state's institutions. He was fired and replaced by a finance officer.

Although lower courts have recognized a right to treatment on the part of involuntarily committed patients, the U.S. Supreme Court has not. The right to treatment recognized in 1974 by the Fifth Circuit Federal Court of Appeals in *O'Connor v. Donaldson* was rejected in 1975 by the U.S. Supreme Court (Weiner, 1982). The court held in this case, however, that states have no right to confine "a nondangerous individual who is capable of surviving safely in freedom by himself or with the help of willing and responsible family members and friends" (Weiner, 1982, p. 462).

The federal district court that decided *Wyatt v. Stickney* has remained active in working for improved levels of care in Alabama's state mental hospitals. Similar cases may therefore force state legislatures to allocate more resources to institutional care of the mentally disordered and to community-based care (Kaufman, 1979). Right-to-treatment cases on behalf of the mentally retarded have had some success in this regard (McGarry & Kaplan, 1973). Right-to-treatment litigation does raise the dangerous possibility that lawyers and judges rather than mental health professionals may begin determining the details of hospital administrative practices and the adequacy of individual treatment plans. If courts intrude too far on the decision-making prerogative of mental health professionals working in state institutions and departments of mental health, even fewer professionals will choose to work there than do now (Robitscher, 1974).

The right of committed patients to refuse treatment is not widely recognized. Since committed patients are deprived of their liberty in exchange for treatment that is presumably in their best interests, to allow them to refuse it would seem contradictory. On the other hand, the state's coercive power must be restrained to prevent capricious application. Committed patients usually are regarded as legally incompetent to decide whether to accept particular treatments, although exceptions are made for electroconvulsive therapy and psychosurgery in a few states on the grounds that these treatments may harm patients or change them irrevocably. Electroconvulsive therapy, however, is much safer than many common surgical procedures; it is not known to cause permanent brain damage, and it brings about well-documented benefits (Avery & Winokur, 1976; Fink, 1979; Janicak et al., 1985). In most states, a committed patient's only grounds for refusing medications is religious principle, recognized by the Second Circuit Federal Court of Appeals in *Winters v. Miller* in 1971. These grounds for refusing were then recognized by the U.S. Supreme Court in the same year.

In Massachusetts, Colorado, and Oklahoma, however, committed mental patients can refuse treatment, except in narrowly defined emergencies, unless they are found incompetent by a judge. If a patient is found incompetent, the judge will decide "whether the patient, if competent, would have consented to the administration of antipsychotic drugs" (Gutheil, 1985, p. 213). Gutheil believes that the failure in Massachusetts "to defer in the average case to medical judgment may have introduced significant delays and impediments to the good treatment of patients in the name of protecting their rights"(p. 216).

In California the 1983 decision by the Federal District Court for the Northern District of California in *Jamison v. Farabee* established a review process when a treating psychiatrist wishes to use neuroleptic (antipsychotic) medication to treat an involuntary patient who has refused medication or who cannot give informed consent. Rather than resorting to judicial review, as in Massachusetts, the California decision requires an outside psychiatrist to examine the patient and the clinical records and then to approve or deny the medication's use. NIMH has funded a study of the implementation of *Jamison v. Farabee*, to identify costs, effects, and problems and their probable causes. After implementation of this ruling the rate at which patients in California successfully refused involuntary medications remained at its historic 1%. About half the patients who successfully refused medication subsequently deteriorated (Hargreaves et al., 1987). Because all laws and judicial policy decisions are social experiments, more frequent empirical investigations of their effects are desirable.

That involuntary treatment is not limited to psychiatric settings is often forgotten. Nonpsychiatric physicians on medical and surgical units of general hospitals use or prescribe restraints, psychoactive and other medications, intravenous fluids, and nursing care for patients who have refused these treatments (Appelbaum & Roth, 1984).

The invocation of an insanity defense during John Hinckley's trial for the attempted assassination of President Reagan stimulated great public and professional interest in this difficult area of law. The Insanity Defense Work Group of the APA subsequently issued a review of the legal history of this concept and an exploration of potential changes in its application. The American Medical Association (1984) and the American Bar Association (Riley & George, 1984) also issued position statements. Whereas the APA and ABA argued for the preservation in criminal trials of a more constrained insanity defense "based on inability to appreciate the wrongfulness of one's conduct at the time of the offense" (Glass,

1985, p. 399) the AMA argued for the abolition of the insanity defense and the enactment of laws "providing for acquittal when the defendant, as a result of mental disease or defect, lacked the state of mind (*mens rea*) required as an element of the offense charged" (AMA, 1984, p. 2967).

The APA group noted that most insanity acquittals are not awarded by juries; they result from concurrence between the prosecution and the defense. Among other issues, the group discussed (1) abolishing the insanity defense, (2) allowing a "guilty but mentally ill" verdict, (3) changing current standards employed in defining the legal concept of insanity, and (4) determining the appropriateness of current dispositions for defendants found "not guilty by reason of insanity" (Insanity Defense Work Group, 1983). Although this point of intersection between psychiatry and the law episodically receives great public attention, the intersection points discussed earlier affect far greater numbers of citizens. Several well-publicized cases in the 1980s and early 1990s focused public attention on physical relationships between patients and their therapists (Appelbaum & Jorgensen, 1991). Several states have passed legislation or are considering bills invoking criminal penalties for such relationships, for which therapists are held responsible. The APA modified its code of ethics to reflect a stricter standard of behavior. This controversial issue is likely to remain the topic of legal and professional debate for some time.

"Mental health" encompasses the entire adaptation of the individual. Legal issues closely interrelate with psychiatric ones. Psychiatrists are often expected to perform a social control role in the process of hospitalizing and treating potentially dangerous patients. At the same time, the legal system is concerned with punishment for wrongdoing and not treatment for illness. Patients have individual legal rights, but when their judgment is impaired, what is their right to treatment? When their judgment is impaired by a mental disorder, who decides what is more important—freedom or health? These questions will continue to be debated within our democracy, both within the medical and legal professions and between them.

Conclusion: Progress in Understanding Mental Illness and the Promotion of Mental Health

Mental health care has grown, diversified, and prospered, especially over the last 35 years. Large state hospitals have been supplemented and supplanted by psychiatric units in general hospitals, new outpatient clinics, community mental health centers, day treatment, halfway houses, and private practitioners. Treatment has become more effective and specific, based on our growing understanding of the brain and behavior. Psychopharmacologic treatment has made possible the shift away from long-term custodial institutions, and psychosocial treatments continue the process of care and rehabilitation in community settings. Recent advances in the biological and behavioral sciences will continue to create improved opportunities for diagnosing, treating, and preventing mental disorders (Institute of Medicine, 1984).

Today as we confront the opportunities of health care reform, we must rethink issues of access, quality, and cost for mental health and substance abuse treatment. As we have seen, the epidemiology is robust, the treatments more and more effective, and as access is expanded through the provision of benefits to those who do not have them, we must develop our delivery system to triage and manage the inevitable increase in demand for care.

Resources are limited so priorities for care must be established and choices made. These choices often depend on the values of the choosers—mental health/ mental illness is a broad area for such discussions in the future. More extensive education of general physicians regarding mental disorders and their treatment is needed. The development of the continuum of care as an approach to serious and persistent mental illness must grow, and an emphasis on the alternatives to the inpatient care are key if we are to contain costs. More day treatment programs, home visits, psychosocial rehabilitation efforts, and residential group homes are needed. Reducing our current two-tier system to one tier will take the sincere efforts of policy makers at state and local levels, but is essential if we are to develop an accountable and a fair system for all Americans.

The growth in our knowledge base and opportunities for new discoveries provides for optimism and hope. Whether this promise can be converted into reality is the next chapter for mental health services as we approach the twenty-first century.

References

American Medical Association, "Report of the Board of Trustees: Insanity Defense in Criminal Trials and Limitation of Psychiatric Testimony." *Journal of the American Medical Association, 251*, 2967, 1984.

American Psychiatric Association, Public Information Office. Washington, DC: American Psychiatric Press, 1993.

American Psychiatric Association, *DSM-IV*. Washington, DC: American Psychiatric Press, 1994.

Appelbaum, P. S., "Standards for Civil Commitment: A Critical Review of Empirical Research." *International Journal of Law and Psychiatry, 7*, 133, 1984(a).

Appelbaum, P. S., "The Supreme Court Looks at Psychiatry." *American Journal of Psychiatry, 141*, 827, 1984(b).

Appelbaum, P. S., & Jorgenson, L., "Psychotherapist-Patient Sexual Contact After Termination of Treatment: An Analysis and a Proposal. *Am J Psychiatry, 148*, 1466–1473, 1991.

Appelbaum, P. S., & Roth, L. H., "Involuntary Treatment in Medicine and Psychiatry." *American Journal of Psychiatry, 141*, 202, 1984.

Avery, D., & Winokur, G., "Mortality in Depressed Patients Treated with Electroconvulsive Therapy and Antidepressants." *Archives of General Psychiatry, 33*, 1029, 1976.

Barchas, J. D. et al. (Eds.), "*Psychopharmacology: From Theory to Practice.*" New York: Oxford University Press, 1977.

Beers, C. W. A., *A Mind That Found Itself*. New York: Doubleday, 1939.

Beigel, A., & Sharfstein, S. S., "Mental Health Care Providers: Not the Only Cause or the Only Cure for Rising Costs." *American Journal of Psychiatry, 141*(5), 668–672, 1984.

Beigel, A., & Sharfstein, S. S. (Eds.), *"The New Economics and Psychiatric Care."* Washington, DC: American Psychiatric Press, 1985.

Beresin, E. V., & Borus, J. F., "Child Psychiatry Fellowship Training: A Crisis in Recruitment and Manpower." *Am J Psychiatry, 146,* 759-763, 1989.

Bergin, A. E., "The Evaluation of Therapeutic Outcomes." In A. E. Bergin et al. (Eds.), *Handbook of Psychotherapy and Behavior Change.* New York: Wiley, 1971.

Bernstein, I. C. et al., "Lobotomy in Private Practice: Long Term Follow Up." *Archives of General Psychiatry, 12,* 10, 1975.

Bockoven, J. S., *"Moral Treatment in Community Mental Health."* New York: Springer Publishing Co., 1972.

Borus, J. F., "Deinstitutionalization of the Chronically Mentally Ill." *New England Journal of Medicine, 305,* 339, 1981.

Brady, J., Sharfstein, S. S., & Muszynski, I. L., "Trends in Private Insurance Coverage for Mental Illness." *American Journal of Psychiatry, 143,* 10, 1986.

Brook, R. H. et al., "Does Free Care Improve Adults' Health?" *New England Journal of Medicine, 309,* 1426, 1983.

Broskowski, A. et al., (Eds.). "Linking Health and Mental Health." In *SAGE Annual Reviews of Community Mental Health* (Vol.2). Beverly Hills and London: Sage Publications, 1978.

Carter, E. W., "Psychiatric Nursing." In H. I. Kaplan & B. J. Sadock (Eds.), *Comprehensive Textbook of Psychiatry* (Vol. l, 4th ed.). Baltimore and London: Williams and Wilkins, 1985.

Center for Mental Health Services. *Mental Health. United States. 1992.* Manderscheid, R.W. & Sonnenschein, M.A., Eds. DHHS Pub. No (SMA)92-1942. Washington, DC, U.S. Government Printing Office, 1992.

Council of State Governments & National Clearinghouse on Licensing Enforcement and Regulation, "State Credentialing of the Behavioral Science Professions: Counselors, Psychologists, and Social Workers." Lexington, KY: Council of State Governments, 1986.

Deutsch, A., "The History of Mental Hygiene." In J. K. Hall et al. (Eds.), *One Hundred Years of American Psychiatry.* New York: Columbia University Press, 1947.

Dorwart, R. A. et al., "A National Study of Psychiatrists' Professional Activities." *American Journal of Psychiatry,* 149:1499–1505, 1992.

"Electroconvulsive Therapy: Consensus Conference," *Journal of the American Medical Association, 254* (15), 2103, 1985.

Estes, C. L., & Wood, J. B., "A Preliminary Assessment of the Impact of Block Grants on Community Mental Centers." *Hospital and Community Psychiatry, 35,* 1125, 1984.

Fink, M., *Convulsive Therapy: Theory and Practice.* New York: Raven Press, 1979.

Fink, P. J., & Weinstein, S. P., "Whatever Happened to Psychiatry? The Deprofessionalization of Community Mental Health Centers." *American Journal of Psychiatry, 136,* 406, 1979.

Foley, H. A., & Sharfstein, S. S., *"Madness and Government: Who Cares for the Mentally Ill."* Washington, DC: American Psychiatric Press, 1983.

Frank, G. F., & Kamlet, M. S., "Direct Costs and Expenditures for Mental Health Care in the United States in 1980." *Hospital and Community Psvchiatry, 36,* 165, 1985.

Frank, J. D., & Frank, J. B., *Persuasion and Healing: A Comparative Study of Psychotherapy.* Baltimore: Johns Hopkins University Press, 1991.

Glass, R. M., "Realities Not Myths." *Journal of the American Medical Association, 253,* 399, 1985.

Goldman, H. H., Cohen, G. D., & Davis, M., "Expanded Medicare Outpatient Coverage for Alzheimer's Disease and Related Disorders." *Hospital and Community Psychiatry, 36*(9), 939, 1985.

Goldman, H. H., & Manderscheid, R. W., "Chronic Mental Disorder in the United States." In R. W. Manderscheid & S. A. Barrett (Eds.), *Mental Health United States,* 1987 (DHHS Pub. No. ADM 87-1518). Washington, DC: U.S. Government Printing Office, 1987.

Gutheil, T. G., "Rogers v. Commissioner: Denouement of an Important Right-to-Refuse-Treatment Case." *American Journal of Psychiatry, 142,* 213, 1985.

Hall, R. C. W. et al., "Physical Illness Presenting as Psychiatric Disease." *Archives of General Psychiatry, 35,* 1315, 1978.

Hargreaves, W. A., *Jamison versus Farabee Implementation: The External Investigator.* Paper presented at the American Psychiatric Association Annual Meeting, Dallas, Texas, May 1985.

Hargreaves, W. A. et al., "Effects of the Jamison-Farabee Consent Decree: Protection for Involuntary Psychiatric Patients Treated With Psychoactive Medication." *American Journal of Psychiatry, 144,* 188–92, 1987.

Hoffman, R. S., & Koran, L. M., "Detecting Physical Illness in Patients with Mental Disorders." *Psychosomatics, 25,* 654, 1984.

Insanity Defense Work Group, "American Psychiatric Association Statement on the Insanity Defense." *American Journal of Psychiatry, 140,* 681, 1983.

Institute of Medicine, *Research on Mental Illness and Addictive Disorders: Progress and Prospects.* Washington, DC: National Academy Press, 1984.

Janicak, P. G. et al., "Efficacy of ECT: A Meta-Analysis." *American Journal of Psychiatry, 142,* 297, 1985.

Jones, J. R., & Vischi, T. R., "Impact of Alcohol, Drug Abuse and Mental Health Treatment on Medical Care Utilization." *Medical Care, 17,* ii–82, 1979.

Kaufman, E., "The Right of Treatment Suite as an Agent of Change. *American Journal of Psychiatry, 136,* 1428, 1979.

Kendall, R. E., "The Concept of Disease and Its Implications for Psychiatry." *British Journal of Psychiatry, 127,* 305, 1975.

Kiesler, C. A., & Sibulkin, A. E., "Episodic Rate of Mental Hospitalization: Stable or Increasing?" *American Journal of Psychiatry, 141,* 44, 1984.

Knesper, D. J. et al., "Mental Health Services Providers' Distribution across Countries in the United States." *American Psychologist, 39,* 1424, 1984.

Koran, L. M. (Ed.), *The Nation's Psychiatrists.* Washington, DC: American Psychiatric Association, 1987.

Koranyi, E. R., "Morbidity and Rate of Undiagnosed Physical Illnesses in a Psychiatric Clinic Population." *Archives of General Psychiatry, 36,* 414, 1979.

Krizay, J., "Federal Employees' Experience as a Guide to the Cost of Insuring Psychiatric Services in the Various States." *American Journal of Psychiatry, 139,* 866, 1982.

Lamb, H. R., "The New Asylums in the Community." *Archives of General Psychiatry, 36,* 129, 1979.

Langsley, D. G., "Prevention in Psychiatry: Primary, Secondary, and Tertiary." In H. I. Kaplan & B. J. Sadock (Eds.), *Comprehensive Textbook of Psychiatry* (Vol I, 4th ed.). Baltimore and London: Williams and Wilkins, 1985.

Lave J. R., & Goldman H. H., "Medicare Financing For Mental Health Care." *Health Affairs*, 9:19–30, 1990.

Lewis, M., & Solnit, A. J., "Residential Treatment." In A. M. Freeman et al. (Eds.), Comprehensive Textbook of Psychiatry, vol. 2. Baltimore, MD: Williams & Wilkins, 1975.

Lishman, W. A., *Organic Psychiatry*. London: Blackwell Scientific Publications, 1978.

Locke, B. Z., & Regier, D. A., "Prevalence of Selected Mental Disorders." In C. A. Taube & S. A. Barrett (Eds.), *Mental Health, United States, 1985* (DHHS Pub. No. ADM 85-1378). Washington, DC: U.S. Government Printing Office, 1985.

Malan, D. H., "The Outcome Problem in Psychotherapy Research." *Archives of General Psychiatry, 29*, 719, 1973.

Mandersheid, R. W., & Witkin, M. J. et al., "Specialty Mental Health Services: System and Patient Characteristics-United States." In C. A. Taube & S. A. Barrett (Eds.), *Mental Health. United States, 1985*. (DHHS Pub. No. ADM 85-1378). Washington, DC: U.S. Government Printing Office, 1985.

McGarry, A. L., & Kaplan, H. A., "Overview: Current Trends in Mental Health Law." *American Journal of Psychiatry, 130*, 621, 1973.

Meltzer, M. L., "Insurance Reimbursement, a Mixed Blessing." *American Psychologist, 30*, 1150, 1975.

Mills, M. J. et al., "Protecting Third Parties: A Decade after Tarasoff." *Am J Psychiatry*, 144:68–74, 1987.

Modlin, H. C., "Psychiatric Social Service Information." In A. M. Freedman et al. (Eds.), *Comprehensive Textbook of Psychiatry* (Vol.2). Baltimore: Williams and Wilkins, 1975.

Mora, G., "Historical and Theoretical Trends in Psychiatry." In A. M. Freedman et al. (Eds), *Comprehensive Textbook of Psychiatry* (Vol. 2). Baltimore: Williams and Wilkins, 1975.

Moore, M. D., "Some Myths about 'Mental Illness.'" *Archives of General Psychiatry, 32*, 1483, 1975.

Morrissey, J. P., & Goldman, H. H., "Cycles of Reform in the Care of the Chronically Mentally Ill." *Hospital & Community Psychiatry, 35*, 785, 1984.

Mumford, E. et al., "A New Look at Evidence about Reduced Cost of Medical Utilization Following Nental Health Treatment. *American Journal of Psychiatry, 141*, 1145, 1984.

Murphy, J., "Psychiatric Labelling in Cross Cultural Perspective." *Science, 191*, 1019, 1976.

Musto, D. A., "Whatever Happened to 'Community Mental Health'?" *Public Interest, 39*, 53, 1975.

Muszynski, S. et al., "Paying for Psychiatric Care." *Psychiatric Annals, 14*, 861, 1984.

Myers, J. K. et al., "Six-Month Prevalence of Psychiatric Disorders in Three Communities." *Archives of General Psychiatry, 41*, 959, 1984.

Narrow, W. E., "Use of Services by Persons With Mental and Addictive Disorders: Findings From the National Institute of Mental Health Epidemiologic Catchment Area Program." *Archives of General Psychiatry, 50*, 95, 1993.

National Advisory Mental Health Council: Health Care Reform for Americans with Severe Mental Illness: Report of the National Advisory Mental Health Council. *Am J Psychiatry*, 150:1447–1465, 1993.

National Association of Social Workers Information Office. Washington, DC, 1993.

National Commission for the Protection of Human Subjects of Biomedical and Behavioral Research. *Psychosurgery* (DHEW Pub. No. OS 77-0001). Washington, DC: U.S. Government Printing Office, 1977.

National Foundation for Brain Research, *The Cost of Disorders of the Brain.* Washington, DC, 1992.

National Institute of Mental Health, *Patterns in Use of Nursing Homes by the Aged Mentally Ill* (DHEW Pub. No. ADM 74-69). Washington, DC: U.S. Government Printing Office, 1974.

National Institute of Mental Health, *Mental Health Services in Primary Care Settings: Report of a Conference April 2–3. 1979.* (DHHS Pub. No. ADM 83-995.) Rockville, MD: U.S. Government Printing Office, 1983 (a).

National Institute of Mental Health, *Mental Health United States: 1983* (DHHS Pub. No. ADM 83- 1275). Rockville, MD: U.S. Government Printing Office. 1983 (b).

National Institute of Mental Health, *Mental Health. United States: 1985* (DHHS Pub. No. ADM 85-0000). Rockville, MD: U.S. Government Printing Office, 1985.

National Institute of Mental Health, *Mental Health United States 1987* (DHHS Pub. No. ADM 87-1518). Washington, DC: U.S. Government Printing Office, 1987.

National Institutes of Mental Health Information Office.

Ochberg, F. M., "Community Mental Health Center Legislation: Flight of the Phoenix." *American Journal of Psychiatry, 133,* 56, 1976.

Office of Demographic, Employment, and Educational Research, APA Education Directorate. *"Profile of All APA Members: 1993."* Washington, DC : American Psychological Association, 1993.

Olfson, M., Pincus, H. A., & Dial, T. H., "Professional Practice Patterns of U.S. Psychiatrists." *American Journal of Psychiatry, 151,* 89, 1994.

O'Toole, A. W., "Psychiatric Nursing." In A. M. Freedman et al. (Eds.), *Comprehensive Textbook of Psychiatry* (Vol. 2). Baltimore: Williams and Wilkins, 1975.

President's Commission on Mental Health, *Report to the President 1978* (Vols. 1–6). Washington, D.C.: U.S. Government Printing Office, 1978.

Rabkin, J., "Public Attitudes toward Mental Illness. A Review of the Literature." *Schizophrenia Bulletin, 10,* 9, 1974.

Reed, L. S. et al., *Health Insurance and Psychiatric Care: Utilization and Cost.* American Psychiatric Association, Washington, DC, 1972.

Regier, D. A. et al., "The De Facto U. S. Mental and Addictive Disorders Service System: Epidemiologic Catchment Area Prospective 1-year Prevalence Rates of Disorders and Services." *Archives of General Psychiatry, 50,* 85, 1993.

Regier, D. A. et al., "The DeFacto U. S. Mental Health Services System." *Archives of General Psychiatry, 35,* 685, 1978.

Reifman, A., & Wyatt, R. J., "Lithium: A Brake in the Rising Cost of Mental Illness." *Archives of General Psychiatry, 37,* 288, 1980.

Riley, W. D., & George, B. J., Jr., "Reform, Not Abolition." *Journal of the American Medical Association, 251,* 2947, 1984.

Robitscher, J., "Implementing the Rights of the Mentally Disabled: Judicial Legislative and Psychiatry Action." In F. J. Ayd, Jr., et al. (Eds.), *Medical Moral and Legal Issues in Mental Health Care.* Baltimore: Williams and Wilkins, 1974.

Rodnick, E. H., "Clinical Psychology." In H. I. Kaplan & B. J. Sadock (Eds.), *Comprehensive Textbook of Psychiatry* (Vol. 1, 4th ed.). Baltimore and London: Williams and Wilkins, 1985.

Roth, L. H., "A Commitment Law for Patients, Doctors and Lawyers." *American Journal of Psychiatry, 136,* 1121, 1979.

Rowley B. D. et al., "Graduate Medical Education in the United States." *JAMA*, 264: 822–832, 1990.

Rubenstone, S. F., "Licensed To Care." *In View*, *3*, 4, 1991.

Schlesinger, H. J. et al., "Mental Health Treatment and Medical Care Utilization in a Fee-For-Service System: Outpatient Mental Health Treatment Following the Onset of a Chronic Disease. *American Journal of Public Health*, *73*, 422–428, 1983.

Sharfstein, S. S. et al., *Health Insurance and Psychiatric Care: Update and Appraisal*. Washington, DC: American Psychiatric Press, 1984.

Sharfstein, S. S., & Magnas, H. L., "Insuring Intensive Psychotherapy." *American Journal of Psychiatry*, *132*, 70, 1975.

Sharfstein, S. S., & Taube, C. A., "Reductions in insurance for Mental Disorders: Adverse Selection, Moral Hazard, and Consumer Demand." *American Journal of Psychiatry*, *139*, 1425, 1982.

Shryock, R. H., "The Beginnings: From Colonial Days to the Foundation of the American Psychiatric Association." In J. R. Hall et al. (Eds.). *One Hundred Years of American Psychiatry*. New York: Columbia University Press, 1947.

Smith, M. L., & Glass, G. V., "Meta-Analysis of Psychotherapy Outcome Studies." *American Psychologist, 32*, 752, 1977.

Stapp, J., Tucker, A. M., & VandenBos, G. R., "Census of Psychological Personnel." *American Psychologist, 40*, 1317, 1985.

Stone, A. A., *Mental Health and Law: A System in Transition*. National Institute of Mental Health (DHEW Pub. 75-176), 1975.

Strecker, E. A., "Military Psychiatry: World War I. 1917–1918." In J. K. Hall et al. (Eds.), *One Hundred Years of American Psychiatry*. New York: Columbia University Press, 1947.

Szasz, T. S., *The Myth of Mental Illness*. New York: Hoeker-Harper, 1961.

Talbott, J. A. (Ed.), *State Mental Hospitals: Problems and Potentials*. New York: Human Sciences Press, 1980.

Talbott, J. A., *Contemporary Social Issues and Decisions That Will Affect the Future Practice of Psychiatry*. Unpublished manuscript, 1985.

Taube C. A. et al., Medicaid Coverage for Mental Illness: Balancing Access and Costs. *Health Affairs*, 9:5–18, 1990.

Tsuang, M. T., & Simpson, J. C., "Mortality Studies in Psychiatry." *Archives of General Psychiatry*, *42*, 98, 1985.

VandenBos, G. R., & Stapp. J., "Service Providers in Psychology: Results of the 1982 APA Human Resources Survey. "*American Psychologist, 38*, 1330, 1983.

Weed, J. A., "Suicide in the United States: 1952–1982." In C. A. Taube & S. A. Barrett (Eds.), *Mental Health United States, 1985* (DHHS Pub. No. ADM 85-1378). Washington, DC: U.S. Government Printing Office, 1985.

Weiner, B. A., "Supreme Court Decisions on Mental Health: A Review." *Hospital and Community Psychiatry, 33*, 1982.

Wells, K. B. et al., Cost *Sharing and the Demand for Ambulatory Mental Health Services*. Santa Monica, CA: Rand Corporation, 1982.

Witkin, M. J. et al., "Specialty Mental Health System Characteristics." In R. W. Manderscheid & S. A. Barrett (Eds.), *Mental Health United States 1987* (DHHS Pub. No. ADM 87-1518) Washington, DC: U.S. Government Printing Office, 1987.

10

Financing for Health Care

James R. Knickman and Kenneth E. Thorpe

A key factor that shapes the delivery of health care in the United States is the evolving system for financing services. The types of services delivered and the organizational approaches to delivering services are heavily influenced by how health care is paid for and the aggregate resources available for health care.

The financing system that has evolved over the past 30 years in the United States involves a complex blend of public and private responsibilities. This system varies substantially from the largely public financing systems that exist in many European countries. An understanding of how health care is paid for is useful for developing an understanding of the general organization of health care in America.

Payment approaches for health care have been undergoing tremendous changes since the early 1980s. The basic approach for reimbursing hospital care has been completely restructured by many payers for care, and payment approaches for physicians and long-term-care providers also are being restructured. As emphasized here, financing approaches vary from provider to provider and from payer to payer, and financing approaches will continue to evolve over time. Thus, this chapter attempts to explain not only the current structure of financing approaches, but also the principles behind the financing system.

In explaining how the American health care financing system operates, this chapter focuses on

- What health care resources buy.
- Where resources come from.
- How health care providers are paid.
- Why health care expenditures have been increasing.

As displayed in Table 10.1, $752 billion, or just over 13% of the gross national product (GNP), was spent for health purposes in 1991. These expenditures represent $2,868 per year for each person. Thus, the health care sector represents a major

TABLE 10.1 Aggregate and Per Capita National Health Expenditures, by Source of Funds and Percentage of Gross National Product, Selected Calendar Years, 1929–1995

Calendar year	Total GNP[a]	Total health expenditures			Private health expenditures			Public health expenditures		
		Amount[a]	Per capita	Percentage of GNP	Amount[a]	Per capita	Percentage of total	Amount[a]	Per capita	Percentage of total
1929	$103.3	$3.6	$29	3.5	$3.2	$25	86.4	$0.5	$4	13.6
1935	72.2	2.9	23	4.0	2.4	18	80.8	0.6	4	19.2
1940	99.7	4.0	30	4.0	3.2	24	79.7	0.8	6	20.3
1960	503.7	26.9	146	5.3	20.3	110	75.3	6.6	36	24.7
1970	982.4	74.7	359	7.6	47.5	228	63.5	27.3	131	36.5
1980	2,631.7	248.0	1,049	9.4	142.2	601	57.3	105.8	448	42.7
1990	5,542.9	675.0	2,601	12.2	390.0	1,502	57.8	285.1	1,098	42.2
1991	5,694.9	751.8	2,868	13.2	421.8	1,609	56.1	330.0	1,259	43.9
1992[b]	5,909[c]	819.9	3,098	13.9[d]	443.5	1,675	54.1	376.5	1,422	45.9
1993[b]	6,259[c]	903.3	3,380	14.4[d]	482.2	1,805	53.4	421.1	1,576	46.6
1995[b]	7,069[c]	1,101.9	4,050	15.6[d]	573.0	2,106	52.0	528.8	1,944	48.0

[a]In billions of dollars.

[b]These figures are projections based on "National Health Expenditures projections through 2030," *Health Care Financing Review*, Fall 1992.

[c]Gross Domestic Product

[d]Percentage of Gross Domestic Product

Source: Adapted from R. M. Gibson et al., "National Health Expenditures, 1983," *Health Care Financing Review*, 6 Winter 1984; R. M. Gibson "National Health Expenditures, 1978," *Health Care Financing Review*, 1, and *Health Care Financing Review*, Fall 1992 (pps. 14 and 19).

element of the American economy. As a component of the economy, health care has been growing at a fast rate over the past 30 years. As a point of comparison, health expenditures totaled only $43 billion in 1965, or 5.8% of the GNP. From 1965 onward, outlays for health rose, on the average, 11.7% each year. Although the rate of increase in costs between 1990 and 1991 was 11.4%, which was much lower than the peak inflation rate of 15.3%, growth in health care expenditures continues to exceed by a wide margin the overall inflation rates prevalent in the American economy. An important element of the study of health care finance, therefore, is analysis to understand the dynamics of spending in the United States and to understand what is being achieved by the ever-increasing health care expenditure levels.

What the Money Buys

National health care expenditures, as measured by the federal Health Care Financing Administration (HCFA), are grouped into two categories: (1) research and medical facilities construction and (2) payments for health services and supplies (see Table 10.2). Personal health care expenses constitute the bulk of the latter—$660.2 billion in 1991. Five types of personal health care expenditures account for over 75% of the 1991 total: 38.4% went to hospitals, 18.9% to physicians, 8.0% for nursing home care, 8.1% for drugs and drug sundries, and 4.9% for dentists' services. The other categories of expenditures are "other professional services," such as podiatry and private speech therapy, 4.7%; "other health services," 1.7%; administrative expenses, 5.8%; government public health activities, 3.3%; and construction, 1.4%. The costs of medical education are not included in these HCFA figures, except insofar as they are inseparable from hospital expenditures and biomedical research.

Where the Money Comes From

Ultimately, the people pay all health care costs. Thus, when we say health care monies come from different sources, we really mean that dollars take different routes on their way from consumers to providers: through government, private insurance companies, and independent plans, in addition to out-of-pocket payments. In 1991 close to 22% of personal health care expenditures were directly out-of-pocket ($144.3 billion). At the same time, the government share was nearly 43% (about $283.3 billion), with the federal government bearing nearly three-fourths of that. Finally, almost 32% was paid through insurance companies ($209.3 billion) (Letsch et al., 1988).

Public Outlays

The 43% of personal health care expenditures transferred by the public sector in 1991 ($283.3 billion) compares with 40% in 1980, 22% in 1965, 22% in 1950, and 9% in 1929. The increase, especially since 1965, is largely a result of greater federal expenditures. Proportionately, state and local government outlays have remained rather constant over time, in the 10 to 13% range. The significant rise in federal spending is accounted for by the Medicare and Medicaid programs, Title XVIII and XIX, respectively, of the Social Security Act.

Medicare. Medicare was inaugurated on July 1, 1966. It provides a range of medical care benefits for persons aged 65 and over who are covered by the Social Security system. The 1972 amendments to the Social Security Act extended benefits to persons aged 65 and older who do not meet the criteria for the regular Social Security program, but who are willing to pay a premium for coverage. In July 1973 benefits were further extended to the disabled and their dependents and those suffering from chronic kidney disease (Russell et al., 1974)

Part A of the program, financed by payroll taxes collected under the Social Security system, provides coverage for care rendered in a hospital, an extended-care facility, or the patient's home. Part B, a voluntary supplemental program that pays certain costs of physicians' services and other medical expenses, is supported in part by general tax revenues and in part by contributions paid by the elderly (Somers & Somers, 1961). Neither Part A nor Part B of Medicare, however, offers comprehensive coverage. Built into the program are deductibles (set amounts the patient must pay for each type of service before Medicare begins to pay) and co-insurance (a percentage of charges paid by the patient). Limitations on the amount of coverage exist as well. Hospital benefits cease after 90 days if the patient has exhausted his lifetime reserve pool of 60 additional days; extended-care facility benefits end after 100 days.

In 1988, Congress passed a bill to substantially expand Medicare coverage. This legislation, the Medicare Catastrophic Act of 1988, set limits on the maximum out-of-pocket costs that beneficiaries were responsible for in the case of hospital care, physician services, and pharmaceuticals.

The Medicare Catastrophic Program, however, was greeted unenthusiastically by many elderly. In the fall of 1989, under heavy pressure from the elderly, Congress repealed the Catastrophic Coverage Act. The program's unpopularity was caused by its financing approach, which passed along the costs of the program to the elderly in the form of new premiums and income-related surcharges to the elderly's federal income tax. The elderly particularly objected to the added income tax, in part because many of the wealthy elderly who were required to pay the maximum tax already had arranged for similar supplementary insurance coverage through private insurance companies.

Quality and cost of care delivered by public programs have been long-standing issues. Medicare amendments passed in 1972 established professional standards review organizations (PSROs) to monitor the quality and quantity of institutional services delivered to Medicare and Medicaid recipients. The 1982 Tax Equity and Fiscal Responsibility Act (TEFRA), discussed below, replaced the PSROs with a "utilization and quality control peer review organization" (PRO) Subsequent legislation (P.L. 98-21) required that hospitals covered under Medicare's new case payment system contract with a PRO by 1984. The new PROs differ substantially from the old PSROs: PROs are to be statewide organizations unless exceptional circumstances pertain; they may be for-profit as well as nonprofit operations; they require participation of only a small segment of area physicians; and they operate under contract with the Health Care Financing Administration, with performance judged against pre-established and quantifiable contract objectives.

As with quality and cost reviews, recent changes in Medicare provisions have radically changed the way Medicare pays for hospital care. The TEFRA legislation of 1982 was designed to provide incentives for cost containment. Most important, TEFRA established a case-based reimbursement system (DRGs, or diagnosis related groups) while also placing limits on the rates of increase in hospital revenues. TEFRA was followed in 1983 by Title VI of P.O. 98-21, which established a prospective payment system. Discussion of the principles of these 1983 amendments is provided later in this chapter.

In the Omnibus Budget Reconciliation Act of 1989 (OBRA 1989), Medicare changed the way physicians are paid. Previously, Medicare payment rates for a service were based on the amounts physicians charged. The new payment system is a national fee schedule that assigns relative values to services based on the time, skill, and intensity it takes to provide them. The relative values are then adjusted for geographic variations of payment. This system went into effect on January 1, 1992.

OBRA 1989 also limited the amount that physicians are allowed to charge patients above the amount that Medicare pays, and implemented a system intended to help Congress limit growth in Medicare expenditures for physician payments. Further discussion of these changes is provided later in this chapter.

Medicaid. Unlike Medicare, Medicaid is a program run jointly by federal and state governments; the name is more or less a blanket label for 50 different state programs designed specifically to serve the poor. Beginning in January 1967, Medicaid provided federal funds to states on a cost-sharing basis (according to each state's per capita income) so that welfare recipients could be guaranteed medical services. Payment in full was to be afforded to the aged poor, the blind, the disabled, and families with dependent children if one parent was absent, unemployed, or unable to work. Four types of care were required to be covered: (1) inpatient and outpatient hospital care, (2) other laboratory and x-ray services, (3) physician services, and (4) nursing facility care for persons over age 21. Legislation enacted in subsequent years added coverage of home health services for those entitled to nursing facility services, and early and periodic screening, diagnostic and treatment services for persons under age 21.

The 1972 Social Security Act amendments added family planning to the list of "musts." States must also now cover the services of rural health clinics, community and migrant health centers, health centers for the homeless, and similar qualified centers, nurse-midwives, and nurse practitioners. Currently, the law specifies another 31 optional services that states may elect to cover. These include prescription drugs, intermediate care facilities for the mentally retarded, optometrists' services, dental services, and eyeglasses. States may place certain limits on the extent to which services are covered. For example, they may limit the number of covered prescriptions or hospital days.

Eligibility for Medicaid is determined by the states within federal guidelines. By and large, Medicaid is available only to very low-income persons. The program also has categorical restrictions; that is, only families with children, pregnant women, and those who are aged, blind, or disabled can qualify.

With few exceptions, recipients of cash assistance are automatically eligible for Medicaid. In addition, most states extend Medicaid to some "medically needy" groups, who meet the nonfinancial criteria for Medicaid eligibility but exceed the income requirements. Individuals with great medical expenses may "spend down" to the medically needy standard. Aged or disabled persons receiving long-term care in institutions or in alternative community-based programs can, in some states, spend down to Medicaid eligibility, and, in others, receive Medicaid if their income is below a federally specified level.

Historically, because of the linkage between Medicaid and welfare eligibility, state variation in eligibility criteria for cash assistance resulted in variable Medicaid coverage across states. However, legislation enacted since the mid-1980s has decoupled Medicaid eligibility from receipt of cash assistance, extending mandatory Medicaid eligibility to numerous groups—chiefly low-income pregnant women and children—and producing greater uniformity in Medicaid eligibility.

Due to the expansions, state Medicaid programs must now cover all pregnant women and children up to age 6 with family income below 133% of the poverty level; children below 100% of poverty who are aged 10 or younger (all poor children under age 19 will be covered by 2002); for a transition period, poor families who lose cash assistance because of earnings from work; for a 12-month period, two-parent families in which the principal earner is unemployed; and disabled persons who lose eligibility for cash assistance due to earnings from work.

Medicaid also pays the Medicare premiums, deductibles, and coinsurance for certain low-income Medicare beneficiaries. Finally, states have the option to cover a variety of other groups.

It should be noted that, even with the expansions, Medicaid covers only some 40% of the poor.

Because of the gaps in insurance coverage for the poor and near poor that are not taken care of by the Medicaid programs, much recent debate and analysis has focused on how to pay for services to individuals uncovered by Medicare, private insurance, or Medicaid. As of 1993, at least 25 states have established bad-debt and charity-care pools to pay for hospital services and, in some cases, physician services for individuals who have no source of payment for their medical care. These programs have developed, in part, to spread the burden of the costs of care to indigents across the hospital system. The pools are generally funded through some form of tax or surcharge on hospital revenues from third parties (Lewin & Lewin, 1988).

Other Public Expenditures. In 1991 Medicare and Medicaid accounted for 76.5% of public outlays for personal health care services. The next-largest expenditure category, state and local government outlays, accounted for 7.2% of the $283.3 billion spent on public programs (Letsch et al., 1988, included here are funds used to operate psychiatric hospitals and other long-term care facilities, as well as acute care general hospitals at the county and municipal levels.

There are four remaining significant personal health care categories for which government monies are spent: (1) federal outlays for hospital and medical services for veterans ($12.1 billion in 1991, 4.3% of public personal health care expenditures); (2) provision of care by the Department of Defense for the armed forces and military dependents (in 1991, $12.6 billion; 4.4%); (3) worker's compensation medical benefits ($16.6 billion; 5.9%); and (4) other federal, state, and local outlays for personal health care ($8.0 billion, 2.8%), including support for maternal and child health programs, vocational rehabilitation, Public Health Service and other federal hospitals, the Indian Health Service, temporary disability insurance, and the Alcohol, Drug Abuse, and Mental Health Administration. In contrast, all government public health activities are recorded as costing only $24.5 billion in 1991. It must be noted, however, that while federal prevention and control operations are included in this figure, excluded are funds expended by other than health departments at the state and local levels for air and water pollution control, sanitation, and sewage treatment (Letsch et al., 1988) The relatively low level of government funding for public health activities deserves special attention in view of the growing recognition of the relationship between the environment and health, and importance of preventive care and health promotion.

Worker's compensation is an insurance system operated by the states, each with its own law and program, that provides covered workers with some protection against the costs of medical care and loss of income resulting from work-related injury and, in some cases, sickness (Congressional Research Service, 1976; Price, 1979a, b; U.S. National Commission on State Workermen's Compensation Laws, 1973.) The first worker's compensation law was enacted in New York in 1910; by 1948 all states had enacted such laws. The theory underlying worker's compensation is that all accidents, irrespective of fault, must be regarded as risks of industry and that the employer and employee shall share the burden of loss.

Finally, public spending for research and facilities construction totaled approximately $14.0 billion in 1991. Public outlays for research totaled $11.7 billion in 1991, with the federal government the source for the vast majority (see Table 10.2).

TABLE 10.2　Aggregate and Per Capita Amount and Percentage Distribution of National Health Expenditures, Selected Calendar Years 1960–1993

Type of expenditure	Aggregate amount ($ Billions)			
	1960	1980	1990	1993
Total	27.1	250.1	675.0	903.3
Health services and supplies	25.4	238.9	652.4	875.9
Personal health care	23.9	219.4	591.5	803.7
Hospital care	9.3	102.4	258.1	358.8
Physicians' services	5.3	41.9	128.8	167.3
Dentists' services	2.0	14.4	34.1	41.0
Other professional services	0.6	8.7	30.7	44.9
Home health care	0.0	1.3	7.6	12.3
Drugs and drug sundries	4.2	21.6	55.6	70.9
Eyeglasses and appliances	0.8	4.6	11.7	13.9
Nursing home care	1.0	20.0	53.3	74.3
Other health services	0.7	4.6	11.5	20.4
Expenses for prepayment and administration	1.2	12.2	38.9	48.0
Government public health activities	0.4	7.2	22.0	24.2
Research and medical facilities construction	1.7	11.3	22.7	27.4
Research	0.7	5.4	11.9	15.7
Construction	1.0	5.8	10.8	11.7

Type of expenditure	Per capita amount ($)			
	1960	1980	1990	1993
Total	142.56	1063.80	2600.15	3380.61
Health services and supplies	133.61	1016.16	2513.10	3278.07
Personal health care	125.72	933.22	2278.51	3007.86
Hospital care	48.92	435.56	994.22	1342.81
Physicians' services	27.88	178.22	496.15	626.12
Dentists' services	10.52	61.25	131.36	153.44
Other professional services	3.16	37.01	118.26	168.04
Home health care	0.0	5.53	29.28	46.03
Drugs and drug sundries	22.09	91.88	214.18	265.34

Source: Health Care Financing Administration, Office of the Actuary, Data from the Office of National Health Statistics.

Private Health Care Expenditures

The bulk of private health care expenditures comes from two sources; individuals receiving treatment and private insurers making payments on the behalf of patients. In 1991 private expenditures totaled $377.0 billion, 57.1% of all personal health care expenditures. In 1965, prior to the advent of Medicare and Medicaid, private expenditures accounted for 76.9% of all personal health care expenditures; in 1935, 82.4%; in 1929, 88.4% (Gibson, 1979). This recent decline in the private share of total expenditures is due primarily to the sharp drop in out-of-pocket payments associated with increased federal spending. In 1965, 53% of personal health care expenditures was paid directly by the patient; in 1991, it was 22%. Yet because of inflation and other factors, the per capita dollar amount paid directly in 1983 was four times what it was in 1965 (Gibson, 1979; Letsch et al., 1988).

Private insurers have paid between 20 and 32% of personal health care costs since 1965. Their share was $45.3 billion in 1978, 27% of the total; in 1991, it was $209.3 billion, or 31.7% of the total.

Before considering private health insurance in any depth, the manner in which the term "insurance" is used in the health care industry should be clarified. "Insurance" originally meant, and still usually refers to, the contribution by individuals to a fund for the purpose of providing protection against financial losses following relatively unlikely but damaging events. Thus, there is insurance against fire, theft, and death at an early age. All of those events occur within a group of people at a predictable rate, but are rare occurrences for any one individual in the group.

When medical insurance began, it was in this tradition. From 1847, when the first commercial insurance plan designed to defray the costs of medical care was organized, to the 1930s, health insurance consisted essentially of cash payments by commercial carriers to offset income losses resulting from disability attributable to accidents. Sickness benefits (cash payments during sickness) began as an extra, a "frill" on accident insurance policies. As with accident insurance, emphasis was on the replacement of income lost, in this instance as a result of contracting certain specified and catastrophic communicable diseases, such as typhoid, scarlet fever, and smallpox (Health Insurance Institute, 1975). With the organization of Blue Cross and Blue Shield, a new policy developed: reimbursing health care costs in general.

Health care utilization is not a rare occurrence. On average, each person in the United States visits a physician five times a year. One of every six Americans is admitted to a hospital at least once a year. Other than coverage for catastrophic illness, a fairly rare event, health insurance has become a mechanism for offsetting expected rather than unexpected costs. The experience of the many is pooled in an effort to reduce outlays for any one individual to a manageable prepayment size. Perhaps the term assurance more appropriately describes the health care payment system that has evolved. In Britain, assurance is used to denote coverage for contingencies that must eventually happen (e.g., life assurance), whereas insurance is reserved for coverage of those contingencies, like fire and theft, that may never occur.

Structure of the Private Insurance Industry. The organization of private insurance in the United States is undergoing dramatic changes. Before 1980 virtually all private insurance was provided by either the national system of Blue Cross and Blue Shield plans or by commercial insurance companies, which offered health care insurance as one of many types of insurance products available to employers. These insurance companies charged employers or individuals annual premiums and generally paid health care providers on what is termed a fee-for-service basis. A set amount, often prescribed by the insurance plan or negotiated between the insurer and the provider, was paid by the insurance company to a provider each time a beneficiary used a covered service.

Starting in the early 1980s, however, a range of new insurance approaches and a range of new relationships between insurers and providers have emerged. Health maintenance organizations (HMOs), which deliver services on a capitated basis rather than a fee-for-service basis, have been expanding rapidly; they accounted for 9% of all private insurance in 1992. Preferred provider organizations (PPOs), which either limit beneficiaries to a set list of physicians and other providers or provide economic incentives to use physicians who have offered discounts to the insurer, are also expanding rapidly; they accounted for 13% of all private insurance in 1992 (see Table 10.3). Point of service plans, which generally require members to go to providers within their networks for certain services but which give them the option to go to nonnetwork providers for other services, generally at a much higher cost, accounted for 16%.

Table 10.3 indicates that fee-for-service insurance still accounts for 62% of the health insurance market. However, 50% of private insurance policies are fee-for-service but use some "managed" care approaches to limit utilization. These approaches include second surgical opinion requirements, preadmission certification review, and length-of-stay reviews.

The growth of insurance plans that do not rely on unmanaged fee-for-service coverage has been a response to the rapid rise in insurance premiums that has faced both employers and individuals. Insurance premiums have been increasing at a rate that far exceeds general inflation rates, and employers have been seeking alternative insurance approaches that can reduce employer costs.

A second major change in the structure of the insurance industry is the growth of self-insured or self-funded health plans. Self-insurance refers to the assumption of claim risk by an employer, union, or other group, whereas self-funding refers to the payment of insurance claims from an established bank or trust account (Arnett & Trapnell, 1984). Self-insurance offers potential advantages to employers: they are exempt from most premium taxes and are able to retain interest on reserves (Arnett & Trapnell, 1984). Moreover, they have generally been exempt

TABLE 10.3   Enrollment in Managed and Unmanaged
            Group Health Plans, 1992

Group plan	Percentage of enrollment
Managed FFS	50%
Unmanaged FFS	12%
HMO	9%
PPO	13%
POS	16%

FFS: fee-for-service insurance

POS: point-of-service

Source: Hay/Huggins Company, 1992, as quoted in *Medical Benefits*, Volume 10, Number 1, January 15, 1993.

from state laws mandating minimum benefits under the Employee Retirement Income Security Act of 1974 (ERISA), however, a U.S. Supreme Court decision ruled that a Massachusetts mandated-benefit law is not preempted by ERISA because it applies to insurance contracts purchased for plans subject to ERISA.

The growth in self-insurance has been significant. In 1992, 67% of companies were at least partially self-insured for their employees health care costs, up from 46% in 1986 (A. Foster Higgins as quoted by Bulinski, 1993). One common operational mode of self-insured plans is the administrative services only (ASO) plan. Under an ASO plan, the insurance carrier handles the claims and benefits paperwork for the self-insured group. Insurance claims are normally paid from an employer bank account.

Blue Cross and Blue Shield. The establishment of payment mechanisms to defray the costs of illness can be traced to the Great Depression. Previously hospitals had sought to assure reimbursement for their services through public education campaigns directed at encouraging their users, middle-income Americans, to put money aside for unpredictable medical expenses (Law, 1974). When hard times proved the inadequacy of the savings approach, attention turned to the development of a stable income mechanism. A model was at hand in the independent prepayment plan pioneered in 1929 at Baylor University Hospital in Texas to assure certain area school teachers of some hospital coverage. Under the plan, 1,250 teachers prepaid 50 cents a month to provide themselves with up to 21 days of semiprivate hospitalization annually.

In the early 1930s nonprofit prepayment programs offering care at a number of hospitals were organized in several cities. The American Hospital Association (AHA) vigorously supported the growth and development of these plans, soon to be named Blue Cross, and the special insurance legislation that was required for their establishment in each state (Law, 1974). The AHA set standards for plans and then offered its seal of approval to plans meeting the standards. A provider-insurer partnership was firmly established; indeed, not until 1972 did national Blue Cross formally separate from the AHA.

Whereas Blue Cross developed as a hospital insurance system, Blue Shield developed independently, beginning in 1939 as an insurer for physician services. These two insurers tend to be financially and organizationally distinct, but they have many similarities and most often work together to provide hospital and physician coverage. Blue Cross and Blue Shield both are local or statewide undertakings organized for the most part under special state enabling acts. In most states a department or commissioner of insurance supervises the "Blues," issuing or approving their certificates of incorporation, reviewing their annual income and expenditure reports, and monitoring the rates subscribers pay into the program and the rates the programs pay to the providers (Law, 1974).

In line with their nonprofit status, both programs, at least initially, were committed to "community rating." Under such a policy a set of benefits is offered at a single rate to all individuals and groups within a community, regardless of age, sex, health status, or occupation of community members. In essence, the rate represents an averaging out of high- and low-cost individuals and groups so that the community as a whole can be served with adequate benefits at reasonable cost (Somers & Somers, 1961). When commercial for-profit insurance companies entered the field, however, they did so with a policy of "experience rating," charging different individuals and population subgroups different premiums, based on their use of services. Low-risk groups could secure benefits at lower premiums. As a result, the Blues began to offer a multiplicity of policies with differing rate and benefits structures, and they generally have adopted experience rating. Had they not, their health insurance portfolios would have been heavily composed of adverse risks (Krizay & Wilson, 1974).

Commercial Insurance. Commercial insurance companies (Aetna, Metropolitan Life, etc.) entered the general health insurance market cautiously. They had realized losses on income-replacement policies during the Depression and were leery of the Blues' initial emphasis on comprehensive benefits. However, a Supreme Court decision recognizing fringe benefits as a legitimate part of the collective bargaining process, following as it did the freezing of industrial wages during World War II, proved too much of a temptation. Business was shopping for insurance carriers, and the commercials responded (Somers & Somers, 1961).

In the main, Blue Cross offers hospitalization insurance; Blue Shield, coverage of in-hospital physician services and a limited amount of office-based care. The commercials offer both. As in the case of the Blues, commercial insurance is primarily provided to groups through employee fringe-benefit packages negotiated through collective bargaining. Individual coverage can be purchased, but it is usually quite expensive or has limited coverage. The commercials also sell major-medical and cash payment policies. The former, directed primarily at catastrophic illness, pay all or part of the treatment costs beyond those covered by basic plans. They are sold on both a group and an individual basis. Cash-payment policies pay the insured a flat sum of money per day of hospitalization and are usually sold directly to individuals, often through mass advertising campaigns. Although the daily cash-payment sum is usually small, it can help defray costs left uncovered by other insurance.

Like the Blues, the commercials are subject to supervision by state insurance commissioners, although such supervision does not include rate regulation. One general requirement is that commercials establish premium rates high enough to cover claims made under the insurance they provide. Solvency of the insurer is the principal aim of insurance commission surveillance in this instance (Krizay & Wilson, 1974).

HMOs. The form of health insurance that is reshaping the way many Americans relate to the health sector is the HMO. HMOs integrate the delivery of health care and insurance for health care. Although there are many different types of HMOs, the essential idea is that an annual payment is made by or for beneficiaries and then a group of providers delivers all covered services for this "capitated" payment. The HMO concept fundamentally changes the traditional approach of paying physicians and other providers on a fee-for-service, "piece-work" basis. An HMO is paid a capitated amount to "maintain" (and when necessary, to restore) the health of an enrollee.

Table 10.4 displays the growth in HMO members between 1976 and 1992, when 41.4 million Americans received care through HMOs. The 1992 membership is almost 7 times that of 1976. The number of HMOs has grown from 174 in 1976 to 546 in 1992.

There are four distinct types of HMOs, which vary in how the fiscal agent relates to the providers of care group (Group Health Association of America, 1986). The traditional type of HMO is a "staff" model in which the fiscal agent employs salaried physicians who generally spend all their time delivering services to the HMO's enrollees. A "group" model is a slight variant of this in that the physicians as a single group contract with the fiscal agent to deliver services. In a "network" type of HMO the fiscal agent has contracts with multiple physician groups to provide services to enrollees; often the physician groups deliver services to non-HMO patients also. The fourth HMO type is the "independent practice association" (IPA) model, in which the fiscal agent contracts with a range of physicians, who work in independent practices or multispeciality group practices to provide services to HMO enrollees. Again, IPA physicians generally provide services to both HMO enrollees and patients with other forms of insurance.

HMOs vary in how they relate to hospitals. Some HMOs own their own hospitals, and others have varying forms of fiscal arrangements with community hospitals. The fiscal arrangements can include some version of a capitation payment or some form of discounted per diem or per case reimbursement mechanism.

TABLE 10.4   Number of HMO Members (In Millions)
1976–1987

Year	As of June	As of December
1976	6.0	na
1977	6.3	na
1978	7.5	na
1979	8.2	na
1980	9.1	na
1981	10.2	na
1982	10.8	na
1983	12.5	na
1984	15.1	na
1985	18.9	na
1986	23.7	25.7
1987	28.6	29.3
1988	na	32.7
1989	na	34.7
1990	na	36.5
1991	na	38.6
1992	na	41.4

na, data not available.

Source: Adapted from Gruber, R., Shadle, M., & Polich, C. L. "From Movement to Industry: The Growth of HMOs," *Health Affairs*, 7(3), p. 198. Group Health Association of America's *National Directory of HMOs Database* and *Health Affairs*, Summer 1988.

The reason for increased enrollment in HMOs in recent years is principally the expectation and claim that HMOs reduce health care costs while providing coverage that has fewer co-payment features and uncovered services. Many studies have found that HMOs, particularly group and staff models, reduce hospital use and total costs (Arnould et al., 1984; Luft, 1978, 1981; Manning, 1984; Roemer & Shonick, 1973; Wolinsky, 1980). Physicians working in HMOs generally have a strong incentive to use resources efficiently because of the capitated payment approach. Most important, HMO providers have strong incentives to avoid hospitalizations. Studies consistently indicate that even after adjusting for demographic differences, HMO patients are hospitalized 15 to 40% less often than fee-for-service patients (Luft, 1981).

PPOs. In addition to HMOs, the other growing form of insurance coverage is that which uses PPOs. As with HMOs, there are many different types of PPOs.

However, the general concept involves beneficiaries using physicians who have agreed to give price discounts to the insurer. The beneficiary usually is provided some incentive to use a preferred provider, in the form of either lower insurance premiums or waiver of cost-sharing requirements.

As indicated in Table 10.3, PPOs accounted for 13% of the private insurance market in 1992. PPOs have been growing, especially in areas where there is significant competition for patients among physicians and other health care providers. In competitive markets insurers are best able to persuade providers to offer price discounts in return for a chance to increase patient volume. A recent survey found that PPOs are often established not by insurers but by groups of physicians interested in maintaining patients in the face of competition from HMOs (de Lissovoy et al., 1986).

Extent of Private Health Insurance Coverage in the United States. Private health insurance coverage for Americans is extensive but far from complete. As of 1992, all but 37.4 million, some 16.7% of the nonelderly population, had some form of health insurance. These latest figures show the continuation of a reversal in the longtime trend toward reductions in the number of the individuals without health insurance (Swartz, 1989).

Although large numbers of individuals have some health insurance, the breadth of their coverage is uneven. An examination of the proportion of total consumer expenditures met by private insurance for various types of care indicates variations in coverage (see Table 10.5). As noted earlier, in 1991 expenditures made through private health insurance amounted to about 32.5% of the total. Table 10.5 translates that percentage for 1991 and prior years into the proportions of expenditures met for the several categories of health care covered by such insurance. It is clear that many individuals have some coverage for drugs, physicians' office visits, and dental care, although the coverage often does not go very far.

One type of service that has very poor insurance coverage is long-term care that is custodial in nature. In discussing Medicare, it was noted that coverage for long-term care that involves rehabilitation has recently been expanded. However, very few long-term care services are for rehabilitation; most are custodial, involving chronic care of the frail elderly. Medicare pays less than 7% of all nursing care costs, and private insurance pays less than 1%.

The current system of financing long-term care relies on out-of-pocket expenditures by the elderly who can afford such expenditures. In most states, after an elderly person becomes impoverished by the costs of services, the state Medicaid program will cover services.

Although private insurance has played a very small role in insuring long-term-care services, in recent years a market for private insurance has been emerging, and the number of policies has been expanding. In addition, numerous proposals have been made for developing an integrated public-private insurance system for

TABLE 10.5 **Percentage of Consumer Health Expenditures Met by Private Health Insurance, 1950–1991, Selected Years**

Year	Total	Hospital care	Physicians' services	Prescribed drugs (out-of-hospital)	Dental care
1950	12.2%	37.1%	12.0%	a	a
1960	27.8	64.7	30.0	a	a
1965	30.5	70.1	34.0	2.4%	1.6%
1966	30.4	71.0	34.0	2.7	2.0
1967	32.8	76.7	36.7	3.5	2.5
1968	34.5	78.8	40.5	3.6	3.1
1969	35.5	77.7	41.1	4.0	3.9
1970	37.2	77.7	43.7	3.9	5.3
1971	39.1	80.9	43.7	4.9	6.3
1972	39.0	76.5	45.8	5.0	7.2
1973	39.0	75.4	46.0	5.6	8.1
1974	41.4	77.3	49.8	6.2	11.0
1975	45.0	82.6	51.3	6.7	15.8
1976	47.0	84.6	53.1	7.9	19.6
1977	45.5	79.3	52.9	7.9	20.2
1981	54.5	82.9	58.9	13.4	34.9
1982	56.2	83.2	60.4	14.6	34.4
1983	56.5	83.5	60.6	14.8	34.9
1984	56.0	80.0	62.6	14.6	35.7
1985	55.5	79.4	62.2	14.8	36.5
1986	55.8	79.4	62.9	15.1	37.4
1987	56.2	79.5	62.9	15.6	37.6
1988	59.4	87.1	70.1	15.6	43.2
1989	61.0	88.6	70.5	15.2	43.7
1990	61.9	90.1	71.6	15.9	44.0
1991	62.9	91.1	72.2	16.9	44.7

a. Coverage insignificant.

Source: Adapted from M. S. Carroll & R. H. Arnett III, "Private Health Insurance Plans in 1977; Coverage, Enrollment and Financial Experience," *Health Care Financing Reviews, 1,* Fall 1979, p. 14; R. M. Gibson, K. R. Levitt, H. Lazenby, & D. Waldo, "National Health Expenditures, 1983," *Health Care Financing Review, 6,* Winter 1984, Table 3; S. Letsch et al., "National Health Expenditures, 1987," *Health Care Financing Review, 10,* Winter 1988. Table 1, *Health Care Financing Review,* Fall 1991, Table 10, p. 8.

long-term care services that would combine private insurance and some public resources now devoted to Medicaid long-term care services (Knickman, 1988).

How the Money is Paid Out

Paying Physicians

As indicated in Table 10.2, physician services account for approximately 20% of all health care expenditures. However, the method used to pay physicians influences not only this 20% of the health care bill but also the large share of health care costs that are controlled largely by physicians' decisions. It is important to emphasize the role of physicians in deciding when a patient uses hospital resources and in prescribing drugs and medical tests.

As already mentioned, methods used by insurers to reimburse physicians are undergoing substantial change. The growth of HMOs and PPOs is changing the ability of physicians to set prices freely. Increased regulation of fees by Medicare also is affecting the way physicians are reimbursed.

Fee for Service. The dominant approach to paying physicians continues to be some variation of a fee-for-service approach. A traditional fee-for-service approach is a simple system in which a physician sets a price for each type of service delivered, and then the patient or the insurer pays this price.

For individuals who have no insurance for physician services, traditional fee-for-service generally is used. Even when an individual has private insurance, fee-for-service rates are generally charged, with the patient paying any share of the rate the insurer judges to be above a stated payment scale. Insurers use a wide range of methods for establishing payment scales for covered services.

The Medicare program's system for paying physicians is based on the fee-for-service approach. Prior to 1992, the system was based in part on a comparison of each doctor's fee schedule for a given type of service with those of other physicians in a community. Medicare never paid an individual physician an amount that exceeded the 75th percentile of charges by all physicians in a community (this was termed the "prevailing" fee). However, the Medicare program also used a cost of living index, termed the Medicare Economic Index, to constrain the growth in the maximum payment it would pay in a community for each type of physician service (Congressional Budget Office, 1986).

In OBRA 1989, Medicare substantially changed its system for paying physicians. Under the new payment system, each physician service is assigned a "relative value" based on the time, skill, and intensity it takes to provide it. The relative values are then adjusted for geographic variations and multiplied by a national conversion factor to determine the dollar amount of payment. This fee schedule, called the "resource-based-relative-value-scale" (RBRVS) system went into effect on January 1, 1992.

This approach was intended to lead to relative increase in payment for cognitive services (i.e., physicals and diagnostic visits) and relative decreases for services that involve procedures. This rebalancing would occur because the previous system led to higher rates for procedures than makes sense based on objective measures involving time, training, or relative expertise. Preliminary evidence suggests, however, that the RBRVS system has led to less change in relative payment rates than originally anticipated.

Preferred Provider Approaches. An alternative to traditional fee-for-service payment approaches is the use of negotiated discounts by physicians or groups of physicians. PPOs used this discounting approach to set reimbursement rates for patients covered by a participating insurer. In many ways, however, the discounting approaches inherent to PPOs are not distinct from fee-for-service approaches but rather a variation on the fee-for-service idea. Physicians continue to be paid on a service-by-service basis but at a somewhat lower rate than is charged for non-PPO patients.

Capitation and Salary. The alternative forms of provider reimbursement are capitation and salary. The latter approach is self-explanatory; its use as a payment mechanism for health professionals is widespread. Certainly, from the employer's point of view, a salary system has the merit of administrative simplicity. When the employer is the government, there is the added benefit of flexibility: The movement of providers into areas of medical scarcity and unpopular jobs is more easily accomplished under a salary system than under other payment mechanisms. From the provider's point of view, he or she has an income protected from sudden fluctuation in supply and demand, has no bill collection problems, and usually receives extensive fringe benefits (Roemer, 1962).

Various types of capitation approaches are used by individual practice associations to compensate physicians. There were more than 300 IPAs across the country in 1992, and the payment approaches used by these organizations vary substantially. Some pay individual physicians using discounted fee-for-service plans, but most put physicians at some financial risk for the costs of their patient's care. Often a physician receives a capitated annual payment for each patient who uses that physician as a primary provider. The capitated payment is meant to cover certain forms of primary care and, depending on the arrangement, some share of specialty care, ancillary services, and hospital care. The physician thus has strong incentives to manage resources efficiently.

Another form of capitation is to have a group of IPA physicians receive some percentage of a fee-for-service rate, with the remaining percentage held in escrow to assure that aggregate health care costs across the group do not exceed targets. The escrow amounts are distributed to the physicians at the end of the year if utilization targets are met.

Paying Hospitals

There are two major approaches to hospital reimbursement: retrospective and prospective; although there are numerous modes of payment within these two categories.

Retrospective Payment. Retrospective rates for payment to hospitals by third-party payers and individuals are set after services are provided. There are two major modes of retrospective payment: charges and cost. Most commercial insurers and some Blue Cross plans reimburse hospitals on the basis of submitted charges. Charges are simply prices set by hospitals. Most hospitals set charges for basic and intensive-care room and board, as well as for each service provided. These prices may or may not reflect the true economic costs of the particular service. Often the variation above cost is a function of patient mix. Charges will exceed actual costs to the extent that a hospital serves a large number of nonpaying patients and to the extent that "cost-based" insurers actually pay amounts that are less than actual costs.

The more sophisticated retrospective payment mode is based on cost. The determination of cost never involves individual patients; rather, it is a matter of negotiation between hospitals and third-party payers as Blue Cross and Medicaid. Cost reimbursement is used when insured patients receive their benefits as service rather than as dollar indemnities. Almost all group health insurance policies in the United States now provide service benefits rather than dollar indemnities. To determine reimbursable costs, third-party payers sum-total hospital costs, decide which costs are "allowable," then, using a formula, reimburse hospitals on a per-patient-day basis.

Prospective Payment. The most significant change in hospital payment methodologies in the last 10 years has been recent expansion in prospective payment services. Of special importance were the changes in the method used by Medicare to pay hospitals. In the Tax Equity and Fiscal Responsibility Act (TEFRA) of 1982, Congress established a cost-per-case basis for hospital payment. TEFRA also placed a ceiling on the rate of increase in hospital revenues that would be supported by the Medicare program.

The 1983 amendments to the Social Security Act further defined the case payment system. These amendments created a revolutionary method of paying hospitals for inpatient care to Medicare patients, one that is based on DRGs. Under this system, hospitals are paid a pre-established amount per case treated, with payment rates varying by type of case. The DRGs measure hospital output by originally classifying patients into 23 major diagnostic categories (MDCs), based on major body systems. The MDCs are divided further into 47 diagnostic groups based on the patient's diagnosis or the surgical procedure used and on age, sex, and other clinical information. One additional group is also used for cases in which diagnosis and surgical procedure do not match (Grimaldi & Micheletti, 1982).

Not all hospitals are included in Medicare's case payment system. Certain specialty hospitals, such as children's long-term care, rehabilitation, and psychiatric hospitals are exempt. So are certain states, such as New Jersey and Maryland, that have approved alternative payment systems. Moreover, certain hospital costs, such as direct medical education and capital-related costs, continue to be reimbursed on a cost basis and are excluded from costs used to calculate case payment rates. There is continuing debate, however, about how to include capital costs in the case payment system.

Payment that an individual hospital receives for treating Medicare patients in a given DRG depends on the DRG's "cost" weight multiplied by a "standardized" average cost for all Medicare patients. The standardization process includes adjustments for differences in wages and teaching intensity. Also, different rates are set for urban and rural hospitals. Payment amounts to hospitals are also adjusted each year by an "update factor," consisting of a measure of the price of goods and services purchased by hospitals. In addition, a discretionary adjustment factor (DAF) accounts for changes in new technology and productivity. Although Congress originally set the DAF at 1 percentage point each year, the Deficit Reduction Act of 1984 capped these adjustments at 0.25%.

Two aspects of this payment system depart significantly from previous methods used to pay for Medicare patients. First, the DRG concept holds that the "best" measure of hospital output is the diagnosis treated rather than individual services provided or length of stay. That is, the basis of payment is the case treated rather than ancillary or routine inputs to hospital care.

Second, unlike retrospective payment methodologies, DRG payments are determined prospectively and are fixed. Although a portion of the initial rates for fiscal year 1984 were determined by historical costs, subsequent rates of increase in the payments are controlled before payment is made. Hence, Medicare now has the ability to control the per-case rate of increase for Medicare patients.

The use of DRGs as a basis for hospital payment transcends Medicare and is spreading rapidly to other payers. At least 21 states, such as Pennsylvania, Utah, Ohio, Michigan, and Washington, have adopted case-based systems to pay for hospital care received by Medicaid patients. Thirty-two states, including Arizona, Oklahoma, and Kansas, employ a DRG system to pay for Blue Cross patients. As of 1993, Maryland is the only state that uses a DRG system for all third-party payers.

Use of classification schemes as the basis for hospital payment assumes that the classifications are clinically meaningful and "reasonably" homogeneous with respect to resource consumption. There is, however, mounting evidence that some of the DRG categories do not satisfy either requirement (Prospective Payment Assessment Commission, 1985). Perhaps the most common criticism of the DRG categories is that they include patients with dissimilar resource needs because they often do not account adequately for differences in patient complexity or severity of illness (Horn et al., 1984). Variation in severity within each DRG category is cause for concern if patient complexity can be assessed before admission to the hospital; this can create an incentive to divert more complex patients to other hospitals. Long-run consequences may include shedding unprofitable DRG "products" and expanding the volume of "profitable" services to ensure hospital financing viability. Changes in hospital service mix may not be entirely undesirable, however, if increased patient volume allows hospitals to eliminate facility duplication and exploit economies of scale. On the other hand, narrowing the scope of services may adversely affect access to care in some cases.

Research concerning the impacts of the new Medicare DRG payment system indicates that the approach is significantly changing hospital utilization patterns. Medicare hospital admissions decreased 15.9% during the first 3 years of the new reimbursement system, and average length of stay decreased 17% (Guterman et al., 1987). Although it is difficult to determine exactly how much of these dramatic reductions in utilization are attributable to DRGs, research studies do document that utilization rates fell much more quickly in states where the DRG system was implemented compared to the states that received waivers to delay or avoid implementation.

The reduction in hospital use has not been without side effects, however. In particular, evidence consistently indicates sharp increases in posthospital use of services, including home health care, and nursing home care, as well as increased readmissions (Guterman et al., 1987). The tighter regulation of Medicare payment rates also may be responsible for part of the rapid growth in cost of private insurance as hospitals shift some of their costs from Medicare to private insurance. That is, higher rates may be charged for individuals with private insurance to compensate for any operating losses associated with care delivered to Medicare patients.

The Rising Costs of Health Care

National spending for health care grew an average of 12.4% per year from 1970 to 1991. In addition, the rate of increase in health care costs has consistently far exceeded the rate of inflation in the general economy. Thus, health care expenses each year account for an increasing share of the nation's GNP.

Several factors have contributed to the rise in medical costs: general inflation in the economy, population growth, the development of new medical technology, and an increased "intensity" of services provided to all patients. Rapid development of medical technology and intensity of medical care services have been encouraged by growth in the extent of health insurance coverage and previous retrospective, cost-based payment systems that rewarded higher reported costs with higher payments (Feldstein, 1971). As insurance coverage increases, the out-of-pocket cost to the patient is reduced, leading to increases in demand for higher-quality medical care and hence to rising prices. The growth in the comprehensiveness of third-party insurance coverage is stimulated in part through federal government tax subsidies (Phelps, 1984). Under current tax law, employer payments to employees for health insurance are not considered taxable income. Because these tax subsidies reduce the price of health insurance, they provide incentives to purchase more health insurance.

Despite the theoretical connection between the extent of health insurance and costs, until recently there was little persuasive empirical evidence that increased health insurance coverage led to greater use of health care services. Some even argued that more comprehensive insurance, especially for ambulatory care, would reduce total spending by encouraging preventive health care and more "appropriate" hospital use (Roemer et al., 1975).

Recent data from the Rand Corporation's Health Insurance Experiment (Newhouse et al., 1981) provide considerable insight into the connection between insurance coverage and utilization. The experiment ran from 1974 through January 1982 and enrolled 7,706 individuals between the ages of 14 and 61 who belonged to 2,756 families. Families were assigned randomly to one of four major types of experimental plans.

1. A "free-care" plan, in which all care was received without charge (i.e., there were no co-insurance or deductible requirements).
2. An individual deductible plan, which imposed a 95% co-insurance rate on outpatient care, up to a maximum out-of-pocket expenditure of $450 per family, with all care beyond that amount (either inpatient or outpatient) free at time of service.
3. A series of intermediate co-insurance plans with cost-sharing requirements of either 25% or 50%.
4. "Income-related catastrophic" plans that included a 95% co-insurance requirement with income-related maximum dollar spending caps.

The results of the experiment were quite robust. Health care spending was almost 50% lower in plans with 95% cost-sharing, compared to those in the free-care plans. Perhaps of more interest was the finding that any cost sharing—even just for ambulatory care services-reduced costs, compared to the free-care plans.

Another important finding from the experiment was that, in general, the reduced utilization of health care due to cost sharing did not affect most measures of health status. However, two exceptions to those findings were slight increases in blood pressure for individuals with high blood pressure at the start of the study, and for individuals who had low incomes (Brook et al., 1983).

The system of third-party reimbursement also has been implicated as a primary factor spurring the recent growth in new medical technology. Although in certain instances new technology has increased the length and quality of life, it is often very costly. As one observer of the system has noted, "with some important exceptions, the norm for hospital care in the United States approximates the maxim, 'If you think it will help, do it'" (Aaron & Schwartz, 1984, p. 7). Since most patients are insulated from the true social costs of medical care, our present system encourages the uses of services that may yield only slight, if any, positive diagnostic information, often regardless of cost. The HCFA, for example, found that the increased per-admission intensity of care accounted for over 20% of the growth in expenditures for community hospital inpatient care over the past 10 years (Freeland & Schendler, 1983).

Although the spread of new technology undoubtedly offers unprecedented medical benefits, some innovations are of marginal value. Further, facilities and services unavailable in the late 1970s or found only in medical centers are now offered in a substantial number of community hospitals. The increase in diagnostic imaging by computerized axial tomography (CAT) has been impressive, more than doubling since 1980 (Office of Technology Assessment, 1981). Similarly, rapid diffusion of magnetic resonance imaging (MRI) has occurred. The medical benefits of CAT scanning are well known; for instance, it has reduced the need for exploratory surgery. Yet growth in new technology has expanded the potential pool of recipients as well as symptoms diagnosed. Thus, although it is true that new technology provides unprecedented medical benefits, the downside is that new technology increases expenditures.

The battle over medical efficacy, new technology, and health care expenditures has escalated with the advent of Medicare's DRG payment system. Under the DRG system, hospitals may become more reluctant to purchase new technologies that add significantly to their operating costs because reimbursement rates will not automatically increase with an expenditure for technology. Moreover, the rate of technological diffusion in the industry will be sensitive to the method ultimately chosen by the HCFA to reimburse hospitals for capital expenditures. Yet, to date, the tremendous growth in new medical technology shows no perceptible signs of abating. Each year new, more expensive technologies with the potential for saving and improving the quality of life appear. Many consider cost increases resulting from advances in and greater use of medical technology as the necessary price of improvements in health care, if not health. Opponents suggest that a substantial portion of the utilization of technology is generally unnecessary. They link a proportion of the increase in ancillary service to physician fear of exposure to malpractice claims. Indeed, small increases in diagnostic accuracy often require substantial increases in the health care bill. This concern has increased interest in redirecting resources into programs—especially public health intervention—with more favorable cost-benefit implications

Some observe that any appreciable reduction in spending can be accomplished only by denying medical benefits (Aaron & Schwartz, 1984). Others note that increased cost sharing may reduce spending and utilization, often without deleterious effects on health status (Brook et al., 1983). Thus, the debate continues surrounding the health implications of recent attempts, such as the expansion of the DRG system, to reduce the rate of growth of health care costs. At the very least, the debate over efficiency, access, and quality will heighten in the coming years.

Conclusion

Money funds the health care delivery system, but the routes dollars take from consumers to providers can be labyrinthine. Some dollars go directly, some via the government, and some through insurance companies. Most health care providers are paid by salary, but some are paid on a piecework basis. Hospitals are paid for services provided in numerous ways. Some insurers base payments on what the hospital charges, whereas others pay on the basis of allowable average costs. Still others, notably Medicare and some Medicaid and Blue Cross plans, pay hospitals on a "case" basis, with the payment rate set in advance.

In the United States in the 1960s and 1970s a health insurance system that emphasized coverage for hospital care, with physician service in hospitals generally being more lucrative than in the office setting, "tilted" the system in the direction of utilization of the most expensive component of the system. Technological change, a significant factor in rising health care costs, was often poorly planned and evaluated, with decisions frequently made on the basis of universal access rather than cost-effectiveness.

The 1980s, however, witnessed a virtual revolution in the financing and structure of medical care delivery. Fundamental changes in the methods used to pay health care providers, growing involvement by employers and employees in direct negotiation with providers, and a projected aggregate surplus of physicians have led to the changes in the structure of the delivery system. Perhaps most notable has been the move from retrospective to prospective modes of payment. Although prospective per-case payment systems are generally restricted to in-patient hospital care, considerable research and development efforts—aimed at designing prospective case payment systems for long-term care, home health care, and outpatient care are currently underway. In some quarters, across-the-board capitation payments may prove feasible.

The 1980s also saw the beginning of dramatic changes in the organization of medical practice. The growth in prepaid group practice, ambulatory surgery, and the "unbundling" of hospital services are indicative of the magnitude of recent changes in the delivery system. New alignments between providers, employers, and employees—in the form of HMOs, PPOs, and self-insurance ventures—also reflect the recent entrance of the consumer into direct financial negotiation with health care providers.

References

Aaron, H., & Schwartz, W., *The Painful Prescription: Rationing Hospital Care.* Washington, DC: The Brookings Institution, 1984.

Arnett, R., II, & Trapnell, G., "Private Health Insurance: New Measures of a Complex and Changing Industry." *Health Care Financing Review,* 6, 2, Winter 1984.

Arnould, R. et al., "Do HMOs Produce Services More Efficiently?" *Inquiry, 21,* 3, Fall 1984.

Brook, R. et al., "Does Free Care Improve Adults' Health? Results From a Randomized Controlled Trial." *New England Journal of Medicine, 319,* 1426, 1983.

Carroll, M.S., & Arnett, R. H., II., "Private Health Insurance Plans in 1977: Coverage, Enrollment and Financial Experience." *Health Care Financing Review, l,* 3, Fall 1979.

Christensen, S., & Kasten, R., "Covering Catastrophic Expenses under Medicare." *Health Affairs, 3,* 5, 79, 1988.

Congressional Budget Office. *U.S. Congress Physician Reimbursement Under Medicare: Options for Change.* Washington, DC: U.S. Government Printing Office, 1986.

Congressional Research Service. *Workmen's Compensation: Role of the Federal Government.* (1B75054). Washington, DC: Library of Congress, 1976.

Davis, K., & Rowland, D., "Uninsured and Undeserved: Inequities in Health Care in the United States." Milbank Memorial Fund Quarterly: *Health and Society, 61,* 149, 1983.

de Lissovoy, G., Rice, T., Ermann, D., & Gabel, J., "Preferred Provider Organizations: Today's Models and Tomorrow's Prospect." *Inquiry, 23,* 7 Spring 1986.

Feldstein, M.S., *The Rising Cost of Hospital Care.* Washington, D.C.: Information Resources Press, 1971.

Freeland, M. S., & Schendler, C. E., "National Health Expenditure Growth in the 1980's: An Aging Population, New Technologies, and Increasing Competition." *Health Care Financing Review, 4,* 3, 1983.

Gabel, J., DiCarlo, S., Fink, S., & de Lissovoy, G., "Employer-Sponsored Health Insurance in America: Preliminary Results from the 1988 Survey." *Research Bulletin.* Washington, DC: Health Insurance Association of America, January, 1989.

Gibson, R. M., "National Health Expenditures, 1978." *Health Care Financing Review, 1,* 1, Summer, 1979.

Gibson, R. M., Levitt, K., Lazenby, H., & Waldo, D., "National Health Expenditures, 1983," *Social Security Bulletin, 6,* 2, Winter 1984.

Grimaldi, P., & Micheletti, J., *Diagnosis Related Groups: A Practitioner's Guide.* Chicago: Pluribus Press, 1982.

Group Health Association of America. *HMO Industry Profile: Trends, 1985–1986* (Vol. 4) Washington, DC: Group Health Association of America, 1986.

Gruber, L. R., Shadle, M., & Polich, C. L., "From Movement to Industry: The Growth of HMOs." *Health Affairs,* 7(3), 197, 1988.

Guterman, S., Eggers, P. W., Riley, G., Greene, T. F., & Terrell, S. A., "The First 3 Years of Medicare Prospective Payment: An Overview." *Health Care Financing Review,* 9(1), 67, 1987.

Health Insurance Association of America. *Sourcebook of Health Insurance Data, 1984 Update.* New York: Health Insurance Association of America, 1985.

Health Insurance Institute. *Source Book of Health Insurance Data, 1974–75.* New York: Health Insurance Institute, 1975.

Hellinger, F., "Recent Evidence on Case-Based Systems for Setting Hospital Rates." *Inquiry, 22,* 1, Spring 1985.

Horn, S. et al., "The Severity of Illness Index as a Severity Adjustment to Diagnosis-Related Groups." *Health Care Financing Review, 5* (Suppl.), 1984.

Hsiao, W., & Stason, W., "Toward Developing a Relative Value Scale for Medical and Surgical Services." *Health Care Financing Review, 1,* 23, 1979.

Knickman, J., "Private Long-Term Care Insurance: Alleviating Market Problems with Public–Private Partnership." *Health Economics and Health Service Research, 9,* 135, 1988.

Krizay, J., & Wilson, A., *The Patient as Consumer.* Lexington, MA: D.C. Health, 1974.

Laudicina, S., "State Health Risk Pools: Insuring the 'Uninsurable.'" *Health Affairs, 7*(4), 97, 1988.

Law, S. A., *Blue Cross: What Went Wrong?* New Haven, CT: Yale University Press, 1974.

Lewin, L., & Lewin, M., "Financing Charity Care in an Era of Competition." *Health Affairs, 6*(1), 47, 1988.

Letsch, S. et al., "National Health Expenditures, 1987." *Health Care Financing Review, 10,* 109, Winter 1988.

Luft, H., "How Do Health Maintenance Organizations Achieve Their Savings?" *New England Journal of Medicine, 298,* 1336, 1978.

Luft, H., *Health Maintenance Organization: Dimensions of Performance.* New York: John Wiley, 1981.

Manning, W., "A Controlled Trial of the Effects of a Prepaid Group Practice on Use of Services." *The New England Journal of Medicine, 310,* 23, June 1984.

McCarthy, C. M., "Incentive Reimbursement as an Impetus to Cost Containment." *Inquiry, 12,* 320, 1975.

Muse, D. N., & Sawyer, D., *The Medicare and Medicaid Data Book,1981* (HCFA Pub. No. 03128). Washington, D.C.: U.S. Department of Health and Human Services, 1982.

Newhouse, J. P. et al., "Some Interim Results from a Controlled Trial of Cost Sharing in Health Insurance." *New England Journal of Medicine, 305,* 1501, 1981.

Office of Technology Assessment. *Policy Implications of the CT Scanner: An Update.* Washington, D.C.: U.S. Office of Technology Assessment, 1981.

Phelps, C. E., "Taxing Health Insurance: How Much Is Enough?" *Contemporary Policy Issues, 3,* 2, Winter 1984.

Price, D. N., "Workers' Compensation Programs in the 1970s." *Social Security Bulletin, 42*(5), 3, 1979a.

Price, D. N., "Workers' Compensation Coverage, Payments and Costs, 1977." *Social Security Bulletin, 42*(10), 18, 1979b.

Prospective Payment Assessment Commission. *Report and Recommendation to the Secretary, U.S. Department of Health and Human Services.* Washington, D.C.: U.S. Government Printing Office, 1985.

Roemer, M. I. "On Paying the Doctor and the Implications of Different Methods." *Journal of Health and Human Behavior, 3,* 4, Spring, 1962.

Roemer, M. I. et al., "Copayments for Ambulatory Care: Penny-Wise and Pound-Foolish." *Medical Care, 13,* 457, 1975.

Roemer, M., & Shonick, W., "HMO Performance: The Recent Evidence." *Health and Society, 51,* 271, 1973.

Russell, L. et al., *Federal Health Spending, 1969–74.* Washington, DC: National Planning Association, 1974.

Somers, H., & Somers, A. R., *Doctors, Patients and Health Insurance.* Washington, DC: The Brookings Institution, 1961.

Swartz, K., *The Uninsured with a Special Focus on Workers*. Unpublished report, The Urban Institute, 1989.

U.S. National Commission on State Workmen's Compensation Laws. *Report*. Washington, DC: U.S. Government Printing Office, 1973.

Wilensky, G., "Filling the Gaps in Health Insurance." *Health Affairs*, 7(3), 133, 1988.

Wolinsky, F., "The Performance of Health Maintenance Organizations: An Analytic Review." *Milbank Memorial Fund Quarterly*, 58(4), 4, 1980.

11

Health Care Cost Containment: Reflections and Future Directions

Kenneth E. Thorpe

Despite vigorous efforts to control health care costs, health care expenditures continue to rise at rates exceeding general inflation. In 1991 health care accounted for 13.2% of our gross national product (GNP), compared to 10.7% just 5 years earlier (Health Care Financing Administration [HCFA], 1988). The sustained rise in health care expenditures has raised a number of concerns. First, public expenditures for health care account for a substantial portion of the federal budget. Thus, recent efforts to reduce the size of the federal budget deficit (estimated at approximately $380 billion in 1993) have focused attention on publicly financed health care programs. Second, recent increases in premiums paid by employers have skyrocketed. Health benefits rose from 2.4% of total compensation in 1970 to 5.8% in 1989, and from 23% of total benefits in 1970 to 36% in 1989 (Employee Benefit Research Institute, 1991). Rates for the 77 Blue Cross and Blue Shield plans nationally increased between 15 and 25% during 1989 (Mullen, 1989). Third, the sustained premium increases are not limited to traditional forms of insurance coverage. Employers deciding to "self-insure" also faced large increases during 1993, averaging approximately 7.4% (KPMG-Pete Marwick, 1993). Perhaps even more distressing is the 86.1% projected rise in rates by health maintenance organizations (HMOs), medical supermarkets widely touted as the consummate cost-containment mechanism, between 1988 & 1993 (Group Health Assoc. of America, 1993).

The continued escalation in health care costs suggests that efforts by third-party payers to lower cost growth have largely failed to achieve their goal. Although some payers have reduced their expenditures over time, spending by others has increased, leaving the overall rate of growth largely unaffected. The factors accounting for the sustained increase in health care costs, the effects of recent public and private sector attempts to control this growth, and an assessment of the future direction of health care cost containment serves as the focus of this chapter.

Factors Accounting for Health Care Expenditure Growth

The United States currently spends over $750 billion, some $2,868 per capita, on health care (HCFA, 1988). This represents an 11.4% rise between 1990 and 1991 alone, a $76.8 billion jump. Four major factors generally account for these large yearly increments: general economy-wide inflation, inflation specific to the health care industry (over and above general rates of inflation), population growth, and changes in the nature and intensity of health care delivery. The relative contributions of these factors to yearly changes in health care costs are discussed below.

Approximately 36% of the yearly rise in health care spending is traced to general inflation (HCFA, 1988). This includes inflation in the price of inputs used in the delivery of medical care (e.g., electricity, material, etc.). Another 9% of the yearly increase is traced to population growth. Thus, approximately 45% of the yearly rise in health care costs stem from general trends in the economy.

About 54%, or $41 billion, of the most recent increase in health care spending is traced to the health care "marketplace." Of this portion, some 25%, or $19.2 billion, of the most recent increase is the result of "real" as opposed to the general level of inflation (noted above) changes in health care prices. This includes rapid growth in wages paid to health care workers, as well as rising interest rates for capital expansion. Finally, the remaining 29%, or $22.5 billion stems from continuous changes in the "intensity" of a health care visit. The intensity of care refers to the volume of medical care inputs used by physicians to treat patients (e.g., ancillary tests, procedures) per visit. Thus, among those factors specific to the health care industry, changes in the intensity of care account for over 50% of the yearly change in expenditure growth.

Two factors commonly thought responsible for the rise in health care costs are the rapid spread of comprehensive health insurance (traced to demand-side distortions) and technological change (a supply-side issue). These factors and their interrelationships are explored below.

Demand Side Distortions

Economists have traditionally identified the spread of health insurance as a primary cause for health care cost growth (Pauly, 1986). The rapid spread of health insurance has generated continued increases in demand for health care, in terms of both volume and perceived quality. The rapid increase in the scope (type of health care insured) and comprehensiveness (the proportion of a health care bill paid by a third party) of health insurance during the 1960s and 1970s has been traced to the tax treatment of health benefits (Manning et al., 1987). In particular, employer contributions for health insurance benefits are exempt from federal and state income taxation. With employer health benefit contributions estimated at $139 billion in 1990, this exemption translated into a $56 billion revenue loss. The tax treatment subsidizes the marginal dollar of fringe benefits employees receive from employers relative to other forms of compensation (e.g., wages), therefore increasing the demand for health insurance relative to other goods.

The tax treatment of health insurance benefits has two consequences. First, individuals purchase more insurance than they would without the tax subsidy. Second, more extensive health insurance results in higher health care spending. With respect to insurance, the tax laws encourage individuals to purchase less preventive care and insure against marginal risks. More comprehensive policies with few cost-sharing obligations also lead to higher spending. The magnitude of the additional expenditures is substantial. One recent experimental study, conducted by the Rand Corporation, examined the impact of insurance on health care spending. Their results indicate the use of services respond to the level of cost sharing. In short, per capita expenditures in plans with no cost sharing were approximately 33% greater than in plans with a 95% co-insurance obligation (Manning et al., 1987). Moreover, relative to a free-care plan, per capita spending among those enrolled in plans with 25% co-insurance was approximately 15% lower. Lower expenditures did not result in measurable reductions in patient health status. For example, for an average individual enrolled in the plan, the Rand study did not detect significant differences in health status across insurance plans during the 3-year tracking period. These findings suggest that low co-insurance obligations result in higher rates of utilization with few measurable short-run health benefits.

Supply Side Factors

Imperfect information and cost-increasing technological changes represent two supply side factors that distinguish the health care industry from more "competitive" markets. These factors, in conjunction with the demand-side distortions noted above, also have contributed to the real changes in medical care prices as well as intensity of medical care over time.

Imperfection Information. Potential consumers of medical care have imperfect information concerning its price and quality. High search costs and extensive health insurance coverage reduce the potential net benefits of searching for lower-cost providers. The importance of search costs and their impact on medical care prices have received much attention. The "increasing monopoly" thesis, outlined by Pauly and Satterthwaite (1981), consists of two observations. First, consumer information concerning physicians and other providers decreases with higher numbers of providers. Second, if search for providers is more difficult, consumers are less price-sensitive, and physicians have more discretion in increasing fees. Thus, according to this thesis, growth in the per capita number of physicians would result in higher prices.

Even with extensive price shopping by consumers, comprehensive health insurance coverage reduces any potential savings resulting from identifying low-cost providers. Thus, both high search costs and extensive health insurance coverage dilute the incentives for consumers to engage in vigorous price shopping.

Further complicating the consumer's task is the lack of information concerning provider quality. Measuring the quality of care provided by individual physicians or hospitals has traditionally been very difficult. Although we have witnessed an explosion of medical outcomes research over the past 10 years, outcome-based measures remain in their infancy. Instead, consumers often have used proxies such as the physician's board certification or a hospital's teaching affiliation as a signal for higher quality. As a result, higher perceived quality is also associated with higher fees and costs. At issue is whether these higher fees and prices reflect unobserved quality differences. Thus, price competition among providers will continue to be limited until consumers are able to compare both price and quality differences accurately.

Despite the informational problems facing consumers, hospitals and physicians do compete. However, the features of the health care delivery system noted above have encouraged competition in perceptions of quality rather than price. This includes both inadequate information on price and quality differences as well as the pervasiveness of first-dollar health insurance coverage. Thus, instead of competing on a price basis to attract patients, hospitals have competed to attract physicians (and through them patients). Hospitals in more concentrated (competitive) markets attempt to attract physicians through specific capital investments. These capital investments include the latest technologies, a broad range of clinical services, and other amenities. Since new technology increases service intensity, quality competition is quite costly. Whether the additional service intensity translates into better health outcomes remains at issue.

That hospitals have traditionally pursued competition in quality, rather than in price, has been the subject of numerous empirical investigations. The results generally conclude that, other factors held constant, hospitals in more competitive markets produce more services and have significantly higher costs (Robinson & Luft, 1985, 1988). Although these results generally held through the mid-1980s, efforts by state governments and other payers to encourage price competition have altered the behavior of hospitals. The more recent role of competition and market structure are discussed below.

Technological Change. The demand side distortions noted above, combined with traditional "nonprice" competition among providers, have created an environment for rapid adoption and diffusion of new technologies. These technologies generally fall into three categories: replacing accepted medical practices (e.g., hip replacement techniques and coronary artery bypass surgery), new therapies (e.g., liver, heart, and other organ transplants), and new imaging devices (e.g., magnetic resonance imaging). Without question, many of these new technologies clearly extend years of active life to many who would have died even 25 years ago. The down side is that many of the new technologies have large price tags.

Although international comparisons of health care delivery systems often raise more questions than they answer, one recent study has attempted to document the role of technology in increasing health care costs (Aaron & Schwartz, 1984). Based on their analysis of the U.S. and British health care systems, Aaron and Schwartz conclude that per capita health care costs would fall 10% if U.S. physicians used 10 key technologies (e.g., hip replacement, computed tomography, intensive care units) and intensive care at (population adjusted) rates similar to their British counterparts. Their analysis did not detect significant differences in health status resulting from the less intensive use of these technologies.

The critical role assumed by technological change (discussed above as increased service intensity) in rising health care costs has generated a growing volume of research focused on practice patterns and the appropriateness of medical procedures. This research has been spurred by international comparisons as well as by large variations in practice patterns documented domestically. One early pioneer, John Wennberg, noted magnitude differences in rates of specific procedures completed by physicians. Fourfold differences in hysterectomy rates, prostatectomies, tonsillectomies, and other common surgical procedures were discovered within and between states (Wennberg, 1984). Subsequent research indicates that these variations are not related to underlying differences in patient characteristics but rather to physician's practice patterns. These large variations among common procedures have resulted in a significant body of research aimed at examining the "appropriateness" of these differences.

Researchers at the Rand Corporation also have been active in examining the appropriateness of various practice patterns. Their studies of four surgical procedures—coronary artery bypass surgery (CABG), carotid endarterectomy, coronary angioplasty, and upper gastrointestinal endoscopy—examined the magnitude of unnecessary procedures and hospitalizations. With respect to CABG, the Rand researchers judged that 44% of the procedures examined were performed for inappropriate reasons (Chassin, 1987). Some 17% of coronary angiographies, used to diagnose blockages in heart arteries, were deemed inappropriate, as were a similar volume of gastrointestinal endoscopies. Eliminating inappropriate surgery would result in continued savings of billions of dollars per year. Although the precise magnitude of the savings remains speculative, if the rates of inappropriate use found in these procedures are extrapolated, reducing unnecessary use could reduce health care spending by over $50 billion per year.

Efforts to Control Rising Health Care Costs: The Early Experience

This section summarizes previous and current efforts by third-party payers to control health care costs. We focus specifically on hospital cost containment, an area attracting most of our cost-control efforts.

Historically, third-party payers have implemented four distinct methods of cost control: control over the inputs used by hospitals, control over hospital admitting practices, limits on hospital payment, and the development of alternative (i.e., competitive) delivery systems. During the 1970s, public payers most actively pursued these cost-containment activities. By the mid-1980s, however, private payers adopted many of the cost-control techniques discussed below.

Limits on Hospital Inputs

Historically, efforts to control the use of inputs by hospitals have focused on capital expenditure decisions. Government has assumed a major role in initially financing and subsequently limiting hospital capital expansion for more than 40 years. The initial role of the government in health planning was to facilitate expansion of the hospital industry. In this capacity, the Hospital Survey and Construction Act (Hill-Burton bill) of 1946 supplied federal funds to underwrite new hospital construction. These funds were allocated to states according to population and state per capita income levels to redress a perceived shortage and maldistribution of hospital beds. Using some simple bed-to-population guidelines, local health planners allocated the funds to expand the nation's hospital bed supply.

In light of the rapid growth in the capacity of the hospital sector, health planning efforts have recently focused on limiting future hospital capital expansions. Although some voluntary efforts preceded, the most comprehensive planning efforts commenced in 1974 with the National Health Planning and Resource Development Act. This act provided federal funding for local health systems agencies (HSAs) and state health planning and development agencies. The health planning act developed because of growing concern over rising hospital costs increasingly linked to facility (both physical plant and technology) duplication. Thus, a primary role of the HSAs was to develop planning recommendations for specific hospital investments exceeding some dollar threshold (often $100,000). Based on the work of the local HSAs, a certificate of need (CON) was usually issued at the state level granting the capital spending. Although health planning agencies reached their peak during the 1970s, HSAs have generally been phased out during the mid-1980s.

In practice, state CON programs differed both in structure and organizational goal. They varied according to four characteristics thought to be related to their potential effectiveness (i.e., their stringency): (1) the program's orientation (i.e., planning/redistribution or cost containment), (2) locus of decision making (state or local), (3) the scope of formalized review standards, and (4) extent of an appeals process exemptions.

Early evaluations of the ability of the CON process to control were quick to question the cost-containment capabilities of the program. Although the CON process appeared initially to reduce the growth rate in hospital beds, it was accompanied by a larger rise in total assets per bed (Salkever & Bice, 1976). Moreover, even those CON programs that, *ex ante*, appeared more restrictive had little impact on total capital expenditures (Joskow, 1981). These results suggest that hospitals merely substituted one form of "unconstrained" capital investment for beds.

Other studies examining the effectiveness of the CON process focused on the diffusion of specific technologies. Those examining the role of the planning process in slowing the diffusion of potentially "duplicative" technologies (e.g., computerized tomography [CT]) and expensive new technologies (e.g., new surgical techniques) into hospitals were also negative (Sloan, Valvona, & Perrin, 1986). Although the CON process may have achieved other objectives, containing capital expenditures and total health care spending was not among them. Although the growing interest in competition among health plans and hospitals contributed, the inability of the CON process to achieve its fundamental goal—slower rates of capital expansion and overall cost growth—ultimately led to its decline.

Regulating the Utilization of Medical Care

This section focuses on public sector efforts to limit the utilization of hospital services. More recent attempts by the private sector to manage the course of a patient's treatment are addressed below.

Efforts to prevent unnecessary and low-quality care delivered to publicly insured patients commenced in 1972 with the advent of professional standard review organizations (PSROs). The goals of the PSRO program, albeit quite broadly defined, were to "promote the effective, efficient, and economical delivery of health care services of proper quality." Thus, the language in the enacting legislation included both cost-containment and quality-enhancement goals. The lack of clear direction in the program's goals likely contributed to the inability of most PSROs to focus their efforts effectively. In practice, PSROs focused primarily on Medicare and Medicaid beneficiaries, although some anticipated a broader spillover to privately insured patients. Despite the broad range of goals articulated under the original act, most PSROs attempted to reduce the length of stay among the Medicare population.

Evaluations of the PSRO program have produced mixed results. On average, the PSROs appeared to reduce total days of hospitalization among Medicare patients by 1.5% (Congressional Budget Office, 1981). PSROs appear to have reduced total days through reductions in length of stay rather than by preventing admissions. Although some studies suggest the PSRO program produced some public sector savings, these costs appear to have been shifted to other payers (Congressional Budget Office, 1981). The impact of the program on the Medicaid population remains unknown. When considering the administrative costs of the program, Medicare savings (through reduced utilization) were nearly offset by the costs of the program. Viewed more broadly, the Congressional Budget Office researchers found that savings to the Medicare program were offset by increases in charges (and expenditures) by private payers. Hence, when administrative costs and charges in total health care expenditures were examined, the PSROs appeared less effective.

The PSROs were replaced with peer review organizations (PROs) in 1984. The PROs differ from their predecessor, the PSROs, in that PROs are awarded on a competitive bidding process, based in part on their ability to achieve specific utilization goals. These goals are developed through negotiations with the Health Care Financing Administration (HCFA) and relate to five objectives (Office of Technology Assessment, Appendix G): (1) to reduce unnecessary hospital readmissions; (2) to assure the provision of adequate care, which, if not given, would cause serious complications; (3) to reduce the risk of mortality associated with specific procedures and conditions; (4) to reduce unnecessary surgery; and (5) to reduce avoidable postoperative or other complications. Negotiations between a PRO and the HCFA define specific performance markers (e.g., reduce readmissions resulting from substandard care by 20% used to evaluate the effectiveness of each PRO).

Starting in 1989, PROs assumed an extended set of responsibilities beyond hospital care, including review of outpatient procedures, home health care, and care provided to military personnel and their families. By 1993, however, the program's effectiveness was in question, especially given its $300 million annual price tag. Starting that year, PROs began adopting a new strategy called the Health Care Quality Improvement Initiative. Under this initiative, PROs shift their focus from identifying individual clinical errors to helping providers improve the mainstream of medical care. The Peer Review Organizations use statistical quality controls to examine variations in both the processes and the outcomes of care. They then share this information with hospitals and physicians, and work with them to interpret and apply the findings.

Hospital Rate Setting (1969–1980)

Attempts to limit payment rates to hospitals represents a third cost-containment strategy. Between 1969 and 1974, 15 states introduced some form of hospital rate-setting program (Coelen & Sullivan, 1981). Although similar in their objectives, these programs differed with respect to a number of key design features, including the unit of payment, the scope of revenue covered (i.e., the number of payers and proportion of total revenue included), and a variety of design issues defining the actual prospectivity of the payments. These technical design features largely determined the restrictiveness of the rate-setting rules and ultimately their effectiveness. A brief description of these programs and their impact on reducing hospital expenditures follows.

Hospital rate setting generally refers to some form of prospective payment (i.e., the determination of payment rates prior to services rendered) by third-party payers. Methods actually used to define the payment rates are, in practice, quite complex. The essential elements include a base year and a trend factor. For example, Medicaid and Blue Cross payments to New York hospitals during 1989 were calculated by using a 1981 base year increased each year by an allowable trend factor. In this case, actual payment rates to hospitals are effectively divorced from individual hospital spending decisions. Thus, the degree of prospectivity built into the rate-setting system depends on the frequency in which the base year is moved. More stringent or restrictive rate-setting programs (such as the New York State program) move the base year infrequently. The trend factor used to define allowable revenue increases is also critical in determining the ability of rate-setting programs to control cost growth. The allowable trend factor could differ by multiple percentage points depending on key design decisions. For instance, trend factors may or may not include allowances for technological change. Moreover, allowed increases in wages may reflect more general wage trends or focus specifically on changes in the health care sector. Beyond these basic elements, most rate-setting programs differ with respect to the unit of payment (e.g., per diem, per case), who sets the rates (e.g., a separate rate-setting authority), and the extent to which historic (base year) costs are subjected to efficiency screens. These efficiency screens often compare each hospital's inpatient costs (after a variety of adjustments) to the mean or median within the state. In more restrictive programs, costs above the mean are "disallowed" and not recognized in developing the base year for subsequent payment. In contrast, less restrictive programs effectively pass-through all historic costs into the base.

Although state rate-setting programs differed with respect to a variety of important design issues, they also shared some common characteristics. First, rate-setting programs generally determined rates of payment prospectively. Second, the prospective rates generally applied only to inpatient operating expenses, leaving physician fees, direct medical education spending, capital, and outpatient expenses unregulated. In addition to the features noted above, state rate-setting programs varied in other respects. Three states—New Jersey, Maryland, and New York—established regulated per diem rates of payment. Elsewhere, rate setting focused on department revenue or total revenue caps. The number of payers within each state participating in the rate-setting program also varied. Prior to 1980 the rate-setting program in one state, Maryland, included all third-party payers. Programs in other states were more limited. Most programs included Medicaid and Blue Cross plans, although some, such as Indiana and Kentucky, covered only Blue Cross plans.

An impressive volume of research has examined the impact of state rate setting on hospital costs (Eby & Cohodes, 1985). The research generally concludes that state rate-setting programs reduced hospital costs, although the effects varied across states. During the 1970s cost growth per day and admission was 2 to 3% lower in states with rate-setting programs. The empirical results also suggest that rate setting reduced hospital expenditures over the long run by 10 to 20% (Sloan, 1983). There is less compelling evidence, however, that rate-setting programs reduced the growth in per capita health care spending. If true, this suggests that any reductions in inpatient hospital costs were offset by similar increases in unregulated sources of revenue. These findings are similar to the experience with PSROs discussed above.

Although implementation of rate-setting programs reduces cost growth on average, their performance varies widely across states. These effects have ranged from none to reductions exceeding 6% per year (Coelen & Sullivan, 1981). Much of the variations across programs stem from important design issues that define payment levels. Key design issues identified from previous studies as associated with their effectiveness include frequency in which the base year is moved, scope of revenue covered, number of payers included, and the construction of the trend factor (Thorpe & Phelps, 1989).

The Process of Cost Reductions

Effective rate-setting programs provide incentives for hospitals to adjust their "behavior" across many dimensions. Most notably, rate-setting programs provide incentives for hospitals to reduce the service intensity of medical care. In an earlier section, increased service intensity was identified as a major factor accounting for real increases in yearly health care costs. Reductions in service intensity are possible through lower staffing levels, a less expensive mix of personnel (e.g., the substitution of licensed practical nurses for registered nurses), slower adoption of new technology, or all of the above. The early literature on rate setting found evidence of adjustment across all dimensions (Cromwell & Kanak, 1982).

More effective rate-setting programs reduced costs by limiting the inputs (most notably technology) used to produce medical care. Hospitals in rate-setting states adopted new technologies at slower rates. Among the diffusion patterns examined were such major expense items as intensive care units, open-heart surgery, coronary artery surgery, obesity surgery, and burn care units (Romeo, Wagner, & Lee, 1984). Moreover, other technologies, most notably imaging devices such as CT, were adopted by hospitals at a slower pace in rate-setting states.

Rate setting also resulted in reduced hospital payroll expenses per patient day (Kidder & Sullivan, 1982). These "productivity" increases were achieved through both reductions in staff per adjusted day and changes in the mix of personnel. In some instances, particularly in teaching hospitals, administrators reduced their ancillary staff component, including intravenous and phlebotomy teams, messenger/transporters, and clerks, among others. Their tasks were generally absorbed by resident physicians, nurses, or both.

Although rate-setting programs during the 1970s achieved some of their goals, some dysfunctional side effects were evident. Rate setting programs that focused solely on the day of care often led to increases in the average length of a hospital stay (Sloan, 1983). In some cases, average hospital occupancy rates also increased. As a result, per capita days of care remained relatively stable after the implementation of rate-setting programs, blunting the full cost-containment potential. As noted earlier, the first rate-setting programs appeared less effective in reducing per capita health care spending. This led many observers to speculate that hospitals merely shifted their fixed costs to other, unregulated payers (often termed cost shifting) or unregulated sources of revenue (e.g, outpatient care) (Eby & Cohodes, 1985). The ability of hospital administrators to escape the full regulatory potential of the rate-setting laws created increased demand for alternative cost-containment strategies. Sharp increases in charges to unregulated payers—who were largely commercial health insurers—created growing allegations that they bore the burden of any cost savings enjoyed by regulated (generally, government) payers (Sloan & Becker, 1984). The growing differential between "costs" reimbursed by regulated payers and "charges" to unregulated payers raised concerns about the overall effectiveness and equity of rate-setting programs. These concerns were largely responsible for the subsequent generation of rate-setting programs, competitive bidding schemes, and alternative delivery systems described below.

Efforts to Control Health Care Costs (1983–present)

Informed by the early experience with hospital rate-setting, attempts to control rising health care costs changed in four important aspects during the mid-1980s. First, private payers and employers increased their efforts to develop cost-containment programs. Second, state governments and Medicare experimented with new approaches to hospital rate setting. Third, both the public and private sector created incentives for hospitals to compete on the basis of price, rather than other dimensions. Finally, the cost-containment debate was extended to physician payment in addition to institutional payment reforms.

Role of Private Payers

Facing sharply rising health insurance premiums during the early 1980s, private payers extended their efforts to control health care costs (particularly, hospital costs) in three important directions. First, private payers and employers increased efforts to "manage" the utilization of health care. Second, dissatisfied with the ability of private health insurance carriers to control costs, a growing number of employers decided to "self-insure." Third, using their purchasing power for leverage, private payers increasingly negotiated rates of payment with health care providers.

Growth in Managed Care

During the early 1980s the HMO concept assumed a prominent role in the health care delivery system. The key features of the HMO concept include (1) serving a defined population voluntarily enrolled in the plan, (2) the assumption of contractual responsibility and financial risk by the plan to provide a stated range of services, and (3) the payment of a fixed annual or monthly payment by the enrollee independent of the actual use of services (Luft, 1981). The intent of the HMO concept was to shift some financial risk to providers (rather than to patients under various cost-sharing schemes). Risk shifting would, in theory, create incentives for the plan to provide appropriate levels of medical care in general and preventive care in particular. Payment of a fixed annual fee also limited the ability of providers to thwart the intent of the cost controls through shifting costs to unregulated payers or costs.

Enrollment in HMOs grew rapidly during the 1980s and early 1990s, increasing to 39.8 million by July 1, 1993, a 340% rise in just 13 years (InterStudy, 1994). "Point-of-Service" (POS) Plans and "Preferred Provider Organizations" (PPOs) are also making impressive enrollment gains. In fact, managed care in its various forms has become the dominant insurance vehicle in the United States. Overall, 58% of employees were enrolled in HMOs, PPOs or POS Plans in 1993, up from 56% in 1992 and 27% in 1988 (Medical Benefits, 1993).

The interest of corporate America in managed-care plans is not without merit. Several studies have documented the wide variation in medical practice patterns, many of which result in costly and inappropriate patterns of medical care (Wennberg, 1984). Estimates of the magnitude of this inappropriate use vary widely. Some estimate that up to 30% of all health care costs result from unnecessary medical and surgical tests, treatments, and procedures (Chassin, 1987).

Among the most popular of the managed-care options is the HMO. The spectacular growth in HMO enrollment noted above was enhanced by their well-documented ability to reduce total health expenditures. Early, nonexperimental experience placed the magnitude of these cost savings between 20 and 40% compared to those enrolled in more traditional health care plans (Luft, 1981). At issue was whether the observed reductions in expenditures stemmed from a different style of medicine practiced by physicians in HMOs, a favorable selection of enrollees, or both. Indeed, there was mounting evidence that healthier, younger individuals were more likely to join HMOs. Thus, the observed savings may simply represent self-selection rather than real savings.

Evidence from the Rand Health Insurance Experiment (HIE) provided insight into the selection issue. Using an experimentally controlled population, the HIE found that, compared to a free, fee-for-service plan, HMOs reduced total expenditures by 29% (Manning et al., 1985). The magnitude of these reductions was impressive, similar to those observed under a 95% co-insurance rate. Thus, the experimental results indicated that HMOs did not require favorable selection to achieve their large apparent cost savings. Remaining at issue, however, is whether these savings represent one-time or continued reductions in health care spending. One early comparison of premium growth among traditional plans with that of HMOs found little difference in rates of increase (Newhouse, Schwartz, Williams, & Witsberger, 1985). If these results are valid, they suggest that HMO savings, although substantial, may be transitory.

Spurred by the studies documenting their effectiveness, selected aspects of HMOs, such as a second surgical opinion, preauthorization of selected hospital admissions, concurrent review, and outpatient surgery and testing requirements, assumed standard roles in many health plans (Jensen, Morrisey, & Marcus, 1987). In some cases, immediate reductions in health care spending resulted. Although evaluations of the cost savings traced to private sector utilization programs are rare, one study provided some early insight. For the large private health insurer examined, hospital utilization review (which included preadmission certification and on-site and concurrent review) reduced admissions 12.3%, inpatient spending 11.9% and total per capita expenditures 8.3% (Feldstein, Wickizer, & Wheeler, 1988). Other, company-specific evaluations have found similar expenditure reductions accompanying the introduction of utilization review programs. Whether these limited programs generate spillover savings (or additional costs) to other payers is not clear.

Growth in the Number of Self-Insured Companies

Frustration over the inability of more traditional third-party payers to control the rise in health insurance premiums led many companies to self-insure. Between 1986 and 1992, the number of firms that were either partially or fully self-insured increased from 46% to 67% (Bulinski, 1993). A number of factors account for the rapid growth in self-insured firms. Self-insured plans are exempt from state mandated-benefit laws that require group health insurance plans to include specific benefits. Many of the mandated benefits receive little criticism. Others, such as chiropractic services, catastrophic coverage, and more esoteric benefits (e.g., wigs, acupuncture), are often criticized and are thought responsible for a portion of the continued rise in health care premiums. The growth in the number of mandated health benefits has been spectacular, rising from approximately 40 in 1970 ("Health Insurance Premiums", 1988) to over 1100 in 1993 (Bulinski, 1993). Thus, some of the continued rise in group health insurance premiums stems from the proliferation of mandated benefits.

In addition to avoiding state benefit mandates, there are additional incentives to self-insure. For instance, self-insured funds are not subject to state premium taxes or to laws governing capital and financial reserve requirements. Moreover, self-insured funds do not contribute to state "risk pools," designed to finance insurance for high-risk, low-income individuals through state taxes.

Growth in the number of self-insured plans is also symptomatic of the longer-term trend away from "community"-rated plans and toward "experience" rating. Built into traditional group health insurance premiums are costs stemming from uncompensated care, insurance company profits, and cross-subsidies of high-cost policyholders. The rising number of uninsured individuals and uncompensated care has accounted for a portion of the yearly increases in health insurance premiums. Firms that self-insure avoid these additional costs, which are built into a typical group health insurance premium. In this sense, self-insuring eliminates any cross-subsidies included in health insurance premiums. However, the move to self-insuring also transfers all (or in some cases most) of the financial risk of catastrophic cases from private insurers to firms.

Despite the benefits accruing to firms that self-insure, the comparative ability of such plans to contain costs remains unproved. One study compared the level and rate of increase in costs among self-insured commercial and Blue Cross plans. The results found no significant differences in expenditures across plans between 1981 and 1985 (Jensen & Gabel, 1988). Moreover, firms self-insuring during this period actually experienced sharper increases in health care spending compared to commercial and Blue Cross plans. Although our experience with self-insured plans is relatively new, their ability to significantly reduce cost growth relative to more traditional payers appears questionable.

Point-of-Service Products

Another important trend is the growing popularity of "Point-of-Service" (POS) plans. These hybrid plans combine key features of HMO and traditional indemnity products. Enrollees are permitted to choose at the point of service whether to use the plan's provider network or seek care from nonnetwork physicians. Typcially, in-panel physicians are paid on a capitated or discounted-fee basis and out-of-panel physicians receive traditional fee-for-service reimbursement.

From the consumer's perspective, free choice of providers is a major selling point for Point-of-Service Plans. However, the reimbursement provisions of these plans are designed to dissuade enrollees from exercising the out-of-network option. Most enrollees in open-ended products pay coinsurance in the 30% range and deductibles of up to $300 for use of out-of-network providers, while services provided in-network are subject to mimimal co-payments. (HMO Industry Profile, 1993). These financial differentials effectively deter out-of-network care. By strongly encouraging, but not requiring, use of in-network physicians, POS Plans aim to reap the benefits of tightly managed care while bypassing its least popular feature; that is, restricted consumer choice.

Growth in PPOs

Finally, private payers and self-insured firms have increasingly used their purchasing power to negotiate payment rates with providers. Under a PPO arrangement, private payers negotiate a discounted rate, often guaranteeing the provider a specified volume of business. For hospitals suffering from low occupancy rates (generally in California, Colorado, and Florida), the arrangements are quite attractive. The number of PPOs increased from 115 in 1984 to 1036 in 1992. More than 57 million individuals are eligible to join a PPO offered through their or a family member's employer.

Although the sponsorships, form, and incentives found in PPOs differ widely, today's PPOs share four common characteristics:

1. PPOs represent an organized network of providers (e.g., hospitals, physicians) available to provide care.
2. Patients enter the PPO network through financial incentives in their benefits, a physician gatekeeper, or both.
3. PPOs negotiate discounts from providers from prevailing market payment rates.
4. PPOs include a variety of managed-care elements, usually including physician gatekeepers, utilization review, and second-opinion programs.

The early PPOs focused on negotiating reduced rates of payment to both hospitals and physicians. Little attention was directed toward including checks on utilization. As a result, early experience with PPOs provided mixed results. Although unit costs fell, the volume of services often increased, reducing the success of the ventures. More recently, insurers have developed hybrid programs incorporating utilization-control features along with negotiated payments. The utilization-control features in these hybrid plans are similar to those found in most HMOs. A central feature of these plans is the use of a "gatekeeper" primary care physician. The primary care physician in essence manages the patient referral process. Most hybrid plans include financial incentives for the gatekeeper to monitor utilization by setting specific targets for hospital admissions, total hospital days, and outpatient surgery. Since these hybrid plans are so new, few empirical analyses have assessed their impact on health care expenditures. One recent study, however, examined the impact of a PPO for a large western company. The study found no discernible difference in spending among these enrolled in the PPO compared to other employees. Whether these results will generalize to other settings remains unknown.

Innovations in Hospital Rate Setting—Growth in Diagnosis-Related Group Payment Systems

Perhaps the most important change in hospital rate setting during the 1980s was Medicare's shift from a retrospective cost-based program to a prospectively determined payment based on diagnosis-related groups (DRGs). Under this system, hospitals are paid a preestablished amount per case treated, with payment rates varying by type of case. The DRGs measure hospital output by originally classifying patients into 23 major diagnostic categories (MDCs), based on major body systems. The MDCs are divided further into more than 470 diagnostic groups based on the patient's diagnosis or surgical procedure used, and on age, sex, and other clinical information.

Three aspects of this approach differ from Medicare's previous payment methodology. First, the payments are determined in advance and are fixed. Second, the unit of payment changed from per day to per admission. Finally, payment rates were eventually divorced from each hospital's own cost experience.

The new payment scheme implemented by Medicare applies only to inpatient, operating costs. Excluded are payments for physicians' services (discussed below), capital (which Medicare continues to reimburse at levels slightly below interest and depreciation expenses), direct medical education (e.g., salaries for attending physicians and residents), and outpatient and emergency departments. Not all hospitals were included in Medicare's case payment system. Some specialty hospitals, such as children's, long-term-care, rehabilitation, and psychiatric hospitals, were exempt. Also exempt were four states (New York, Massachusetts, Maryland, and New Jersey) receiving waivers from the HCFA to develop their own experimental payment programs. However, by 1993, only Maryland retained its waiver.

Payment that an individual hospital receives for treating Medicare patients in a given DRG depends on the DRG's "cost" weight (i.e., its cost relative to an average Medicare admission) multiplied by a "standardized" average cost for all Medicare patients. The standardization process includes adjustments for interhospital differences in wages, teaching status, and amount of care provided to low-income patients. Different rates are also set for urban and rural hospitals. In addition, payment amounts to hospitals are adjusted each year by a trend factor, consisting of a measure of the price of goods and services purchased by hospitals and a discretionary adjustment factor to account for changes in new technology and productivity.

The original plans called for a gradual phase-in of the case payment system over 3 years. In the first year (1984), 75% of a hospital's per-case payments were to be based on its own cost experience. This level gradually declined over time, and by 1988 payment rates (known as prices) to hospitals were based on national "standardized" average costs per admission. Movement to a pricing system divorced payment rates from each hospital's costs.

Medicare's experience with the DRG system has produced mixed results. Initially, hospitals responded quite dramatically to the altered incentives created by the DRG payment system. The payment of a fixed price per admission provided hospitals clear incentives to reduce costs. Any savings stemming from these reductions could be retained by the hospital. The new opportunity to earn short-term profits resulted in impressive changes during the early years of the program. During the first year of the program (federal fiscal year 1984), inpatient expenditures declined as the number of full-time equivalent (FTE) employees fell 2.3%, reversing the trend of earlier years. Although lengths of stay among the elderly had been falling for years, the DRG program accelerated the decline. Finally, total admissions fell 2.6% during the first year of the DRG program, again reversing a long trend toward increased admissions.

Falling lengths of stay, admissions, and employment levels resulted in slower hospital expenditure growth. Total Medicare inpatient operating costs decreased 6 percentage points during the first year of the program. Inpatient cost per admission increased slightly, approximately 1.3%, significantly below the 4.7% update factor allowed during the first year. With cost growth slower than increases in revenue, hospital operating margins rose sharply. By 1984 the median hospital's margin was 11.3%, the highest in nearly two decades (AHA, 1988).

Unfortunately, the expenditure reductions were short-lived. Many of the trends observed in the initial year of the program were reversed in subsequent years. Total Medicare operating costs increased 3% during fiscal year 1985 and 6.5% during 1986 (see Table 11.1). The latter increase was cause for concern, as it exceeded the allowed increase in revenues (e.g., the trend factor) by 6 percentage points. Although the factors accounting for the more recent rise in Medicare spending are unknown, hospitals may simply have reinvested large portions of their "profits" back into hospital operations. If true, this would account for the cost growth bubble observed in fiscal year 1986.

Lengths of stay also increased during 1986 and 1987, although admissions continued to fall. However, since the average acuity of patients admitted to hospitals increased, adjusted (for case mix) lengths of stay did not rise. In contrast to the initial decline, total hospital employment increased during 1986 and 1987. The bulk of the increase occurred in hospital outpatient departments, with employment levels on the inpatient side continuing to fall.

The new DRG payment system also provided strong incentives for hospital administrators to "unbundle" services. This included encouraging physicians to complete tests and procedures outside the hospital (which are not subject to the payment controls) Moreover, recent changes in medical technology, most nota-

TABLE 11.1   Percent Change in Medicare Inpatient Expenses, Hospital Staffing, and Hospital Volume, 1980–1987

Year	Medicare inpatient expenses	Total inpatient expenses	Total hospital FTEs[a]	Length of stay	Admissions
1980	—	16.8%	4.7%	−0.1%	6.7%
1981	—	18.4	5.4	−0.1	3.0
1982	—	15.6	3.7	−2.3	4.1
1983	—	9.6	1.4	−4.5	4.7
1984	−4.4%	3.5	−2.3	−7.6	−2.6
1985	3.0	4.1	−2.3	−2.0	−5.2
1986	6.5	7.1	0.3	0.3	−1.2
1987	—	6.1	0.7	1.1	0.4

[a]FTEs, full-time equivalent employees.

Source: American Hospital Association, National Panel Survey. Prospective Payment Assessment Commission, Annual Report to Congress.

bly surgical procedures, have accelerated the trend toward outpatient care. These incentives and changes in technology resulted in substantial increases in Medicare's spending for outpatient services. For instance, by 1987 Medicare expenditures for outpatient services increased 21%, more than five times the rate of increase observed for inpatient expenditures (Physician Payment Review Commission, 1988). The large increase in outpatient department expenditures blunted the full cost-containment potential of the DRG program.

In addition to the most recent rise in Medicare spending, the DRG program had uneven impacts on hospital expenditure growth. As discussed above, a central element of the new system was the use of predetermined "prices" for hospital payment. These prices were based on national average Medicare costs per discharge standardized for teaching status, share of low-income patients treated, wage rates, and urban/rural location. Because payments were no longer based on historic hospital costs, payments to some hospitals were lower and others higher than their average costs. Hospitals with payment rates set lower than average costs were thought less efficient and were the initial targets of the regulatory program. However, large numbers of hospitals initially benefited from the program because payment rates exceeded their average costs.

Use of the pricing methodology led to an uneven response by hospitals to the DRG payment system. On average, total inpatient costs growth was initially attenuated under the DRG system. To a more modest extent, the DRG system reduced the rate of increase in total (both inpatient and outpatient) expenditures through 1986. The reduced growth in costs, however, was generally limited to those hospitals with payment rates set below costs. Among these hospitals, inpatient cost growth was over 4.4 percentage points lower than the overall average

(Feder, Hadley, & Zuckerman, 1987). In contrast, compared to the most tightly constrained hospitals, expenditures for hospitals least constrained were some 7 percentage points higher. Thus, the redistributive effect of the pricing system limited the full cost-containment potential of the DRG program.

Throughout the 1980s reforms of the DRG system focused on a variety of "technical" adjustments to the payment rates as well as adjusting the methodology used to reimburse for capital expenses. Until 1992, Medicare reimbursed hospitals a percentage (less than 100) for all depreciation and interest spending. Failure to include capital payments in the prospective payment system likely reduced the potential effectiveness of the DRG program. A capital pass-through ensured that hospital spending decisions were insensitive to interest rates or less costly methods of expansion. Moreover, the pass-through also provided incentives for hospitals to inefficiently substitute capital for labor.

In FY 1992, a 10-year phase-in of prospective payment for hospital capital costs began. When fully implemented, Medicare will reimburse capital costs much as it now pays for operating costs under the DRG program. Payment will be based on standardized national average costs per discharge, adjusted for teaching status, share of low-income patients, wage rates, and urban/rural location. (These adjustments are not identical to their operating costs counterparts.)

Growth and Subsequent Decline in All-Payer Rate-Setting Programs

State experiments with innovative hospital rate-setting programs expanded during the 1980s. Until then, most state rate-setting programs set prospective per diem rates for Medicaid and Blue Cross plans. In some cases, commercial payers were also included. However, Medicare payments to hospitals were outside the prospectively determined rates. Beginning in 1977, Maryland obtained a waiver from the HCFA allowing the state to develop its own payment rules for Medicare. This allowed the state to include all sources of third-party inpatient revenue under the state's rate-setting rules. Three other states—New Jersey, Massachusetts, and New York—subsequently obtained Medicare waivers during the early 1980s. Like Maryland, each state included Medicare payments within its historic rate-setting programs.

The genesis of these four all-payer systems was complicated. They included concern over both continued escalation in hospital costs within these states as well as issues regarding the equity of payment rates facing private payers. As discussed below, use of the rate-setting process to achieve both cost reductions and distributional objectives distinguished the all-payer approach from previous efforts (Thorpe, 1987). Each state adopting the all-payer approach had previous rate-setting programs covering some portion of inpatient revenues. Although these programs were often successful in reducing cost growth among some payers (and in the case of New York, all payers), costs among unregulated payers continued to climb. Price controls on Medicaid and Blue Cross plans created incentives for hospitals to increase charges—often referred to as cost or charge shifting—to unregulated commercial payers. As a result, the difference between charges and costs for commercial payers escalated rapidly during the late 1970s and early 1980s. Thus, protecting commercial payers against cost shifting assumed an important role for all-payer systems.

Growth in the number of uninsured individuals over this period created another set of pressures. Between 1979 and 1984 the number of individuals without health insurance increased 20% to more than 34 million individuals (Congressional Research Service, 1988, Table 4.7). Growth in the number of individuals without health insurance increased the volume of bad debt and charity care provided by hospitals. For those hospitals unable to recover such costs through commercial payers (through increased charges) or state and local governments (in the case of public hospitals), a serious deterioration of operating margins resulted. Deteriorating hospital financial conditions, combined with the growing number of uninsured patients, created pressures on state governments to provide some financial relief.

The growing demands of the commercial insurance industry to limit legislatively the difference between charges and costs (e.g., the differential), combined with the mounting requirements of hospitals to finance uncompensated care, presented a dilemma. Limiting the size of the differential would eliminate one traditionally passive method of financing a portion of uncompensated care. Thus, some alternative and more explicit financing method would be required. Moreover, the growth in the differential created a common perception that commercial payers were assuming an unfair burden in financing care for the uninsured (Meyer, Johnson, & Sullivan, 1983). Thus, to distribute the costs of uncompensated care more evenly, each state developed some type of uncompensated-care pool. Although methods of collecting revenue and distributing it to hospitals differed across states, the burden of financing uncompensated care was more widely distributed.

Finally, experience with the "partial" payer approaches used by most state rate-setting programs during the 1970s provided mixed results. As noted above, cost growth among regulated payers was often attenuated, although per capita cost growth was generally stable. Thus, the all-payer approach was also designed to provide a uniform inpatient revenue cap, reducing the ability of hospitals to escape the intent of the regulatory controls. Although the programs provided a comprehensive inpatient rate cap, payment methods for outpatient services in each state were largely left intact.

The four state all-payer programs described above generally achieved their intended results. Relative to the "unwaivered" states, the all-payer states were able to reduce total cost growth. Inpatient costs per admission were 2 to 3 percentage points lower between 1982 and 1985 in waivered states relative to unwaivered states (Schramm, Renn, & Biles, 1986). More impressive perhaps was the 2-percentage-point reduction in total costs per admission (adjusted for outpatient visits).

Lower cost growth among the all-payer states was achieved through reductions in labor, rather than reduced admissions or length of stay. The number of FTE personnel in the waivered states grew at significantly slower rates than observed elsewhere (Schramm et al., 1986). Thus, the comprehensive regulatory controls appeared to increase the productivity of hospital care. Fewer labor inputs per patient day were also accompanied by slower rates of technological diffusion. As noted in an earlier section, slower adoption rates were especially pronounced in New York. Although growth in hospital personnel in all-payer states proceeded at a significantly slower pace, changes in average length of stay between the waivered and unwaivered states revealed few discernible differences.

The all-payer states were also successful in limiting the differential between private charges and costs. Each state enacted a statutory limit on the magnitude of each hospital's allowed difference between costs and charges. In New York this reduced the differential from a statewide average of 30% to less than 15% by 1985 (Thorpe, 1987). Similarly, the all-payer program in Massachusetts reduced the magnitude of the differential by 1.4% in its first year and steadily lowered it to approximately 7.5% by 1985. The magnitude of the differential in these states was significantly lower than the national average of 25% (AHA, 1988).

Finally, the regulatory approach adopted by the all-payer states raised a significant volume of revenue to finance hospital uncompensated care. More than $300 million was raised each year in New York and Massachusetts, with similar amounts (relative to total state hospital costs) in the other states. The pool revenues allowed financially strained hospitals to maintain, and often increase, the volume of care they provided the medically indigent. Moreover, the significant influx of revenues raised by the pools improved the operating margins of many hospitals. In New York, for example, the magnitude of the statewide hospital operating deficit was over $600 million less during the experiment relative to deficits projected without the pools (Thorpe, 1987). Thus, the redistributive goals of the all-payer programs were largely fulfilled.

The success of the all-payer programs in simultaneously reducing cost growth and internally redistributing revenues to fiscally distressed facilities ironically led to their near elimination. Hospitals in each state were quick to compare the expected revenue under their waivered systems with revenues expected under the national DRG program (Hospital Association of New York State, 1985). For instance, the hospital association in New York State projected a $400 million influx of Medicare revenues in 1986 should the state switch from its waivered system to the DRG program. Similar projections of higher revenues flowing to the waivered states also were developed in other states. In partial response to industry interests in switching to the DRG program, New York and Massachusetts did not extend their waivers, thus joining Medicare's DRG payment programs. New Jersey renewed its waiver once, but in 1989 it also joined the Medicare DRG system.

Growth in Competitive Bidding

A final payment innovation during the 1980s was the growth in competitive bidding schemes designed to create incentives for providers to compete on a price
basis. As discussed in an earlier section, competition among providers in the health
care industry has traditionally occurred along nonprice dimensions (e.g., service
intensity, technology, and amenities). Those interested in promoting price competition were quick to highlight the shortcomings of the regulatory approach
(Enthoven, 1981). According to this school of thought, vigorous price competition
among health care plans and providers would provide the only "practical" solution to the health care cost crisis.

While other states moved to increase the scope of hospital revenue regulated,
others moved to competitive bidding. The California Medi-Cal program implemented the most notable bidding scheme, known as selective contracting, in 1983.
Under this program hospitals would submit price bids to the state contracting "czar"
to provide services to Medi-Cal beneficiaries. Except in emergencies, hospitals
not receiving contracts could not receive payment from the state. Two other state
Medicaid programs followed California's lead: Illinois in 1985 and, most recently,
Washington State.

The early experience with selective contracting in California has produced
favorable results (Melnick & Zwanziger, 1988). In contrast to earlier research
results that found higher cost growth in the most competitive markets, the opposite held for California hospitals after the implementation of selective contracting. Between 1983 and 1985, real (adjusted for general inflation) inpatient
costs increased an average of 1% for hospitals in less competitive markets,
compared to an 11.3% decrease among hospitals in more competitive markets
(Melnick & Zwanziger, 1988). In keeping with the empirical results noted above,
the state estimated savings exceeding $1 billion during the selective contracting
program.

Both the selective contracting program implemented in California and the all-
payer rate-setting systems discussed above were able to reduce cost growth. Still
at issue is their relative ability to contain costs. Is competitive bidding the salvation or the imposition of more comprehensive and binding rate-setting programs?
Recent studies provide at least an initial insight. Based on a national study, all-
payer rate regulation reduced cost growth by 16.3% in Massachusetts, 15.4% in
Maryland, and 6.3% in New York between 1982 and 1986 relative to a set of
control states (Robinson & Luft, 1988). Cost growth in New Jersey was similar to
that observed among the control states. In comparison, cost growth among California hospitals using the selective contracting strategy was 10.1% lower compared to states without rate-setting or competitive bidding. Thus, based on these
results, it appears that, on average, the more comprehensive rate-setting programs
and selective contracting have similar impacts on cost growth. Whether the longer-
term performance of these decidedly different approaches is similar requires continued monitoring.

Reform of Physician Reimbursement

During much of the 1980s, efforts to reduce health care costs often focused on payments to institutions (especially hospitals), rather than payments for physician and outpatient services and hospital capital. After implementing the DRG system, however, policymakers turned their attention to reforming the way in which Medicare pays physicians. This attention was justified/merited. Between 1975 and 1987, total Medicare expenditures for physicians increased an average of 18% annually (Physician Payment Review Commission, 1988). Also, although expenditures for physician services accounted for less than one-quarter of all spending, physicians potentially influenced over 70% of all health care spending.

Medicare's traditional method for reimbursing physicians was based on the "customary, prevailing, and reasonable" (CPR) reimbursement system, a methodology that was typical of the fee-for-service methods used by most third-party payers. Under the CPR method, payments for each service performed were based on the lower of the physician's historic charge, the billed charge, or an average charge of similar physicians in the area. Payment rates were also limited to yearly increases in the Medicare Economic Index. This system was roundly criticized as inflationary and complex. In addition, it provided higher payment rates (relative to costs) for specialists and those performing complex procedures (relative to those performing more cognitive tasks). This structure was frequently cited as influencing physicians' specialty choices. The apparent "surplus" of surgeons and subspecialists projected over the next 20 years has often been traced to this payment system.

Two options were frequently advanced to address both the cost-growth and the specialty-choice issues. The first payment option was to expand the number of physicians paid on a capitated basis. The role of capitation in addressing cost growth was addressed earlier. The second option was a new fee schedule for physicians.

In the 1989 Budget Act, Congress chose the second option. It mandated the implementation of a specific type of fee schedule, called a resource-based relative value scale (RBRVS), starting in 1992. This particular relative-value scale has three components: a measure of total "work" by the physician, an allowance for practice costs, and an allowance for the cost of malpractice insurance. Each service is assigned a given number of relative value units, or RVUs. These RVUs are then multiplied by a national conversion factor to determine a dollar amount of payment for that service.

A major objective of the RBRVS was to develop a more equitable method of reimbursing physicians. In contrast to the CPR, two services that require the same amount of work, practice expense and malpractice expense should be reimbursed at the same level (except for an adjustment to account for different price levels in different geographic areas). This was intended to eliminate the distortive effect that the CPR has on specialty choice and service mix.

In the 1989 Budget Act, Congress also made two other changes to the way that physicians are reimbursed for services they provide to Medicare paients. First, limits were placed on the amounts that physicians could charge patients above a Medicare-approved amount. In 1992, doctors were not allowed to charge more than 20% more than the Medicare-approved amount. From 1993 on, this percentage dropped to 115%.

The final reform was the creation of the Medicare Volume Performance Standard (MVPS). The MVPS is a target rate that Congress sets annually to reflect its view of the appropriate growth rate in Medicare spending for physician services. It is intended to take into account both general cost inflation and acceptable increases in volume and intensity of services provided.

Under the CPR system, payment rates each year were updated by the amount of the Medicare Economic Index. The MVPS simply adds another "layer" to this process. After a year has ended, the MVPS rate of increase in spending and the actual rate are compared. If the MVPS is lower than the actual rate of increase (i.e., spending grew at a higher level than Congress considered appropriate) then the next year's increase (normally the MEI) is decreased by the amount of the excess. If the MVPS is higher than the actual rate of spending, then the annual update is increased by the amount of the shortfall.

An MVPS was first set in 1990, and it first impacted the amount of the annual payment update in 1992. Actual expenditures exceeded the MVPS in 1990, but in 1993 all expenditures were below the MVPS. However, because of other influences on volume (including the responses to significant payment rate reductions that were also part of Medicare Physician Payment Reform) it is presently difficult to conclude how well the MVPS has controlled expenditure and volume growth.

Summary and Conclusions

Despite 20 years of regulatory controls, health care spending continues to grow relative to the GNP. The inability to reduce the national rate of expenditure growth continues to frustrate both public and private payers. Indeed, despite growing efforts to reduce costs, health care spending now accounts for 13.2% of the GNP, up from 9.1% in 1980. Even though the United States spends more on health care as a percentage of GNP than does any other industrialized country, more than 37 million Americans remain uninsured. Frustration over the sustained rise in health care costs and a 23% increase in the number of uninsured since 1979 has increased interest in more fundamental changes in our financing system. For the first time in decades, polls report that most Americans want a fundamental shift in the direction of U.S. health policy. Indeed, a poll taken at the beginning of the Clinton administration indicated that nearly 7 out of 10 Americans expected substantial progress from the new president on health care issues (Washington Post/ABC News, 1993). This mounting sentiment for change will likely continue, creating pressure for more innovative methods of addressing health care cost issues.

The continued rise in health care costs indicates that our attempts to address the problem have failed. This failure may be traced to a mismatch between the underlying problem and previous interventions. Our earlier discussion indicated that the fundamental force driving up health care costs was the diffusion of new technologies. Of the estimated sevenfold real increase in health care spending since 1950, new technologies and practice patterns account for up to 90% of the growth (Manning et al., 1987). Innovations in medicine have been nothing short of remarkable. Our capacity to increase average life expectancy and its quality reflect these developments. The growth in transplant capacity, diagnostic imaging, and drugs represents a few of these medical innovations. If this increase in spending had generated commensurate increases in benefits, then the "problem" of health care cost growth would be illusory. In short, that we spend over 13% of our GNP in the health care sector may simply reflect societal preferences to direct limited resources to health rather than to other areas.

At the center of the debate over the growth of health care costs is whether the same level of health could be purchased for less. A growing body of research indicates that substantial savings could be achieved without significant changes in the health of our population. Critical examination of the "appropriateness" of various medical procedures indicates that health care spending could be reduced by $50 billion without a deleterious impact on health. At issue is the appropriate intervention to address the underlying problem of health care cost growth. The push of new technology suggests that more centralized, rather than fragmented, approaches underlie any solution. This would require the multiple public and private payers to reach some consensus concerning a comprehensive strategy to address the technology issue. One promising proposal is the development of a national technology assessment commission empowered to conduct clinical trials of new technologies before they are widely diffused. Another would move us closer to the Canadian budget-cap system. Although the precise path is not evident, what is clear is that failure to match the next generation of interventions with the technology and costly variation in practice pattems will continue to thwart our efforts to contain costs.

References

Aaron, H., & Schwartz, W., *The Painful Prescription: Rationing Hospital Care.* Washington, DC: Brookings Institution, 1984.
American Hospital Association. *National Hospital Panel Survey.* Chicago: AHA, 1988.
Bulinski, C., "Self Insurance Showdown." *Managed Healthcare*, October, 1993. pp. 42–44.
Chassin, M., "Does Inappropriate Use Explain Geographic Variation in the Use of Health Care Services? A Study of Three Procedures." Santa Monica, CA: Rand Corporation, 1987 (N-2748).

Coelen, C., & Sullivan, D., "An Analysis of the Effects of Prospective Reimbursement Programs on Hospital Expenditures." *Health Care Financing Review*, Winter, 1, 1981.

Congressional Budget Office. *The Impact of PSROs on Health Care Costs: An Update of CBO's 1979 Evaluation*. Washington, DC: U.S. Government Printing Office, 1981.

Congressional Research Service. *Health Insurance and the Uninsured: Background Data and Analysis*. Washington, DC: U.S. Government Printing Office, 1988.

Cromwell, J., & Kanak, J., "The Effects of Hospital Rate-Setting Programs on Volume of Hospital Services." *Health Care Financing Review*, 4(2) 47, 1982.

Eby, C., & Cohodes, D., "What Do We Know About Rate-Setting?" *Journal of Health Politics, Policy and Law*, Summer, 299, 1985.

Employee Benefits Research Institute: Issue Brief, No. 118, Washington, September 1991.

Enthoven, A. C., *Health Plan*. Reading, MA: Addison-Wesley, 1981.

Feder, J., Hadley, J., & Zuckerman, J., "How Did Medicare's Prospective Payment System Affect Hospitals?" *New England Journal of Medicine*, *317*, 867, 1987.

Feldstein, P., Wickizer, T., & Wheeler, J., "The Effects of Utilization Review Programs In Health Care Use and Expenditures." *New England Journal of Medicine*, May 19, 1988, pp. 1310–1314.

Freeland, M., & Schendler, C. E., "National Health Expenditure Growth in the 1980s: An Aging Population, New Technologies and Increasing Competition." *Health Care Financing Review*, March, 1, 1983.

Fuchs, V., *Who Shall Live?* New York: Basic Books, 1974.

Gabel. J. et al., *Trends in Managed Health Care*. Washington, DC: Health Insurance Association of America, 1989.

Group Health Association of America. "HMO Industry Profile: 1993 Edition," Washington, DC: Author, November 1993.

Group Health Association of America. "Member Year-End Surveys (1989–1993), and GHAA Annual HMO Industry Survey," Washington, DC: Author, (1988).

Health Care Financing Administration. *HHS News*, November 18. Washington, DC: Health Insurance Association of America, 1988.

"Health Insurance Premiums to Soar in '89." *Wall Street Journal*, p. B1, October 25, 1988.

Hospital Association of New York State. *Modelling Alternative Reimbursement Systems*. Albany, NY: HANYS, 1985.

Interstudy. *National HMO Census, 1987*. Excelsior, MN:, 1988.

The InterStudy Competitive Edge Industry Report, 3(2), 1994.

Jensen. G., & Gabel, J., "The Erosion of Purchased Health Insurance." *Inquiry*, 25(3), pp. 328–343, 1988.

Jensen, G., Morrisey, M., & Marcus, J., "Cost Sharing and the Changing Pattern of Employer-Sponsored Health Benefits." *Milbank Memorial Fund Quarterly*, 65(4) 521, 1987.

Joskow, P., *Controlling Hospital Costs: The Role of Government Regulation*. Boston: MIT Press, 1981.

KPMG–Pete Marwick Survey of 1003 Firms, 1993.

Kidder, D., & Sullivan, D., "Hospital Payroll Costs, Productivity and Employment Under Prospective Payment." *Health Care Financing Review*, 4(2) 89, 1982.

Luft, H., *Health Maintenance Organizations: Dimensions of Performance*. New York: John Wiley, 1981.

Manning, W. et al., *A Controlled Trial of the Effect of a Prepaid Group Practice on the Utilization of Medical Services.* Santa Monica, CA: Rand Corporation, 1985.

Manning, W. G. et al., "Health Insurance and the Demand for Medical Care." *American Economic Review, 77*(3), 251, 1987.

Medical Benefits, 10(22), 1–2, November 30, 1993.

Melnick, G., & Zwanziger, J., "Hospital Behavior under Competition and Cost-Containment Policies." *Journal of the American Medical Association, 260*(18), 2669, 1988.

Meyer, J., Johnson, W., & Sullivan, S., *Passing the Health Care Buck: Who Pays the Hidden Cost?* Washington, DC: American Enterprise Institute, 1983.

Mullen, P., "Big Increases in Health Premiums." *Health Week*, December 27, 1988, p. 1.

Newhouse, J. P., Schwartz, W., Williams, A., & Witsberger, C., "Are Fee-For-Service Costs Increasing Faster than HMO Costs?" *Medical Care, 23*(8), 960, 1985.

Office of Technology Assessment. *Medicare's Prospective Payment System: Strategies for Evaluating Costs, Quality and Medical Technology* (OTA-H-262CDC). Washington, DC: U.S. Government Printing Office. October 1985.

Pauly, M., "Taxation, Health Insurance and Market Failure in the Medical Economy." *Journal of Economic Literature*, 629, 1986.

Pauly, M., & Satterthwaite, M., "The Pricing of Primary Care Physicians' Services: A Test of the Role of Consumer Information" *Bell Journal of Economics*, 488, 1981.

Physician Payment Review Commission. *Annual Report to Congress, 1988*. Washington, DC: U.S. Government Printing Office, 1988.

Physician Payment Review Commission. *Annual Report to Congress 1993*. Washington, DC: U.S. Government Printing Office, 1993.

Prospective Payment Assessment Commission. "Medicare and the American Health Care System—Report to Congress, June 1993." Washington: U.S. Government Printing Office. June, 1992, pp. 62, 80.

Robinson, J., & Luft, H., "The Impact of Hospital Market Structure on Patient Volume, Average Length of Stay, and the Cost of Care." *Journal of Health Economics*, 4(4), 333, 1985.

Robinson, J., & Luft, H., "Competition, Regulation and Hospital Costs, 1982–1986." *Journal of the American Medical Association*, 2676, 1988.

Romeo, A., Wagner, J., & Lee, R., "Prospective Reimbursement and the Diffusion of New Technologies in Hospitals." *Journal of Health Economics*, 3(1), 1, 1984.

Salkever, D., & Bice, T., "The Impact of CON Controls on Hospital Investment." *Milbank Memorial Fund Quarterly*, 54, 185, 1976.

Schramm, C., Renn, S., & Biles, B., "New Perspectives on State Rate-Setting." *Health Affairs*, 5(3), 22, 1986.

Sloan, F., "Rate Regulation as a Strategy for Hospital Cost Control: Evidence from the Last Decade." *Milbank Memorial Fund Quarterly, 61* (Spring), 195, 1983.

Sloan, F., & Becker, E., "Cross-Subsidies and Payment for Hospital Care." *Journal of Health Politics, Policy and Law*, Winter, 670, 1984.

Sloan, F., Valvona, J., & Perrin, J., "Diffusion of Surgical Technology: An Exploratory Study." *Journal of Health Economics*, 5(1), 31, 1986.

Thorpe, K. E., "Does All-Payer Rate Setting Work? The Case of the New York Prospective Hospital Reimbursement Methodology." *Journal of Health Politics, Policy and Law, 12*(3), 391, 1987.

Thorpe, K. E., & Phelps, C. E., *Regulatory Intensity and Cost Growth. Journal of Health Economics*. Boston: Harvard School of Public Health, 1989.

Washington Post/ABC News Poll of 1510 randomly selected adults on January 14–17, 1993. Published in the Washington Post on January 19, 1993.

Wennberg, J. E., "Dealing with Medical Practice Variations: A Proposal for Action." *Health Affairs*, Summer, pp. 6–32, 1984.

12

The Government's Role in Health Care

Charles Brecher

Government is a major force shaping the health care industry. It spends over $330 billion or more than four of every ten dollars spent on care; it employs about 1.6 million people to deliver health care directly, and it regulates private providers by determining who shall be entitled to practice medicine and what the standards for that care shall be. Without an understanding of what government does, and why, students would be ignorant of an important part of what happens in health care.

This chapter provides an introductory perspective on the nature of government's role. The first section identifies the key questions to be addressed and presents some concepts essential for answering them. The second section describes the functions governments perform, and the third analyzes why government health care policies change. The final section considers alternative views of what government's role ought to be in the future.

Key Questions and Concepts

In light of the vast and diverse nature of government activities, some particular perspective should be chosen for considering the role of the public sector. Three distinct, but not mutually exclusive, approaches to the subject can be taken.

The first is descriptive. It asks simply, what is government's role? Much of this chapter will be devoted to answering this question.

A second approach seeks to go beyond knowing what government currently does to understanding what causes government to act in certain ways. It asks, why does government do certain things? It is based on a recognition that government activities vary among units of government (the United States' public sector role differs markedly from that of Great Britain) and over time (the public sector role today in the United States is markedly different from what it was 25 years ago).

A third approach considers not what is, but what might be. It asks whether government's role conforms to some normative standard of what is a desirable set of public activities. Since reasonable individuals differ over the best role for government, the answers to this question vary widely. Yet it is possible to reach some judgements after making explicit the value assumptions which underlie them.

The next three sections of this chapter examine these three types of questions in successive order. But to answer them in a sophisticated fashion, it is necessary to use a few key concepts. One set relates to the fragmented nature of American government; a second set relates to the multiple possible roles government can play.

Multiple Governments

In the United States there is no single government, rather there are multiple governments with distinct roles in a federal system. The nation has one national government entity, but 50 states and 84,955 units of local government within the states. (See Table 12.1.) Not all these units are involved in health care, but many are. The federal government and virtually all the states play some role in health care financing and delivery. Of the local governments, many of the 3,043 counties and some of the larger cities are involved in health care activity and most of the 14,422 school districts also have some health education and health delivery functions.

The federal nature of American government has important implications for how the key questions identified above can be answered. Descriptive questions need

TABLE 12.1   Governmental Units in the United States, 1992

Type of Government		Number of Units
U.S. Government		1
State Governments		50
Local Governments		84,955
County	3,043	
Municipal	19,279	
Township	16,656	
School District	14,422	
Special District	31,555	

Source: U.S. Department of Commerce, Bureau of the Census, *1992 Census of Governments*, Vol. 1, Table A, p. VI (Washington: U.S. Government Printing Office, 1993).

to be answered separately for each level of government; the answers to causal questions may vary among units of government; and normative arguments about the proper role for government need to specify not just what government should do, but which level of government should do it.

Potential Roles. In any industry, including health care, government activity can be considered along three dimensions—financing, delivery, and regulation. The extent of government activity can vary along each dimension and units of government most active on one dimension need not be active on another. Moreover, the same roles are played in varying degrees by the private sector.

Government financing of an activity typically takes the form of levying a tax to raise funds and then appropriating the funds to purchase or provide the service. However, financing may be separated from delivery. Tax funds can be used to purchase care from the private sector or to pay the salaries of civil servants employed to provide care. As will be seen, American governments follow both courses. It is also worth noting that governments can provide care without financing it. Governmental units established to provide care can and do operate without appropriations of tax dollars; they can "earn" revenues from private purchases or from insurance programs sponsored by other organizations. Examples of such arrangements in health care include some local public hospitals, which operate without direct governmental subsidies.

Regulation is the setting of standards for those engaged in the delivery of care. Regulations include licensing of occupations as well as facilities, setting standards for the process of care, and imposing restrictions on capital investments. The extent to which governmental entities engage in each form of regulation, and the particular standards they set, may vary.

It is worth noting that these roles are not unique to the public sector. Obviously private individuals and firms engage in the financing and delivery of care; they also engage in regulation. Private insurers set standards for receipt of payment and engage in utilization review; private health maintenance organizations (HMOs) set standards for practice by their physicians and monitor utilization. Thus, there is tremendous potential variation in the way in which roles are divided both between the public and private sectors and among units of government within the public sector.

What Are the Governments' Roles?

The key concepts of federalism and multiple potential roles can be combined to create a framework for describing governments' roles. As summarized in Figure 12.1, the federal government plays a major role in financing health services, serves as a direct deliverer only for selected specialized populations, and engages in some important regulation. The states show tremendous variation in their roles,

FIGURE 12.1 Summary of Governments' Major Health Care Roles

	Financing	Delivery	Regulation
Federal	Large role through Medicare and Medicaid; other categorical programs.	Operates facilities for veterans and Indians	Sets standards for Medicare providers; prohibits discrimination by providers; determines what drugs and devices may be sold.
State	Funds Medicaid, mental health, medical education and public health programs.	Operates mental hospitals, health departments and medical schools.	Regulates insurance industry; licenses facilities and personnel; establishes health codes.
Local	Subsidizes public hospitals; funds local health departments.	Operates county and municipal hospitals; operates local health departments.	Establishes local health codes.

but an aggregate summary is: they play a substantial role in financing; they are important direct providers of mental health and professional education services; they vary widely in regulatory activity but typically license providers, set standards for insurers, and are otherwise the dominant source of restrictions on the private sector. Similarly local governments vary in their health activities but they typically provide relatively little funding, especially for general medical care, and establish few local regulations. However, many cities or counties operate hospitals and clinics to insure access to care for poor residents. This summary description provides an introduction to a more detailed analysis of the ways in which government units perform each role.

Governments as Financers

More complete information about the public sector's financial role is presented in Table 12.2. In 1991 (the latest year for which data are available), government was the source of almost 44% of all expenditures for health care. Within the public sector the federal government played the largest role accounting for over two-thirds of all government spending.

The trend in governments' financing role is a sharp increase from the early 1960s to the mid-1970s and relative stability since. In 1965 government accounted for

TABLE 12.2 National Health Expenditures, Selected Years 1965–91

Amount (*dollars in billions*)	1991	1990	1985	1980	1975	1970	1965
Total	$751.8	$675.0	$419.0	$248.1	$132.7	$75.0	$41.9
Private	421.8	390.0	244.0	142.9	76.4	47.2	30.9
Public	330.0	285.1	175.0	105.2	56.3	27.8	11.0
Federal	222.9	194.5	123.1	71.0	37.0	17.7	5.5
State & Local	107.1	90.5	52.0	34.2	19.3	10.1	5.5
Percentage distribution							
Total	100.0%	100.0%	100.0%	100.0%	100.0%	100.0%	100.0%
Private	56.1	57.8	58.2	57.6	57.5	63.0	73.8
Public	43.9	42.2	41.8	42.4	42.5	37.0	26.2
Federal	29.6	28.8	29.3	28.6	27.9	23.6	13.2
State & Local	14.2	13.4	12.4	13.8	14.5	13.5	13.0

Source: Data for 1985 and earlier from Health Care Financing Administration, U.S. Department of Health and Human Services press release November 18, 1988; data for 1990 and 1991 from Suzanne Letsch et al., "National Health Expenditures, 1991" *Health Care Financing Review,* (Winter 1992) Vol. 14, No. 2, pp. 1–25.

just 26% of health care spending, but by 1975 the figure was 42%. It remained at about that level through most of the 1980s, but approached 44% in 1991. The recent stability and latest modest increase in share of funding has occurred in the context of rapid increases in total spending causing the absolute amount of public spending to rise dramatically. Between 1980 and 1991, public spending jumped from $105.2 billion to $330.0 billion or 214%.

Much of the public spending is accounted for by two programs—Medicare and Medicaid. The passage of these two programs in 1965 and their subsequent implementation explains much of the trend in government spending. Nonexistent in the early 1960s, these two programs accounted for $216.7 billion in spending in 1991 or 66% of the government total.

Medicare is a two-part program designed to help pay the medical care costs of the elderly. (Certain disabled individuals also have been made eligible). Part A covers most hospital and some nursing home care; part B covers physician care and some other out-of-hospital services. Part A benefits are financed primarily through a payroll tax; Part B is financed through a combination of federal general fund appropriations and premiums paid by elderly enrollees. Both parts are administered by the federal Health Care Financing Administration (HCFA), a division of the Department of Health and Human Services.

Medicaid is a joint federal-state program to pay for medical care of the indigent. The federal legislation authorized the federal government to reimburse states for cost of providing such care. In the years following enactment in 1965 most states established such a program with Arizona being the last to do so in 1982. The states must cover persons receiving public assistance and may cover other persons with low income. States must provide certain basic services including hospital care, family planning, skilled nursing care and physician services; they have the option of receiving federal reimbursement for additional services. Benefit structures vary widely because of the extent to which states include the optional benefits and because states' provision of the mandatory services vary in the number of days of hospital or nursing home care covered and the rate at which they pay for the benefits. Thus, in effect, Medicaid is 50 different programs having different eligibility criteria and different benefit structures. The share of the poor covered by the program varied from 104% in Hawaii to just 17% in South Dakota, and the average cost per beneficiary varied from $2,897 in New York to $793 in West Virginia. (Ruther et al., 1990, p. 97.)

Both Medicare and Medicaid are modeled on private insurance programs; few of the benefits are provided directly by government agencies, most are purchased from private vendors. Medicare Part A pays hospitals directly at rates established by the federal government. (The basis for setting the rate was shifted from per diem to per admission in 1983.) Part B pays physicians directly if they agree to accept government-established fees or reimburses patients for the established amounts if they choose to pay the provider directly. Medicaid only pays providers directly, but the basis for setting rates varies widely among the states. Some states have adapted the Medicare payment standards; others have established less generous rates; still others have been imaginative in designing innovative payment schemes to encourage more efficient delivery. Arizona, for example, relies almost exclusively on capitation to apply for acute care and is extending the concept to long-term care benefits; New York has designed a Resource Utilization Group (RUGs) patient classification system to pay for nursing home care that builds upon the experience of the Diagnosis Related Groups classification system for acute care.

Because the states have so much discretion in designing their Medicaid programs, it is important to note that the aggregate spending figures cited earlier understate the role of state governments. Although they raise only 43% of the $75.2 billion of Medicaid expenditures, state governments substantially control the entire sum including the federal portion. (Congressional Research Service, 1993). In this sense the states control expenditures amounting to about one-quarter of all public expenditure for health care.

The benefit structures of the Medicare and Medicaid programs strongly influence the distribution of government spending among different types of health care services. While 44% of the total, government spending is under 35% of spending for physician services and over 56% of hospital expenditures. The relatively generous payment for hospital care by Medicare and the heavy use of hospitals by the elderly makes government the predominant source of hospital revenues. In contrast the more uniform use of physician services among age groups and the less generous role of Medicare in paying for the elderly's doctor bills leaves the bulk of physician services paid for from private sources. Slightly more than half (53.9%) of all nursing home care is paid for by government, and within the public sector Medicaid dominates. It accounts for 47% of nursing home expenditures compared to Medicare's 4%. The restrictions on eligible nursing home care under Medicare have kept its share of nursing home payments in check.

Governments as Deliverers

In assuming a strong role in financing health care, governments have typically followed an insurance model and avoided operating medical care facilities and employing physicians and other providers. However, there are important exceptions to this pattern. Each level of government has assumed responsibility for delivering either certain types of care or more comprehensive care to a specific subset of the population.

The federal government selected three population groups for which it funds and delivers services—veterans, native Americans, and merchant seamen. The medical care program operated by the federal Veterans Administration (VA) is one of the largest health delivery systems in the world. Its 1991 spending for health care programs including the operation of 172 medical centers, 127 nursing homes, and 169 clinics was nearly $12.8 billion (Department of Veterans Affairs, 1991).

The VA program has evolved through a special Congressional concern for veterans. In addition to providing pension and cash disability benefits, Congress sought to provide veterans health care. Like hospitals generally, the VA's hospital system initially grew as an extension of homes for the aged and disabled. Homes were authorized for indigent and disabled Civil War veterans, and after World War I this system was expanded to include a separate hospital system. After World War II the system was dramatically expanded and integrated with more advanced medical technology through a program of affiliations with medical schools. About 40% of the VA hospitals were built between 1946 and 1966, many near medical schools. In 1965 nursing home benefits were broadened and the system was expanded accordingly, although much VA nursing home care is purchased from private homes rather than provided in VA operated facilities. (Congressional Budget Office, 1984.)

Initially VA medical care benefits were limited to those who developed conditions during their wartime service. A 1924 law broadened eligibility to include those who suffer from a condition likely to have been linked to military service even if it did not require treatment or become evident until later. Subsequently any veteran who testified he was unable to pay for care became eligible, and in 1970 benefits were extended to any veteran past age 65 regardless of income or nature of condition. It was estimated that in 1990 the number of veterans over age 65 would total about 7.2 million, more than twice the number in 1980. The aging of World War II and Korean war veterans and the extension of benefits to all veterans over age 65 has and will continue to markedly increase the number of people eligible for VA care.

However, the VA system is not based on an insurance model with benefits funded as an "entitlement." Instead each year Congress appropriates a fixed sum to the VA for provision of care to its constituents. To live within its budget, the VA has established priorities for deciding who should receive what. The priority system has become complex, making distinctions based on whether or not the veteran has a service-related condition, his or her household income, and the type of service required. In brief, veterans with service-related disabilities receive highest priority, indigent veterans also receive priority, and the lowest priority is given to nonpoor veterans with health conditions not derived from their military service. Also VA hospital and VA outpatient care are provided with a higher priority than nursing home or community hospital care. A recent advisory commission questioned how the VA could continue to perform its mission adequately without changes in structure and financing, as well as a revised priority system (Commission on the Future Structure of Veterans Health Care, 1991).

The wisdom of continuing to operate a separate public health care system for veterans has been questioned. A prestigious 1977 report from the National Academy of Sciences recommended the gradual integration of VA facilities with the nation's general medical care system (National Academy of Sciences, 1977). However, this policy is opposed by VA employees, veterans relying on the system, and medical schools benefiting from their affiliations with the VA hospitals. Together, these constituencies have been politically strong enough to thwart any efforts to dismantle the system despite recommendations from outside bodies.

A second group to whom the federal government provides care directly are Native Americans living on reservations. Expenditures in 1991 by the federal Indian Health Service (IHS), a division of the Department of Health and Human Services, totaled $1.4 billion (General Accounting Office, 1993). The agency funded 50 hospitals, 158 health centers, and numerous other clinics to serve nearly 1.1 million Indians (Indian Health Service, 1993).

Federal involvement in health care for Indians dates from the early 1800s, but the current program traces its origins to the Snyder Act in 1921. It provided a relatively open-ended authorization, which was used by the Bureau of Indian Affairs in the Department of the Interior. The Bureau gradually expanded its commitment and in 1955 a separate unit to provide care to Indians was established within the Public Health Services (PHS). Significant new funding and staff followed the Indian Health Care Improvement Act of 1976.

Since there is no "mainstream" system serving Indians, the need for a separate federal system seems self-evident. However, there are efforts to integrate the IHS facilities into the larger medical system through referrals. Since many of the IHS facilities are necessarily in rural areas and have low volume, they often refer cases to other providers for specialized care. Almost one-fifth the IHS budget is spent for care at private facilities that is not available at the IHS facilities (Wagner, 1988). In addition, the 1976 legislation gave tribal governments the right to assume responsibility for operating IHS facilities. Tribes wanting to do so can contract with the IHS for operation of hospitals and clinics. In 1991, eight of the 50 hospitals, 93 of 158 health care centers, and numerous other clinics were managed by tribes under these contracts and grants, and they comprised over $450 million or nearly one-third of the IHS budget. The IHS seems committed to promoting tribal self-determination, and the policy of tribal management of health facilities is consistent with this goal.

A third federal delivery system, that for merchant seamen, has been largely dismantled. The federal responsibility in this area dates from the 1798 act creating the Marine Hospital Service. Subsequently, responsibilities of care for foreigners in quarantine were added and in 1889 a separate quasimilitary personnel system, known as the commissioned corps, was established within the federal Public Health Service. To provide this care separate PHS hospitals were constructed. However, the PHS expanded its responsibilities in other areas after World War II including research and control of communicable diseases. The PHS hospitals became vestigial organs as the need for care of seaman and foreigners declined. Eventually budgetary pressures led to the PHS hospitals being either closed or transferred to private control. However, the commissioned corps of the PHS remain a group of federal employees who engage in health care activities. Few provide direct personal care; they primarily work in communicable disease control.

Despite its disengagement from delivery of personal health care, the PHS remains an important federal agency within HHS. It operates the National Institute of Health, a major source of funding for research and of intramural research. Its Center for Disease Control is the nation's major source of intervention in control of communicable diseases; its Food and Drug Administration regulates these substances; its Health Resources and Services Administration and its Alcohol Drug Abuse, and Mental Health Administration have as their major activities the distribution to states and to private organizations of federal grant funds to expand the capacity of the health care system.

In general the federal government has restricted its role as direct provider at the same time that it has expanded its commitments as a financer. The PHS hospitals have been eliminated; the IHS is relying more on private contracting and management by tribal organizations; the VA also is increasing its reliance on private purchase of care, although it remains strongly committed to maintaining a separate delivery system including VA hospitals affiliated with medical schools.

State governments are involved in the direct provision of medical care in three important ways—the operation of state mental hospitals, the conduct of medical education, and the maintenance of state (or often combined state and local) health departments. States' roles in the provision of mental health services dates from the late nineteenth century movement to identify insanity as a medical or mental condition requiring treatment rather than confinement in either poor houses or prisons. The reformers successfully encouraged state governments to create mental institutions, usually in remote areas, where the ill could be removed from sources of stress and receive available treatment. However, the facilities were underfunded and became notorious "snake pits" providing only minimal treatment and low quality food and shelter. The poor conditions together with the availability of drug treatment in the 1950s led to a movement toward "deinstitutionalization." The population of state mental hospitals peaked in 1955 and has been declining since (Mechanic, 1987).

The initial impetus for deinstitutionalization was accelerated in the 1960s through expanded federal financial resources for alternative modes of care or, at least, residence. The federal Community Mental Health Centers Act in 1963 funded outpatient care in facilities located closer to patients' previous homes; the Medicaid and Medicare programs funded psychiatric care and nursing home care for many previously supported in state facilities by state appropriations; the federal Supplemental Security Income program passed in 1972 provides direct cash benefits for the aged and disabled that permitted many to reside in private homes rather than be placed by their relatives in state institutions (Clarke, 1979). As a result of these medical and policy changes the population in state mental hospitals dropped from 558,000 in 1955 to under 87,000 in 1991 (American Hospital Association, 1992).

Despite the shrinkage, state mental hospitals remain major institutions in the American health care system. In 1991 these 219 hospitals accounted for 97,480 beds. Their budgets totaled over $7.0 billion and they employed about 165,000 workers (American Hospital Association, 1992). These hospitals are often a major source of employment within state government, and their historic location in small communities often makes them a dominant source of employment for communities with little other major economic activity. As a result of these political pressures as well as a serious need to upgrade the facilities, employment at state mental hospitals has not shrunk at a pace anywhere near that of their bed capacity.

A major problem associated with the deinstitutionalization of the mentally ill has been a lack of corresponding investment in outpatient care for those sent home or not admitted. States have tended to rely on local government to provide the outpatient care and have not typically shifted resources to the localities to assist them in meeting the expanded need. There is poorly planned, coordinated or supervised outpatient care for many of the mentally ill. As a consequence, they too often end up on the streets, homeless and unmedicated. States vary widely in the extent to which they have undertaken themselves or in cooperation with localities a system of outpatient mental health services, and in some states the design and implementation of such a system remains a major policy failure (Blum & Blank, 1989).

States are also important supporters of medical education, and because medical education has a significant clinical component this requires states to become involved in direct delivery of care. In the 1992 academic year, state and local appropriations approached $2.7 billion and comprised nearly 11% of total revenues for all medical schools (Krakower et al., 1993). State governments, through their public university systems, sponsor 73 of the nation's 127 medical schools (Jolly et al., 1988). Often the state medical schools have a general medical care hospital attached to them, which also is operated by the state.

These state general care hospitals typically combine two roles. They provide medical students access to patients, and they provide the medical school faculty a place to admit private patients. The two roles are sometimes quite divergent; the patients with whom medical students obtain clinical training are typically poor and dependent on the state subsidy to the hospital for their access to care; the faculty's private patients are often commercially insured and their fees provide the faculty with a significant source of private income. In some instance the two roles are performed satisfactorily at the same facility, but often the state's general hospitals serve only one of these functions. Where it is primarily a source of clinical experience for students, the medical school typically lacks an affiliation with a large voluntary hospital; where it is primarily a source of income for faculty, the medical school typically has an affiliation with another hospital (often public) that has a large patient volume, but the faculty do not use that facility as the preferred site for their private patients.

State health departments are another area of direct government provision. In this area it is often difficult to distinguish state from local efforts. The relations between states and localities in structuring a public health department are often complex; some states establish subunits that are identified as local entities while others primarily fund local governments to conduct activities. However, it is clear that the combined network of state and local health departments provide a significant volume of medical care along with engaging in regulatory and other public health activities (Miller & Moos, 1981). The personal care delivery is typically oriented to maternal and child health, vaccinations and other communicable diseases control activity, and treatment for chronic conditions. While sometimes available to all citizens, the state health department services are more typically targeted to low-income residents (Davis & Millman, 1983).

Health departments provide these services directly because they believe the services would not otherwise be available. Even when other agencies or programs fund services, there may not be delivery capacity available in a community in the private sector. Reluctance or an inability of private practitioners to treat indigent (even Medicaid enrolled) patients with multiple disabilities, psychiatric, or substance abuse problems, and the need to have outreach services for many poorly educated potential patients often justify continued health department provision of personal services.

The major remaining form of government involvement in direct delivery of care is local governments' operation of general care hospitals. The last comprehensive examination of these hospitals in the late 1970s found they comprised over one-third of all community hospitals, nearly one-quarter of all community hospital beds, and 28% of such hospital outpatient department visits. Moreover, they account for a major share of health professions' education including a disproportionate share of graduate medical education (Commission on Public General Hospitals, 1978). A more recent effort to examine the significance of these hospitals by the National Association of Public Hospitals found that its 100 member hospitals accounted for disproportionately large volumes of residency training, outpatient services, care of AIDS patients, care to the uninsured and trauma care (Gage et al., 1991).

The most troubled and widely publicized of these public institutions are those located in the nation's largest cities. A mid-1980s survey found that 48 of the 100 largest cities had a local public hospital and another 23 had a state government hospital (Altman et al., 1989). These urban public hospitals are often characterized by political controversy because of their staffing and financing arrangements, but they play a major role in providing care to the urban indigent. Cities with public hospitals were found to provide more care to the uninsured poor then those without, although private hospitals did increase somewhat their uncompensated care in areas that lacked a public hospital (Thorpe & Brecher, 1987).

Governments as Regulators

The ability to regulate private behavior is inherent in government authority and is not derived from the public sector's role as financer. Government legally can call the tune, even when it does not pay the piper. In its role as regulator of otherwise private behavior, the government is generally seeking to protect the consumer. Because private individuals have little basis on which to determine if a seller of medical goods or services is competent and honest, the government sets standards for such providers. Many government regulatory activities derive from this distinct legal authority (Levin, 1980).

Government's major role as financer is a second source of regulatory activity. As a purchaser of care, the government has set standards that providers must meet before public funds will be paid to them. The setting of such conditions for participation in public programs is another type of regulatory activity. Because Medicare and Medicaid are the leading sources of public financing, they have also been the major source of this type of regulation.

The leading example of federal regulation intended to protect consumers in otherwise private transactions is the role of the Food and Drug Administration. This agency's authority dates from the 1906 Pure Food Act, which responded to scandals arising from the unsanitary methods used to produce some food products (Grabowski & Vernon, 1983). Regulatory authority was extended to drugs and cosmetics by 1938 legislation, this time in response to the death of more than 100 children due to a drug company's use of a toxic chemical in creating a liquid form of sulfanilamide. The FDA was given authority to set standards that pharmaceuticals must meet before being marketed.

Important amendments to the law were passed in 1962, again following large-scale tragedy. Limited testing of thalidomide in the United States, and more widespread use in Europe, revealed its use among pregnant women led to the birth of deformed babies. The well-publicized tragedy led Congress to establish extensive requirements for premarket testing of drugs.

The standards for drug testing, which the FDA now administer, are a source of controversy. It is believed that they provide little or no additional protection over the prior 1962 standards, but they add substantially to the cost of developing new drugs and the time required before they can be widely used (Statman, 1983). As a result, the United States often lags behind other countries in the use of new drugs and American pharmaceutical firms are at a disadvantage in developing new products. The spread of AIDS and a consequent sense of urgency in developing treatments for AIDS produced additional pressures to alter the extensive premarket requirements (Panem, 1988). In 1991, amid much controversy, the FDA permitted more widespread use of a previously experimental drug used in AIDS treatment and thereby set a precedent for more rapid use of other experimental drugs (Arno & Feiden, 1992).

Another form of consumer protection regulation is the licensing of health care practitioners and facilities. This licensure activity is conducted by state governments. The scope of state licensure authority varies, but virtually all states require that physicians, nurses, optometrist, chiropractors, and podiatrists meet state standards to obtain a license before practicing in that state. Some states recognize the licenses granted by other states in order to facilitate mobility among professionals, but this is not always the case.

Although the principle of licensure as a form of consumer protection is well established, its practice by state governments has been criticized on two grounds (Begun, 1981). First, the standards are not well enforced. The record of state agencies in locating and disciplining practitioners who violate professional standards is poor. Relatively few licenses are revoked each year despite evidence of more widespread professional misconduct. Second, licensing sometimes seems to protect the "turf" of selected professionals and thereby thwarts more effective delivery of care. Physicians have been accused of using state laws to prevent nurses, physician assistants, and optometrists from assuming broader responsibilities in delivery of care. Reforms designed to make state licensing efforts more effective include the appointment of more consumers and nonphysicians to the state boards setting and enforcing licensing standards.

State government regulation of the insurance industry is another example of consumer protection efforts. Initial public regulation of the insurance industry was intended to protect consumers from firms, particularly life insurance firms, that might sell policies and then disappear with the premium income before paying benefits. To protect consumers, firms were required to establish reserves for future benefit payments and meet other standards.

These regulatory requirements have been applied to private sales of health insurance as well. In addition, some states have extended their scope of regulation to include minimum benefit standards. These requirements were initially designed to protect consumers from believing they were well protected when benefits were actually very poor. Thus minimum numbers of days of hospital inpatient coverage and other standards were set for health insurance products. This concept has been extended by some states to require certain types of benefits or prohibit certain types of exclusions such as maternity benefits for pregnancy or alcoholism treatment.

The states' ability to regulate private health insurance has been constrained by the federal Employee Retirement Income Security Act (ERISA). Originally passed in 1974 as a measure to protect the pension benefits of private sector workers, ERISA has had two important consequences for state-level insurance regulation. First, it effectively exempts employers who choose to self-insure from minimum benefit standards as well as premium taxes. As a result, many large firms now self-insure rather than purchase group health insurance. Second, it prohibits states from mandating that employers provide health insurance to their workers. (The state of Hawaii has a unique exemption). As a result, state efforts along this line, such as that in Massachusetts in 1988, took the form of "play or pay" arrangements that did not directly mandate insurance coverage, but instead levied a tax on those employers who did not provide health insurance of a minimum standard.

Federal government regulations established for participation in the Medicare and Medicaid programs in some ways complement state regulations and in other ways expand the scope of government regulations. The complementary nature of the two types of activity is evident in the standards set by the federal government for providers; they generally defer to state licensing requirements and recognize physicians, hospitals, and other providers licensed by a state as eligible.

The federal government has also relied on state governments to implement its regulatory program for hospital capital investments. Between 1974 and 1986 the federal government required that a hospital or nursing home receive approval from a state planning agency before making a major hospital investment in order for that capital expense to be reimbursed by Medicare and Medicaid. The federal government abandoned this form of regulation in 1986, but some states continue to regulate the capital investments of providers in their borders despite the absence of federal requirements to do so and of federal funds to underwrite the effort. Both the aborted federal programs and the continuing state programs are justified not on grounds of consumer protection, but on grounds that excessive capital investment, especially in hospital bed capacity, leads to unnecessary costs that will be financed by government funds and by private consumers through higher insurance premiums.

Federal Medicare and Medicaid regulations also work independently of state governments. A particularly dramatic example was the requirement that hospitals and nursing homes desegregate in order to be eligible for funds under the programs. When the legislation passed in 1965 many facilities in the south remained racially segregated, and there were no state laws prohibiting this. The federal requirements for racial integration of hospitals (for patients and medical staff) were widely perceived as helping to speed integration in the south.

A final form of Medicare and Medicaid regulation worth noting are the programs' utilization review requirements. Beginning in 1972 the federal government authorized and financed independent organizations to review hospital services for which federal funds were sought to determine if they were medically necessary. The organizations, originally called Professional Standards Review Organizations (PSROs), regulated the quality of care by reviewing hospital records to see if more care than necessary (i.e., a longer length of stay) was provided or if the entire admission itself was unnecessary. At the peak of the program there were 182 regional PSROs operating, and the program received $150 million in federal appropriations (Lohr & Brook, 1984).

The program was substantially revised in conjunction with changes in the Medicare program that shifted hospital payments from a per diem to a per admission basis. The new payment approach was expected to provide hospitals with economic incentives to lower lengths of stay, so regulation of this aspect of hospital utilization was de-emphasized. Instead greater attention was given to assuring the accuracy of diagnostic information (since the payment per admission varied with the type of condition treated) and verifying the medical necessity of the entire admission. Accordingly, PSROs were reorganized into a smaller number of Peer Review Organizations (PROs), and these entities were expected to review hospital services with emphasis on minimizing inaccurate diagnostic data and unnecessary admissions.

The requirements for review of hospital stays by PSROs and PROs have subjected physicians to far more scrutiny of their practice than was previously the case. These requirements, together with trends in malpractice litigation, have obliged physicians and hospital personnel to be more diligent and detailed in making entries in medical records and to document the reasons for medical decisions more extensively than before. These requirements are associated, often unfavorably, with government regulations.

Causes of Change and Variation

The previous section illustrates that governments' roles change over time and vary among places. In the past quarter century major new federal programs have been enacted and significantly modified several times; the practices of states and localities in financing and delivering services and in regulating providers vary widely. For example, as noted, Medicaid is in many ways 50 different state programs rather than a single, uniform national program.

Explaining change and variation in government activity is a major focus of political science, and political scientists have applied their conceptual tools to the analysis of health policy. Two broad (and hence not entirely accurate) types of theoretical explanations are the Marxist approach and the interest group (or pluralist) approach (Marmor, 1983). Both theories see change arising from conflict within society, but they differ over the sources of those conflicts. Marxists see the conflicts as essentially economic and as between two inherently hostile economic groups (or classes)—those who own means of production (capitalists) and those who work for them (labor). The public sector is seen as serving the interests of capitalists in the United States and other noncommunist nations. Fundamental change can occur only after violent revolution places control of the government in the hands of the labor class. Pending such revolutionary change, reforms are made by the ruling capitalist class only as necessary to appease workers to insure peaceful compliance with government rules that serve capitalist interest.

Interest group theory sees conflict arising from a more diverse set of interests than only economic positions. Individuals perform multiple social roles and may belong to numerous social groups. Those groups have diverse interests and their efforts to promote their particular goals through government action draws opposition from other groups. The groups and their competing interests have many different sources beside economic class including place of residence, ethnic identity, religious beliefs, and occupational roles. Decisions of government are seen as shaped by the relative influence different groups bring to bear on elected officials (Truman, 1960).

In American society variations of interest group theory have proved more useful than Marxist theory for explaining change and variation. The emergence of a large "middle class" with substantial influence and income derived from service as opposed to capital-intensive manufacturing industries, the effectiveness of elections in promoting the interests and legislative agenda of labor organizations as well as middle class citizens, and the concentration of social and economic problems among an "underclass" that is largely outside of the world of regularized work have reduced the relevance of classic Marxist theory and led its revisionists to adopt modifications that closely approximate variations of interest group theory. Thus, the concept of changing or different balances of influence among competing groups is a more useful conceptual framework for analyzing American health care policy.

Changes in Federal Policy

From a broad perspective, federal health care policy can be seen as divided into three periods. Prior to 1960 the federal government avoided large-scale participation in the financing of personal health care services; from 1960 to the mid-1970s the federal role expanded rapidly; from approximately 1975 to 1992, the federal role was relatively stable with some efforts at contraction. Since the election of President Clinton, there is an expectation that the federal role will again expand.

These shifts in policy can be related to broad shifts in patterns of interest groups influence. In the first two periods, the same types of groups were active but their relative influence shifted; the third period is associated with the partial withdrawal of one type of interest and the emergence of a new, influential group. The prediction of a possible new phase is related to the emergence of additional new influential groups as well as greater strength of others.

For much of this century national health care politics was a battle between proponents of national health insurance and its opponents (Marmor, 1973). Proponents included most working Americans who promoted their cause through union political activity. Their cause was championed by the Democratic party. Opponents were many physicians and other providers including hospitals who feared the consequences of government involvement in their income flow, private insurance companies who feared a loss in their market for health insurance, and business organizations who feared the tax burden associated with a government funding program.

Until 1960 the opponents were highly successful. Efforts to include a health insurance program in the original 1935 Social Security Act were dropped by President Roosevelt because he feared strong physician opposition would jeopardize the entire program. Post World War II efforts to add national health insurance to the nation's social security system by President Truman led to a large-scale, well-funded campaign against it by the American Medical Association and organizations representing businesses. The victory of a Republican in the 1952 presidential election led to an 8-year period of little action or prospect for change in federal health care policy.

The presidential election of 1960 saw a revival of interest in federal efforts. This time the Democrats, supported by labor organizations, advocated hospital insurance for the elderly only, rather than immediate enactment of a universal system. The Democratic presidential candidate won, but the legislation that emerged from Congress reflected major compromises with more conservative legislative leaders. The Kerr-Mills Act of 1961 established a program to pay for the medical expenses of the poor elderly that was closely linked to joint state-federal welfare programs rather than a broader program linked to federal Social Security.

The landslide victory of the Democrats in the 1964 national elections made possible the passage of broader legislation. The 1965 amendments to the Social Security Act added Titles 18 and 19, Medicare and Medicaid. As described earlier, these programs provide relatively comprehensive health insurance for the elderly and opportunities for states to create relatively extensive programs for the indigent.

In response to the initial success of Medicare, the opponents, including physicians and many business leaders, changed their position on national health insurance. By 1974 Democrats and Republicans in Congress appeared to have reached agreement on programs that would cover all Americans through a combination of Medicare for the elderly, a more uniform national version of Medicaid for the poor, and mandatory employment based insurance for others (Rivlin, 1974). However, the impending impeachment of President Nixon diverted Congressional attention and improved prospects for the Democratic party in the 1976 elections undermined the compromise and ended prospects for national health insurance.

From the mid-1970s to 1992, federal efforts focused on controlling the rising cost of Medicare and Medicaid rather than expanding their scope. As noted earlier, this shift was first evident in 1972 with the creation of utilization review organizations for the programs. The health planning legislation of 1974 established a system of regulation for capital investments also intended to promote efficiency. The federal Health Maintenance Organization Act of 1973 sought to promote these organizations because they also were viewed as cost-saving delivery mechanisms.

The election of a Democrat to the White House in the 1976 elections did not lead to renewed pressure for national health insurance. Instead, President Jimmy Carter sought to create an effective mechanism for controlling hospital costs before expanding government financing of the industry. His 1977 proposal for a national system of price controls for hospitals was defeated in Congress due to strong lobbying efforts by the hospital industry (Hughes et al., 1978). Initiatives to redefine the administration's position after this defeat never came to fruition, but led to exploration of greater emphasis on competition among providers as a means for cost control.

The triumph of conservative Republicans in the 1980 national elections, and the reelection of President Ronald Reagan in 1984, gave greater energy to efforts to curb spending under Medicare and Medicaid as well as virtually all other forms of domestic federal policy. Health policy, like most domestic policy, became a subtheme of budget policy. Expenditure reductions for Medicaid were sought by measures that limited growth in federal reimbursement to states and that gave states greater freedom in structuring their programs. States pursued some of these options and innovated in designing new ways to pay providers to encourage efficiency, but the states relied on other policies as well. Specifically, states reduced enrollment in the program by failing to adjust Medicaid income eligibility limits for inflation. As a result, the share of the poor covered by Medicaid nationwide fell from 74% in 1979 to just 59% in 1984 (Holahan & Cohen, 1986).

Reagan administration efforts to curb Medicare spending led to the new prospective payment system in 1983. This changed the basis on which Medicare pays hospitals from cost reimbursement based on average per diem costs to a national price system that establishes standardized rates for different categories of hospital admissions. Under the new system the federal government has been able to curb Medicare benefit payment growth and better control expenditures under Part A.

The apparent success of the prospective payment system for hospitals led to new efforts to revise the payment system for physicians. Rapid increases in Medicare Part B expenditures led to a freeze on physician fees in 1984 and 1985 (Holahan & Etheredge, 1986). With the recognition that a freeze was not a viable long-term policy, Congress created a Physician Payment Review Commission in 1986. The Commission made recommendations for a new system for paying physicians in 1989. Legislation establishing a national fee schedule and expenditure targets for Medicare was adopted that year and became effective in 1991. The intention is to slow the rate of growth in Part B spending and to narrow disparities in income among physician specialties (Smith, 1992).

The shift in emphasis of federal policy from a period of expansion in federal financing to one of cost control was linked to changes in patterns of interest group influence. In the initial two periods, the battles were largely between groups seeking expansion of federal policy and those opposed; the dormant period of 1935–1960 resulted from stronger influence by the opponents, while the expansion from 1960 to 1974 represented greater influence by the proponents. However, the post-1974 shift to cost control has seen a new actor become prominent and develop new relations with the old opponents.

The new actors in federal health politics are bureaucrats administering the federal programs. Lodged in the Health Care Financing Administration and the Office of Management and Budget, these professionals administer programs on behalf of taxpayers. They bargain with providers in a pattern political scientist

Lawrence Brown calls "technocratic corporatism" (Brown, 1985). Professionals hired by the government interact with representatives of provider organizations to shape health policy. This pattern was evident in the creation of the prospective payment system in 1982 and in the revisions of physician payments under Medicare in 1989. In health care politics in the period of cost-containment were battles between professionals representing taxpayers and the providers of services (Smith, 1992).

The prospects for a new period of expansion in health care politics is linked to the emergence of another type of interest group (Tierney, 1987). Consumer groups (other than labor unions) have been organized and gained in strength. These groups include organizations such as Ralph Nader's Health Research Group. But by far, the most influential new consumer group is the elderly—Medicare beneficiaries—represented by the powerful American Association of Retired People (AARP). Although founded in the 1950s, AARP grew rapidly in the 1980s to have a membership of over 27 million and an annual budget of $185 million by 1987 (Kosterlitz, 1987). In 1992, it reported membership of 32 million and revenues of $387 million. Because its members have direct economic dependence on the federal government through cash social security benefits as well as Medicare, they vote in national elections at high rates and give great attention to domestic policy positions including health care issues.

The influence of the AARP is evident in recent significant changes in Medicare, the passage of the Medicare Catastrophic Coverage Act of 1988 and its repeal a year later. At a time when budget deficits were leading to expenditure reductions for most federal programs and when tax increases were politically unacceptable, Congress nonetheless passed a program that extended benefits at an added annual costs projected at $10.6 billion. The new benefits were passed largely due to the effective lobbying efforts of the AARP. However, in a compromise with the Reagan administration, the AARP agreed to phase in the new benefits and finance them with higher premiums and a new surcharge on the personal income tax liability of the elderly. When the elderly began to pay the price before receiving all the benefits, many objected loudly. Especially disgruntled were the wealthier elderly, who paid more income tax, and they are a key segment of AARP's membership. As a result, in 1989, with AARP's tacit consent, the catastrophic benefits were repealed in exchange for dropping the higher taxes (Kosterlitz, 1988a).

Variations in State Policy

The substantial variation in health care activity among the states is related to three sets of factors—levels of economic development, general political culture, and patterns of interest group activity. The first two are general state characterisitics, while the third is distinct for the health care arena.

Studies of a wide range of state policies have demonstrated that states with higher levels of income and urbanization tend to be more active (Gray et al., 1983). In general, per capita spending by states for most functions rises with average per capita income. Wealthier states provide their citizens with relatively more public services than poorer states. This generalization applies to health care.

However, the relationship between economics and state government activity is influenced by political forces. The degree of party competition in states, the division of responsibility between states and their localities, and the balance of political values among citizens between moralistic and traditionalistic values have been found to be important influences on state expenditure levels for a variety of services including health.

Finally, the nature of interest group activity also shapes state health policy. The principal competing interests within state capitols typically are provider groups, business groups concerned with tax levels, local government officials involved in financing or delivering care, and, more recently, state employees analogous to the federal "technocrats." However, the relative influence of these groups and the resulting policies vary widely among states.

The different patterns of state health politics are illustrated by important decisions for State Medicaid programs during the 1980s in Arizona, California, and New York. Arizona was the last state to establish a Medicaid program, a decision not reached until 1982 (Brecher, 1984). The absence of a program was largely due to sentiment among conservative business interests; they felt state taxes should not be increased to finance health care for the poor, rather this should be either a private concern or one of local governments. The pressure to change this policy was from local government officials who faced great difficulty in financing local programs when statutory limits were placed on local revenues from the property tax. To obtain federal aid for care for the indigent, the local officials successfully pressured the state legislature for a Medicaid program. Health care provider groups played little role in shaping the program, which mandated enrollment in capitation programs.

In California the same interests interacted differently. California established a relatively generous Medicaid program early, and its expenditures increased rapidly. The program was supported by local officials and health care providers with little opposition. However, a state budget crisis in the early 1980s led to major reforms in which the business community played a strong role. The reforms changed the way the state pays hospitals for its Medicaid enrollees with the intention of lowering payments to hospitals and altered the distribution of financial responsibility between the state and localities for care to the indigent in a way that obliged localities to do more. These changes resulted from business interest intervention in a policy area previously left largely to the localities and the providers. As one observer put it: "With the passage of this remarkable legislation, the relationship among interest groups, units of state and local government, and private medical care systems were changed, perhaps permanently. The California

Medical Association and the California Hospital Association, previously undisputed winners of the legislative game, had been crowded off the board by pressures from the budget, by the newly activated business coalitions, and by the insurance companies" (Bergthold, 1984, p. 213).

In contrast, Medicaid reforms in New York in the 1980s were more responsive to providers', particularly hospitals', concerns (Brecher, 1986). In 1975, in response to state and local budgetary pressures, New York began to regulate tightly payments to hospitals on a prospective basis. The hospitals did not respond with necessary expenditure reductions and soon faced severe operating deficits. After several years of such deficits, many hospitals were facing contraction or bankruptcy. In response, the state established a new payment system that included extra revenues for hospitals providing care to the uninsured poor. This substantially improved the financial position of the providers (although it did little to improve coverage for the uninsured poor). Providers obtained additional concessions after the federal government switched Medicare to a prospective payment basis. The state abandoned its waiver under Medicaid in order to permit hospitals in the state to participate in the new federal program because the state hospital association had calculated members' revenues would be greater under the new federal system than under the continued state controlled system (Thorpe, 1989).

As these examples suggest, a state's health policy is shaped by more than the state's levels of economic development. Competition between local officials, providers, business groups, and others leads to a wide range of compromises. Within the federal system, states respond to these competing pressures in different ways, with widely differing benefits for the interests represented as well as for the low-income consumers who are often unrepresented at the bargaining tables.

Values and Policy Preferences

The political competition among interest groups produces divergent policies in different states and localities, and leads to a steadily changing federal policy. How does one judge whether one policy is better than another or whether proposals for change should be judged as steps forward or backward?

The answer inevitably obliges a citizen to consider his or her personal values. Often, choices about the governments' roles are choices between competing values. In a broad sense, the conflicting values are typically efficiency and equity. Efficiency often requires that rewards or benefits be linked to economic output, while equity seeks to ensure that all citizens receive some minimum standard of goods and services regardless of their economic output. When a proposal for government action enhances (or reduces) both efficiency and equity, it clearly is preferable (or undesirable). But when proposals promote one value while reducing another, citizens must make more difficult choices.

The proposal made by President Clinton in the fall of 1993 for large-scale change in the nation's health care system exemplifies the difficult choices to be made in national health care policy. The President's proposal would significantly change government roles as financer and regulator, while making fewer changes in the government's delivery role. In each case, important choices between equity and efficiency values arise.

The Clinton proposal, called the Health Security Plan, would restructure the health care industry by creating two new types of entities—health alliances and certified health plans. Alliances are state-created bodies to serve as large-scale purchasers of care. All nonexempt individuals (primarily the elderly remaining in Medicare and people employed by firms with 5,000 or more workers) would purchase their care through an alliance. Alliances would accept bids from competing plans. The certified plans would offer a nationally established benefit package for a fixed premium. The plans would guarantee the benefits and have arrangements with hospitals, physicians, and other providers to deliver the care. Individuals could choose from among several plans with which their alliance had negotiated arrangements.

The new plan would assure services to virtually all residents, including most of those now uninsured. This would be accomplished financially by requiring employers to make payments typically equal to 7.9% of their payroll expenses. The employer payments would be supplemented by federal payments to subsidize the cost of coverage for the unemployed. In addition, because the new plan would replace Medicaid, states would be required to make payments approximately equal to their current expenditures for Medicaid. The benefit package for all those enrolled, including those formerly in Medicaid or uninsured, would be equal permitting its proponents to assert, "The Health Security Plan guarantees every American and legal resident health coverage that can never be taken away."

As this brief description suggests the plan would significantly change governments' roles. As a financer, the major change is a new program of federal subsidies for the unemployed and a shift for states from a partner in financing Medicaid to a fiscal obligation based on previous Medicaid expenditures. Much financing would continue to be by employers on behalf of employees, but all employers—even those now not offering group insurance—would be required to make payments. In exchange for the mandates to make payments, employers would have their contributions capped at 7.9% of payroll, a figure below that now paid by some employers. In addition, some small and low-wage employers would be eligible for federal subsidies for the cost of insuring their workers.

Governments' regulatory roles would also be changed. While insurance regulation is now in the hands of the states, it would be shifted to the federal government. A newly established National Health Board, consisting of seven members appointed by the President, would set benefit standards for the plans. It also would establish quality measures based on outcome data that each plan would be required to report to the public annually.

The plan also uses regulatory authority to guarantee cost-containment objectives. Its intent is to have the price competition among plans keep premiums charged to alliances low, presumably by encouraging efficiency within the plans' operations. However, if these market forces do not curb growth in premiums, the federal agency may set and enforce caps on the rate of premium increases. Under certain conditions, health alliances would not be permitted to pay premium increases above the capped rate.

The President's plan involves bold changes in financing and regulation, but much less change in government's role as deliverer. It would not eliminate the defense, veterans, or Indians' health service delivery roles of the federal government. However, extending coverage to the uninsured could indirectly alter the delivery role of local governments. Local public hospitals may find the demand for their services eroded. They would presumably remain the major source of care for undocumented aliens (whom the Health Security plan does not cover), but this mission alone may not sustain these institutions. More likely, to survive, public hospitals would be obliged to transform themselves into providers or plans that compete effectively, based on their special sensitivity to the needs of minority and low-income populations.

The desirability of changes in governments' role such as those in the Clinton plan is a function of the different values individuals attach to equity and efficiency. Proponents of the plan, and other reforms like it, attach a high value to its promotion of equity by extending coverage to almost all residents. The current problem of about 35 million Americans lacking health insurance and thereby not always receiving adequate care would be solved. In addition, advocates argue the plan would promote efficiency by curbing the rate of growth in national health expenditures through some combination of its competitive pressures and regulatory authority.

Opponents of the plan see its threats to efficiency as outweighing its equity gains. They argue the required employer contributions will be a burden to employers of low-wage workers, and will destroy many low-wage jobs. Some firms will no longer be able to compete at the higher labor costs and will go out of business. They also argue that the federal capping of premiums and regulation of benefits will have adverse effects. Limiting premiums is believed to lead to slower innovation in the development and deployment of new life-saving technology, leading to an undermining of the United States' position as a leader in advancing high-technology medicine. Similarly, the regulation of benefits may be used to slow the availability of new procedures that emerge and new devices that are developed.

Decisions on the relative merits of reforms such as those proposed by President Clinton will be made by Congress in 1994 and subsequent years. The votes will have significant impact on the roles governments play in this vast sector of the economy, and will reflect the nation's values as citizens and members of Congress weigh their concerns for equity with the perceived risks to efficiency.

References

Altman, S. H. et al., *Competition and Compassion.* Ann Arbor: Health Administration Press, 1989.

American Hospital Association. *Hospital Statistics*, 1991–92 edition. Chicago: American Hospital Association, 1992.

Arno, P. S., & Feiden, K. L., *Against the Odds: The Story of AIDS Drug Development, Politics and Profits.* New York: Harper Collins Publishers, 1992.

Begun, J. W., *Professionalism and the Public Interest*, Cambridge: The MIT Press, 1981.

Bergthold, L., "Crabs in a Bucket: The Politics of Health Care Reform in California." *Journal of Health Politics, Policy and Law*, 9(2), 203–222, 1984.

Blum, B., & Blank S., "Mental Health and Mental Retardation Services." In G. Benjamin & C. Brecher (Eds.) *The Two New Yorks.* New York: Russell Sage Foundation, 1989.

Brecher, C., "Medicaid Comes to Arizona," *Journal of Health Politics, Policy and Law*, 9(3), 411–425, 1984.

Brecher, C., "Progress in New York State Hospital Payment Policy." *Bulletin of the New York Academy of Medicine*, 62(1), 115–123, 1986.

Brown, L. D., "Technocratic Corporatism and Administrative Reform in Medicare." *Journal of Health Politics, Policy and Law*, 10(3), 579–600, 1985.

Clarke, G. J., "In Defense of Deinstitutionalization." *Milbank Memorial Fund Quarterly*, 57(4), 461–479, 1979.

Commission on the Future Structure of Veterans' Health Care, U.S. Department of Veterans Affairs. *The Price of Freedom is Visible Here*, Report of the Commission, November 1991.

Commission on Public General Hospitals, *Readings on Public General Hospitals.* Chicago: Hospital Research and Educational Trust, 1978.

Congressional Budget Office. *Veterans Administration Health Care: Planning for Future Years*, April, 1984.

Congressional Research Service. *Medicaid Source Book: Background Data and Analysis.* Washington, DC: U.S. Government Printing Office, 1993.

Davis, E. M., & Millman, M. L., *Health Care for the Urban Poor*, Totowa, NJ: Rowman and Allanheld, 1983.

Department of Veterans Affairs. *Annual Report of the Secretary of Veterans Affairs*, Fiscal Year, 1991.

Gage, L. S. et al., *America's Safety Net Hospitals.* Washington, DC: National Association of Public Hospitals, 1991.

Grabowski, H. G., & Vernon, J. M., *The Regulation of Pharmaceuticals.* Washington, DC: American Enterprise Institute, 1983.

Gray, V., Jacob, H., & Vines, K. N. (Eds.), *Politics in the American States: A Comparative Analysis.* Boston: Little, Brown and Company, 1983.

Holahan, J. F., & Cohen, J. W., *Medicaid: The Trade-Off Between Cost Containment and Access to Care.* Washington, DC: Urban Institute Press, 1986.

Holahan, J. F., & Etheredge, L. M., *Medicare Physician Payment Reform: Issues and Options.* Washington, DC: Urban Institute Press, 1986.

Hughes, E. F. X. et al., *Hospital Cost Containment Programs: A Policy Analysis.* Cambridge: Ballinger Publishing Company, 1978.

Indian Health Service, Public Health Service, U.S. Department of Health and Human Services. *Trends in Indian Health: 1992*, 1993.

Jolly, P., Taksel, L. & Beran, R., "U.S. Medical School Finances." *Journal of the American Medical Association*, August 26, *260*(8), 1077–1135, 1988.

Kosterlitz, J., "Test of Strength." *National Journal*, October 24, pp. 2652–2657, 1987.

Kosterlitz, J., "Graying Armies." *National Journal*, March 12, pp. 664–668, 1988a.

Kosterlitz, J., "Catastrophic Coverage a Catastrophe." *National Journal*, November 19, pp. 2949, 2952, 1988b.

Krakower, J. et al., "U.S. Medical School Finances." *Journal of the American Medical Association*, September 1, *270*(9), 1085–1091, 1993.

Lohr, K. N., & Brook, R. H., *Quality Assurance in Medicine: Experience in the Public Sector*. Santa Monica: The Rand Corporation, October, 1984.

Levin, A. (Ed.), *Regulating Health Care*. New York: Academy of Political Science, 1980.

Marmor, T. R., *The Politics of Medicare*. Chicago; Aldine, 1973.

Marmor, T. R., *Political Analysis and American Medical Care*. New York: Cambridge University Press, 1983.

Mechanic, D., "Correcting Misconceptions in Mental Health Policy." *Milbank Quarterly*, *65*(2), 203–230, 1987.

Miller, C. A., & Moos, M., *Local Health Departments: Fifteen Case Studies*. Chapel Hill: American Public Health Assocation, 1981.

National Academy of Sciences. *Study of Health Care for American Veterans*. Washington, DC: U.S. Government Printing Office, 1977.

Panem, S., *The AIDS Bureaucracy*. Cambridge: Harvard University Press, 1988.

Rivlin, A. M., "Agreed: Here Comes National Health Insurance." *New York Times Magazine*, July 21, 1974.

Ruther, M. et al., *Medicare and Medicaid Data Book, 1990* U.S. Health Care Financing Administration, HCFA Publication No. 03314.

Smith, D. G., *Paying for Medicare: The Politics of Reform*. New York: Aldine de Gruyter, 1992.

Statman, M., *Competition in the Pharmaceutical Industry*. Washington, DC: American Enterprise Institute, 1983.

Thorpe, K. E., "Health Care." In G. Benjamin & C. Brecher, (Eds.) *The Two New Yorks*. New York: Russell Sage Foundation, 1989.

Thorpe, K. E., & Brecher, C., "Access to Care for the Uninsured Poor in Large Cities: Do Public Hospitals Make a Difference?" *Journal of Health Politics, Policy and Law*, *12*(2), 313–324, 1987.

Tierney, J. T., "Organized Interests in Health Politics and Policy Making." *Medical Care Review*, *44*(1), 89–118, 1987.

Truman, D., *The Governmental Process*. New York: Alfred Knopf, 1960.

United States General Accounting Office. *Indian Health Service: Basic Services Mostly Available, Substance Abuse Problems Need Attention*, HRD-93-48, April 1993.

Wagner, L., "Blending Old Traditions with Modern Medicine." *Modern Health Care*, August 26, pp. 22–28, 1988.

13

Planning for
Health Services

Roger Kropf

Introduction

Planning involves selecting and carrying out a series of actions designed to achieve stated goals. It could be argued that such planning should take place for health services at every level—national, state, and local.

In fact, the history of planning for health services in the United States shows great disagreement about whether national or even state planning for health services is necessary, and what the role of government should be. Some of the issues are:

- Who should define the goals? The federal government? State or local government? Consumers? Hospitals? Physicians?
- What actions can government prevent or force anyone to take in order to achieve a goal? For example, can it prevent a hospital from being built?
- Do the actions of individual hospitals and physicians, unregulated by government, lead to the achievement of goals for the community such as improved health?

Government at both the national and state levels has given different answers to these questions since the end of World War II.

The process of planning health services in the U.S. as we approach the middle of the 1990s is largely in the control of private hospitals (both not-for-profit and for-profit) and physicians. In certain communities, health maintenance organizations and public hospitals are also important. Private companies that manufacture medical equipment and drugs must also plan for the development, production, and distribution of their products. Organizations that have created systems or networks of hospitals and physicians to provide services to employers and Medicare and Medicaid recipients under "managed care" contracts have a growing influence. Such organizations are unevenly distributed across the U.S., with the greatest concentration in California and the Midwest, but are expected to increase in number and size rapidly because of proposals by the Clinton Administration to reform the health care system.

The role of government in planning the quantity and location of services is very limited. The Reagan and Bush Administrations and many states viewed government as another purchaser of health care in what was expected to be a marketplace controlled by supply and demand. Only in the areas of medical research and the fight against major diseases such as AIDS was there a consensus in Congress and the Reagan and Bush Administrations that the federal government must act forcefully and commit substantial resources, although there were disagreements about how much money to spend in a time of large budget deficits.

The Clinton Administration has taken the position that government has a role in defining the basic package of services that all Americans should receive, and in setting targets for the growth of total health care expenditures. It has not proposed a role for the federal government in planning the type, size, and location of resources that should be available. This remains an issue for the competitive marketplace to decide, although the federal government would be more active in determining the nature of the contractual negotiations that would occur, for example, how consumers would be organized to bargain with providers.

Overview

The process of planning hospital services will be described, since hospitals are the most numerous and most active planners of health services in any community. Within the hospital community a debate continues about the importance of "strategic" planning and marketing. Both will be defined and the differences between them will be examined.

A range of techniques for planning health services will then be described to convey what planners and managers actually do, regardless of whether they work in a hospital, for a private physician's group, or in an HMO.

Planning—Politics and Analysis

Planning is not a science where conclusions emerge solely from mathematics, computers, and data. Nor should it be a political process where the conclusions depend solely on which groups or individuals have the most money or influence. Regardless of whether planning is carried out in a for-profit hospital or state gov-

ernment, planning needs to involve both politics and analysis. The analysis needs
to educate those making decisions, while politics determines what actions are
feasible.

Those who take the position that planning has nothing to do with politics or
nothing to do with analysis often become disillusioned with planning. For those
who hold that politics should not be involved in planning, the failure to achieve a
plan for political reasons leads to disillusionment with the planning process. For
those who see no real role for analysis, the failure of programs when facts are
ignored makes planning seem irrelevant. The best chance for success comes when
informed decision-makers take actions that are feasible within the political environments in which most managers operate.

For this reason, both planning techniques and the politics of planning will be
stressed in this chapter. The two are not contradictory, but equally important for
those who plan health services.

National Health Planning In The Clinton Administration (Circa 1993)

President Clinton clearly articulated during his campaign that health care expenditures were a major problem not only because of the contribution of federal expenditures to the deficit, but because high health care costs were hurting the
competitiveness of American business. Despite high expenditures, the existing
system for financing health care was also not providing all Americans with the
security of knowing that they would receive needed services. Reform of the health
care system became a priority.

Some of the assumptions of previous administrations in regard to planning were
accepted by the Clinton Administration. The federal government would not create a plan for the volume and location of services that should be provided, including how many hospitals should exist and where, or the number of physicians that
should practice in various cities and states. The federal and state governments
would not become the sole payor, as in Canada and Great Britain. A free, competitive market (although operating under some new rules) would make resource
allocation decisions.

Some assumptions were challenged. The federal government would take additional steps to assure that the free market resulted in lower costs. For example,
small businesses and individual consumers would be organized into purchasing
cooperatives that would bargain with providers—a central tenet of a plan for reform articulated by Prof. Alain Enthoven of Stanford University.

The federal government would also set limits on the increase in premiums for
health insurance, and therefore constrain health care expenditures without government becoming involved in choices on the use of resources. By defining a
minimum set of services to be included in all insurance policies purchased by

Americans, the federal government would also stimulate or retard the growth of certain services, for example, encourage preventive care.

The Clinton Administration also proposed direct federal regulation of the number of residencies available in various medical specialties with the stated objective of increasing the number in primary care. Government intervention was justified on the basis of market failure, that is, that an increasing demand for primary care had not resulted in an increase in the number of primary care physicians being trained.

In summary, the federal government would continue not to plan the size and location of health services, but would use its authority to redefine the conditions that influenced the planning decisions of private, for-profit and not-for-profit providers.

The Clinton Administration's assumption that government shouldn't develop plans for the size and location of hospitals and other services will be challenged by some states that continue to believe in direct government planning. New York State is likely to be a prominent example. The idea that thousands of hospitals and physicians acting independently in response to the current system of financing will produce a better result than conscious planning is a matter of faith rather than fact.

For some, the concept of central government control is so repugnant and frightening that the cost of a free market system in inefficiency is a small price to pay for freedom. For others, the loss in efficiency is too high. So far, those in the latter group are a minority in the Congress and state legislatures, and the free market system of planning (or not planning) receives at least tacit support.

Americans want health services that produce better health, low taxes, and a government that does not often tell people what they can and can't do. They want government to be a prudent buyer with tax-payers money. All of this requires planning in a general sense. The major questions are who shall do the planning and how will we decide when the desires of individuals and private organizations need to take a second place to what government believes is needed to reach widely shared goals.

The answers may change as we understand the positive and negative impact of the free market model for health reform that is enacted.

Hospital Planning in the United States

The history of hospital planning since World War II will be described in this section in order to show how private organizations have responded to a changing environment and federal legislation. While other organizations plan health services, hospitals have a longer history of formal planning so that changes in their behavior over the last 40 years can be assessed by looking at the plans they produced and how they carried out the planning process (Kropf & Goldsmith, 1983). Hospital planning also affects every community in the U.S. Other organizations that have a long history of formal planning (e.g., some HMOs such as Kaiser-Permanente in California) have been concentrated in specific regions of the U.S., and serve a much smaller percentage of Americans.

Hospital Planning Responds To A Changing Environment

Hospital planning in the 1950s and 1960s reflected the emphasis on construction and modernization that was made possible by the availability of federal funds under the Hill-Burton Act and its successors. Hospital planning was facilities planning, and building design and construction were the focus of planning.

With the passage of Certificate-Of-Need legislation by many states in the late 1960s and 1970s, emphasis began to shift to the documentation of the need for hospital services in the community and in a particular hospital. CON legislation required that state approval be obtained for the construction of most health facilities. Hospital planning had to combine both community and facilities planning.

The shift in emphasis by the federal government to control of hospitals through reimbursement, the repeal of many state Certificate-Of-Need laws, and the failure of Congress to pass a national health planning act again altered hospital planning in the 1980s. At the same time, hospital admissions began to decrease, and lengths of stay continued to decline—a trend that started in the 1970s (Moss & Moien, 1987). The number of admissions to community hospitals dropped by 15% between 1981 and 1991. Average length of stay decreased by 6%. The result was a decline of 13 percentage points in occupancy rates, from 76% in 1981 to 66% in 1991 (American Hospital Association, 1992).

Hospital managers now searched for a way to fill the empty beds. Facilities planning had taken for granted that whatever services were available would be used. Community planning assumed that government would grant a franchise to the "best" hospitals, limiting supply, and that services would then be used. In the new environment, neither approach seemed relevant.

Hospital managers searching for something new and relevant could draw on two management approaches that had been developed in the general business community—"strategic" planning and marketing. Both assumed that firms competed for customers in a market where supply often exceeded demand and where rapid technological change continually produced new products. They both therefore fit the new environment faced by hospitals.

Strategies in the 1980s and 1990s. Strategic planning requires that managers use resources to put their organization in a favorable position in the marketplace. Such a position might be (1) having the largest share of the demand in a market, (2) being the most technologically advanced company whose products command a higher price, or (3) being a high volume, low-price company, which is very profitable.

The major strategies used by hospitals during the 1980s and early 1990s to achieve a favorable market position are *vertical integration, horizontal integration*, and *diversification*.

An "integrated" firm includes a number of businesses that are related either because they produce the same product or service ("horizontal" integration), or carry out a number of stages in the manufacturing process ("vertical" integration). Marriott is a horizontally integrated corporation because it owns a number of hotel chains. General Motors is vertically integrated because it owns companies that produce components for automobiles as well as assembling, marketing, and financing the purchase of automobiles.

There are many advantages and disadvantages to vertical and horizontal integration (Porter, 1980; Harrigan, 1985; Smith & Reid, 1986). In the hospital industry, horizontal integration was viewed as potentially advantageous because a chain of hospitals might be able to purchase supplies and services at a volume discount, would be able to hire specialized staff at the corporate level to increase expertise, would be able to raise capital less expensively on the securities markets, and would be able to market hospital services under a single brand name in a number of communities.

A vertically integrated health care "system" could include outpatient or office services for routine and preventive care, diagnostic services to detect disease, and treatment services to cure patients. Nursing home care and rehabilitation and mental health care might also be included. The potential advantages of a vertically integrated system are that the consumer—both patients and referring physicians—would never have to leave the system to get the health services needed. Revenues would be kept in the system while the patient's care was managed to assure that the needed services were provided.

Diversification simply meant adding services not usually found in a hospital. This might include home care, physical fitness centers, prevention and detection services provided at the workplace, or residential drug and alcohol treatment services. The potential advantage of diversification is that revenues are not lost to other organizations. The hospital's reputation in the community would provide it with an advantage over companies that might move in and offer the same services.

Horizontal integration proved the easiest strategy to carry out. Chains of for-profit hospitals (such as Hospital Corporation of America) grew, with growth financed by investors who thought they saw a profitable trend in the hospital industry. Chains of not-for-profit hospitals also emerged, and actually remain the most numerous. Some of the chains, however, simply involved agreements to cooperate (e.g., in purchasing supplies) rather than actual ownership of all the hospitals by a single company. The largest "multi-hospital system" of not-for-profit hospitals, Voluntary Hospitals of America (VHA), was formed when hospitals agreed to invest in a new corporation that would start new businesses (and return profits to investors), negotiate favorable purchase agreements with suppliers and take other actions that would benefit hospital investors. VHA doesn't own any hospitals, however.

Vertical integration was far less common in the 1980s. The examples that are most widely known—the Kaiser-Permanente Medical Plans, the Cleveland Clinic Foundation, the Mayo Clinic—were all formed much earlier. Even in these organizations the full continuum of services is not provided. Long-term nursing home care, for example, is rarely provided by these organizations.

Diversificaton was more common than vertical integration. Hospitals diversified and provided those services which market analysis showed might be profitable.

As hospitals entered the 1990s, considerable disillusionment developed with all three of these strategies. While volume purchasing has resulted in real savings to chains of hospitals, the other advantages of horizontal integration are less apparent. Several hospital chains have sold off hospitals to raise capital and improve their profitability. Doubts about whether the additional expertise is worth the extra costs of a central corporate office are being expressed. As profits have fallen, both for-profit and not-for-profit chains are paying more to raise capital. Managers of profitable community hospitals that have a healthy share of a local market are not sure that remaining independent will hurt them in the long-run, a common assumption in the early 1980s. While joining a group of hospitals to obtain discounts on supplies and services still makes a lot of sense, selling the hospital to a chain is now more difficult to justify to Boards of Trustees.

Hospitals have lost considerable money trying to start HMOs, the most common attempt at vertical integration. Diversification into other businesses has frequently resulted in long periods during which the new businesses had to be subsidized and smaller profits than had been expected (Freudenheim, 1988).

Professional journals and lecturers at conventions have begun to discuss whether a new strategy is needed—a "back-to-basics" strategy. Hospitals, it is argued, should seek to provide the traditional range of inpatient and outpatient services, but with a new emphasis on quality, measured both in improved health and higher levels of patient and physician satisfaction (Kropf, 1990; Kropf & Szafran, 1988; Peterson, 1988; Perry, 1988; Grossman, 1991). This would make them attractive to employers and other purchasers of services, as well as to HMOs and other managed care organizations (e.g., managed care divisions of large insurance companies).

While this may seem attractive to many groups within a hospital, it will not be an easy strategy to pursue. Most hospitals have always believed they provide high-quality services. Unless they can document and communicate to patients and physicians that they in fact provide higher quality services, they may be left investing in improvements that don't produce significant changes in volume. Some dimensions of quality are very difficult to measure and others are subjective. Proving that a hospital offers higher quality services may be very difficult, although the goal is admirable. Whether it produces the bottom-line results that hospital managers are seeking isn't clear.

There has been increased interest in vertical integration as well. Rather than offering themselves as contractors to managed care organizations—and providing discounts—some hospitals and hospital systems have sought to create vertically integrated health care systems that can provide most healthcare services.

This opens up the possibility of contracting directly with employers and government (to serve government employees or beneficiaries of programs such as Medicaid). In addition to greater profits, this offers greater security, since the contracts are held directly by the healthcare system and not by an HMO or insurance company—which can choose to contract with another organization.

Since long-term inpatient care is rarely a covered benefit, this has primarily meant that hospitals have to increase the variety, volume, and location of ambulatory services, including primary care and home care. A major decision that has to be made is the relationship that the hospital wishes to have with physicians, and especially primary care physicians. Some hospitals have emphasized the purchase of physician practices, others have sought to build primary care facilities and staff them with physicians on salary. Others have sought to create a separate corporation in which physicians can become investors. These vertically integrated systems face competition from for-profit corporations that have spent millions of dollars purchasing medical groups, partly to secure managed care contracts. They also face competition from vertically integrated HMOs like Kaiser-Permanente. Many hospitals, especially not-for-profit hospitals that cannot issue stock, are in the position of having far less access to capital than such competitors.

Focus On Marketing Tactics. In military jargon, a strategy is an idea that results in winning a war, while tactics are actions that win battles. A military strategist isn't alarmed about losing a battle if an effective strategy continues to be implemented.

A number of hospitals, alarmed at actual or projected drops in patient volume and revenues, have pursued advertising, sales and other tactics of marketing in an attempt to reduce anxiety and produce better end-of-the-year results. The results have been disappointing for many hospitals. Marketing experts have countered that hospitals have neglected market research and overlooked the development of market strategies in the pursuit of tactics to produce quick results. They have also criticized the tactics as inappropriate for the kinds of problems that hospitals were actually facing (Powills, 1986).

For many hospitals, marketing meant advertising. For a smaller number, it meant sales through sales forces paid on a commission basis.

Many hospitals—for the first time—began advertising their "products." Marketing professionals already knew, based on years of experience in a variety of businesses, that advertising alone doesn't produce large increases in demand. In order to achieve a change in the behavior of customers, repeated exposure to the message is necessary (Robertson, 1984). Advertising campaigns that reach large numbers of people with a message many times are very expensive. Some hospital managers appear to have thought that a few ads in the newspapers would produce a significant increase in demand. When the increase didn't occur and bills for thousands of dollars of advertising arrived, the result was disillusionment with marketing.

Notably missing was an emphasis on market research prior to deciding on strategy and tactics. American industry spends huge resources on market surveys in an attempt to understand consumer behavior. Hospitals have spent much more on advertising than market research. Consultants and marketing professionals report little concern in hospitals about the concepts that underlie much of marketing strategy, particularly market position (how consumers perceive a product in relation to competitors).

What explains this approach to marketing? It may partly be that some senior managers of hospitals do not have experience in other industries and were trained in academic programs which placed little emphasis on marketing because of the very different environment hospitals faced in the 1960s and 1970s.

Hospitals are also relatively small organizations that cannot compete in salary and career advancement with major industries for trained marketing professionals. Hospital staff placed in charge of marketing either had no formal training in marketing, or have come from sales and public relations positions in other industries.

The research and strategy-development skills and knowledge are available in marketing firms, but at a cost that far exceeds what hospitals have wanted to pay. For example, a "focus group" involving a 1 to 2 hour discussion among 6 to 8 consumers, a full transcript and an analysis of significant comments would cost a hospital $5,000 to 10,000 if done by a professional marketing firm.

The development of a marketing strategy, including careful and professional market research, a consensus among hospital decision-makers on the position which the hospital should seek to obtain in the market, product and personnel changes to implement the strategy, and a multi-year advertising and public relations campaign to communicate to the desired market is both time-consuming, expensive, and likely to result in conflict in the complex, highly political environment of a hospital.

It is perhaps not surprising then that some hospital managers without previous experience and training in marketing would opt for tactics such as advertising rather than market strategy development and implementation.

What Should Hospital Planning Include? The hospital industry arrived at the end of the 1980s without a widely accepted model for how hospital planning should be carried out. It would have been possible at the end of the 1970s to have described what a hospital plan looked like and what a hospital planner did. At the end of the 1980s there is far greater diversity but also a great deal of frustration among hospital managers. Just what should hospitals be doing? More marketing?

More strategic planning? In the 1990s, the question was whether health care systems as opposed to hospitals should be the appropriate object of planning. Did it make any sense to plan only for acute and tertiary care services?

In an industry composed of so many organizations, different answers will be given to this question. We are likely to see considerable anxiety among hospital managers about whether their hospital is doing the right thing.

To understand the choices facing an individual hospital, it is important to understand what strategic planning and marketing are, as well as the differences between them.

Strategic Planning

Strategic planning involves the allocation of resources in a way that leads an organization in a direction that is believed will achieve its long-range goals. It involves selecting among alternative use of resources and among alternative goals. It involves forecasting future conditions and where an organizaton will wind up under alternative scenarios about the future (Kropf & Greenberg, 1984).

The major debates about strategic planning, both in the hospital and other industries, concern (1) who should carry out the strategic planning process, (2) whether a plan is necessary or desirable and (3) whether the term "strategic management" would be a more appropriate description of what managers need to do in turbulent environments.

Numerous case studies have shown that planning must involve the real decision-makers to result in changes in the organization's behavior. While no one will argue that planning isn't a responsibility of boards of directors and the President or CEO of a company, the reality is that planning as an organizational function in large organizations often becomes the name of a department headed by a middle-level staff person. When this occurs, considerable time and money can be spent on activity about which the Board and senior executive is only vaguely aware. The result is often wasted effort. The middle-level staff member doesn't understand what the Board/President wants and will accept, while the Board/President isn't interested in what the planning department produces.

Reinforcing this message is research which shows that many plans are not implemented because they are incorrect and irrelevant by the time they are produced. In industries where the environment changes weekly, a plan that took 2 years to prepare is rarely useful. The central role of forecasting in the development of plans is being questioned, since forecasts of many variables are highly suspect.

It is now frequently argued that strategic planning should be one of the day-to-day activities of top managers. Mintzberg (1987) has coined the term "crafting strategy" using an analogy to the way a potter creates a vase or bowl. Based on day-to-day contact with the reality in which the organization operates, the senior manager crafts the strategy of the organization, rejecting one idea for another as events unfold.

The term that has emerged for this dynamic, flexible style of strategic planning carried out directly by the senior manager is "strategic management." It responds to the major criticisms of strategic planning, but at the same time leaves open some questions. How does the senior manager locate and draw conclusions from the vast amount of data about the organization and its environment and still get all his/her other jobs done? Is there a role for staff? How does the manager communicate the content and rationale for the organization's strategy to key decision-makers such as the Board? Is a written plan necessary or desirable?

In seeking the answer to the question of what hospital planning should become, the concept of strategic management needs to be carefully considered. It suggests that hospital managers are going to have to incorporate more long-range thinking into their daily activities, that they are going to have to develop information systems that are responsive to the needs of senior managers and that communication about what the hospital's strategy is as it develops is going to have to become a formal activity.

Marketing

It is easy to exaggerate the differences between strategic planning and marketing by emphasizing the tactics of marketing, especially advertising, public relations, and sales. On the other hand, popular textbooks used at graduate business schools have titles like "strategic marketing" and "strategic market management." The point is that marketing, like strategic planning, requires a vision of where the organization wants to go in the future and requires a plan for getting there.

The rationale for both marketing and strategic planning is that an organization will not automatically achieve its goals and objectives—and will not meet customer needs and desires as effectively—unless a formal process of selecting among alternative uses of resources is carried out.

A major difference is the points from which strategic planning and marketing often begin. Strategic planning begins by asking what the organization's mission and goals are. Marketing begins by asking what the needs and desires of consumers are. Both must consider these two issues at some point. Both proceed in ways which are very similar until the question of tactics arises. Marketing may turn more frequently to its well-developed tactics, including advertising, while strategic planning may consider more frequently alternatives suggested by economics, for example, diversification, and horizontal and vertical integration.

This suggests another difference between strategic planning and marketing, that is, their theoretical roots. Marketing professionals are far more likely to use the terms and concepts of human psychology, while strategic planning draws on those of economics. For example, Kotler and Clarke (1987) use Maslow's hierarchy of needs to understand which of the individual's basic needs may be served by a product. They note that it would be futile to offer activities such as jogging and exercise classes to the poor who lack food and shelter. Activities such as these will more likely appeal to those seeking to fulfill the higher social esteem and self-actualizing needs.

Michael Porter (1980), a prominent writer on strategic planning, focuses on what he calls the "value chain" to explain why organizations and individuals purchase goods and services. The value chain is the series of activities that the purchaser must go through, for example, travel to where a service is provided. By increasing the value of the good or service at any point along the chain, the chances that the purchase will be made are increased. For example, providing a physician with the report of an x-ray procedure faster adds value to the service, since the physician wishes to inform a patient, especially about any negative results. The value chain concept can be applied to a range of health services (Kropf & Szafran, 1988; Kropf, 1990). It should be noted, however, that Porter has simply borrowed the concept of "value-added" from economics (i.e., that manufacturing involves the addition of value at each step of the process), and made the assumption that people are primarily motivated by their calculation of the monetary value of the services they purchase.

The theoretical roots of strategic planning and marketing are therefore different. Both processes, however, draw upon a wide range of concepts and techniques from many disciplines.

Techniques for Planning Health Services

Techniques are needed to produce the information to be used by decision-makers and to manage the process of decision-making by the individuals who must agree before action is taken.

Information is needed about the needs and desires of the people to be served, other organizations who provide health services and the general environment in which the health care organization must operate—especially what actions government and other third-party payors are likely to take.

In this section a number of techniques for investigating the needs and desires of consumers are presented. Techniques are presented for:

- describing the *health* of the population,
- describing what people *desire*, regardless of need, and
- describing *past utilization* of health services.

Techniques for managing part of the process of decision-making in a group are then presented. These include:

1. A technique for determining perceptions of the *strengths, weaknesses, opportunities*, and *threats* facing an organization. Agreement on these subjects is necessary before a group can decide on how to allocate resources.
2. The Nominal Group Process, a technique for assuring that all viewpoints are heard by the group prior to making a decision. This is likely to increase the chances that a plan of action will be successfully implemented.

Measuring Health Status

The extent to which people are healthy or ill is valuable information for planning. Much has been written, however, about the difficulties of defining health and illness, as well as the methodological and cost problems of measuring the extent of health or illness in a population (Goldsmith, 1972; Berg, 1973).

For example, if we define health as the absence of organic illness (e.g., the absence of infection, cancer, malfunction of an organ or body system), this would leave out the feeling of well-being that many individuals associate with "feeling healthy." An overweight individual who gets little exercise and felt lethargic can still be "healthy," that is, free of organic illness. Even if we expand our definition to include body weight and muscle tone characteristics considered ideal, it would leave out the perception of well-being that many individuals associate with good health.

On the other hand, if we expand the definition of health to include other dimensions, for example, "emotional well-being," how do we define and measure what is good health? Such a definition would lead us to define health as what is perceived by the individual to be positive, which is highly subjective and vastly different from person to person.

Regardless of whether good health is defined in terms of the absence of disease and/or a feeling of physical and emotional well-being, the problems of measurement remain. How do we know in the absence of extensive medical testing if an individual is free of organic disease? Individuals free of symptoms may be at high risk of a heart attack, for example, because of blocked arteries. Determining physical and emotional well-being would require extensive interviews that are costly to carry out.

While the debate continues on how to measure health status, individuals involved in planning health services continue to rely on measures that are believed to be closely related or correlated to the level of health, for example, the rate of infant mortality, total mortality, and mortality from specific causes that are preventable or treatable (Dever, 1980). Measures that use the death rate require data that are available from public records for almost all deaths in a community.

The reliance on death rates, however, is particularly troublesome for health care organizations which are seeking to become more responsive to consumer demand. Such organizations are likely to rely more on data concerning the use of health services, rather than data on deaths, as an indication of both need and demand for health services (Rice & Creel, 1985; Tseng, 1983). When the investment (and the risk) is large enough, surveys and other forms of consumer research are more likely to be undertaken to determine with more certainty how consumers feel about their health, and what services they want.

Consumer Analysis—Understanding What Physicians and Consumers Want

Until the 1980s, individuals responsible for planning health services at all levels paid surprisingly little attention to the subject of what consumers' and physicians' wants and desires were in regard to health services. Planning for health services focused on the question of need. Most health care professionals accepted the idea that what the consumer wanted was at best a secondary consideration to getting consumers the services that physicians and other professionals thought they should have.

The competitive environment described earlier produced a great change in this attitude among some health services managers whose organizations faced significant underutilization. The issue now became how to determine what consumers desired so that their organization could provide it. A significant number of pregnant women, for example, wanted alternatives to the hospital labor and delivery rooms that they didn't, in the minds of many obstetricians, "need." A number of hospitals, however, established birthing centers and other new arrangements for labor and delivery to win a greater share of patients in the community.

Since a physician's advice has a major impact on the decisions made by consumers, what referring physicians wanted also became a major concern. Hospitals developed a range of programs in response, including courier services for test reports to get them to physicians faster, more formal arrangements for providing specialty consultations and even links to the hospital's computer to allow the sharing of information (Kropf, 1990).

In order to understand what its consumers (including physicians) wanted, hospitals and other healthcare organizations looked at the techniques being used by other industries which had made analysis of consumer desires and behavior a major part of their planning processes (Ross et al., 1987; Berwick & Weinstein, 1985).

Market Segmentation. A fundamental concept in marketing is the *market segment* (Kotler & Clarke, 1987). This is a group of individuals who are distinguished by one or more characteristics believed to affect their purchasing behavior. Consumers may, for example, be segmented by age, and the over-70 market segment identified as behaving differently. Within this over-70 segment, those with high income can be segmented and offered different services, such as luxury accommodations while in a hospital.

Several important points need to be made. Market segmentation is based on consumer research. Second, segments need to be determined for specific products or services, since it is purchasing behavior we are trying to predict.

Consumer Research. In order to identify market segments, research must be conducted to determine how consumers behave, and the attitudes, knowledge, and beliefs which may affect that behavior.

Telephone, mail, and personal interview surveys are frequently used to gather data. Formal discussion groups called "focus groups" are a popular way of gathering preliminary data to be used in preparation for more formal research.

Analysis. Computer technology has had a major impact on the ability of an analyst to follow a line of questioning. General purpose programs for analyzing survey data such as Statistical Package for the Social Sciences or SPSS (SPSS, Inc., 1988) are available to assist the analysis. Several firms such as HBO & Company in Atlanta, and the Sachs Group in Evanston, Illinois have developed computer systems which allow the analysis of market-related data and which produce tables, maps and graphs that combine census data, data on utilization from bills and survey research data. For example, a map could be produced that showed the number of people in each zip code that had cardiac surgery during the last year to assist in deciding on the location of an ambulatory cardiac rehabilitation facility.

Impact. Analysis of consumer behavior, attitudes, knowledge, and beliefs is changing the way in which some health care organizations plan for new services. For some organizations, the major question has become "What do our consumers want?" rather than "What do consumers need that we want to offer?" How many organizations have changed their way of thinking is hard to tell, but the number of new programs being offered that emphasize life-style change, disease detection, and alternatives to traditional hospital care suggest that some organizations have changed their behavior.

The Analysis of Health Services Utilization

Data Sources. The number and type of health services used by consumers is critically important information for planning. The necessary data are usually obtained from national surveys, bills, and related forms that are completed in order to receive payment, and special surveys undertaken at the local level (Kropf & Greenberg, 1984).

The most important national surveys are undertaken by the National Center for Health Statistics within the U.S. Department of Health and Human Services. The National Health Interview Survey, for example, provides self-reported data on the physician and hospital services used by individuls in approximately 40,000 households. Data is available for over 20 years, allowing the planner to look at trends over time—which is extremely important for forecasting.

Since NCHS surveys are samples of the entire U.S. population, they cannot in most cases provide local data (i.e., for an individual city, town, county, or state). Data from bills and related forms can be aggregated to provide such data. In states such as New York and Massachusetts, state government requires that hospitals submit a copy of the hospital bill and a discharge abstract for each patient in a form that can be read by a computer. The number of times that people in an individual area are hospitalized and the reason can be determined. Only a minority of states require that such data be submitted, however, so the only national data source on hospitalization comes from the Medicare program, and this covers only people over the age of 65. The U.S. Department of Health and Human Services has, however, been reluctant to release this data to anyone but those doing research because of concerns about the violation of the confidentiality of patients.

In order to collect data on a range of topics other than hospital stays, private organizations, and local government sometimes pay for surveys that are conducted over the telephone or through the mails, and more rarely in individual households Such surveys are, however, expensive.

In summary, local data on how many and which type of hospital inpatient services consumers use is available in a minority of states, although the federal government possesses such data for all states for Medicare recipients. Local data on what occurs outside of the hospital is scarce for all age groups, since no state has yet mandated that physicians or insurance companies submit copies of bills for services outside the hospital. The federal government has not made local data on the services used by Medicare recipients outside of the hospital available to hospitals and other organizations which plan health services.

Tools for Analysis. Computer technology has vastly changed how the data described above can be analyzed (Kropf & Greenberg, 1984; Dever, 1980). The major impact has been to allow the analyst to follow a line of questioning as information is received rather than being forced to accept a fixed series of tables. As each question is raised the computer allows the analyst to ask for tables and graphs. In response to this new information, new questions can be raised, for which new tables and graphs are requested.

Mobile Mammography for the Corporate Customer: A Case Study in Planning

To illustrate how the techniques that have just been described might be used, the situation faced by an organization—a hospital or a physician group practice—wishing to establish a mobile mammography screening program aimed at employees of corporations will be discussed (Kettlehake & Malott, 1988).

Mobile mammography screening is an attractive option for some organizations seeking to increase their volume of patients. This is because it:

1. brings the organization into contact with women who may not have personal physicians and will use the organization for other services,
2. can locate women who have cancer and therefore need specialized services which the organization can offer,
3. increases the visibility of the organization to all those who come into contact with the promotional materials for the program,
4. can enhance the public image of the organization, and
5. can serve as the entry point into a corporation, resulting in later sales of other services.

Mobile mammography screening involves the use of specialized x-ray equipment placed in vans and driven to an office or factory location, or portable equipment which is set up inside a building. Employees are offered the opportunity to register and receive a mammogram, which is read by radiologists. The report is then returned to the woman's personal physician, or an appointment is made with a physician affiliated with the sponsoring healthcare organization. The role of employers is to offer the opportunity to employees by allowing access to employees, for example, use of company internal mail, and facilities. The employer may or may not subsidize the cost of the mammogram.

Health Status. It is estimated that approximately one in nine women will develop breast cancer at some time during their lives. It is estimated there were 150,000 new cases of breast cancer detected in 1990. In 1989, 42,837 women died of the disease (National Center for Health Statistics, 1992).

Analysis of data on breast cancer mortality suggest that annual screening of women over 50 could reduce mortality by 30% or more when followed by appropriate treatment (Kolata, 1988). The evidence on the impact of routine screening on women 40–49 is mixed, with some experts suggesting that the cost is not justified for women who have no symptoms and whose mother or sister(s) have not had the disease (Kolata, 1988). Current guidelines from the American Cancer Society suggest that a baseline mammogram be taken between age 35 to 39 to facilitate the detection of later changes, that a mammogram be taken every 1 to 2 years for women ages 40 to 49, and every year for symptomless women age 50 and over.

An organization considering offering such a service could use data from death certificates collected by all states to determine the number of women who die from breast cancer and their ages in particular towns, cities, and counties.

Consumer Analysis. The ACS guidelines suggest that market segmentation by age is essential. Women under 35 need to be advised that mammography is not advisable. The message communicated to women 35 to 39, 40 to 49, and over 50 will be different because of their differing professionally defined needs. The next question is what other segmentation of the market should be undertaken.

The organization could hold one or more focus groups to suggest what differences in attitudes, beliefs, and desires exist among women in each age group. Since a large amount of research suggests that the use of preventive services is strongly related to education and income, the organization may also wish to investigate (through focus groups or surveys of samples of women) the differences among women in various employment categories within the organization (e.g., managerial, clerical, manufacturing).

The purpose of focus group research is to suggest topics that should be explored in more formal personal interviews, or mail or telephone surveys. How much research is carried out will depend on the size of the investment to be made, the willingness of the corporation to allow customization of the program to fit the desires of groups of workers and prior experience in offering screening programs.

Some of the results of research might be that (Seago, 1986):

- younger patients express a greater desire for the procedure;
- higher-paid, better-educated workers have greater knowledge of the procedure;
- most women have a friend or relative who has had a mammogram and told them what to expect.

If survey research is undertaken and yields a large number of responses, the organization or a consultant will probably analyze the data using a computer program to examine the relationship between responses. For example, does age or employment category better explain differences in the expressed desire for the service?

The impact of this kind of consumer analysis can be on the content of promotional material. Simplified descriptions of the need for the procedure and how it will be carried out could be distributed to lower-paid, less-educated women who need basic information. Higher-paid, better-educated women can be given materials that focus on the qualifications of the organization, the amount of radiation that will be exposed to and other subjects that are shown to be of interest to this group.

Consumer analysis can also have an impact on how the service is provided. Only female staff may be used because of concerns expressed about being seen by men (Seago, 1986), and because it is assumed that women nurses and technicians will be viewed as more sympathetic to the anxieties and concerns of women.

Analysis of Utilization. One of the problems faced by an organization that considers offering this service is the absence of data on the number of women in local communities who have had a mammogram.

Data from the National Hospital Discharge Survey for 1991 show that 156,000 women were discharged with "malignant neoplasm" or cancer of the breast listed as the first diagnosis (National Center for Health Statistics, 1992). Local data on hospital utilization is available in those states where hospitals are required to submit discharge abstracts to state government. This allows the organization not only to determine the number of discharges, but the age and place of residence of the woman, and what percentage of these patients were treated in each hospital in the community, and outside of the area.

Data from the National Health Interview Survey for January–June 1985 indicate that 34% of women age 30 to 44 practice breast self-examination once a month or more. Thirty-seven percent of women 45 to 64 do so (Thornberry et al., 1986). This suggests that a substantial majority of women do not follow current ACS guidelines. The ACS estimates that only 28% of women over 40 have annual mammograms, and that an additional 14% have mammograms every 2 to 4 years. The ACS does not have data on how many of these women are over 50 (Kolata, 1988).

Other Planning Tasks. This discussion of the information that may be collected as part of the planning process for this service is not meant to suggest that data collection and analysis is the only task to be undertaken. The current activities of competitors must be examined. The willingness of the Board or owners of the organization to devote resources must be determined. The willingness of employers to promote the use of this service must be assessed. Equipment, personnel, and supplies must be obtained.

Asking questions about what the needs and desires of consumers are has been stressed because it is a task which many health care organizations are less familiar with.

Before any action can be taken, however, the decision-makers in any organization must agree on many issues, including the best way to allocate resources.

Group Process Techniques

Decisions are made by people and not computers. The highest quality information is useless if it has no impact on the thinking of the individuals who must approve the allocation of resources.

Planning health services involves the selection of a process for arriving at a decision on how resources are to be spent and for what. Since it is rare in health care organizations that a single individual has the sole authority to allocate major resources, the techniques for arriving at a decision that are most relevant are techniques used with groups.

The final method for decision-making is often the vote of a board of directors or trustees. The question is how this group of individuals arrives at decisions about what the major facts are, what the options are, and which options are most attractive given the mission, goals, and capabilities of an organization.

SWOT Analysis. A simple technique for moving closer to a consensus on the current environment is a Strengths-Weaknesses-Opportunities-Threats or SWOT analysis (Peters, 1985). The decision-making group can be asked to meet for an extended period of time (e.g., a weekend) to discuss these four topics with an experienced discussion leader brought from outside the organization to facilitate the discussion.

Decision-makers can be asked during a series of meetings to define:

1. What are the major *strengths* of the organization?
2. What are its major *weaknesses*?
3. What *opportunities* in the environment should the organization take advantage of?
4. What *threats* exist to the achievement of the organization's mission and goals?

Consensus on the answers to these topics in a short period of time is highly unlikely. Each individual is likely to have a different level of knowledge of the "facts." If they agree on the facts, they may not agree on the implications of those facts.

For example, decision-makers may arrive with different ideas about the extent to which their competitors' hospital beds are full or empty. When given the best estimate, they may still disagree on what the numbers imply their own organization should do.

The job of the discussion leader is to help the members of the group define the information they need, apply it to their situation, expose the differences in values and beliefs that explain differences in opinion and lead the group over time to a consensus on what needs to be done. There are certainly no fixed rules for carrying this process to a successful conclusion, and some organizations may never reach the required consensus. Over the years, however, consultants and professional planners have developed some techniques that appear to facilitate at least part of the decision-making process.

The Nominal Group Process. The Nominal Group Process is one such technique (Spiegel & Hyman, 1978). Research by sociologists and psychologists has shown that some individuals will not speak in a group discussion. Other people will use the situation to express their views and attempt to dominate the group. The end result is that the group does not reach a consensus because (1) the opinions of some members have never been revealed and opened to scrutiny or (2) opinions are rejected simply because they are voiced by members whose attempt to dominate the group is resented by others.

The Nominal Group Process seeks to solve the problem by asking each member of the group to write a response to one or more specific questions on index cards. The question might be one of the four listed above for a SWOT analysis. The discussion leader then goes in clockwise order around the room and asks each participant for a response, for example, a strength of the organization. The group is asked not to comment until the end of the process. Each response is written on a large piece of paper and posted for everyone to see. A number of rounds is completed until all responses are out in the open. The discussion leader then leads the group in a discussion, for example, of which responses are similar and which are believed to be true or not true. The virtue of this process is that each person contributes, their contribution is not evaluated until all responses are known, and no one can dominate the discussion until everyone's opinion is known.

Although the technique isn't perfect, it offers advantages over an unstructured discussion that have made it popular with planners. Other techniques are available to fit different objectives and environments (Spiegel & Hyman, 1978).

Should We Merge With Metro?: A Case Study In Board Decision Making

To understand how these decision-making techniques might be used, let us consider the situation faced by the Board of Directors of a small, rural HMO that was faced with a major decision.[1] It had received an inquiry from Metro Health Plan, one of the nation's largest HMOs, concerning a merger. The HMO was not-for-profit and consumer-controlled (i.e., a majority of the board were members who were not physicians, nurses or other providers of health services). The HMO had experienced slow growth in the 10 years it had been in operation, and operated in only 3 sites all located within a 10-mile radius of each other.

The Board decided to hire an experienced consultant to lead them in a weekend retreat to consider the offer. The consultant recommended that they meet for the first 4 hours and carry out a SWOT analysis. Table 13.1 shows the list produced by the end of the session.

A consensus was reached that the strengths, weaknesses, opportunities, and threats listed in Table 13.1 summarized the situation faced by the HMO. The Board then went through another Nominal Group Process to reach consensus on its options, which included a merger with Metro, a merger with a smaller HMO in a rural part of the state, and a conversion to a for-profit corporation in order to possibly sell stock to raise capital.

Eventually, the Board voted for a merger with Metro Health Plan.

---

[1]This case was prepared for teaching purposes, based on a situation actually faced by a rural HMO.

TABLE 13.1   SWOT Analysis for a Rural HMO

Strengths
- Loyalty of current members
- High level of employee satisfaction
- Stable financial condition
- High quality of service as perceived by both providers and consumers

Weaknesses
- Stagnation in membership growth
- Limited ability to borrow funds for expansion
- Limited range of expertise in current administration (e.g., no attorney on staff)

Opportunities
- Become the largest high-quality, rural HMO in the state by remaining independent and:
  a. using its current reputation for quality and consumer satisfaction to market the plan in adjacent communities;
  b. being the first HMO to start operations in a number of rural areas in the state; and
  c. using the knowledge of its board and members to design facilities and programs that would appeal to rural communities.
- Join a much larger organization whose resources would allow the HMO to dominate an expanded market area.
- Merge with another HMO and develop a statewide HMO that would locally controlled but have sufficient resources to growth and dominate an expanded market area.

Threats
- Metro or another HMO would enter rural communities first and sign up members who would be reluctant to change plans later
- The HMO could not expand fast enough and compete with other HMOs because of the lack of capital and management expertise.

The Future of Health Services Planning

The role of the federal government in deciding on the volume and location of health services that will be provided to Americans is likely to remain limited. It is unlikely, for example, that the federal government will seek any role in determining the number and location of MRI (Magnetic Resonance Imaging) scanners, even though costs are in excess of $1 million dollars per scanner and major metropolitan areas are believed to have an excessive number. Even those members of Congress and the Clinton Administration who feel regulation is needed appear willing to let the states and market demand deal with this issue.

Planning at the federal level is likely instead to focus on the control of total health expenditures by stimulating competition among providers. The Clinton

Administration's health reform proposal, released in September of 1993, also calls for controls on the premiums charged by health alliances using a national inflation factor intended to reduce increases to an amount equal to the Consumer Price Index by 1999.

The model of planning being accepted could be compared to national economic planning in the U.S. (e.g., at the Federal Reserve Bank), where the purpose of regulation is to assure that broad goals are achieved (e.g., growth in the economy) without undesirable side effects (e.g., high inflation). The major difference is that the Clinton Administration, unlike the Federal Reserve Bank, wants to control what is purchased and by whom. The major goal is to assure that all Americans are insured for at least a basic set of benefits.

This is a new form of federal planning in the U.S. The Clinton Administration accepts the need for some form of central planning, but recognizes that it would be impossible for the central government to directly control the delivery of health services. As the President's proposal moves through Congress, the debate is likely to be whether it gives too much authority to government for making resource allocation choices, or whether it doesn't go far enough to assure that the broad objectives of universal access to desirable services are met.

The Clinton Administration has accepted the same solution as the Hill-Burton Act to forge a compromise—a role for the states in planning. But the health care reform proposal made by the Clinton Administration would give states far greater authority than that earlier legislation. For example, states would certify health plans and establish one or more regional health alliances responsible for providing health coverage to residents in every area of the state. A state could establish a single-payer health care system rather than alliances offering multiple plans. A single-payer system is one in which the state makes all payments to health care providers with no intermediaries or health plans assuming financial risk. Some states are likely to use this and other options to increase their authority, while other states are likely to accept a more limited set of goals.

The extent to which state government is involved in planning health services is likely to continue to vary dramatically. States with a long tradition of actively pursuing solutions to health problems (e.g., New York, Massachusetts, Hawaii) are likely to continue to plan and to implement those plans.

Another way in which the Clinton reform proposal differs from a centralized national planning approach is in the authority given to the private organizations that will establish health plans and make the actual decisions on the volume and location of services to be provided. These private organizations could be existing insurance companies and HMOs, new organizations (either nonprofit or investor-owned), and provider organizations such as hospitals and medical groups. Dramatically different predictions have been made about what will occur. Advocates of a national single-payer system have argued that the Clinton proposal will result in the consolidation of ownership of health plans by a few major insurance companies such as Aetna, Metropolitan Life, and Prudential. Others have argued that health care is a local business and multiple organizations will contract with alliances to provide health services.

At the local level, hospitals are likely to retain a role as a major planner of health services in most communities. Most hospitals will, however, participate in larger organizations developed to win a greater share of the managed care contracts being offered by insurance companies and HMOs. This prediction is based on a number of assumptions.

The first assumption is that the major insurance companies (e.g., Aetna, Prudential, MetLife) will continue to subcontract with providers for most services, rather than attempting to buy the hospitals and hire the physicians needed, as Kaiser-Permanente does in most of the areas it serves. This seems a reasonable assumption, since the capital required to purchase a national network of providers is enormous and insurance companies have little experience in actually operating hospitals.

The second assumption is that hospitals will dominate the networks they belong to because of their expertise, capital, and community support. Hospitals will, however, need to learn how to plan a wider variety of services and work with other organizations such as nursing homes to create a system of care. They will also need to develop positive working relationships with physicians and help them develop more organized and integrated forms of practice. Group practices and the number of salaried physicians are likely to grow.

Other predictions have been made. Some experts have argued that a small number of large, national, integrated health care systems will dominate health care—a prediction reminiscent of the one made about hospital chains a decade earlier. The financial problems of Humana, Hospital Corporation of America and other large chains that attempted to develop horizontally integrated systems of hospitals suggest that this scenario will be difficult to achieve. Regional integrated networks are being formed in some states, including California, Minnesota, and Michigan. This may result in more centralized, multi-city and even multi-state planning, but is unlikely to affect more than a minority of Americans and will be concentrated in specific regions of the U. S. where economic conditions, significant market share for managed care, and the existence of organizations with the necessary experience make it profitable.

Americans will continue to face the same questions that have arisen over and over again in regard to health planning:

- Should government be directly involved in planning a health care system that is largely in private hands? If so, what decisions should government make? What means of control are preferable?
- What should be the relative authority of the federal, state and local governments?
- What role should citizens/consumers in local communities have?

References

American Hospital Association. *Hospital Statistics: A Comprehensive Study of U.S. Hospitals.* Chicago: AHA. 1992.

Berg, R. L. (Ed.), *Health Status Indexes.* Chicago: Hospital Research and Educational Trust, 1973.

Berwick, D. M., & Weinstein, M. C., "What Do Patients Value? The Willingness to Pay for Ultrasound in Normal Pregnancy." *Medical Care, 23*(7), 1985.

Dever, G. E. A., *Community Health Analysis: A Holistic Approach* Rockville, MD: Aspen Publishers, 1980.

Freudenheim, M., "Hospital Ventures: Some Successes." *The New York Times.* Tuesday, August 23, p. D2, 1988.

Goldsmith, S. B., "The Status of Health Status Indicators." *Health Services Reports, 87,* 212, 1972.

Grossman, J. H., "Emerging Medical Quality Management Support Systems for Hospitals." In Couch, J. B. (Ed.), *Health Care Quality Management for the 21st Century.* Tampa, FL: American College of Physician Executives, 1991.

Harrigan, K. R., *Strategic Flexibility.* Lexington, MA: Lexington Books, 1985.

Kettlehake, J., & Malott, J. C., "Mobile Screening Mammography for the Corporate Customer." *Radiology Management 10,* 2, Spring, 1988.

Kolata, G., "Doubts Increase on Need for Early Mammogram." *The New York Times,* March 11, 1988.

Kotler, P., & Clarke, R., *Marketing for Health Care Organizations.* Englewood Cliffs, NJ: Prentice-Hall, 1987.

Kropf, R., *Service Excellence In Health In Health Care Through The Use Of Computers.* Ann Arbor, MI: American College Of Healthcare Executives, 1990.

Kropf, R., & Goldsmith, S. B., "Innovation In Hospital Plans." *Health Care Management Review, 8,* 2, 1983.

Kropf, R., & Greenberg, J. A., *Strategic Analysis for Hospital Management.* Rockville, MD: Aspen Systems, 1984.

Kropf, R., & Szafran, A., "Developing A Competitive Advantage in the Market For Radiology Services." *Hospital And Health Services Administration,* Summer, 1988.

Mintzberg, H., "Crafting Strategy." *Harvard Business Review,* July–August, 1987.

Moss, A. J., & Moien, M. A., "Recent Declines in Hospitalization, United States, 1982–1986. *Advance Data from Vital and Health Statistics.* No. 140. DHHS Pub. No. (PHS) 87-1250. Public Health Service. Hyattsville, MD: September 24, 1987.

National Center for Health Statistics. "Health, United States, 1991." Public Health Service, Hyattsville, MD., 1992.

Perry, L., "The Quality Process: Hospitals Begin To Emphasize Quality in Devising Strategic Plans." *Modern Healthcare,* April 1, 1988.

Peters, J., *A Strategic Planning Process For Hospitals.* Chicago: American Hospital Association, 1985.

Peterson, K., *The Strategic Approach to Quality Service In Health Care.* Rockville, MD: Aspen Publishers, 1988.

Porter, M., *Competitive Strategy.* New York: Free Press, 1980.

Powills, S., "Hospitals Call A Marketing Time-Out." *Hospitals,* June 5, 1986.

Rice, J., & Creel, G., *Market-Based Demand Forecasting for Hospital Inpatient Services.* Chicago: American Hospital Association, 1985.

Robertson, T. S., & Wortzel, L. H., "Consumer Behavior and Health Care Change: The Role of Mass Media." *Advances in Consumer Research*, Volume 5, 1984.

Ross, C. K. et al., "The Role of Expectations in Patient Satisfaction With Medical Care." *Journal of Health Care Marketing, 7,* 4, 1987.

Seago, K., "Breast Imaging Centers and Patient Emotions: Niceness Counts." *Applied Radiology,* November/December, 1986.

Smith, H. L., & Reid, R. A., *Competitive Hospitals: Management Strategies.* Rockville, MD: Aspen Publishers, 1986.

Spiegel A. D., & Hyman, H. H., *Basic Health Planning Methods.* Rockville, MD: Aspen Systems, 1978.

SPSS, Inc. *SPSS-X User's Guide.* Chicago: SPSS, Inc., 1988.

Thornberry, O. T. et al., "Health Promotion and Disease Prevention, Provisional Data from the National Health Interview Survey: United States, January-June 1985."*Advance Data From Vital and Health Statistics.* No. 119. DHHS Pub. No. (PHS) 86-1250. Hyattsville, MD: Public Health Service. May 14, 1986.

Tseng, S., "Community Demand Analysis for Hospital Ambulatory Care Services" in Meshenberg and Burns, *Hospital Ambulatory Care: Making It Work.* Chicago: American Hospital Association, 1983.

14

Improving Quality of Care

Beth C. Weitzman

"There are differences in the quality of care given by physicians and hospitals. We can measure those differences and that information should be conveyed to the public."

Rarely does a statement provoke as much heated debate as the above issued by Dr. William L. Roper, administrator of the Health Care Financing Administration in 1988 (*NY Times*, 1988). But then again, few health care issues have engendered as much controversy as have recent discussions of the assessment and improvement of the quality of care. Although it is agreed that quality health care is desirable, and despite substantial advances in the field, there continues to be much disagreement about its definition, its measurement, and methods for promoting its occurrence.

Quality of care problems are diverse and as new quality assessment tools have become available, new problems have been identified. They include excessive or inappropriate surgery, variable outcomes of surgical procedures, inappropriate diagnosis or treatment of common acute conditions, and excessive or inappropriate use of prescription drugs (Lohr et al., 1988). Such problems may be classified as overuse, underuse, or misuse of medical care (Chassin, 1991). Whether one is discussing the relative merits of fee-for-service and capitated payment systems, the increased role of nonphysician providers, or the introduction of new technologies, questions of quality must be addressed.

Historically, there has been surprisingly little concern about the quality of care provided. "Do no harm," taken from the Hippocratic Oath, served as the guiding principle. However, soaring health care costs and government financing of health care coupled with increased consumer dissatisfaction and malpractice litigation have contributed to a growing concern about quality. Furthermore, the field has been bolstered by new management models for approaching questions of quality improvement and control.

This chapter will begin with a brief review of the early history of quality assessment and assurance. Definitions and methods of measuring quality health care will then be explored. This will be followed by a discussion of the strategies for promoting the quality of health care services, including the recent introduction of the methods and philosophy of Continuous Quality Improvement (CQI).

History of Quality Assessment and Assurance

It is only within recent decades that the concern with quality became a focal issue for the health care community. The stage for this discussion, however, was set well over a hundred year ago. In the early 1860s, Florence Nightingale helped lay the groundwork for medical care evaluation by suggesting a uniform format for collecting and presenting hospital statistics (Christoffel, 1976). At the turn of the century a Boston surgeon, Dr. Ernest Codman encouraged the collection and evaluation of systematic information on the end results of patient care activities (Christoffel, 1976). Entitled "end result analysis," it was introduced at Massachusetts General Hospital in 1900 and featured a careful analysis of cases for which treatment was unsuccessful. Like many current approaches, end result analysis featured data collection on large numbers of patient outcomes and a recognition that a poor outcome might result from a range of factors. Codman's ideas failed to gain widespread acceptance in the earliest years of the Twentieth Century, a period characterized by rapid gains in medical science, growth in medical professionalism, and limited consumer knowledge.

Despite the initial lack of enthusiasm for end result analysis, one of the foremost agencies for quality assurance—the Joint Commission on Accreditation of Healthcare Organizations (JCAHO)—traces its inception back to Codman's original proposal (Roberts, 1987). Dr. Edward Martin believed the American College of Surgeons should be established to implement and introduce Codman's end result idea. In 1917, the College established and published the Minimum Standard for Hospitals which contained the first formal requirements for the review and evaluation of the quality of patient care. Quality of care in hospitals that participated in the Hospital Standardization Program improved noticeably (Shanahan, 1983). In 1951, the American College of Surgeons joined with the American College of Physicians, the American Hospital Association, the American Medical Association, and the Canadian Medical Association to establish the Joint Commission on Accreditation of Hospitals (JCAH). JCAH's function was to oversee the Minimum Standards: by this time over one-half of all hospitals in the United States were approved (Roberts, 1987).

In the mid-1970s, the JCAH commenced a period of dramatic change in its approach to quality. Whereas earlier standards "referred in general terms to assessing and improving the quality of care" and relied on retrospective audits, standards adopted in 1975 required hospitals to ensure "optimal" care by thorough, continuous evaluation (Joint Commission, 1991). By the early 1990s, the Joint Commission moved further away from retrospective audits toward a method which emphasized a system of continual assessment and improvement. During this time period, in recognition of the growing diversity of health care provider settings, the JCAH also broadened its scope and, in the mid-1980s, became the Joint Commission for the Accreditation of Healthcare Organizations.

During the past few decades, government has also played an increasingly active role in regard to health care quality. With the funding of hospital facilities through the Hill-Burton Act and, more dramatically, with the enactment of Medicare and Medicaid in the 1960s, the federal government became a major source of health care dollars. Quality standards for participation in these federal programs were established. By the 1970s, due to the large federal deficit and increasing federal expenditures, cost containment and its relationship to quality emerged as key issues in health care (Thurow, 1985). Through the introduction of new initiatives such as utilization review, emphasis was placed on the elimination of the overuse of medical procedures; overuse occurs when the risks of the service outweigh the benefits (Chassin, 1991). The quest for quality became tied to the drive to contain costs. As the federal government makes decisions about future methods of financing and delivering care, critical questions of quality will need to be addressed.

Traditionally the focus of quality assurance programs has been on hospital care both because it is so expensive and because hospitals are more amenable to organizational constraint (Donabedian, 1985). Only recently have such programs been widely applied to ambulatory care. Yet, it is care outside of the hospital setting which is growing most rapidly; the quality issues specific to ambulatory and long-term care are likely to take center stage in coming years.

The Definition of Quality

According to *Webster's Seventh Collegiate Dictionary*, quality may be defined as "degree of excellence" or "superiority in kind." This concept of quality is certainly not unique to health care. As consumers we must assess the quality or degree of excellence of a broad range of products and services. Whether we are selecting a restaurant, purchasing an article of clothing, or making a reservation with an airline, consumers—like providers—use available information to try to identify the best quality product, relative to its cost. Yet in few cases is this assessment of quality more difficult than in regard to health care. Many have concluded that, given the complexity and diversity of health care services, there is not one quintessential definition of quality, but rather several legitimate definitions. Yet, planners, managers, and policy makers must work from some definition that is consensually accepted before quality of care can be assessed and promoted.

The Components of Quality

In defining quality, widely agreed upon components do, indeed, exist. Quality care aims to promote, preserve, and restore health; it is delivered in an appropriate setting, in a manner that is satisfying to patients. Quality refers to the extent to which the improvements in health status that are possible are, in fact, realized. It is not an assessment of the state of medical science but rather an assessment of the application of existing knowledge (Donabedian, 1980).

In trying to define and measure precisely what can be called quality care, there is a dilemma or tension between focusing on that which is unacceptable or poor quality care and that which is optimal or highest quality care. For many purposes, good quality care is seen as that which is free of incidence or evidence of poor quality; this is a standard which focuses on minimal requirements for quality. Such definitions are often employed because they are easy to use and measure. In other cases, the definition aims to characterize that which is an optimal or ideal standard of high quality. Often this sort of definition can be difficult to use in a meaningful way. Further, operationalizing the concept of "optimal care" may be elusive because there can be a wide gap between the actual level of quality that is achieved and the level of quality that is possible (Laffell & Berwick, 1992).

Competing Definitions. Health care quality can be defined in relationship to (1) the technical aspects of care, (2) the interpersonal relationship between practitioner and patient, or (3) the amenities of care. Research has indicated that one's role in the health care delivery process is likely to influence how one defines quality. Traditionally, quality of care has been defined by clinicians and primarily in terms of the technical delivery of care—"the application of the science and technology of medicine, and of the other health sciences, to the management of a personal health problem" (Donabedian, 1980, p. 4). From early in the development of medical practice in the U.S., and especially since the beginning of the Twentieth Century, society has delegated the establishment of quality standards to the medical profession (Caper, 1988). Even though most quality assurance efforts have been aimed at institutions (especially hospitals) the standards for these institutions have typically been developed by physicians. Peer review—a member of a profession being responsible for assessing the work of colleagues within that same profession—has been placed at the center of quality assessment and assurance efforts. The medical profession's peer review efforts have emphasized the scientific aspects of quality; appropriate drug prescription, postoperative infection rates, and accuracy of diagnosis are among the measures of quality that have been used.

In contrast to the physician's emphasis on the technical aspects of care, most patients tend to focus on interpersonal aspects of care in assessing quality. Lacking technical expertise, clients most typically judge the quality of technical care indirectly, by evidence of the practitioner's interest in, and concern for, the patient's health and welfare (Donabedian, 1985). Also, patients may assume technical competence, especially in university-affiliated settings, and thus assess quality in terms of the interpersonal relations and the amenities of care (Donabedian, 1985). Research has indicated that patients use such indicators as length of visit and the time spent in counseling as indicators of the physician's quality (Ware et al., 1978). Hospital quality is often assessed in regard to the care and concern demonstrated by the nursing staff, although consumers appear more likely to choose a hospital if it is affiliated with a medical school (Luft et al., 1990). Of note, different aspects of quality may be of greater or lesser importance to different types of inpatients (e.g., surgical versus medical). For example, in one study, nursing satisfaction mattered a good deal to medical patients, while pain control and room satisfaction were most important to surgical patients (Cleary et al., 1989).

Up until most recently, patients' assessments of the quality of care have typically been overlooked or dismissed as too subjective and unreliable. However, the importance of client satisfaction and of the interpersonal relationship to medical outcomes and overall quality must be considered. First, there is a significant body of research indicating that the quality of the patient–practitioner interaction may be a major contributor to treatment success, through greater patient compliance and return for care (Cleary et al., 1989; Danziger, 1986; Svarstad, 1986). Second, comparisons of the viewpoints of clients and practitioners suggest that there is a great deal of similarity between the two (Donabedian, 1980). Finally, the viewpoint of patients must be understood because client satisfaction is, in itself, an important component of the quality of care. Clients' assessments of quality guide them through the competitive market of health care providers. That quality must be defined by the consumer is a central principle of the movement toward Continuous Quality Improvement.

Administrators, nurses, and other health care personnel emphasize different aspects of quality from that stressed by physicians and patients (Donabedian, 1980). Administrators, for example, tend to focus on the amenities of care, perhaps because this is the area over which they have greatest control. Nurses present something of a middle ground—looking both to indicators of technical competence and interpersonal relations. As health care becomes more of a team effort, and as more nonphysician professionals begin to practice independently, the entire focus of quality of care must broaden (Lohr et al., 1988). Definitions of quality in health care can no longer be left solely to physicians and cannot emphasize the technical management of care to the exclusion of its other dimensions. Furthermore, whereas there has been a tendency to define quality in terms of the attributes of facilities and clinicians and of their behavior (Donabedian, 1980), there is growing recognition of the need to define quality in terms of the consequences of care.

Quality of Care vs. Quantity of Care. More care does not necessarily equal better care. Sometimes, however, quality of care may be confused with quantity of care; consumer ratings of quality do reflect, at least in part, how many services are received (Davies & Ware, 1988). Yet closer examination reveals that although there are times when more care does equal better care, there are also times when more is not better but is worse.

The precise relationship between inputs and benefits is not clear in health care. When care received is insufficient to bring about the realizable benefits in patient health and welfare, the care is clearly poor in quality because of quantitative inadequacy (Donabedian, 1980). Underuse occurs when the benefits of an intervention outweigh the risks, yet it is not used (Chassin, 1991). Such inadequacy is exemplified by an incomplete vaccination series; more care is needed before benefits can be realized. In under developed areas of third-world nations, and in some of our own nation's poorest communities, more is almost definitely better (Maxwell, 1985). In these cases, where the existing quality of care is low because of the inadequate quantity of care, improving quality necessarily costs money. Eventually, however, a point is reached where increments in services are unlikely to improve the quality of care. Care can become excessive and even harmful; such care is costlier but of equal or poorer quality.

There are many good examples of care that may be simply excessive or unnecessary. Annual pap smears (Benedet et al., 1985) and routine use of fetal sonograms in low-risk pregnancies (Luthy et al., 1987; McCusker et al., 1988) have been criticized on these grounds. Such care is excessive, but with little attendant risk. It is wasteful in that it is costlier but without corresponding increases in quality (Donabedian, 1980). Costs for unnecessary care are hard to justify; resources could be better spent elsewhere.

There are other situations where additional care is not only excessive or wasteful, but also harmful. According to some, routine chest and annual dental x-rays are examples of care which is more intensive and expensive yet of poorer quality. Such "ritualistic" care may appear to be of good quality, since additional services are being provided, but offers no real benefit to the patient and introduces potential danger to the patient's physical well-being.

Overuse of many procedures, including those that are highly invasive, has been well documented. In a study of Medicare patients it was found that 17% of angiographic procedures and 32% of carotid endarterectomies were inappropriately performed (Brook et al., 1990); both procedures are associated with a fair degree of risk. In another example, the use of the intensive care unit as a precautionary measure was found to lengthen hospital stays and result in lower patient satisfaction, without any improvement in medical outcomes (Eagle et al., 1990). Eliminating the use of these unnecessary and potentially detrimental medical procedures and practices has been the focus of many cost containment programs such as "second surgical opinions" and utilization review. Several studies have shown that some cost containment efforts do actually improve the quality of care. Despite concerns that the introduction of Medicare's prospective payment system in 1984 would result in patients being discharged "quicker and sicker," it was found that the processes of care in the hospital were improved and mortality rates were unchanged or lower (Rogers et al., 1990).

In addition to unnecessary and excessive care, sometimes care is produced inefficiently. In these cases, reducing the costs of care can be achieved, not by reducing the quantity or intensity of care, but rather by producing it more efficiently. Substitution of a nurse-practitioner for a physician or the use of ambulatory rather than in-patient surgery are two examples of strategies aimed at maintaining quality while reducing costs.

The risks, as well as financial costs, associated with treatment have often been ignored or glossed over by the medical community. When risks are not considered it is easy to mistake quantity for quality care. Alternatively, Thurow suggests that the medical community's traditional reliance on the principle of "do no harm" should be converted to one of "employ a treatment only when you are sure that it will make a noticeable improvement" (1985).

In contrasting the quality of care with the quantity of care, individual and societal needs should be distinguished. There may be times when the extra "unit" of health care cannot be justified in terms of the social good, even if the individual believes it can be justified in terms of personal good. In the debate over annual mammograms for young women, part of the discussion focuses on whether the yield from additional screening (identification of women with positive x-rays) is sufficient to justify the cost. The overall costs are weighed against the overall risks; but for the individual woman whose cancer has gone undetected, one would presume this cost benefit ratio to be different.

Donabedian's "unifying" model represents an effort to bring together the issues of costs, benefits, and risks in assessing the quality of care (1980). At first, benefits of care increase rapidly while the risks of such care remain small. As more services are added, however, the increase or marginal benefits become smaller while the increases or marginal risks become greater. Theoretically, the optimal point—perfect quality—is reached when the benefits minus the risks is greatest (see Figure 14.1). Increased monetary costs may eventually be accompanied by poorer quality, as risks begin to outweigh benefits. Since it is difficult to objectively identify the "optimal" point in Donabedian's model—where benefits are maximized and risks are minimized—individual consumers, providers, and policy makers must routinely make their own assessments of the tradeoff between quality and quantity of care. In trying to assess benefits relative to risk, one must consider the likelihood and magnitude of the potential benefits and risks. Unfortunately, our knowledge of risks and benefits tends to be very limited. We may have some sense of the risks and benefits to large groups, but possess extremely limited ability to project the risks and benefits in individual cases (and, therefore, medicine must often be practiced as an "art" and not a "science"). Our ability to make such assessments for groups or individuals is dependent on the availability of accurate information on the risks and benefits associated with procedures and treatments. Only by linking care with its consequences can informed decisions be made.

FIGURE 14.1 Some Hypothetical Relationships Germane to the Definition of the Quality of Medical Care

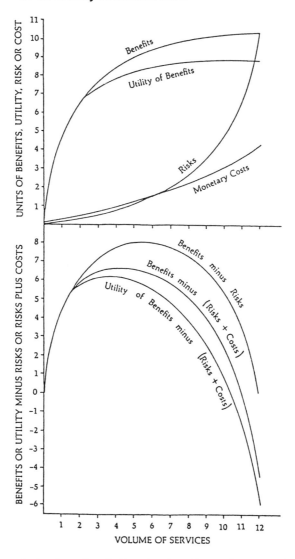

Used with permission from Avedis Donabedian, *The Definition of Quality and Approaches to Its Assessment*, Volume I of *Explorations in Quality Assessment and Monitoring*, Ann Arbor, MI: Health Administration Press, 1980, pg. 9.

The relationship between the quantity and quality of care is of critical importance to policy makers as they decide on the relative merits of various health care reimbursement systems. The incentive structure built in to traditional fee-for-service medicine encourages greater use of services; its quality risk is overuse. More recent reimbursement schema, which work on a capitated basis, run the risk of underuse; providers earn more by doing less. With changing economic incentives, we may experience new and different problems with the quality of care.

Measuring Quality

Structure, Process, and Outcome

Defining what is meant by the term "quality" is only the first step toward assessing the delivery of health care. Appropriate variables must be identified for assessing the degree to which quality is present. Structure, process, and outcome are the three most commonly defined approaches to gathering information on the presence or absence of the attributes that constitute or define quality. Structure has been defined as "the relatively stable characteristics of the providers of care, of the tools and resources they have at their disposal, and of the physical and organizational settings in which they work" (Donabedian, 1980, p. 81). We may view structure as those things that exist prior to, and separate from, interaction with patients. Structural indicators that are commonly used include board certification for physicians, nurse/bed ratios for hospitals, and availability of laboratory facilities for HMOs. Structure is an indirect measure of quality; it is useful to the degree that structure can be expected to influence the direct provision of care.

Process concerns the set of activities that go on between practitioners and patient. Process may be seen as the object of assessment. Process measures may be used to assess the quality of the technical management of care (e.g., was the appropriate laboratory test ordered?), as well as the interpersonal aspects of care (e.g., was the medical history taken in a sensitive and caring manner?). Process may be viewed as what is done to patients, while outcomes are what happens to them (Hogness, 1985). Outcome refers to a change in a patient's current and future health status that can be attributed to antecedent health care (Donabedian, 1980). Outcome measures include mortality rates, postoperative infection rates, and rates of rehospitalizations.

The Causal Model. Before we can use structure, process, or outcome measures to assess quality, it is important that we understand something about the relationship among all three. The underlying *causal model* in most quality assessments is that structure influences the process of care, which has an impact on the outcome of care. In other words, the basis for the judgement of quality is what is known about the relationship between the characteristics of the structure and processes of the care that is delivered and their subsequent impact on the health and welfare of individuals and of society. Most definitions of quality assume that the application of the appropriate process of care will maximize patient outcomes (Lohr et al., 1988). However, the validity, or justifiability, of this inference must be established; there is considerable disagreement about cause and effect in health care.

Scientific research methods, especially those of program evaluation and medical research, are used to establish the links between particular structures and processes and the desired outcomes. Scientific methods are used to test whether changes in health status (outcome) are really the result of the care given. Are board-certified physicians (structure) more likely to make appropriate use of laboratory tests (process)? And does the appropriate utilization of laboratory tests have an impact on patient recovery (outcome)? Do second surgical opinion programs (structure) influence the use of surgery (process)? And does this have an impact on patient health (outcome)? Once the relationships between structure, process, and outcome are established, we can focus on one area of measurement and have greater confidence that it is, in fact, providing a good indicator of quality.

"Structure . . . is relevant to quality in that it increases or decreases the probability of good performance" (Donabedian, 1980, p. 82) Despite the fact that structure has been a commonly used indicator of quality, there is only limited information about the relationship between structure and performance. There is some evidence, for example, that large urban teaching hospitals may provide better medical care than smaller, rural hospitals (Keeler et al., 1992). In contrast, one study found that larger hospitals—once we control for the volume of surgery—are associated with poorer surgical outcomes (Luft, 1980). Overall, however, we know relatively little about when and how structural indicators (e.g., board certification for physicians or bachelor's degrees for nurses) influence the processes and outcomes of care. Structure is, at best, a crude measure of quality since it can only address general tendencies. Information on structural indicators are, however, generally easy and inexpensive to access and measure, whereas information on the process and outcomes of care are often unavailable, incomplete, or expensive. Therefore, in those cases where there is sufficient information to link structural characteristics with health care outcomes, structure can provide an important measure of quality in health care.

As already noted, process is the most direct measure of quality. A great virtue of process evaluation lies in the broad clinician involvement and education which is a consequence and may subsequently result in improved practices (Blum, 1974). Process measures tend to be more timely than outcome measures. But their validity as a measure is limited to the extent that their relationship to outcomes has been well established. When the link between process and outcome has been validated, process indicators become an important tool for assessing and assuring quality in a direct and timely fashion. Since we know that immunizations are critical to the promotion of children's health, we know that completed immunization series (or lack of completion) provide a valid process indicator for assessing the quality of pediatric practice.

Too often what is described as high quality care has not been demonstrated to have much of an impact on the health status of the patients. The Congressional Office of Technology Assessment has estimated that only 10 to 20% of clinician practices are supported by randomized controlled trials (Eddy & Billings, 1988). In other words, for most health care practices there is a lack of scientific evidence of the efficacy of the treatment. For example, in a study in which process and outcome criteria were separately applied for evaluating the quality of hypertension care, there was no statistically significant association detected between process and outcome (Nobrega et al., 1977). Despite low physician compliance with established criteria, the outcome of care among these hypertensive patients was rather good. This reminds us that the use of process criteria, in the absence of a scientifically tested causal model, can result in the perpetuation of ineffective practice.

While the validity of elements of process depends on the contribution of process to outcome, outcomes tend to be inherently valid since change in health status and patient well-being is the ultimate goal of health care. When high-quality care is delivered, we expect improvement in such outcomes as mortality, morbidity, or social functioning. But before outcomes are used to make inferences about the quality of care, it is necessary to establish that the outcomes can be attributed to that care. Intervening factors must be ruled out; were the changes in health really the result of the care that is provided? Would the improvement in the patient's health have occurred without the treatment? Conversely, poor outcomes must not be simplistically attributed solely to current failures of the health care organization or process (Blum, 1974).

The release of hospital-based mortality rates by the federal government's Health Care Financing Administration (HCFA) has been criticized on these grounds; many argue that there is insufficient evidence to attribute the mortality to poor hospital performance. Rather, differences in the patient mix (one aspect of structure) may be the reason for many of these differences. Although HCFA had acknowledged that "preventable deaths" would be a more valid indicator of quality of care (Roper & Hackbarth, 1988), they began "to measure the performance of individual physicians by seeing how well their patients do" (*NY Times,* 1988, p. 1). However, in 1993, when Bruce Vladeck was appointed administrator of HCFA, he decided to withhold the data because there was "something lacking in the methodology" (*Medicine and Health*, 1993). This debate reminds us that in the absence of strong scientific evidence, the use of health outcomes, such as mortality, as an indicator of quality of care, may be misleading.

Formulation of Criteria and Standards

Whether one decides to approach the assessment of quality via indices concerning structure, process, or outcome, specific criteria or standards must be formulated. Before we can assess or monitor the quality of care, the abstract construct of quality must be translated into concrete variables and those variables must be made measurable or "operationalized." Differences in structure, process, or outcomes across practitioners, institutions or regions do not, in and of themselves, indicate the appropriate level or highest quality of care. Rather these standards must be established through scientific study or consensus.

Measurement is critical to the assessment and improvement of quality for it is through measurement that we can make precise comparisons of benefits and risks. In selecting appropriate quality measures, note that no single indicator can capture the entire concept of quality or even any major component of it. Indeed, there may be certain aspects of quality that are all but impossible to measure. It is, therefore, superior to use multiple operational definitions or measures that can account for the broadest understanding of quality. For example, in a study comparing costs and benefits of hospice and conventional care for terminally ill cancer patients, a broad range of criteria and measures had to be developed, including measures of pain, symptoms, activities of daily living, as well as patient and family satisfaction (Kane et al., 1984). Any single measure would have provided an incomplete and misleading assessment of the quality of care provided.

Furthermore, criteria and standards change over time; this is integral to the philosophy of quality improvement. Whereas an "optimal"—and, therefore, set—level of quality was implicit to earlier work in the field of quality assurance, more recent activities have stressed a changing standard.

In conducting quality assessment activities, the criteria or measures that are selected must be both valid and reliable. Reliability concerns the accuracy of observed score; how well does the measure reflect the true score? Reliable measures do not fluctuate randomly from one moment to the next; this is called test-retest reliability. Reliable measures yield the same results regardless of who is making the rating; this is called inter-rater reliability. Mortality data tends to be highly reliable, whereas psychiatric and social assessments do not.

The validity of a measure concerns how well it really reflects the concept being assessed. A reliable measure is not necessarily a valid one; although mortality data are considered highly reliable, they may be an invalid indicator of quality of care. The validity of a measure may be considered in terms of its correlation or convergence with other measures of the same concept; if several different measures of the same concept all lead to the same conclusions we can have greater confidence that the individual measures are valid. If we were trying to rate physician performance we might include a review of lab tests ordered, an assessment of the medical histories taken, and a judgement of quality of the medical record; if all three measures led to the same conclusion about the physician's performance we would have greater confidence about the validity of any one measure. Validity of measures may also be considered in terms of their ability to distinguish between cases that are known to differ and in terms of their predictive power.

The scientific validity of a measure is based on a demonstrated causal relationship, as described above. However, in the absence of a scientifically demonstrated relationship "normative validity" is often substituted. Normative validity rests on the presence of professional consensus (e.g., agreement among physicians), so it could also be called consensual validity (Donabedian, 1980). In conducting an assessment of the quality of care, process elements are often used when there is general agreement that certain procedures are appropriate for certain situations, even though there is no "scientific proof" of appropriateness (Donabedian, 1980). The problem with relying on measures that have normative validity, as compared to scientific validity, is that it can lead to the perpetuation of ineffective process. Process measures, which typically possess normative or consensual validity, evaluate conformity to a given standard of performance but do not evaluate the adequacy of the standards themselves (Flood & Scott, 1978).

As a result of the lack of information linking process to outcomes, there is also a tendency to apply the criterion of potential benefit. In this framework a practice is considered appropriate if it *might* have benefit (Eddy & Billings, 1988). The appeal of the criterion of potential benefit's appeal is that it is easy to apply and it deals smoothly with the uncertainty that surrounds many practices. As an example, rather than limit the use of fetal monitors to high-risk deliveries, in some hospitals all pregnancies are monitored since it can be difficult to assess risk and there may be some rare cases where otherwise unidentified problems would be found. Unfortunately, the criterion of potential benefit translates easily into "when in doubt, do it."

Explicit or implicit criteria may be used in operationalizing a variable. Implicit criteria include unguided, individual judgments of quality or unstructured observations. Quality assessments—particularly peer reviews—often rely on the implicit judgement of physicians who may review a medical record or observe a patient encounter and, without any stated guidelines, make an assessment of quality. This can be contrasted with explicit criteria, which are preformulated and provide the rater with clear guidance in making an assessment. In some cases the criteria may fall in between the two extremes; record review with guidance provides an example of guided or structured implicit criteria (Donabedian, 1985).

Sources of Information

In trying to measure and promote the quality of health care, one can use existing, administrative records or data may be gathered through interviews, observations, or record review. Data sources and collection methods may be compared in terms of costs, acceptability, reliability, and validity (Gerbert, 1988). Generally, the method becomes more expensive and less feasible if it requires information that is not routinely collected. On the other hand, routinely gathered data may not have quality assessment as its primary focus; the available information may be only an indirect and incomplete measure of quality.

Administrative Data and Computerized Systems. Administrative data on health care institutions and providers are regularly compiled by a range of public and not-for-profit agencies and are often available in computerized form. Such administrative data typically represent structural indicators of quality. These measures—number of beds, number of RNs, number of board-certified surgeons—have become a routine part of accreditation and certification procedures (discussed in greater detail below).

Routinely collected data on insurance claims, drug prescriptions, and malpractice suits may provide information on the process of care. Their disadvantage is that quality can be measured only in relatively narrow terms. Yet, these data—if properly organized—can permit relatively inexpensive, large scale quality assessment activities. Recognizing the potential benefit of such a system of information, a General Accounting Office (GAO) report suggested that "a centralized medical malpractice information system would help identify recurring problems, including problems with individual medical care providers, and focus attention on needed corrective and preventive actions" (Baines, 1987). The National Practitioner Data Bank, operated by the Department of Health and Human Services, was opened in 1990. Insurance companies must report information on medical malpractice payments to the Data Bank. Similarly, health care organizations, state medical and dental boards and professional societies are required to report adverse professional actions (such as actions against a practitioner's license). It is too early to assess this national data bank as a source of information regarding the quality of care.

The Medical Record. Medical records are the most commonly used source of information on the quality of the process of care. Record review or chart audit have been an integral part of many quality assurance and cost containment programs, such as utilization review. Access is the most attractive characteristic of the medical record. The information is routinely gathered; using it for quality assessment involves limited additional expense or time.

Ideally, the medical record provides information on patient symptoms, on the tests and procedures that were undertaken, and on the patient's progress. The medical record should provide an accurate and detailed report of the medical process. Unfortunately, in reality, medical records rarely reach the ideal standard. They tend to be incomplete. Medical record keeping is local and uses practice-specific terminology; this fragmentation means that information on diagnosis, treatment, and outcomes cannot be linked across settings (Lohr et al., 1988). Problems with the medical record are especially acute in ambulatory care settings where practitioners are less likely to be subject to institutional constraints. Rating the process of care based on the medical record can be questionable given the incomplete nature of reporting practice.

In the case of patients who have died, autopsy reports have been traditionally used to help improve medical practice and assess the quality of care. Was the diagnosis correct? Is there indication that medical practice contributed to the cause of death? In recent years, however, the rate of autopsy has dropped and information from those that are performed is not routinely fed back to physicians (Landefeld & Goldman, 1989). As a result, an important source of information on the quality of care may be lost.

Observations of Process. Another method of obtaining data on the process of care is via direct observation. Several studies have been undertaken to observe, and in some cases videotape, the physician–patient interaction. Since the observation allows actual viewing of the process of care, and the videotape provides a record of that process, it has often been assumed that this method would provide a perfect report of the care provided. Instead, videotaped observations have been found to be difficult to standardize, time-consuming, and costly (Gerbert et al., 1988). Of even greater importance, even if such time and cost concerns were eliminated, recent studies have indicated that the "videotaped observation does not adequately capture the content of visits to the physician in areas of medication regimen, patient signs and symptoms, tests and treatments recommended, and patient education" (Gerbert et al., 1988, p. 530). Finally, there has been limited discussion about the degree to which observation biases the process of care. That is, does a provider (and a patient) change his or her practice style (behavior) when under observation?

Patient and Practitioner Interviews. In addition to chart or record audit and direct observation, information may be obtained by directly interviewing providers and patients. The provider is probably the most accurate source of reported information regarding the process of care (Gerbert et al., 1988). But physician interviews are a very expensive source of information and may not be a good source of information on the nontechnical aspects of care. In contrast, getting information from consumers of care may be no more expensive and, under many circumstances, is less expensive than traditional sources, such as the medical record (Davies & Ware, 1988).

There is good evidence that the information reported by patients is valid and reliable. The consumer seems to be able to distinguish poor quality from high-quality care, especially for common problems. Most crucially, the consumer is probably in the best position to rate the interpersonal aspects of care. Despite these strengths, information on patient satisfaction has typically been gathered for marketing purposes, and "is seldom used as a basis for developing health care protocols or making changes to improve the quality of care" (Prehn et al., 1989, p. 74).

Methods of Assessment

Researchers in the area of quality assessment have developed a broad range of techniques and methods for conducting quality assessments. Overall, methods may be characterized in terms of those that assess the quality of care relative to a positive standard (i.e., what should have been done or what should have occurred) and those that assess it relative to a negative standard (i.e., what should not have been done or what should not have occurred). In regard to the former, we are trying to define and measure good quality care while in the latter we are looking for evidence of poor quality care. Generally it is agreed that it is easier to define and identify cases of poor quality than high quality. For example, we can look for interventions that are either obsolete or so rarely indicated that their mere use is reason enough to question the quality of care (Donabedian, 1985). Prescription patterns can be especially useful after drugs that are ineffective or hazardous have been identified.

Assessments which focus on unnecessary or inappropriate care can be conducted prospectively (that is, before care is provided) or retrospectively (after care is provided). For example, if we are interested in using unnecessary surgical procedures as an indicator of poor quality of care, second surgical opinions would provide a prospective means of approach (how often does the second opinion contradict the first physician's recommendation?). Tissue analysis provides a retrospective method of using the same indicator, unnecessary surgery (how often does the tissue analysis indicate that a healthy organ was removed?). Assessments which have focused on the use of inappropriate techniques and interventions have found poor quality of care to be concentrated; that is, a very small percentage of physicians tend to account for a large proportion of poor quality care delivered (Donabedian, 1985).

Utilization review is another example of quality assessment and assurance that identifies cases of poor quality or inappropriate care. Inappropriate hospital utilization may arise from inappropriate admissions, delayed discharges, or extra days during which services are not fully provided (Donabedian, 1985). Utilization review tends to emphasize the "overstay," and not the "understay" as an indicator of poor quality.

Williamson's health accounting method focus on "achievable benefits" rather than process indicators of quality care (Donabedian, 1985). Acceptable outcome standards are set for patient groups and, if there are substantial failures, corrective action is to be taken. Stress is placed on those areas of care which are most likely deficient and most amenable to change.

"Prospective Outcome Analysis" is another method, or system, which has been suggested for using outcomes to assess quality (Blum, 1974). It also sets positive standards for overall outcomes. Aimed at institutional self-assessment as a means of quality assurance, a medically expert committee selects the most important conditions to be studied based on such criteria as prevalence, cost, and danger and establishes standards or best expectations of specified outcomes for selected conditions. If the outcomes on a sample of cases are significantly worse than expected the committee then does a critical analysis of each case with a poor outcome. The institution continues to check outcomes against its standards until the desired outcome is reached.

The thrust of Continuous Quality Improvement is to integrate methods of measurement and assessment with those of change and improvement; CQI is based on the concepts of Total Quality Management (TQM). The Deming Cycle—plan, do, check, act, and analyze—is named for the creator of TQM (Gabor, 1990). As applied to health care quality, TQM emphasizes the results of care from the patient's point of view (Laffell & Berwick, 1992). CQI uses reliable statistical methods to raise the norm of performance, rather than to weed out "bad apples" (Joint Commission, 1991). The goal is to obtain more uniform, or predictable, results through the analysis of process (Gabor, 1990).

Promoting Quality: Assurance and Improvement

Measuring or assessing the quality of care does not, unfortunately, result in immediate improvements in that care. Simply defining what is meant by "high-quality" care does not guarantee its implementation. Practice guidelines are established, yet little attention is paid to helping practitioners implement those guidelines (Laffell & Berwick, 1992). Quality promotion activities—including assurance and improvement—are intended to translate the concepts and findings of quality assessment into programs that will promote the delivery of higher-quality care. The emphasis shifts from quality measurement to quality control and improvement.

Efforts to encourage the delivery of high-quality care take place at the local and at the national level. They are geared both at individuals and at institutions. Currently, professional associations, health care institutions and organizations, government, private external quality review organizations, and group purchasers of care all play a role in trying to promote quality care.

Organizational Considerations in Promoting Quality

In order to assure good quality care, we need to know something about changing or modifying the behaviors of providers and the organizations in which they practice. And organizational change creates strains and tensions; it raises conflict between the norms of professional freedom and bureaucratic autonomy (Hetherington, 1982).

Professional autonomy may represent one of the most important impediments to health institutions becoming more fully accountable for the care they provide. Physicians have traditionally operated as free agents within the hospital structure.

As quality assurance activities have grown, the hospital (as well as other health care organizations) has imposed new restrictions and requirements upon physicians. Resistance is an expected by-product of these changes. In recent years, as the accountability obligations of health institutions have been formalized, the potential for conflict between institutional goals of self-regulation and the autonomy requirements of clinicians has grown.

Despite resistance and the obstacles posed by the tradition of autonomy, it is possible to improve the quality of care and to hold clinicians and organizations accountable for the care given. Even within the context of a change-resistant environment, we know a great deal about the ways in which health care delivery can be shaped or modified. For example, we know that quality promotion activities are more likely to succeed when professionals have played an active role in developing and administering the regulations. There is also evidence to suggest that to change physician behavior, information must come from a credible source (e.g., a professional organization) and should be backed with financial incentives (Ball, 1988). Furthermore, it is easier to change behavior when there is considerable consensus about what constitutes quality care. In one study, researchers attributed the success of an on-site educational program to reduce inappropriate use of x-ray pelvimetry to the considerable consensus surrounding the use of this procedure (Chassin & McCue, 1986). Institutional commitment to change may also play a role in modifying providers' behaviors. Slenker et al. (1985) looked at the impact of establishing procedural guidelines for physicians, nurses, and allied health professionals in the diagnosis and treatment of cancer. Factors contributing to program success were hospital commitment to the program, ready availability of guidelines, and mandatory participation in the educational program.

Within the CQI framework, organizational change must begin with commitment at the very top of the organization (Berwick, 1988). There is recognition that quality improvement requires resources and that the methods of quality measurement must be taught and learned. Finally, the proponents of quality improvement argue that traditional assurance methods, which attempt to identify and discipline an unruly few, are antithetical to true improvement, which must emphasize change in the overall system and its processes. In this model, fear must be replaced by shared commitment and trust.

Quality Assurance Mechanisms

Licensing, accreditation, and certification, three general approaches to quality assurance, are similar in that they assess an individual's or institution's ability to provide quality care on the basis of meeting established criteria at a particular time. The underlying assumption of these approaches is that education and current knowledge, as measured by a written examination, are good predictors of future performance. Or, in the case of health care organizations, that the presence of certain equipment, personnel, and organizational arrangements promises the delivery of high-quality care over an extended period of time. In the past, these approaches aimed to ensure quality by guaranteeing the presence of certain fundamental, structural characteristics of the institution or individual.

In contrast, a number of other approaches have attempted to promote quality by reviewing specific instances of provider-patient interaction. These approaches, which have been used by Peer Review Organizations and are typified in malpractice litigation, tend to focus on the processes and outcomes of care.

Licensing. Licensing may be distinguished from all other quality assurance activities because licensing is backed by the force of law. Under the United States Constitution the states have been empowered to license both individuals and institutions. That is, the states are permitted to restrict certain activities (e.g., the performance of surgery or a dental exam) to those individuals and institutions it has determined to possess acceptable standards. Numerous health professions and occupations are currently licensed by one or more states, as are a broad array of health care facilities.

In licensing individuals, the state enters into a compact with a professional group. The professional group assumes responsibility for controlling the quality of work provided, while the state grants the professional group the right to control entry into the professional group, and in many cases, to define the content of that work. Some of the occupations that are licensed by all states include medicine, dentistry, pharmacy, nursing, nursing home administration, and podiatry. In some states occupations such as laboratory technicians, midwives, and psychologists are also licensed. Generally, the profession (e.g., nursing) establishes standards based on educational attainment, experience, and performance on a written exam. Once a license is granted, it is traditionally valid for life; in the absence of egregious conduct licenses are rarely suspended or revoked.

The use of licensure as a method of ensuring quality is a source of great controversy. There is ample evidence that rather than protecting the public, licensure protects the professional group and its members from competition and public scrutiny. Licensing makes it difficult to change occupations within the health care sector, or to move from one state to another. For example, as a result of licensing restrictions, the most qualified labor-room nurse may not be able to take responsibility for a baby's delivery. Most significantly, there is little evidence to indicate that the criteria used in licensing actually predict the quality of care to be delivered.

Even if the criteria used for licensing were valid, it is unreasonable to expect that they would be valid throughout a person's life. In a dynamic field, knowledge at the time of graduation from medical school is unlikely to be a good indicator of knowledge 20 years later. As a result, licensing for life is giving way to periodic reevaluation.

The issues posed by licensing are especially complicated in the case of physicians. Physicians are in an unusual professional position; they do not merely control their own work but are also the dominant professional group throughout the health care arena (Freidson, 1970). This position of professional dominance has effectively shielded doctors from public scrutiny and accountability. There is a growing belief that the public has not been well served by this isolation.

One area of "self-policing" that has received considerable attention is the disciplinary actions of the state medical boards that are responsible for licensure. Although increasing in number, such disciplinary actions continue to be the exception. One study indicated that the number of reprimands and censures have grown. Revocations and suspensions of licenses, however, remain relatively constant, despite an increase in the number of practicing physicians (Kusserow et al., 1987). That is, the rate of suspending licenses has actually decreased. In this study it was also found that most reports to state medical boards are provided by consumers and law enforcement agencies and not by health care professionals, hospitals, or peer review organizations.

Licensing of facilities is usually accomplished directly by a state agency, for example, the state health department. All states license hospitals (short and long stay, general and/or psychiatric), nursing homes, and pharmacies; many also license such facilities as homes for the mentally ill or developmentally disabled (Wilson & Neuhauser, 1987). Certain services—such as ambulances and home health care—are also licensed in some states. Institutional licenses may be granted for a period of one or more years. The criteria for licensing typically emphasize structural elements like bed/nurse ratios and the presence of appropriate equipment. Licensing boards for institutions tend to be less completely dominated by providers from the regulated institution than for those of individuals.

Accreditation and Certification. Although licensing is critical to understanding the role of government in the assurance of quality, volunteerism has long characterized the primary approach to quality assurance in health care (Luke & Modrow, 1983). Voluntary self-regulation is reflected in both accrediting bodies such as the JCAHO and in professional certification boards. Accreditation is limited to institutions, while certification applies to individuals.

The basic principles of accreditation are similar to those of licensure; it is assumed that if the institution meets certain standards of physical and organizational structure, then good quality care will be delivered at that time and will continue into the future. In the case of accreditation, groups of like institutions or organizations with mutual interests come together to set up an organization, establish standards and proceed to inspect and "accredit" themselves on a periodic basis. Although accreditation is not a legal procedure, there are often strong legal and financial incentives for undergoing accreditation. For example, state education departments will not recognize diplomas from medical schools that are not accredited.

The JCAHO is, perhaps, the oldest and best known of the accrediting bodies in health care. As already noted, recent changes in the Joint Commission's accrediting standards are reflective of shifts in the approach to quality taken throughout the field. Traditionally reliant on minimal structural standards, in 1966 JCAH's Board of Commissioners voted to rewrite the standards to raise them from "minimal essential" to "optimal achievable" standards and, in 1975, numerical requirements for audit were established to ensure optimal care (Shanahan, 1983). In 1979, new standards were issued which eliminated the numerical audit requirement and directed hospitals to develop a hospital-wide program that integrated all quality assurance activities (Roberts, 1987). In 1987, the Joint Commission embarked on its Agenda for Change, which represented a refocusing of its own standards and greater emphasis on quality improvement through better measures and a system of feedback. In its 1992 Accreditation Manual for Hospitals, the Quality Assurance chapter was renamed Quality Assessment and Improvement, symbolizing the JCAHO's full adoption of the CQI model (Joint Commission, 1991).

Accreditation also plays a critical role in medical education. Medical schools are accredited by the Liaison Committee on Medical Education. The American Medical Association and the Association of American Medical Colleges are equally represented on the committee. Separate accrediting bodies review postgraduate medical education and accredit residency programs. Training for other health care occupations also takes place in accredited programs or schools; accreditation is carried out by a range of boards and agencies representing such fields as dentistry, medical technology, and health services administration.

Certification, like accreditation, represents a form of voluntary self-regulation. And although certification is not backed by law, there are incentives which encourage individual practitioners to seek certification. For example, some third-party payers will only reimburse visits to certified social workers. Of great consequence, most hospitals limit privileges to board-certified specialties. Certification uses standards of education, experience, and achievement on examinations to determine qualification.

A great diversity of health care occupations have certifying bodies. In nursing alone, there are 23 different organizations which offer certification in nursing or one of its subspecialties (Scofield, 1988). These include the American Nurses Association, the Oncology Nursing Certification Corporation, and the Association of Operating Room Nurses.

PSROs and PROs. Professional Standard Review Organizations (PSROs) were established by the 1972 amendments to the Social Security Act. They represented a major step toward institutionalizing peer review of physician care and the quality of care provided outside of the hospital setting. The purpose of the law was to involve local practicing physicians in the ongoing review and evaluation of health services covered by Medicare, Medicaid, or the Maternal and Child Health Programs of the Department of Health and Human Services. PSROs were charged with the dual role of quality assurance and utilization review (which had previously been the function of medical staff review committees). Most PSRO activity focused on utilization review, rather than overall quality assurance, and cost containment became the hallmark of the PSRO's own measure of success. Established in 195 geographic areas, the efficacy of PSROs as a tool for quality assurance was limited by physician protectionism, lack of concern for the nontechnical aspects of care, and overemphasis on cost containment.

Peer Review Organizations (PROs) went into operation in 1984, as the successor to the PSROs. Unlike PSROs, PROs review only Medicare; Medicaid review was now left to the states. PROs are limited to one per state. Physician-based organizations were given a prominent role in the control of the PROs. Under the PRO system, disciplinary procedures are simplified and review functions cannot be delegated to hospitals. In 1987, PROs were also given responsibility for reviewing HMOs participating in the Medicare program (U.S. GAO, 1991).

PROs are awarded fixed-price contracts that specify, in numerical terms, the results to be achieved. For example, some of the PROs' objectives focus on reducing inappropriate admissions, while others focus on reducing admissions overall. Because of the specific nature of the objectives, PROs were given an increased incentive to actually try to change physician behavior. The results, however, have thus far been disappointing. A review of medical records for hospitalized Medicare patients found that approximately 18% of them had received below standard care; yet the PRO had found only 6.3% (Rubin et al., 1992). Further, there has been limited follow through in cases where the PROs have identified weaknesses and made recommendations; for example, the General Accounting Office found that HCFA was unwilling to enforce compliance with the PRO recommendations for HMOs (U.S. GAO, 1991).

Malpractice Litigation. Malpractice litigation may also be seen as an approach to quality assurance. Malpractice focuses on extreme cases of poor quality care, rather than trying to assure ongoing high standards of care. Using malpractice as a tool for quality assurance shifts the focus away from frequent but low cost errors, toward infrequent and high cost ones. Malpractice is not an effective tool for trying to control the over prescription of antibiotic drugs, for example, since the damages accrued to any one individual are generally not of the magnitude to instigate a legal suit.

Recent studies have suggested that malpractice litigation may not be an effective tool for identifying problems in the quality of health care. In reviewing a random sample of patients discharged in New York State in 1984, researchers found that in approximately 1% of the cases there was evidence of an adverse event which was caused by negligence (Localio et al., 1991). Yet, malpractice claims were filed in few of these cases; the researchers estimate that only 1.5% of negligent events lead to claims. Given the relative rarity of malpractice claims, only very incompetent physicians could be identified in this way (Rolph et al., 1991).

Despite empirical evidence suggesting that malpractice claims are relatively infrequent, malpractice litigation is seen as a growing problem in the United States, which has threatened the solvency of some institutions and the practice of some physicians. It is not clear, however, the degree to which the malpractice "crisis" is a function of a more litigious society, dishonest practices by insurance companies, declining patient-provider relations, or the unwillingness of the medical profession to engage in effective quality control, especially in regard to disciplining those physicians responsible for a significant share of practice error.

A number of solutions to the malpractice crisis are currently being tested. These include tort reforms which have been implemented in several states. For example, Virginia gives immunity to providers who render emergency care without pay (Burda, 1987). New York State has tried to limit malpractice premiums and has considered establishing a "medical indemnity fund" for future medical expenses over $100,000 (Fuchsberg, 1988). Other suggestions have included upper limits on the dollar amount that can be awarded for pain and suffering and shorter statutes of limitations. Both consumer and attorney groups have fought such restrictions on malpractice litigation, arguing that tort reform begs the question of reducing the incidence of malpractice.

By contrast, the use of "early warning systems" to identify potentially compensable hospital events has proven to be a successful method of averting liability claims. Such systems have helped hospitals to identifying recurring problems and to diffuse some situations (Burda, 1986).

As already noted, the federal government has become involved in the malpractice debate through the establishment of the National Practitioner Data Bank under the Health Care Quality Improvement Act of 1986. Congress enacted this legislation in order (1) to moderate the incidence of malpractice, (2) to allow the medical community to demonstrate new willingness to weed out incompetents, and to (3) improve the base of timely and accurate information on medical malpractice (Waxman, 1987). The act requires hospitals to request information from the Data Bank whenever they are hiring, granting privileges, or conducting periodic reviews of a practitioner (U.S. GAO, 1992). The use of a mandatory, national data bank should help close the loopholes that permitted interstate movement and continued participation in Medicaid and Medicare for practitioners who had been disciplined in a particular state or institution.

Economic Approaches. Third-party payers have also initiated a number of activities which may be viewed as approaches to quality assurance. Although such activities are often primarily concerned with cost containment, they serve a quality assurance function to the degree that they reduce unnecessary or excessive use of care. Second surgical opinion programs, preadmission review, and DRGs all aim to reduce costs by eliminating unnecessary or excessive care. In addition to third-party payers, employers and unions who must foot the bill for insurance premiums have also begun playing a role in this dual area of cost containment/ quality assurance.

Unfortunately, there is limited reason to be optimistic about the potential of these cost containment efforts to enhance quality. Economic solutions seem to impact as much on appropriate care as they do on inappropriate care (Brook, 1988). Evidence from the RAND Health Insurance Experiment, suggests that cost sharing for inpatient and outpatient care reduces the use of effective and presumably needed services about as much as it lowers the use of ineffective or unnecessary services (Lohr et al., 1988). Before cost containment efforts can be expected to have a positive impact on quality, economic solutions must be coupled with medical solutions. Some argue that medicine must begin to be codified (in what Brook has termed a "gourmet cookbook") and physicians must be rewarded for appropriate medical practice (Brook, 1988). Recent history suggests, however, that those who pay for care, whether governmental or private, may be more interested in cost containment than in quality assurance (Lohr et al., 1988). There is growing debate about whether financial incentives to shift or control expenditure will lead to the under provision or under use of needed and appropriate services and, in turn, to adverse effects on health outcomes and patient well-being (Lohr et al, 1988).

The Promise of Quality Improvement

This chapter has already reviewed many of the essential concepts presented by the adherents of Total Quality Management, or as it is also known, Continuous Quality Improvement. To the degree that this framework truly becomes the modal approach to quality in health care we may see some dramatic shifts in the activities surrounding quality promotion.

There are six principal ideas which drive this framework (Gabor, 1990). First, quality should be defined by the consumer. Second, variation in the process of care must be understood and reduced. Next, top management must be committed to improvement. The fourth principle states that change and improvement must be continuous; it must be all encompassing and involve all members of the organization. Fifth, in order to succeed, training and education of all employees must be ongoing. Finally, trying to measure the contribution of individual employees is usually destructive.

Whereas the quality assurance methods discussed above—such as licensure or certification—have relied on set minimal standards, CQI encourages change and growth. Whereas PROs have relied on punitive actions to enforce their recommendations, CQI requires collaboration, cooperation, and compromise. If CQI were to fulfill its promise, the delivery of high-quality care would be the central goal of all players in the health care field. The use of sophisticated methods of measurement and statistical analyses would be the everyday tool of managers, who would feed information back to practitioners in order to help them enhance their manner of care. The promise made by CQI is noble; its ability to transform the health care delivery system is still uncertain.

References

Baines, D. P., "DOD Health Care." Statement given by the General Accounting Office before the U.S. House of Representatives Subcommittee on Military Personnel and Compensation, July 21, 1987.

Ball, J. R., "Physician Payment: Why Money Doesn't Buy Quality." Presentation made at the Association for Health Services Research. San Francisco, CA: June 27, 1988.

Benedet, J. L. et al., "Cervical Cancer Screening: Who Needs a Pap Test? How Often?" *Postgraduate Medicine, 78*, 8, 1985.

Berwick, D. M., "Quality Assurance and Measurement Principles: The Perspective of One Health Maintenance Organization." in Hughes, E. F. X. (Ed.), *Perspectives of Quality in American Health Care*. Washington, DC: McGraw-Hill's Healthcare Information Center, 1988.

Blum, H. L., "Evaluating Health Care." *Medical Care, 12*, 12, 1974.

Brook, R. H., "Physician Payment: Why Money Doesn't Buy Quality." Presentation made at the Association for Health Services Research. San Francisco, CA: June 27, 1988.

Brook, R. H., "Quality—Can We Measure It?" *New England Journal of Medicine, 296*, 3, 1977.

Brook, R. H. et al., "Predicting the appropriate use of carotid endarterectomy, upper gastrointestinal endoscopy and coronary angiography." *New England Journal of Medicine, 323*, 17, 1990.

Burda, D., "Law." *Hospitals*, May 20, 1986.

Burda, D., "New Tests Reform." *Hospitals, 61*, 8, 1987.

Caper, P., "Defining Quality in Medical Care." *Health Affairs, 7*, 1, 1988.

Chassin, M. R., "Quality of Care—time to act." *Journal of the American Medical Association, 266*, 24, 1991.

Chassin, M. R., & McCue, S. M., "A Randomized Trial of Medical Quality Assurance." *Journal of the American Medical* Association, *256*, 8, 1986.

Christoffel, T., "Medical Care Evaluation: An Old Idea." *Journal of Medical Education, 51*, 2, 1976.

Cleary, P. D. et al., "Patient assessments of hospital care" *Quality Review Bulletin, 15*, 6, 1989.

Danziger, S. K., "The Use of Expertise in Doctor-Patient Encounters During Pregnancy." In Conrad P. & Kern R. (Eds.), *The Sociology of Health and Illness*, New York: St. Martin's Press, 1986.

Davies, A. R., & Ware, J. E., Jr., "Involving Consumers in Quality of Care Assessment." *Health Affairs, 7*, 1, 1988.

Donabedian, A., *Explorations in Quality Assessment and Monitoring (Volume I): The Definition of Quality and Approaches to its Assessment*. Ann Arbor, MI: Health Administration Press, 1980.

Donabedian, A., *Explorations in Quality Assessment and Monitoring (Volume III): The Methods and Findings of Quality Assessment and Monitoring*. Ann Arbor, MI: Health Administration Press, 1985.

Eagle, K. A. et al., "Length of stay in the intensive care unit: effects of practice guidelines and feedback." *Journal of the American Medical Association, 264*, 8, 1990.

Eddy, D. M., & Billings, J., "The Quality of Medical Evidence: Implication for Quality of Care." *Health Affairs, 7*, 1, 1988.

Flood, A. B., & Scott, W. R., "Professional Power and Professional Effectiveness: The Power of the Surgical Staff and the Quality of Surgical Care in Hospitals." *Journal of Health and Social Behavior, 19*, 3, 1978.

Freidson, E., *Profession of Medicine*, New York: Harper and Row, 1970.

Fuchsberg, A., "Editorial: Ralph Nader Calls on Governor Cuomo to Stand Tall." *Trial Lawyers Quarterly, 19*, 20, 1988.

Gabor, A., *The Man Who Discovered Quality*. New York: Penguin Books, 1990.

Gerbert, B., "Validity of Patient Report: A Comparison with Other Methods of Physician Quality Assessment," presentation made at the Association for Health Services Research conference. San Francisco, CA: June 28, 1988.

Gerbert, B. et al., "Agreement among physician assessment methods: Searching for the truth among fallible methods." *Medical Care, 26*, 6, 1988.

Hetherington, R. W., "Quality Assurance and Organizational Effectiveness in Hospitals." *Health Services Research, 17*, 2, 1982.

Hogness, J. R., "What About the Patient." *New England Journal of Medicine, 313*, 11, 1985.

Joint Commission on Accreditation of Healthcare Organizations, *An Introduction to Quality Improvement In Health Care*, Illinois: JCAHO, 1991.

Kane, R. L. et al., "A Randomised Controlled Trial of Hospice Care." *The Lancet*, 1, 8382, 1984.

Keeler, E. B. et al., "Hospital characteristics and quality of care." *Journal of the American Medical Association, 268*, 13, 1992.

Kusserow, R. P. et al., "An Overview of State Medical Discipline." *Journal of the American Medical Association, 257*, 6, 1987.

Laffell, G., & Berwick, D. M., "Quality in Health Care." *Journal of the American Medical Association, 268*, 3, 1992.

Lagoe, R. et al., "Ambulatory Surgery Utilization by Age Level." *American Journal of Public Health, 77*, 1, 1987.

Landefeld, C. S., & Goldman, L., "The Autopsy in Quality Assurance: History, Current Status, and Future Directions." *Quality Review Bulletin, 15*, 2, 1989.

Localio, A. R. et al., "Relation between malpractice claims and adverse events due to negligence: Results of the Harvard Medical Practice Study III." *New England Journal of Medicine, 325*, 4, 1991.

Lohr, K. N. et al., "Current Issues in Quality of Care." *Health Affairs, 7*, 1, 1988.

Luft, H. S., "The Relationship Between Surgical Volume and Mortality: An Exploration of Causal Factors and Alternative Models." *Medical Care, 18*, 9, 1980.

Luft, H. S. et al., "Does quality influence choice of hospital?" *Journal of the American Medical Association, 263*, 21, 1990.

Luke, R. D., & Modrow, R. E., "Professionalism, Accountability, and Peer Review." In R. D. Luke, J. C. Krueger, & R. E. Modrow, *Organization and Change in Health Care Quality Assurance*. Baltimore, MD: Aspen Publications, 1983.

Luthy, D. A. et al., "A Randomized Trial of Electronic Fetal Monitoring in Pre-Term Labor." *Obstetrics and Gynecology, 69*, 5, 1987.

Maxwell, R. J., "Resource Constraints and the Quality of Care." *The Lancet*, 2, 8461, 1985.

McCusker, J. et al., "Association of Electronic Fetal Monitoring during Labor with Cesarean Section Rate and with Neonatal Morbidity and Mortality." *American Journal of Public Health, 78*, 9, 1988.

Medicine and Health, 47, 25, June 21, 1993, p. 4.

NY Times, "US Plans to Rate Doctors Treating Medicare Patients," 6/12/88, p. 1.

Nobrega, F. T. et al., "Quality Assessment in Hypertension: Analysis of Process and Outcome Methods." *The New England Journal of Medicine*, 296, 3, 1977.

Prehn, R. A., Mayo, H., & Weisman, E., "Determinng the Validity of Patient Perceptions of Quality Care." *Quality Review Bulletin*, 15, 3, 1989.

Roberts, J. S., "A History of the Joint Commission on Accreditation of Hospitals." *Journal of the American Medical Association*, 258, 7, 1987.

Rogers, W. H. et al., "Quality of care before and after implementation of the DRG-based proposective payment system: a summary of effects." *Journal of the American Medical Association*, 264, 15, 1990.

Rolph, J. E. et al., "Malpractice Claims Data As a Quality Improvement Tool; II. Is Targeting Effective." *Journal of the American Medical Association*, 266, 15, 1991.

Roper, W. L., & Hackbarth, G. M., "HCFA's Agenda for Promoting High-Quality Care." *Health Affairs*, 7, 1, 1988.

Rubin, H. R. et al., "Watching the Doctor-Watchers: How Well Do Peer Review Organization Methods Detect Hospital cAre Quality Problems? *Journal of the American Medical Association*, 267, 17, 1992.

Scofield, R., "Certification: What Does It Mean?" *Current Concepts in Nursing*, 2, 1, 1988.

Shanahan, M., "The Quality Assurance Standard of the JCAH: A Rational Approach to Patient Care Evaluation." In Luke et al., *Organization and Change in Health Care Quality Assurance*. Baltimore, MD: Aspen Publications, 1983.

Slenker, S. E. et al., "Increasing Physicians' and Nurses' Compliance with Treatment Guidelines in Cancer Care Program." *Journal of Medical Education*, 60, 11, 1985.

Svarstad, B. L., "Patient-Practitioner Relationships and Compliance with Prescribed Medical Regimens." In L. H. Aiken & D. Mechanic (Eds.), *Applications of Social Science to Clinical Medicine and Health Policy*. New Brunswick, NJ: Rutgers University Press, 1986.

Thurow, L. C., "Medicine Versus Economics." *New England Journal of Medicine*, 313, 10, 1985.

U.S. General Accounting Office, *Medicare: PRO Review Does Assure Quality of Care Provided by Risk HMOs* (GAO:HRD-91-48). Washington, D.C.: U.S. GAO Human Resources Division, 1991.

U.S. General Accounting Office, *Practitioner Data Bank: Information on Small Medical Malpractice Payments* (IMTEC-92-56). Washington, D.C.: U.S. GAO Information Management and Technology Division, 1992.

Ware, J. E. et al., "The Measurement and Meaning of Patient Satisfaction." *Health and Medical Services Review*, 1, 1, 1978.

Waxman, H. A., "Medical Malpractice and Quality of Care." *New England Journal of Medicine*, 316, 5, 1987.

Wilson, F. A., & Neuhauser, D., *Health Services in the United States. Second Edition with 1987 Revisions*. Cambridge, MA: L. Ballinger Publishing Company, 1987.

15

Technology Assessment in Health Care

H. David Banta

Technology assessment (TA), defined simply, refers to evaluating technology for its effects. Within the health field, the effects of primary concern are health benefits (efficacy) and financial costs. At the same time, broad social implications of both specific technologies and medical technology in general become more and more apparent (Banta, Behney, & Willems, 1981, pp. 137–156). The rather definitive Institute of Medicine (1985) report defined TA as follows: "any process of examining and reporting properties of a medical technology used in health care, such as safety, efficacy, feasibility, and indications for use, cost, and cost-effectiveness, as well as social, economic, and ethical consequences, whether intended or unintended" (p. 2).

Technology assessment is also sometimes considered as a type of policy research (Banta & Luce, 1993; Office of Technology Assessment, 1982). In this formulation, the goal of technology assessment is to provide policymakers with information on policy alternatives, such as allocation of research and development funds, formulation of regulations, or development of new legislation. Whether this more specific definition or the more general one is used is not particularly important. It *is* important to realize that medical technology can be evaluated very much from a clinical perspective, or from the standpoint of the broader society as part of a decision-making process. This chapter will emphasize the second sense, that is, as a form of policy analysis.

Technology is broadly defined in this chapter. Galbraith (1977) states that technology "means the systematic application of scientific or other organized knowledge to practical tasks" (p. 31). In other words, technology is not merely machines. All commentators on technology agree on this point. For example, Mesthene (1977) supports this broad definition, saying, "It is in this broader meaning that we can best see the extent and variety of the effects of technology on our institutions and values. Its pervasive influence on our very culture would be unintelligible if technology were understood as no more than hardware" (p. 158). Because of these considerations, medical technology has been defined as "the drugs, devices, and medical and surgical procedures used in medical care, and the organizational and supportive systems within which such care is provided" (Office of Technology Assessment, 1978a). However, systems of care are the subject of this entire book. For that reason, the discussion in this chapter will be dealing primarily with clinical technology, that is, the drugs, devices, and procedures of medical care.

The Value of Medical Technology

Medical technology has transformed the face of modern medicine within the recent past (Banta & Gelijns, 1987b). A wide variety of infectious diseases now can be prevented and/or treated. Many chronic diseases also have become controllable, and rates of conditions such as heart disease are falling in this country. Modern medicine has a panoply of diagnostic technologies. Thus there is no real question that medical technology has contributed greatly to the health of the population of the United States and the rest of the world.

At the same time, it is important not to overestimate the benefits of medical technology. McKeown's analysis, discussed in Chapter 2, shows that medical care historically has had a limited impact on death rates. At the same time, many technologies of benefit have other effects besides preventing death. For example, the growing use of hip joint implants leads to restored function and diminished pain (National Institutes of Health, 1982).

It is important to remember the broad spectrum of disease and the possible applications of technology. Much of health care is taken up with psychological problems and physical complaints that have no immediate visible cause. Simple technology may be effective in these conditions. Whether or not caring is a technology is a matter of definition, but counseling patients and achieving their cooperation with therapy surely is a technology, under the definition just given. Bryce (1991) has argued that "soft" technology, such as social supports, requires the same standards of scientific evaluation that are required for such technologies as CT scanners and advanced surgical procedures.

Many other factors influence health besides technology, as discussed in Chapter 2. Health must include how one feels about life. What are the effects of racism in a society on one's feeling healthy, or how does one react to a high unemployment rate? At the personal level, studies have demonstrated direct associations between employment rates and mortality rates (Brenner, 1977). Such factors fall outside the direct responsibility of the health care system but must be considered in promoting health. An important factor is people's own behavior, which can be influenced by health and medical care (Russell, 1986). There is no necessary conflict between technological interventions and attempts to control one's own life and health, but in a society that overvalues technological procedures and pays little attention to the general social and cultural context such conflicts seem to occur frequently. Providers need to keep in mind that the health of the client is at stake; it is up to the client to make the important decisions.

Concerns about Medical Technology

The greatest concern about technology, at least within the policy arena, is the costs that its use engenders. During the 1970s and early 1980s, health care costs rose at an average rate of about 15% a year (see Chapter 10), almost double the rate of general inflation. Expenditures in the Medicare program rose even faster (Office of Technology Assessment, 1984c). The percentage of the gross national product going to health care rose from 6.0% in 1965 to 13.4% in 1991 (OECD, 1993). This may be contrasted with the average for all Organization for Economic Cooperation and Development (OECD) countries (24 industrialized countries with capitalist economies) of 7.8% in that year.

A number of analyses have examined the contribution of medical technology to rising costs. Estimates of the effect of technology on per diem hospital cost increases range from about 33% to 75%, depending on the definition of technology, the period of time, and method of calculation (Banta & Gelijns, 1987b). An analysis by the Office of Technology Assessment (1984c) found that increases in service intensity (a partial measure of new technology) contributed 24% to the rise in hospital costs during the period between 1977 and 1982.

Scitovsky and McCall (1979) traced the change in costs of treating 11 conditions at a large medical clinic, over time. Between 1951 and 1964 the real costs of treating fell for only two conditions: otitis media and pregnancy/delivery. From 1964 to 1971, the real cost of treating 5 of 11 conditions fell, but aggregate costs rose. The general increases in diagnostic tests and therapeutic procedures per diagnosis were especially striking. Laboratory tests per case of perforated appendicitis, for example, rose from 5.3 in 1951 to 31.0 in 1971. Scitovsky (1982) subsequently updated her work to 1981. She found that the net effects from 1971 to 1981 were cost-saving in eight conditions, cost-raising in seven, and neutral in one. The largest differences were in breast cancer and myocardial infarction, where new "big-ticket" technologies increased costs considerably. The other large difference was in the increasing use of cesarean section with its high costs. Showstack et al. (1982, 1985) had similar results in their research, emphasizing the important role of intensive treatments for the critically ill in rising costs.

These rising costs have raised questions about the benefits being derived from the increased use of technology. Early studies assumed that more services were synonymous with better-quality care; however, recognition has grown that many technologies are used extensively in situations where they may not be appropriate. The focus of the debate has shifted away from analysis of technology and medical expenditures in overall categories to the benefits and costs of specific technologies applied in particular circumstances. One problem with this literature is that analysts study past technologies. New and future technology can, in many cases, be cost-reducing (see the case of surgery described later in this chapter). The challenges facing the health care sector, with its aging population and growing rates of chronic disease, can only be faced with new technology (Banta & Gelijns, 1987a). Changing the structure and incentives in the health care system might encourage cost-reducing technology, such as that of home care, and costs could possibly be controlled. What is certain is that without such changes, costs will continue to rise.

How much benefit is gained under what circumstances remains relatively unknown. Concerns have been raised about the benefits of a great many modern technologies that are used routinely in the United States. For example, questions have been raised about electronic fetal monitoring (Banta & Thacker, 1979) and other obstetric practices (Chalmers et al., 1989). The most-quoted case of lack of benefit is gastric freezing, which came into widespread use in the 1960s as a treatment for peptic ulcer, promoted by a renowned surgeon and a commercial enterprise, and then just as quickly fell out of use when it turned out to be dangerous and of no benefit (Fineberg, 1979). A number of surgical treatments for coronary artery disease were developed and used widely before the advent of bypass surgery (Preston, 1977). The rising rate of cesarean sections mentioned above is probably without significant benefit, as is much of intensive care (OTA, 1984b). Particularly expensive and useless procedures are focused at the extremes of life, in very small babies and in very old adults near death.

A greater problem may be technologies that are overused. The computed tomography (CAT) scanner, described later in the chapter, seems to be one case. A technology is typically assessed early, if informally, and if the assessment is positive, it diffuses further into use. At the same time, it is used with more and more indications and with different conditions. Some common technologies that are overused include laboratory tests, many x-rays, gastroendoscopy, many surgical procedures, intensive care units, many drugs (antibiotics are a dramatic example); and many procedures in obstetrics, such as Caesarean section.

At the same time, all technologies are associated with risks. In many cases, these risks are small and perhaps can be ignored if benefits are significant. The risks of many medical technologies are also significant, however, and one is often left with the impression that they are not sufficiently taken into account. Drug risks have been most publicized, as in the cases of thalidomide and estrogen use during pregnancy (Dowling, 1970; Lambert, 1978). Although the risks of these drugs were dramatic, the more typical risk is probably similar to that which often accompanies drug treatment for hypertension: dizziness, impotence, and general tiredness.

Surgery is obviously associated with risks, including mortality and morbidity from such causes as thrombophlebitis (clots in the leg veins). However, many risks are not so obvious, as in the case of carcinogenic effects of x-rays and certain drugs.

Finally, while costs and benefits are the most obvious and direct effects of medical technology, many technologies are also associated with important social consequences. Perhaps the most important social question today is how to provide decent medical care to everyone, given the limitation of resources for the health care arena. At the same time, the ethical questions surrounding the lack of access that many people have today to such care are important to consider. Another important social question concerns the overall role of medical technology in the health care system, given its tendency to depersonalize care. Finally, specific technologies raise serious ethical questions. How does one turn off a respirator when a patient's brain appears to be dead? What is the impact on quality of life of renal dialysis three times a week for as long as the patient lives? The rapid pace of change in the area of genetics, with genetic screening and the possibility of genetic engineering, raises a variety of social and ethical issues (Holtzman, 1989). These concerns all need to be more effectively addressed by the society. Technology assessment is one tool for improving society's ability to deal with such issues. The sections that follow briefly describe the process and methods of technology assessment. The interested reader may consult a series of Office of Technology Assessment publications for more details (OTA, 1976, 1978a, 1980, 1982, 1984a). A textbook published in 1993 also provides an overview (Banta & Luce, 1993).

Evaluating Efficacy and Safety

Efficacy and safety are the basic starting points in evaluating the overall utility of medical technology. If a technology is not efficacious, it should not be used, and if its efficacy is unknown, statements about its value cannot be made. In addition, speaking of financial costs has relatively little meaning without knowledge of efficacy. The question of interest is how much benefit is derived from the cost incurred.

Efficacy may be defined simply as health benefit, but its evaluation requires attention to four factors: (1) the benefits to be achieved, (2) the medical problem giving rise to use of the technology, (3) the population affected, and (4) the conditions of use under which the technology is applied (OTA, 1978a).

The question of benefits is not as simple as it seems at first. Outcomes have usually been measured in terms of mortality and morbidity; however, psychosocial and functional factors have become recognized as important outcomes. As mentioned in Chapter 3, the measurement of health status has progressed greatly in the last few years.

Each technology is associated with a range of outcomes. This may be illustrated by the case of diagnostic technologies, such as CAT scanners, which can be examined at five levels (Fineberg et al., 1977):

1. *Technical capability*: Does the device perform reliably and deliver accurate information?
2. *Diagnostic accuracy*: Does use of the device permit accurate diagnoses?
3. *Diagnostic impact*: Does use of the device replace other diagnostic procedures, including surgical exploration and biopsy?
4. *Therapeutic impact*: Do results obtained from the device affect planning and delivery of therapy?
5. *Patient outcome*: Does use of the device contribute to improved health of the patient?

Often those using diagnostic technology seem to be most interested in the diagnostic outcome, while the outcome for the patient is surely the most important factor. At the same time, evaluating the impact of various diagnostic technologies on patient outcomes is very difficult. Definition and measurement of benefit are often difficult for other classes of technologies as well. For example, coronary bypass surgery may extend life in some patients but is used to relieve chest pain in others. Likewise, technologies are addressed to different medical problems and populations. And, as indicated previously, the outcome of application of a technology is partially determined by the skills, knowledge, and abilities of physicians, nurses, and other health personnel and by the quality of the drugs, equipment, and institutional settings. Similar surgical procedures, for example, can have quite different outcomes, depending on the skill and experience of the surgeon.

Efficacy is differentiated from *effectiveness*. *Effectiveness* is the benefit achieved by the use of a technology under average or community conditions, while efficacy is a measure of benefit under ideal or experimental conditions of use. Thus, a technology with demonstrated efficacy in a university hospital may turn out to be ineffective in the community setting, for a number of reasons. There have, however, been few studies of effectiveness.

Safety, like efficacy, is a relative concept, since no technology is ever completely safe or efficacious. A safe technology does not cause undue harm. It requires value judgments, however, to determine what is undue or acceptable. As with efficacy, the medical problem to which the technology is applied must be defined, the population affected must be specified, and the conditions of use must be stated.

The measurements of efficacy and safety often require quite different study methods. In assessing efficacy, a study is usually oriented to a limited number of specific benefits. The measurement of safety, however, usually involves a study design that is able to identify a broad range of risks, some of which are unknown or unexpected. Side effects of technology often occur in a small percentage of individuals and may occur far in the future.

There are methodological principles that guide the design, conduct, and interpretation of any particular study. Randomized clinical trials (RCTs) are considered the most definitive experimental method for evaluating the efficacy of a technology. An essential element of an RCT is randomization. Patients in an RCT are assigned randomly to one of at least two groups: (1) a study group, of which there may be several, in which subjects are exposed to the experimental treatments, and (2) a comparison group, in which subjects are exposed to a control condition. The control condition can be either no treatment, the then-current standard treatment, or a variation of the experimental treatment. If effects are observed in the experimental group and not in the comparison group, the effects can be attributed to the treatment technology.

In many cases, RCTs are difficult to organize and expensive to carry out. This situation has led to alternative methods of evaluating efficacy. Control groups can be formed retrospectively, for example. However, one always has to be cautious in interpreting such studies.

As mentioned already, examination of safety requires alternative methods, especially observational studies and applications of epidemiology. Case control studies, in which individuals with particular conditions are compared to others without the particular condition, are particularly useful for investigating the relationship between a commonly used drug and a rare adverse event.

It should be stressed that study design depends on multiple factors, including the developmental stage of the technology, the purpose of the study, ethical considerations, the population available, and budget constraints. Seldom is assessment a one-time event. A single study seldom establishes a clear relationship between a suspected cause and a particular effect. Ideally, a strategy of assessment should be laid out so that each new study builds on the previous ones, toward a total assessment of the technology.

Evaluating Costs and Cost-Effectiveness

While costs alone can be evaluated, such studies have little meaning without knowing the benefits derived from the investment. This section, therefore, will concentrate on evaluating cost-effectiveness. *Cost-benefit analysis* is probably a more familiar term than *cost-effectiveness*; however, cost-benefit analysis requires putting all costs and benefits into the same units, usually money, so that the answer is a ratio. Since health outcomes such as life or death are hard to express in such terms, cost-benefit analysis has lost favor in the health area during the past few years. Cost-effectiveness analysis allows one to express effectiveness in different units from costs. For example, the result of a study might be stated in terms of years of life saved per $1,000 investment.

Cost-effectiveness analysis is gaining more and more visibility as a potential help to policymaking (Banta & Luce, 1993). Policymakers have long referred to the need to understand more about the cost-effectiveness of interventions in the health care areas. In response the cost-effectiveness literature has rapidly increased in size (Elixhauser et al., 1992). Nonetheless, there are still relatively few high-quality cost-effectiveness analyses and little evidence that they have made much impact on health policy.

There are a number of reasons why this is so. As mentioned, few good cost-effectiveness analyses have been performed. The Office of Technology Assessment (1980) found that studies by recognized experts were inadequate with respect to the relevancy/usefulness of the results, the validity of the methods, the tenuousness (or error) in the key assumptions, and the validity of the data used. At the same time, like a good RCT, a high-quality cost-effectiveness analysis is expensive and takes time. Policy decisions do not necessarily wait on formal analysis. Thus, OTA concluded that, formally applied, this analytical method could often be too complex, expensive, and time-consuming if used routinely in public-policy decision making.

Nevertheless, the logic behind using cost-effectiveness analysis is important in decision making. Simpler, "back-of-the-envelope" analyses are common within the policy setting and clearly have influenced decision making. OTA (1980) has developed a set of principles of cost-effectiveness analysis that should be used in all situations, whether the analysis is long and expensive or short and cheap:

1. Define problem.
2. State objectives.
3. Identify alternatives.
4. Analyze benefits/ effects.
5. Analyze costs.
6. Differentiate perspective of analysis.
7. Perform discounting.
8. Analyze uncertainties.
9. Address ethical issues.
10. Interpret results.

If these 10 principles are followed consistently, one can have more confidence that one's conclusions are valid.

Evaluating Social Concerns

The social aspects of medical technologies are some of the most difficult to evaluate. There are several reasons for this. It is difficult to tell in advance which of the thousands of medical technologies will have serious social implications and for whom. At the same time, there has been little interest overall in this form of evaluation, so methods have not been developed and defined (Banta & Gelijns, 1987a; Banta & Luce, 1993; Institute of Medicine, 1985).

Clearly, the relationship between medical technology and social values is reciprocal. Technologies affect values, as when technology allowed the definition of "brain death" to supersede the earlier standard life endpoint: heart stoppage. Society still has not been able to grapple effectively with the issue of what to do for a person whose heart and lungs are artificially supported but whose brain is "alive." At the same time, values affect medical technology and its development, use, and evaluation. Social values and technology interact in a very broad sense. For example, what value does society place on health, on innovation, on financial security, on technology itself? It often seems that the present society overvalues technology and undervalues human supports and caring.

Specific technologies also have social effects, as well as being subject to broad social forces. The most visible social impact is on costs. How will society cope with the ever-increasing cost of health care? Will we decide to use some formal criterion such as "social worth" to decide who shall have access to expensive life-saving technologies? Every technology is fed into a delivery system that historically discriminates, in terms of access and distribution, against poor people, minorities, the aged, and other groups. Thus, technological advances can be in part the cause of, in part the catalyst for, and in part the mechanism for continued inequities.

U.S. society has not dealt with such issues effectively and indeed often seems overtly to avoid dealing with them. There are few, if any, examples of a broad technology assessment done of a medical technology, for purposes of policymaking. Perhaps the best example is a study done of the artificial heart by the National Institutes of Health in 1972 (National Heart and Lung Institute, 1973). That report analyzed the broad social consequences of having a workable heart. According to NIH staff close to the decisions, the report helped lead to an emphasis on left-ventricular assist devices and a deemphasis of the totally implantable heart. In 1979, the Health Care Financing Administration delayed the decision on whether or not to pay for heart transplants through the Medicare program until a broad study of the consequences of the technology could be completed by Batelle (Evens et al., 1984). With the growing concern about such social consequences, this field of inquiry seems certain to grow and develop.

The Process of Technology Assessment

Until now this chapter has dealt with original research aimed at evaluating medical technology. Research results often do not affect policy or clinical decisions very directly, however, as policymakers and clinicians do not tend to read research reports and often lack the skills to interpret them, in any case. To assure that assessment results affect decisions on technology requires a more systematic approach.

The components of a medical technology assessment process can be seen as including four stages of assessment (OTA, 1982):

1. *Identification*: Monitoring technologies, determining which need to be studied, and deciding which to study.
2. *Testing*: Conducting the appropriate analyses or trials.
3. *Synthesis*: Collecting and interpreting existing information and the results of the testing stage, and usually making recommendations or judgments about appropriate use.
4. *Dissemination*: Providing a synthesis of the information to the appropriate parties who use medical technologies or make decisions about their use.

A decision to conduct a technology assessment clearly must be preceded by the identification of technologies that should be assessed and the setting of priorities among candidates for assessment. Identifying technologies for assessment is done by a number of federal and private organizations; however, there is no one program or agency with this responsibility.

Testing includes stimulating, requiring, funding, or conducting studies. Shortcomings in this area center around four issues: (1) the quality of methods used in assessment; (2) the level of financial support, particularly for controlled clinical trials; (3) the relative appropriateness of the questions and technologies being studied; and (4) the number of personnel qualified to conduct such research. Again, existing activities are rather limited in scope, but two of the most important are found in the Food and Drug Administration (FDA) and the National Institutes of Health (NIH).

Synthesis of information is a necessary step to providing a convincing and responsible basis for decisions made during all phases of a technology's life cycle. This activity falls into two broad areas: (1) synthesis of the results of individual research studies and (2) synthesis of a body of research findings with various concerns such as risk or social, ethical, or cost factors. The first type of synthesis addresses questions of safety, efficacy, or effectiveness and is oriented toward clinicians. The American College of Physicians' Clinical Efficacy Program is an excellent example of a private program that does such synthesis. The second type is more policy-oriented and often seeks to set guidelines or standards for medical practice or health policy. A pioneer in synthesis studies in the United States is the Office of Technology Assessment (OTA), a part of the U.S. Congress. Another program worth noting is the Consensus Development Program of the National Institutes of Health (Jacoby, 1985). The NIH program uses synthesis of the literature but also includes a multidisciplinary group as part of the process that attempts to arrive at a consensus and give recommendations on the specific technology. It has examined more than 80 technologies. The Office of Health Technology Assessment (OHTA) of the U.S. Public Health Service also does synthesis studies, primarily to guide the Medicare program in its coverage decisions.

A very visible type of synthesis in the United States is developing practice guidelines (Field & Lohr, 1992). Stimulated by rising costs, organizations such as professional associations, insurance companies, government agencies, and others are actively working to develop guidelines. Eddy (1991) is skeptical about the value of guidelines as a control procedure because of the need for information on outcomes and patient preferences, both of which are lacking. Practice guidelines are part of an active strategy of the Agency for Health Care Policy and Research (AHCPR), founded by Congressional act in 1989.

Finally, dissemination deals with questions of who should have the highest priority in receiving information. At a minimum, information must reach decision makers involved with the technology in various aspects of its use. This means industry officials, clinicians, policymakers, and/or the general public. Unfortunately, communication activities are highly flawed and have actually been cut back in recent years. Little is known about how technology is adopted or how information is acquired and used (Thier, 1988).

The Institute of Medicine (1985) estimated that the entire U.S. expenditure for medical technology assessment in 1984 was $1.3 billion, or about 0.3% of the national health expenditure. The federal government invested about $450 million, including $250 million for clinical trials (primarily from the NIH) and $100 million to 150 million for health services research (IOM, 1985). The greatest expenditure was by the drug industry, which must fund clinical trials to obtain approval of its products and which also funds postmarketing surveillance activities; the estimated expenditure from this source is about $700 million. Less than $50 million is spent on activities devoted to synthesis and interpretation of primary evaluative data (IOM, 1985). Its analysis of this issue led the Institute of Medicine (1985) to conclude that funding for medical technology assessment should be increased by $300 million "by instituting new contributions from payers and providers for health care" (p. 6).

Some Examples of Technology Assessment

The Computerized Axial Tomography (CAT) Scanner

The CAT scanner is a diagnostic device that combines x-ray equipment with a computer and a cathode-ray tube to produce images of cross-sections of the human body. Following its development in the late 1960s, the CAT scanner was hailed as the greatest advance in radiology since the discovery of x-rays, and it was rapidly accepted. The scanner was of concern to policymakers from the beginning, however, because of its rapid spread and use and the expenditures associated with that use.

The first technology assessment done in the health area by OTA was of the CAT scanner (OTA, 1978b). The first draft of OTA's evaluation was widely circulated in late 1976, but diffusion of scanners during 1977 and 1978 was nevertheless very rapid. The main conclusion of OTA's draft was that little research had been done on evaluating possible improvement in health outcomes resulting from the introduction of CAT scanning. As noted earlier in the chapter, this is a critical issue in evaluating diagnostic technologies. OTA's final report, published in 1978, included a comprehensive analysis of federal government policies that could be used to control the spread of scanners. Reports on CAT scanners also have been done by the Institute of Medicine (1977), the Consensus Development Program (National Institutes of Health, 1981), and institutions in a number of other countries. The scientific literature is also very extensive.

These studies and reports seem to have had a limited impact in the United States. One reason for this is that the profits associated with using a CAT scanner were extremely high in the early years. OTA estimated average profits per machine in 1976 to vary from $51,000 to $283,000, with an investment for the scanner itself that averaged around $500,000 (OTA, 1978b). In addition, the CAT scanner did give the medical care system a diagnostic tool that was unique. However, in other countries that have more effective methods for controlling the spread of technology, its introduction and use expanded much more slowly. For example, in 1979 the United States had 5.7 scanners per million population, while the Netherlands had only 1.4 per million (Banta & Kemp, 1982). By 1990, the US had 26.8 scanners per million population, compared to 10.6 in Sweden, 7.3 in the Netherlands, and 7.2 in France.

Thus, an early lesson for assessors was that the assessment itself might make no difference to the subsequent adoption and use of a technology. A more important factor might be the effectiveness of government programs, such as those planning for the purchase and siting of medical machines.

The Electronic Fetal Monitor

Electronic fetal monitoring (EFM) of the fetal heart rate during labor and delivery was developed as an alternative to auscultation by stethoscope (fetoscope). It was introduced into obstetric practice during the 1960s and spread rather quickly. By 1980 it was used in 48% of deliveries in the United States (Placek et al., 1984).

By 1977, EFM had become controversial because it tended to replace a human being (usually a nurse or midwife) with a machine. Many women did not like this change, and the women's movement made such depersonalization an issue. Because of this controversy, an RCT was initiated at the University of Colorado, Denver (Haverkamp et al., 1976). The trial, while small, found no benefit to the fetus from EFM, compared with auscultation. At the same time, other trials were underway. By 1986, nine controlled clinical trials had been completed in six countries, including one involving 35,000 women from Dallas (Leveno et al., 1986), with no benefit except a decrease in the occurrence of neonatal seizures of unknown significance in the EFM group (Thacker, 1987). In addition, the use of EFM adds considerably to costs. Much of this increase was due to increased rates of surgical deliveries, especially Cesarean sections, confirmed by pooled data from the nine trials (Thacker, 1987).

EFM was the subject of recommendations in the report of the U.S. Preventive Services Task Force (1989), in a synthetic review of obstetric technologies Chalmers et al. (1989), and in a report of the Candian Task Force on the Periodic Health Examination (1989). Despite consistent recommendations that auscultation is an acceptable alternative, there is no evidence that practice has been modified. Still, in 1989 the American College of Obstetrics and Gynecology recommended to its members a policy that monitoring with intermittent auscultation is acceptable in both low- and high-risk pregnancies (Cogan, 1988). The negative assessments have also been reported in many news articles and magazines.

The main lesson from the EFM case is that assessment itself does not (rapidly) change behavior. Other mechanisms are needed.

Nonetheless, EFM has continued to be used. Why? There are a number of reasons. One is that younger obstetricians have all been trained to use the machine, and many have limited auscultation skill. Another is that malpractice suits have been brought against obstetricians who did not use EFM with their patients. From the standpoint of the policymaker, there are few ways to affect the use of EFM. The machine itself is relatively inexpensive and too small an item to be subject to direct health planning, and FDA's mandate is too limited to allow it to remove EFM from the market.

Surgical Practice

Surgery has existed at least as long as written history. Historically, much of surgery was setting bones or suturing wounds. The sanitary revolution of the late 1800s, with its resulting antisepsis, along with improvements in anesthesia and nursing care, led to a great expansion of surgery.

Surgery has not often been formally assessed. Surgery developed as an empirical art. For modern, high-technology surgery, assessments have been more common. But common surgical procedures such as hysterectomy, appendectomy, prostatectomy, and cholecystectomy (removal of the gall bladder) have only been informally assessed. Surgeons have not been very oriented to assessment and funding agencies have generally not devoted resources to the assessment of surgery.

It can also be very difficult to assess surgery. Patients are often referred for a specific surgery for a specific problem, or they seek that procedure on their own. Entering a clinical trial of surgery requires the patient to agree to accept an invasive procedure without choice, or alternatively, to forego a procedure that he or she may wish to have done. For example, in the case of alternatives to conventional cholecystectomy, as will be described below, patients have demanded the new procedure.

Surgery is costly, but little information is available to compare its cost-effectiveness to alternatives.

Surgery has changed rapidly since World War II. One major change has been that it has become less invasive, through such advances as microsurgery and better anesthesia techniques. However, the real revolution in surgery has followed the introduction of endoscopes, introduced first as diagnostic tools. Endoscopy, such as upper gastrointestinal endoscopy, is quite profitable to the physician who uses it (Showstack & Schroeder, 1981). This is part of the reason, no doubt, that studies have found high rates of inappropriate use of endoscopy. For example, Kosecoff et al. (1987) found in a study of U.S. hospitals, that 17% of such endoscopies were inappropriate and almost 11% equivocal (not clearly demonstrated to be beneficial).

Nonetheless, over time the endoscope has changed the process of surgical therapy. Endoscopes can be used in any of the orifices of the body, and can also be inserted through small incisions, as in the case of the laparoscope (abdomen) and arthroscope (joints). At least 100 surgical procedures are now being done by endoscope (Banta, 1993). The case of the laparoscope and gall bladder surgery can illustrate the issue of assessment.

Laparoscopic cholecystectomy was first done in France in 1987. It spread outside France very quickly, stimulated by presentations and publications of the group of F. Dubois (1990). The first procedure in the United States was done in 1988. Most surgeons were skeptical, but when people needing gall bladder surgery learned that an alternative to invasive gall bladder surgery was available, they demanded it. By 1993, perhaps as many as half of cholecystectomies in the United States were done by laparoscope, and estimates are that as many as 90% of these surgeries will be done by laparoscope in the future.

Laparoscopic cholecystectomy was not scientifically assessed. It was only after several years of diffusion that retrospective studies showed that the method was at least as safe and effective as conventional therapy in most cases (Southern Surgeon's Club, 1991; Cuschieri et al., 1991). In 1992, an NIH Consensus Development Conference (1992) concluded on the basis of clinical experience that laparoscopic cholecystectomy "provides a safe and effective treatment for most patients with symptomatic gallstones." At the same time, the Conference recognized certain problems, such as excessive procedures because of treatment of asymptomatic gall stones and the fact that the outcome of the procedure is highly dependent of the training and experience of the surgeon.

Endoscopic surgery can be quite cost-saving in relation to ordinary surgery. Laparoscopic cholecystectomy, for example, is associated with a shorter stay in hospital and earlier return to normal activities. It can even be done in most cases without an overnight stay in hospital (Southern Surgeon's Club, 1991). Peters et al. (1991) compared patient costs with laparosopic cholecystectomy with costs of a group made up of the previous 58 standard cholecystectomies done in their institution. Operating time was an average 122 minutes, with a range of 45 minutes, compared with 78 minutes (range 30 minutes) for standard cholecystectomy. The mean hospital stay for patients was 27.6 hours (surgical cholecystectomy is associated with about 5 days in hospital). The average patient returned to normal activity in 12.8 days, with a range of 6.8 days. The hospital charges for the laparoscopic group averaged $3,620, with a range of $1,005, while the hospital charges for the standard cholecystectomy group were $4,252, with a range of $988. Physician fees were not included in these estimates, and the authors made no attempt to value the early return to work or other activity.

The case of endoscopic surgery shows that procedures that are less invasive, but that are not necessary superior to conventional procedures, are rapidly diffusing into practice in the United States without careful assessment. While laparoscopic cholecystectomy has turned out to be a positive case, it could have been a literal disaster.

Pneumococcal Vaccine

In 1978, a new vaccine against the pneumococcus, aimed at the prevention of pneumococcal pneumonia, was marketed. The vaccine had been approved by FDA on the basis of proven efficacy in experimental studies, but many groups and individuals were cautious about widespread use of the vaccine because it had not been tested in high-risk groups such as the elderly. In 1979, OTA published a cost-effectiveness analysis of the vaccine, in which it was concluded that the Medicare program would incur a net cost per elderly beneficiary vaccinated of about $5 if the program covered 100% of the vaccination cost and that each vaccination would produce a gain of .004 healthy days of life. If 21.5% of the population were vaccinated, Medicare would spend about $26 million over the lifetimes of those vaccinated, and 22,000 years of healthy life would result. Since Medicare does not pay for all medical expenses of the elderly, however, the actual results would be even more favorable. This analysis led to a congressional act in 1981 providing for coverage of the vaccine under the program. The findings of a reanalysis by OTA in 1984, using the actual experience of the Medicare program, were similar to those of the earlier study (OTA, 1984d). Nonetheless, only about 25% of the high-risk target group has received the vaccine. This indicates that, while financial coverage for technology is important, it is not the only factor in use.

Another important lesson from this case is that technology assessments are more likely to be directly influential when a specific policy decision is involved. Cost-effectiveness analysis has been widely applied in the case of vaccines, probably because immunization programs are developed by the government and are funded with public monies. Other than the pneumococcal vaccine, Medicare, by law, has never covered preventive measures from the time of its passage in 1965 to the mid-1980s. Congress has incrementally added coverage of influenza vaccine, hepatitis B immunization for high-risk beneficiaries, and of biannual screening mammographies. Based on OTA analyses, however, Congress did not cover cholesterol screening and screening for colorectal cancer.

Impact of Technology Assessment

Evaluation is not a new area of medicine, but the RCT is a product of this century. Other forms of assessment are even newer. For example, a random sample of articles from general medical journals found no RCTs in 1946, while 5% of the articles were reports of RCTs in 1976 (Fletcher & Fletcher, 1979). The literature on the impact of technology assessment is small and focuses on the impact of RCTs. By the mid-1970s, the literature had begun to grow, and in 1983 OTA reviewed the literature on the impact of RCTs on policy and practice (OTA, 1983).

Most authors conclude that the impact of RCTs on medical practice has been less than optimal or that their impact is exceedingly slow to develop. The literature as a whole demonstrates great variation in the use of RCTs and in their influence in different medical areas. Recent articles have identified some of the reasons for lack of influence of RCTs, including (1) poor quality of many RCTs, (2) poor dissemination of the results of RCTs, (3) lack of an overall system for assessing medical technologies, (4) less-than-optimal use of RCTs in policy decisions, and (5) different traditions and practices in different areas of medicine (internists are more accustomed to such evidence than surgeons, for example).

Assessments have also had a limited impact on policy. In part, this is related to the small efforts aimed at producing information for policymaking (that is, synthesis activities). In part it is related to the lack of primary data. For example, the Office of Health Technology Assessment (OHTA) assessed 26 technologies for the Medicare program in 1982 and found that randomized clinical trials were available for only 2 (IOM, 1985).

What, then, is the value of technology assessment in health care? Although it is difficult to document, one important use is what might be called "strategic," in which the analysis includes consideration of what the individual, the group, or the organization is attempting to achieve (Smits et al., 1984). An example might be the repeated conclusions of the Office of Technology Assessment during the 1970s that the nature of the payment system for technology was one of the most important policies leading to inappropriate use of medical technology. Such reports surely helped prepare the way for policy changes in the payment system in the Medicare program, including the development of the Diagnostic-Related Groups (DRG) program, a change from retrospective cost reimbursement to prospective payment. More recently, the Congress has expressed its faith in the value of assessment information by establishing AHCPR, which both sponsors extramural research for the study of technologies and conducts assessments through its Office of Health Technology Assessment (OHTA). AHCPR has a central task to support medical outcomes research. AHCPR's budget in 1992 was $120.2 million.

Technology assessment also can be used as part of operational decisions. It has a long-established role in the area of drug regulation as part of the premarketing approval process. A newer role is as a part of payment decisions. As mentioned above, OHTA does studies to guide the Medicare program in its coverage decisions. This function is more visible in other countries, with their centralized payment systems. It is now common in European countries not to allow technologies to be paid for until they have been assessed. In the United States, the decentralization of the payment system has led to many programs, especially in Blue Cross/ Blue Shield and private insurance companies, to establish their own health care TA programs. When decisions have been based on technology assessment information, they seem to have saved the organizations much more than the cost of the assessments (Perry, 1982).

It would be premature to say that health care technology assessment has demonstrated its own cost-effectiveness. It may be too early to ask for such evidence because investments have been small and activities have begun to be rationally organized only during the past decade. Nonetheless, experience thus far is promising enough to lead a number of groups and individuals to support an expansion of such activities, along with the development of national systems (Banta & Gelijns, 1987a; Relman, 1980; IOM, 1985).

Experiences of Other Countries

Other countries have had experiences with medical technology similar to those of the United States (Banta et al., 1994). Although other countries have not experienced increases in cost as dramatic as those of the United States, all European countries are concerned about the ever-growing investment in health care. This concern has led to rapid changes in policies toward medical technology (Banta et al., in press). Countries with national programs for health care technology assessment include Canada, Australia, the United Kingdom, Sweden, and France.

Until fairly recently, the major involvement of governments in medical technology was to promote a new technology's development and adoption actively, through such means as funding biomedical research and technology development or assuring payment for the technology under a national health plan. In recent years, however, governments have become more and more concerned with whether or not new technologies were being used efficiently. Without making a judgment about the efficacy of the technology, governments have intervened to encourage greater efficiency in the production and use of a technology. This has been a major orientation of health planning, for example. With increasing concerns about the cost-effectiveness of technology, governments also have begun to question and test the benefits of medical technologies. A number of governments, especially those in Western Europe, now have new programs to assess medical technology, and funds available are increasing rapidly. Finally, some governments have gone further, by limiting the diffusion of technologies to a level that strikes a balance between the benefits to be gained and the costs of achieving them. England is an example of a country that seems to have moved to this stage.

Summary and Conclusions

The major problem with technology assessment in medicine in the United States is the lack of a system for doing so that would assure timely, high-quality assessment. In 1978 Congress passed legislation establishing the National Center for Health Care Technology, which was a step in that direction. The center was a victim of Reagan administration budget cuts, however, and ceased to exist in 1981 (Perry). Subsequently, a Council on Health Care Technology was established at the U.S. Institute of Medicine to coordinate efforts in health care technology assessment, but the Council too ceased to exist in 1991 after difficulties in obtaining funds. AHCPR has increased support and visibility of health care technology assessment in the United States, but it has no mandate to coordinate national efforts. AHCPR does have a mandate, however, to improve access to technology assessment information, a welcome step.

The result is that the United States has a bewildering array of formal health care technology assessment program. Each class of institution, whether it be government, insurer, or provider, is assessing technology for its own constituency (Banta & Luce, 1993). Until 1993, all efforts to develop a coordinated and consistent national policy toward health care technology assessment in the United States have failed.

References

Banta, D., Behney, C., & Willems, J., *Toward Rational Technology in Medicine: Considerations for Health Policy.* New York: Springer Publishing Co., 1981.

Banta, H. D. (Ed.), *Minimally Invasive Therapy in Five European Countries.* Amsterdam, The Netherlands: Elsevier, 1993.

Banta, H. D., & Gelijns, A. G., *Anticipating and Assessing Health Care Technology: Vol. 1. General Considerations and Policy Conclusions.* Boston: Martinus Nijhoff Publishers. 1987a.

Banta, H. D., & Gelijns, A. G., "Health Care Costs: Technology and Policy. In C. J. Schramm (Ed.), *Health Care and Its Costs: Can the U.S. Afford Adequate Health Care?* (pp. 252–274). New York: W. W. Norton, 1987b.

Banta, D., & Kemp, K. (Eds.)., *The Management of Health Care Technology in Nine Countries.* New York: Springer Publishing Co, 1982.

Banta, H. D. & Luce, B., *Health Care Technology and its Assessment, An International Perspective.* Oxford: Oxford University Press, 1993.

Banta, H. D., & Thacker, S., "Assessing the Costs and Benefits of Electronic Fetal Monitoring." *Obstetrical and Gynecological Survey, 34,* 627, 1979.

Banta, H. D. et al. (Eds.), *Health Care Technology in 8 Countries.* Washington, DC: Office of Technology Assessment (in preparation).

Brenner, M. H., "Health Costs and Benefits of Economic Policy. *International Journal of Health Services, 7,* 581, 1977.

Bryce, R., "Support in pregnancy." *International Journal of Technology Assessment in Health Care*, 7, 478–484, 1991.

Cameron, J. & Gadacz, T., "Laparoscopic cholecystectomy." *Annals of Surgery, 213*, 1, 1991.

Canadian Task Force on the Periodic Health Examination. "Periodic health examination, 1989 Update: 4. Intrapartum electronic fetal monitoring and prevention of neonatal Herpes Simplex." *Canadian Medical Association Journal, 141*, 1233, 1989.

Chalmers, I., Enkin, M. & Keirse, M. (Eds.), *Effective Care in Pregnancy and Childbirth.* Oxford: Oxford University Press, 1989.

Cogan, J., "ACOG considers new guidelines for monitoring and labor." *Obstet Gynecol News*, 23, 43, 1988.

Cuschieri, A., Dubois, F., Mouiel, J. et al., "The European experience with laparoscopic cholecystectomy." *American Journal of Surgery, 161*, 285, 1991.

Dowling, H., *Medicines for Man.* New York: Alfred A. Knopf, 1970.

Drummond, M., Stoddart, G., & Torrance, G., *Methods for the Economic Evaluation of Health Care Programmes.* Oxford: Oxford Medical Publications, 1987.

Dubois, F., Icard, P., Berthelot, G., & Levard, H., "Coelioscopic cholecystectomy, preliminary report of 36 cases." *Annals of Surgery, 211*, 60, 1990.

Eddy, D., "Designing a practice policy, standards, guidelines and options." *Journal of the American Medical Association, 266*, 3077, 1991.

Elixhauser, A., Luce, B., Taylor, W., & Reblando, J., "Health care cost-benefit and cost-effectiveness analysis from 1979 to 1990: a bibliography." Submitted for publication, 1992.

Evens, E. W. et al., *The National Heart Transplantation Study: Final Report.* Seattle, WA: Battelle Human Affairs Research Centers, 1984.

Field, M., & Lohr, K. (Eds.), *Guidelines for Clinical Practice.* Washington, DC: National Academy Press, 1992.

Fineberg, H., "Gastric Freezing—A Study of Diffusion of a Medical Innovation." In Committee on Technology and Health Care, *Medical Technology and the Health Care System.* Washington, DC: National Academy of Sciences, 1979.

Fineberg, H. et al., "Computerized Cranial Tomography: Effect on Diagnostic and Therapeutic Plans." *Journal of the American Medical Association, 238*, 224, 1977.

Fletcher, R., & Fletcher, S., "Clinical Research in General Medical Journals." *New England Journal of Medicine, 301*, 180, 1979.

Galbraith, J., *The New Industrial State.* New York: New American Library, 1977.

Haverkamp, A. et al., "The Evaluation of Continuous Fetal Heart Rate Monitoring in High-Risk Pregnancy." *American Journal of Obstetrics and Gynecology, 125*, 310, 1976.

Holtzman, N., *Proceed with Caution, Predicting Genetic Risks in the Recombinant DNA Era.* Baltimore: The Johns Hopkins University Press, 1989.

Institute of Medicine. *Computed Tomographic Scanning.* Washington, DC: National Academy of Sciences, 1977.

Institute of Medicine. *Assessing Medical Technology.* Washington, DC: National Academy Press, 1985.

Jacoby, I., "The consensus development program of the National Institutes of Health." *International Journal of Technology Assessment in Health Care, 1*, 420, 1985.

Kosecoff, J., Chassin, M., Fink A. et al., "Obtaining clinical data on the appropriateness of medical care in community practice." *Journal of the American Medical Association*, 258: 2538–2542, 1987.

Lambert, E. C., *Modern Medical Mistakes*. Bloomington, IN: Indiana University Press, 1978.

Leveno, K. J., Cunningham, F. G., Nelson, S., Roark, M., Williams, M. L., Guzick, D., Dowling, S., Rosenfeld, C. R., & Buckley, A., "A Prospective Comparison of Selective and Universal Electronic Fetal Monitoring in 34,995 Pregnancies." *New England Journal of Medicine, 315*, 615, 1986.

Mesthene, E., "The Role of Technology in Society." In A. Teich (Ed.), *Technology and Man's Future*. New York: St. Martin's Press, 1977.

National Heart and Lung Institute. *The Totally Implantable Artificial Heart*. A Report of the Artificial Heart Assessment Panel. Bethesda, MD: National Institutes of Health, 1973.

National Institutes of Health. Consensus Development Conference Statement. *Computed Tomographic Scanning of the Brain*. Bethesda, MD: National Institutes of Health, 1981.

National Institutes of Health. Consensus Development Conference Statement. *Total Hip Joint Replacement*. Bethesda, MD: National Institutes of Health, 1982.

Office of Medical Applications of Research, U.S. Department of Health and Human Services. *NIH Consensus Statement 10*(3): 1–26. *Gallstones and Laparoscopic Cholecystectomy*. Bethesda, MD: National Institutes of Health, 1992.

Office of Technology Assessment. *Development of Medical Technology: Opportunities for Assessment*. Pub. No. OTA-H-34. Washington, DC: U.S. Government Printing Office.

Office of Technology Assessment. *Assessing the Efficacy and Safety of Medical Technologies*. Pub. No. OTA-H-75. Washington, DC: U.S. Government Printing Office. 1978a.

Office of Technology Assessment. *Policy Implications of the Computed Tomography (CT) Scanner*. Pub. No. OTA-H-56. Washington, DC: U.S. Government Printing Office, 1978b.

Office of Technology Assessment. *A Review of Selected Federal Vaccine and Immunization Policies*. Pub. Nn. OTA-H-96. Washington, DC: U.S. Government Printing Office, 1979.

Office of Technology Assessment. *The Implications of Cost-Effectiveness Analysis of Medical Technology*. Pub. No. OTA-H-126. Washington, DC: U.S. Government Printing Office, 1980.

Office of Technology Assessment. *Strategies for Medical Technology Assessment*. Pub. No. OTA-H-181. Washington, DC: U.S. Government Printing Office, 1982.

Office of Technology Assessment. *The Impact of Randomized Clinical Trials on Health Policy and Medical Practice*. Pub. No. BP-H-22. Washington, DC: U.S. Government Printing Office, 1983.

Office of Technology Assessment. *Intensive Care Units (ICUs)—Clinical Outcomes, Costs, and Decisionmaking*. Pub. No. BP-HCS-28. Washington, DC: U.S. Government Printing Office, 1984b.

Office of Technology Assessment. *Medical Technology and the Costs of the Medicare Program*. Pub. No. OTA-H-227. Washington, DC: U.S. Government Printing Office, 1984c.

Office of Technology Assessment. *Update of Federal Activities Regarding the Use of Pneu-

mococcal Vaccine. Pub. No. OTA-TM-H-23. Washington, DC: U.S. Government Printing Office, 1984d.

Organization for Economic Cooperation and Development. "Latest OECD health expenditure data for 1991 on diskette." Press release. Paris, 1993.

Perry, S., "The Brief Life of the National Center for Health Care Technology." *New England Journal of Medicine, 307,* 1095, 1982.

Peters, J., Ellison, E., Innes, J. et al., "Safety and efficacy of laparoscopic cholecystectomy: A prospective analysis of 100 initial patients." *Annals of Surgery, 213,* 3, 1991.

Placek, P. et al., "Electronic Fetal Monitoring in Relation to Cesarean Section Delivery for Live Births and Stillbirths in the U.S., 1980." *Public Health Reports. 99,* 173, 1984.

Preston, T., *Coronary Artery Surgery: A Critical Review.* New York: Raven Press, 1977.

Relman, A. S., "Assessment of Medical Practices." *New England Journal of Medicine, 303,* 153, 1980.

Russell, L. B., *Is Prevention Better Than Cure?* Washington, DC: The Brookings Institution, 1986.

Scitovsky, A. A., "Estimating the Direct Costs of Illness." *Milbank Memorial Fund Quarterly/Health and Society, 60,* 4623, 1982.

Scitovsky, A., & McCall, N., "Changes in the Cost of Treatment of Selected Illnesses. 1951–1964–1971." USDHEW Pub. No. (PHS) 79-3216. Hyattsville, MD: National Center for Health Services Research and Bureau of Health Planning, 1979.

Showstack, J. A., Hughes Stone, M., & Schroeder, S. A., "The Role of Changing Clinical Practices on the Rising Costs of Hospital Care." *New England Journal of Medicine. 313,* 1201, 1985.

Showstack, J., & Schroeder, S., Office of Technology Assessment Background Paper # 2: *Case studies of Medical Technologies, Case study #8: The cost-effectiveness of upper gastrointestinal endoscopy.* Washington, DC: U.S. Government Printing Office, 1981.

Showstack, J. A., Schroeder, S. A., & Matsumoto, M. F., "Changes in the Use of Medical Technologies, 1972–1977: A Study of 20 Inpatient Diagnoses." *New England Journal of Medicine, 306,* 706, 1982.

Smits, R. E. H. M., Leyten, A. J. M., & Guerts, J. L. A., *The Possibilities and Limitations of Technology Assessment—in Search of a Useful Approach.* The Hague, The Netherlands: Staatsuitgeverij, 1984. (Summary in English.)

Southern Surgeons Club. "A Prospective Analysis of 1518 Laparoscopic Cholecystectomies." *New England Journal of Medicine, 324,* 1073, 1991.

Thacker, S., "The efficacy of intrapartum electronic fetal monitoring." *American Journal of Obstetrics and Gynecology, 156,* 24, 1987.

Thier, S., "Future Developments in the Transfer of Technology Assessment Information." *International Journal of Technology Assessment in Health Care, 4,* 109, 1988.

U.S. Preventive Services Task Force. (1989). Guide to Clinical Preventive Services: An Assessment of the Effectiveness of 169 Interventions. Baltimore: Williams and Wilkins, 1989.

16

Governance and Management

Anthony R. Kovner

Put simply, governance in health care organizations (HCOs) is the system for making important decisions, and managers are the group responsible for implementing those decisions. Governance and management are important, as health care is being provided increasingly in large organizations, where these functions are partitioned among trustees, managers, and clinician leaders. In small HCOs, such as some doctor's offices and nursing homes, owners and operators often govern, manage, and provide care.

This chapter is divided into two parts. The first, on governance, covers how power is distributed; it describes the role, structure, and function of governing boards, and it examines current issues and approaches toward more effective governance. The second part of this chapter is on management; it describes what managers do and how they are trained; it examines the managerial contribution to HCO performance, and it explores important current issues in management.

Governance

Governance is direction, control, and exercise of authority. Authority is the power or admitted right to command or act. The difference between the concepts is this: governance describes those who have power and how it is exercised; authority explains the bases of such power. Governance may be dominated by a few individuals or by many; it may be exercised in an authoritarian or in a democratic way. Those who govern have the final say and are accountable for what an HCO does.

How the governance of HCOs is viewed depends on how one views their mission. HCOs may be seen as existing primarily to satisfy those who use or consume their services, those who own or work in the organization, or some combination of both. Those who govern make decisions that affect organizational policy or, by not making decisions, they allow others to influence what the HCO chooses to do and how. HCOs are dependent on the resources they require to achieve their purposes and survive. Such resources include patients, clinicians, facilities, and legitimacy. Governance influences the supply of resources as well as their allocation and use. Health care is increasingly provided by organizations rather than by solo practitioners. How HCOs are governed influences the futures of those who work in and are served by them.

Level of Analysis

There are several levels at which health care policy can be determined. Decisions can be made at the national level that affect local activities. For example, as a result of the Medicare legislation of 1965, general hospitals provided older Americans with more inpatient services per capita than previously and with more health care financing relative to other age groups. This decision was, in essence, determined not by each general hospital but by the elected representatives of the American people, who would now have government collect and reimburse more adequately for inpatient services provided to the elderly. Decisions affecting HCOs are also made at the level of the clinician or the consumer.

Here governance will be examined at the level of the HCO rather than that of the industry or the individual provider. HCOs are defined as organizations engaging in the direct provision of health care. By this definition, a hospital, a nursing home, and a group practice are included, but an insurance company, a drug company, and a government regulatory agency are not. Within the HCO the focus is at the level at which policy is determined rather than that at which policy is implemented.

Policy and Administration

The content of policy decisions varies widely among HCOs. What are policy decisions for one HCO are administrative or routine decisions for another. For example, the duties of family health workers in a community health center may be a policy decision, whereas the operation of a laundry facility with other centers is not. The reverse may be true for an urban general hospital, because the objectives of the two HCOs are different. Policy decisions are those that affect objectives. If an objective of a community health center is to provide primary care to a local population, the way in which family health workers are trained is likely to affect the objective, whereas lowering the cost per pound of laundry done does not. If a hospital objective is to reduce operating losses for certain diagnostic related groups (DRGs), however; then, sharing laundry services with other hospitals may involve policy, whereas reconfiguration of the duties of health care workers in the ambulatory care department does not.

Certain types of organizational decisions usually involve policy. Such decisions include long-range planning, the allocation of resources, and the selection and evaluation of top management. Decisions in these areas all have an important effect on organizational objectives. Long-range plans determine which programs will be provided at what level by the HCO and therefore how resources will be allocated. For example, the need for inpatient beds in a large mental hospital may decrease because of improved methods of treatment. This results in a long-range planning decision to emphasize rehabilitative rather than custodial care. Changing organizational objectives, however, often causes conflict within an organization. A new priority of rehabilitative care may be resisted by mental hospital staff because behavior that had been acceptable and perhaps even desirable when custodial care was a primary objective of the mental hospital is unacceptable and undesirable when rehabilitative care becomes a primary objective.

Organizational objectives are also often affected by the allocation of resources. For example, a group practice may weigh its salary structure heavily in favor of senior partners, thereby influencing the kinds of physicians attracted to the group and hence the ability of the group to attract new patients. The group is therefore able to increase revenues primarily by providing additional services to those already using its services. If a hospital increases its budgetary allocation for management or social services, this may indicate that the hospital no longer places the same emphasis on meeting the needs of physicians in their private practice and that it will place a higher priority on coordination of services or meeting the service needs of the disadvantaged.

Another type of policy decision concerns the selection and evaluation of top management, including supervising clinicians in their managerial role. The interests and enthusiasms of a hospital chief of surgery may conflict with those of the governing board. The chief may wish to raise money to invest in facilities and staff to perform open-heart surgery, whereas the board's long-range plan is to establish a prepaid group practice to provide primary and secondary care. Alternatively, the board may place heavy emphasis on the provision of tertiary care, but the chief of surgery may prefer that department to perform a high volume of simple surgical operations.

Governance and Management

Although those who govern are supposed to make policy and those who manage are supposed to administer policy, there is no clear-cut boundary between governance and management. In practice, those who manage are often key participants in governance, as they have the necessary time and information to define a problem or to limit the policy alternatives. This is, in large part, what those who manage are paid to do. On the other hand, those who govern the organization often carry out policy or manage as well, as they have the power and the will to do so.

A more useful distinction between governance and management may therefore involve the importance and nature of the decisions for the HCO. Decisions involving who governs and those involving organizational mission are governance, not management, decisions. Decisions regarding day-to-day operations, such as who should do what and when in the operating room or the personnel office are management decisions.

Governing Boards

This section focuses on HCO governance through a detailed look at the structure and function of HCO governing boards. We shall look at HCOs in which there is a specialized structure such as a board, a group, or a committee that determines policy and in which a substantial number of policy decisions are made by the HCO. These *two conditions* are generally found in general hospitals, health maintenance organizations (HMOs), and large group practices and nursing homes.

The Legal Basis of the Governing Board

In HCOs there is generally a governing body of designated persons who have legal responsibility for the conduct of the organization. Corporations are required to make such designations as a condition of incorporation by the state in which their home office is located.

Hospital or nursing home bylaws usually outline the purposes of the organization, the composition and duties of the governing board, the requirements for meetings of the board and notice of meetings, the duties and nature of corporate officers and the method of their selection, the nature and purpose of board committees, and how the bylaws can be amended. A physicians' partnership agreement may typically include the responsibilities of partners, how net income is shared and losses borne, disability provisions, termination of a partner's agreement, and the composition of the executive committee or board and its functions.

The legal powers of the governing board, suggested in a model constitution and bylaws for voluntary hospitals published by the American Hospital Association (1981) are the following:

> The general powers of the corporation shall be vested in the governing board, which shall have charge, control and management of the property, affairs, and funds of the corporation; shall fill vacancies among the officers for the unexpired terms; and shall have the power and authority to do and perform all acts and functions not inconsistent with these bylaws or with any action taken by the corporation. [p. 11]

These bylaws could be those of any corporation, health care or otherwise, for-profit or not-for-profit.

In theory, the governing board has the responsibility for making policy for the organization. In practice, the power and function of governing bodies in HCOs varies widely, depending on the HCO's history, key resources required for the HCO's survival and growth, the nature of the local power structure, and so forth. Policy in various areas may be formulated and decided on by different groups in different organizations. For example, questions of capital funding may be decided by the board of the multiunit organization of which a hospital is only a part; the scope of services may be decided by the hospital governing board; clinician educational programs may be decided on by the professional staff, and issues of local marketing and community relations decided by management.

The role of the governing board in the HCO is more ambiguous when there are no shares to be sold as in business, it is more complex in HCOs where the medical staff are not employees.

Selection of Board Members

The functions and powers of a governing board are influenced by its composition and its method of selecting members. When a hospital or a group practice is first established, the governing board usually consists of the founders, those who are contributing key resources to begin the enterprise. Officers are selected by the members of the governing board. In the case of investor-owned institutions, this is done formally by voting of shares. In nonprofit organizations and large partnerships, all full members generally have an equal vote. The board members themselves select additional members or replacements, or they are chosen from larger corporate bodies whose membership may be self-selected by those making a contribution of a certain sum to the corporation. In consumer-dominated HMOs or neighborhood health centers, some or all members of the governing board may be elected by health plan subscribers or residents of areas served by the organization.

In 1989 approximately 43% of the average hospital board's membership had backgrounds in business or finance. About 23% of board membership was made up of health care professionals, particularly of physicians (HRET, 1990). There was a wide difference in board composition by the type of control. Unsurprisingly, government and religious hospitals had a greater proportion of governmental officials and religious officers on their boards. Osteopathic hospitals had a greater proportion of doctors on their boards.

Board members may be "insiders"—HCO managers or clinicians—or "outsiders" chosen for some special expertise, status, or access to resources. The type chosen will depend, in large part, on the functions and role of the board. If the primary function of the board is to raise money or give advice and counsel to the chief executive officer (CEO), then outsiders are more likely to be selected. If the primary function is to decide policy, then the directors should have detailed knowledge of HCO operations and environment, and insiders may be preferred. Governance of hospitals has been dominated by outsider trustees, governance of nursing homes by manager outsiders, and governance of group practices by insider physicians.

A sample job description for hospital boards and board members is given in Table 16.1.

Except in large investor-owned HCOs, most board members are not paid for their time, although Witt (1987) and Kovner (1985) suggest they should be. Board members serve for a variety of reasons: community service or fiduciary responsibility, status, access to medical care, or because they believe their skills and experience are vital to HCO mission attainment.

TABLE 16.1 Sample Position Description for the Hospital Board of Directors

---

General functions
  Establish and maintain the organization's mission
  Act as trustee for the assets and investments of the shareholders or owners in the nonprofit corporation
  Select, advise, and audit the CEO.
  Grant physicians staff priviliges and ensure that quality medical care is provided.
  Provide broad direction for the affairs of the hospital and ensure the development and growth of the institution's services.
Specific duties
  Prepare for board and committee meetings by whatever study and preparatory work are necessary to deliberate intelligently with co-directors
  Attend meetings of the board and committee appointments
  Execute board assignments on time.
  Maintain confidentiality and security regarding hospital information
  Contribute positively to board discussions, assisting the board in reaching conclusions
  Serve as a consultant to the CEO and, with his or her approval, to others in the organization
  Acquire a working knowledge of those functional activities for which he or she has committee assignments
  Develop a broad knowledge of today's hospitals and future trends in health care
  Be alert to new program opportunities and assist the organization on specific programs when requested
  Avoid interference in hospital operations
  Avoid conflict of interest whenever an issue arises, and abstain from board discussions when matters in which he or she has a personal interest are being considered

---

Adapted from J. Witt, *Building a Better Hospital Board.* Ann Arbor, MI: American College of Healthcare Executives, 1987, pp. 64–65.

Board Structure and Function

Governing boards vary in internal structure and function. Information is not generally available concerning the number of boards with restrictions on terms of office and mandatory retirement age, nor concerning the length and frequency of meetings or the nature of participation by few of many members. In regard to size, governing boards range from fewer than 10 to more than 200 members. A 1989 American Hospital Association (AHA) survey revealed that the average hospital board consisted of approximately 14 members. Not-for-profit hospitals averaged about 17 members, and boards of investor-owned and public hospitals had 8 and 10 members, respectively (HRET, 1990). Witt (1987) suggests that no board, no matter how large the hospital, should have more than 15 members and that hospitals with revenues of $20 million or less should have no more than 5 to 7 members.

Board committees are generally of two types: standing, or permanent, committees, and special committees, which are discharged on completion of a task. Typical standing committees for a hospital board are executive, finance, medical staff, nominating, and long-range planning. Executive committees usually have power to act between regular meetings of the governing board. A large group practice may have a separate committee on personnel, which is concerned with defining responsibilities and benefits of partners, a committee on hospital relations, and one concerned with recruiting physicians. Focusing on large business corporations, Mintzberg (1983) has suggested the following seven functions for governing boards.

1. Select the chief executive officer.
2. Exercise control during a crisis.
3. Review managerial decisions and performance.
4. Co-opt external influences.
5. Establish contracts and raise funds.
6. Enhance the organization's reputation.
7. Give advice and technical assistance.

A significant omission from this list is "make strategic decisions." Mintzberg argues that part-time board members know less than full-time managers and that deferring too many decisions to the board raises questions about the ability of top managers to run the organization.

The Changing Role of the Board

Views of the role of governing boards differ and are changing. More than 35 years ago, Burling, Lentz, and Wilson (1956) stated that the governing board in a hospital has a responsibility to provide and maintain the hospital to serve a community need according to the wishes of the donors. Underwood (1969) has viewed the governing board as a referee between the interests of the hospital administrator and the medical staff. Pelligrino (1972) has seen the governing board as designated by the community to oversee the process of medical care within the hospital. Perloff (1970) has viewed the responsibility of the board as creating an environment in which health care workers can provide services to patients. To Umbdenstock (1987), the board must be the "organization's conscience, constantly assessing proposed directions . . . in light of what these steps mean for the implementation of a mission to serve and care for all" (p. 12). He divides work between the board and the CEO as follows: "whereas the board is concerned primarily with whether or not the hospital will do something, the administrator is responsible for how it will be done once the board gives the go-ahead" (Umbdenstock, 1983, p. 12). Some HCOs such as veterans hospitals or state mental hospitals do not have any governing boards; they are managed by administrators reporting to state officials and legislatures.

There is probably no one best way to allocate functions between board and management. Rather, what is important in any particular HCO is clarification and agreement as to who in the organization decides what on the recommendations of whom. Otherwise, the political cost of making timely strategic decisions is too high, and the probability of implementing such decisions is too low.

Relation to Medical Staff. In general hospitals, the governing body delegates to the medical staff the authority to evaluate the professional competence of staff members and applicants for staff privileges. Medical staff bylaws, rules, and regulations are subject to governing board approval, which according to the Joint Commission on the Accreditation of Health Care Organizations, shall not be unreasonably withheld. The Joint Commission also mandates that the governing board "requires the medical staff . . . to implement and report on the activities and mechanisms for monitoring and evaluating the quality of patient care, for identifying opportunities to improve patient care, and for identifying and resolving problems" (JCAHO, 1993, p. 27).

The bylaws of hospital governing boards deal with medical staff principally in three areas: (1) organization, appointments, and hearings for medical staff, (2) medical care and its evaluation, and (3) medical staff bylaws. The board's bylaws may include paragraphs dealing with organization and bylaws *of a medical and dental staff.* The AHA's suggested bylaws approach the problem of hospital appointment by recommending the following:

> The governing board shall consider recommendations of the medical staff and appointment to the medical staff, in numbers not exceeding the hospital's needs, physicians and others who meet the qualifications for membership as set forth in the bylaws of the medical staff. Each member of the medical staff shall have appropriate authority and responsibility for the care of his patients, subject to limitations as are

contained in these bylaws and in the bylaws, roles and regulations for the medical staff and subject, further, to any limitations attached to his appointment. (AHA, 1981)

The bylaws then deal with the appointment procedure and the renewal of appointments without formal reapplication (hospital appointments are generally made for a period of 1 year). Then a paragraph may be devoted to opportunity for a hearing if any change is proposed in the appointment to assure due process and afford full opportunity for the presentation of all pertinent information. A key paragraph in the second section dealing with medical care and its evaluation suggests that "the medical staff shall conduct an ongoing review and appraisal of the quality of professional care rendered in the hospital, and shall report such activities and their results to the governing board" (AHA, 1981, p. 18). With regard to medical staff bylaws, the AHA suggests that only those bylaws adopted by the governing board shall become effective.

In hospitals, physicians commonly expect governing boards to keep the organization financially solvent, to avoid "interfering" with the practice of medicine or curbing physicians' freedom, and to respect the contribution physicians make as practitioners. Some of the expectations commonly held by hospital governing boards for physicians include showing loyalty to the hospital by admitting their patients, practicing good medicine, understanding that the hospital is not merely a doctor's workshop, and acknowledging that they as physicians may lack the information to make certain important decisions, such as scope of services or compliance with government regulations.

Some of the reasons that physicians' expectations are not met include the following: Boards increasingly believe that the practice of medicine can have an important impact on hospital solvency; other clinicians, such as nurses, have claims that conflict with those of physicians; and board members may feel that some physicians' benefits from hospital practice far outweigh their contribution to the hospital's objectives.

Some of the reasons that boards' expectations are not met include the following: Some physicians compete against the hospital with which they have a primary affiliation; some physicians do not always meet the standards of adequate medical practice; and some physicians may feel that the medical staff should be a separate organization contracting at arm's length with the hospital to provide medical services.

Lack of Consensus on Board Role. As HCOs become larger and more complex and as the environment in which they function becomes more competitive, consensus on the role of the governing board tends to break down. And many HCOs may have difficulty in adapting to changed requirements for survival and growth. In response to public discontent with the cost and responsiveness of hospitals, some may urge governing boards to assume a legislative role, making policy in a way analogous to governmental legislatures and representing the consumers of services, or to assume merely an advisory role, ceding decision-making power to top executives who can presumably "get things done."

In the face of increasing change, the governance function may become more critical to accomplishment of HCO performance objectives The leadership of medical group practice, for example, may become increasingly specialized, with some clinicians devoting increasing time to, and developing expertise in nonclinical functions such as adapting to competition from HMO, interfacing with government agencies, keeping practicing physicians aware of the pressures facing the group, and the appropriate alternative organizational responses necessary for group survival and growth.

Current Issues

Some current key governance issues include the following: (1) Who should own HCOs? (2) To what extent does board performance need to be improved? (3) What kind of autonomy should HCOs have? (4) How and to what extent should HCOs be accountable to those whom they serve and whom they potentially serve?

Preferable Ownership Patterns

With the increasing role of government in the health care sector of the economy, ownership of HCOs has become an issue. Should HCOs be owned by government or by for-profit or by nonprofit corporations? A separate question, also a current issue, is whether or not there are sufficient significant differences between not-for-profit and for-profit ownership of HCOs to justify tax exemption for the former (Gray, 1986; *Utah County v. Intermountain Health Care, Inc.*, 1985).

There is insufficient evidence to make categorical statements regarding the effect of ownership per se on the cost or quality of medical care. Those who argue against for-profit ownership maintain that the motivation of proprietary owners is profit rather than community service. For-profits concentrate on providing only those services that are profitable, leaving the not-for-profits and public HCOs to provide care for those who lack adequate insurance. A corollary argument is that for-profit HCOs build facilities only in expanding high-income communities, leaving not-for-profit and governmental HCOs to provide services to the urban and rural poor; the monies allocated to shareholders of for-profit HCOs could be better reinvested in the delivery of services; and health care is of lower quality in for-profit HCOs than in nonprofit or governmental HCOs.

Counterarguments have been made in favor of for-profit ownership: Even allowing for profit, these HCOs are more efficient because of the profit incentive, and they pay taxes; consumers should be charged the costs of the services they use rather than overcharging certain consumers because others cannot pay, as is the case in nonprofit HCOs; for-profits can respond more quickly and more flexibly in meeting community demand; and the quality of care provided in most for-profits is adequate and in some for-profits is higher than that provided in certain HCOs under nonprofit or governmental auspices.

Regarding governmental ownership, the following arguments are made in its favor: Total costs and unit costs are lower, signifying greater efficiency; everyone gets treated similarly, based on health needs and regardless of income or disease status; and the quality of care is not lower than that provided in HCOs under other auspices. The following arguments are opposed to government ownership: Primary emphasis is in keeping total costs low rather than upon providing adequate health care; governmental management is bureaucratic and inflexible; and, the quality of care is lower in governmental HCOs.

Arguments in favor of nonprofit ownership are the mirror image of those made in favor and against for-profit and governmental HCOs. Those in favor of not-for-profit HCOs praise their high quality of care and the high level of community service; those opposed cite the high cost. For specific nonprofit HCOs, opponents add that the quality of care is low and the community services nonexistent. This has led to the suggestion that there ought to be clearly articulated standards for what it means to deserve the special "voluntary" description whether these standards are sponsored and regulated by the Joint Commission on the Accreditation of Health Care Organizations, the Internal Revenue Service, or the hospital or health care industry (Seay & Vladeck, 1987).

In order to evaluate these arguments, research must be conducted relating ownership to performance. To do such research it is required that conditions other than ownership, such as size of the HCO, be held constant. Also required is a greater consensus about adequate and effective performance in various HCOs.

The Extent of Organizational Autonomy

To what extent should an HCO be allowed to determine what services to provide to whom at what price? This issue relates to the role of the governing board, regardless of the type of ownership, and to the scope and depth of its powers. The powers, or autonomy, of HCO governing boards have been shrinking since 1960. Federal and state governments have passed legislation forbidding discrimination against patients who seek admission or persons seeking employment and invalidating a requirement that staff physicians of a voluntary hospital be graduates of a medical school approved by the AMA and members of the county medical society. They have removed the exemption of hospitals from state labor laws, specified standards to be met by HCOs in order to be licensed by a state or reimbursed by Medicare, and forbidden construction of hospitals, nursing homes, and related facilities in some states without prior approval by state planning authorities. More recent limitations on the autonomy of HCOs that have been enacted by government include limiting payment for new technology under Medicare and Medicaid; imposing requirements for community services for hospitals to retain not-for-profit status; requiring, in West Virginia, community representation on governing boards; and capping revenues in some states or limiting reimbursement under Medicare (by DRGs) to average payments for length of stay regardless of cost.

There is no simple answer to the question of HCO determination of services, prices, and population served. Too little autonomy for the HCO board will result in withdrawal of high-quality individuals from leadership positions and of voluntary energies that have been a strength of not-for-profit HCOs. Excessive standardization and centralization of decision making in governmental bureaucracies will result in decreased HCO innovation and eventually in decreased productivity. On the other hand, too much autonomy for HCOs may have been responsible, at least in part, for the present situation of uneven age-adjusted mortality and morbidity rates by race and income, overutilization of hospitals and underutilization of long-term care, uneven productivity and service, and high cost. One suggestion for appropriate centralization and decentralization is the regionalization of HCOs. However, that is also subject to similar criticisms of involving too much or too little centralization.

Accountability to Those Served

Whatever the scope of HCO activities and their regulation by government, what should be the extent and nature of governing board accountability to users and potential users of services? Some of those who advocate more formal accountability argue that this can be assured only by a governing board controlled by consumer representatives. Opponents argue that such control will lead to ineffective decision making at the board level and eventual withdrawal of community resources from health care. The opponents ask, furthermore, what evidence there is that the newly chosen representatives will be any more accountable. In what ways would they be more accountable and to whom? Consumers desire health care that is reasonably priced, accessible, provided in a humane, personal way, and technically of high quality. The great majority do not wish to make policy for HCOs, either directly or indirectly through their representatives, as long as they can obtain satisfactory health care. Advocates respond that consumers will not obtain satisfactory health care until governing boards are dominated by consumer representatives.

Regardless of the debate at the governing-board level, appeal mechanisms should be available for consumers at the level at which services are received, especially in large HCOs. In many HCOs consumers lack voice when they are dissatisfied with the manner of the provider, the wait for services, and the explanations they receive about what is wrong and about the alternative courses of treatment and their pertinent costs and benefits. They may be told to seek service elsewhere, or they can sue for malpractice. Consumers who are poor or institutionalized lack even these often-unsatisfactory alternatives. Proposals have been made and implemented regarding a variety of appeal mechanisms—the special board committee, the externally appointed ombudsman, the patient advocate—all specialized mechanisms for helping the patient who is unfairly treated by the HCO. Other, more general mechanisms include consumer advisory councils, focus groups and market surveys, and holding the chief executive personally accountable for responding to consumer complaints. As with all solutions, there are difficulties in implementing appeal mechanisms and limitations to their usefulness. To whom does the consumer appeal if he or she is dissatisfied with the response of the appeal mechanism, which may be, after all, a creation of the HCO? Appeal mechanisms may be costly in relation to the benefits obtained by the consumer. And there are many aspects of care that consumers (and providers) find objectionable but about which little can be done at the level of the HCO, such as obtaining high-quality accessible outpatient service for the uninsured. Finally, appeal mechanisms may serve only as buffers that satisfy the occasional vocal complainant but do little to change the system of care that may be the cause of much more unspoken dissatisfaction among many.

Management

This part will focus on what managers do in HCOs, how they are trained, their contributions to effective HCO performance, and current issues in health care management.

The Organization of Managerial Work in HCOs

In simple organizations such as the physician's office, clinicians themselves perform managerial functions such as billing patients or contracting with an outside vendor to bill patients (see Figure 16.1). In a group practice the hiring, paying, and firing of physicians is done by clinicians who manage and who also practice medicine. Other work such as billing is supervised by nonclinician managers. In the large hospital or HMO, specialized staff managers support clinician and nonclinician managers. Specialized departments include human resource, finance, security, and marketing, among others. In multiunit organizations of several hospitals, nursing homes, and/or group practices, the manager of the individual HCO reports to the division manager of a geographical area such as the northeastern United States. Division managers, in turn, are accountable to corporate headquarters management. In these large organizations certain management functions are divided among headquarters, divisions, and HCOs. Headquarters functions may include legal services, construction, capital financing, and corporate public rela-

FIGURE 16.1 Organization of Managerial Work in HCOs

A. Doctor's office

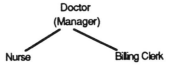

B. Group Practice

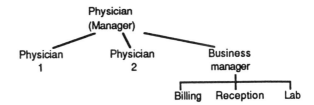

C. Hospital

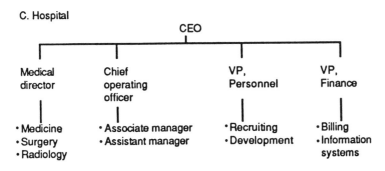

D. Multiunit hospital corporation

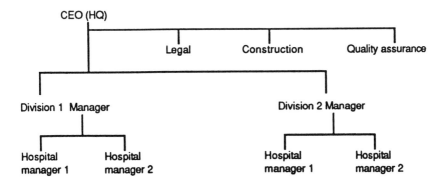

tions. Other functions, such as quality assurance and production standards, are partitioned among the three organizational levels.

A relatively new development in the organization of managerial work in HCOs is the concept of product-line management. The large hospital or group practice can be reorganized into several product lines, such as women's health services, emergency care, cancer care, and rehabilitation services, each with its own manager and budget. The logic behind such reorganization is that these services can be more effectively managed as separate "businesses" than as parts of a large HCO. Whether or not this is really so is unproven. (For a comparison with traditional organization, see Figure 16.2.)

What Managers Do

Positions and Functions

A job or position description is one way of looking at the work that managers do. The position description of an outpatient manager in a hospital is shown in Table 16.2.

Implicit in this job description are managerial functions, each of which comprises a group of activities. Longest (1980) views the basic managerial functions as

- Planning, which involves the determination of objectives.
- Organizing, which is the structuring of people and things to accomplish the work required to meet the objectives.
- Directing, which is the stimulation of members of the organization to meet the objectives.
- Coordinating, which is the conscious effort of assembling and synchronizing diverse activities and participants so that they work toward the attainment of objectives.
- Controlling, in which the manager compares actual results with objectives to provide a measure of success or failure.

Managerial Roles

Another way of conceptualizing what managers do is in terms of roles, which are aspects of behavior that can be isolated for analytical purposes, such as leading, or handling disturbances. Managers settle conflicts, inspire other workers, and represent the organization to outside groups. An individual manager's roles can thus be abstracted. This helps in understanding how managers contribute to organizational effectiveness and the constraints and opportunities they face in their work.

Because of the fragmented authority structure of many HCOs, managers often

FIGURE 16.2 Traditional versus Product-Line Organization

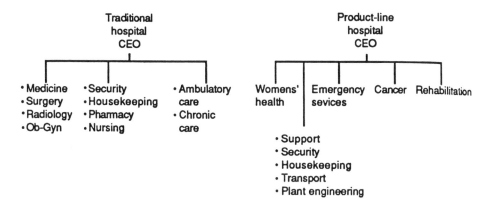

must lead by persuasion rather than by directive. Leadership is a relational rather than a personal characteristic, and therefore effectiveness as a leader is measured by what followers do rather than by how managers behave. The health care manager, especially in public and voluntary organizations, is constantly involved in testing the positions of others inside and outside the HCO and in confronting claimants for organizational resources. The manager must constantly persuade physicians, nurses, and others that the organization has good reasons for not doing what they want or for doing what they object to. External regulatory agencies may compel or allow certain actions desired by claimants. What claimants want may not be equitable. Some claimants may demand unequal treatment because the organization is unequally dependent on them.

An example of this is the demand by a hospital department head of inhalation therapy, supported by the chief of pulmonary medicine, for an increase in salary beyond the general guidelines for department heads. Either the hospital administrator must deny the request and convince these two individuals that the denial is fair, or the administrator must approve the request and convince other department heads that the increase *is* fair, or at least that the decision was arrived at fairly.

Disturbances in HCOs sometimes involve life-and-death issues, such as providing emergency services to victims of a natural disaster, responding to a bomb threat, or confronting deranged employees or aggrieved relatives. In such cases, managers must act quickly and appropriately, as if they know what to do. Managers should plan in detail their responses to possible emergency situations and should test their responses before emergencies occur.

Even when a life-and-death issue is not involved, patients and their families often have intense feelings about what is happening—for example, about death and dying or about diagnosis of infectious disease. It is the manager's job to deal with conflicts and problems that arise in treating such patients and in disturbances

TABLE 16.2   Position Description of Outpatient Manager

Title of Direct Supervisor: *Assistant V.P. for Ambulatory Care*

Purpose

To manage the administrative staff and functions and to coordinate the professional, clerical, and support services of all nonpsychiatric units in the Outpatient Department for the purpose of optimizing delivery of ambulatory patient care.

Description of duties

- Manages day-to-day operations of all ambulatory, medical/surgical, Ob/Gyn, adult and pediatric clinics, subspeciality clinics, private ambulatory service for related services.
- Supervises a staff of approximately 30 clerical and supervisory employees; hires, fires, takes disciplinary action.
- Plans and oversees training and orientation of employees; evaluates performance on a periodic basis; establishes standards, goals, and performance criteria; initiates personnel action as appropriate.
- Determines staffing needs and establishes schedules to ensure appropriate administrative coverage.
- Prepares, maintains, and controls the administrative operating capital budget for the Outpatient Department; designs and installs appropriate expense and manpower controls to measure budget adherence; makes adjustments as necessary and coordinates allocation of resources with other related cost centers.
- Plans and requisitions supplies and services for Outpatient Department.
- Collaborates with nursing, medical and administrative staff to formulate and implement policies for the Outpatient Department.
- Establishes and coordinates systems and procedures that support efficient delivery of medical and support services to the patient and that maintain quality patient care.
- Updates Outpatient Department procedural manuals; distributes information to staff.
- Evaluates all systems and procedures periodically for appropriateness and efficiency in meeting goals.
- Coordinates functions of and serves as a liaison with the hospital departments providing services to the Outpatient Department, such as pathology, radiology, and medical staff administration, to ensure effective and smooth interdepartmental operations.
- Investigates, reviews, and responds to patient complaints.
- Develops periodic statistical analyses and prepares departmental reports.
- Oversees environmental matters; coordinates with support departments to insure proper maintenance of Outpatient Department facilities.
- Assists Assistant Vice President for Ambulatory Care in preparing grant proposals; prepares all budgetary aspects of proposals.
- Participates in outside activities, including conferences and workshops.
- Represents hospital center in dealings with community groups and outside agencies, such as the Association for Ambulatory Care and the Hospital Association Ambulatory Care Project.

(continued)

TABLE 16.2 *Continued*

- Ensures that the Outpatient Department complies with standards of agencies such as JCAHO and the city Department of Health.
- Manages Outpatient Department's quality-assurance program.
- Assists the Assistant Vice President in performing other related duties and projects as needed.

Education required
    B.A./B.S. degree with courses in management; master's degree preferable.
Experiences and/or skills required
    A minimum of 3 years experience in an ambulatory care administrative position, preferably in a hospital setting; experience in third-party reimbursement systems and budgeting.

---

among workers of different backgrounds and skills in a labor-intensive organization. Kovner (1984) has reconceptualized managerial roles into four sets: motivating others, scanning the environment, negotiating the political terrain, and generating and allocating resources.

Motivating Others. Managers spend a great deal of their time recruiting and retaining managerial and supervisory staff and in making decisions about rewards and promotions, work procedures, and development and training. To carry out these activities they use communications and analytical skills. Managers assist subordinates in doing what is required and in doing what subordinates want to do, within organizational limits. This can be difficult if managers have not recruited subordinates (and recruitment is more of an art than a science). An excellent batting percentage in recruitment may be more like .600 than .850.

An example of motivating others is managerial development and training. Managers in new organizations or in new positions in existing organizations must be developed and trained by their supervisors. Such development and training can assist in the subordinate's learning process. Managers can aid those who work with them by identifying the skills that must be learned and the experience that must be acquired for effective job performance. Seniors can also help juniors become more aware of their own values, how they are perceived by others, and how the values of others affect their job performance in this position in this HCO.

Scanning the Environment. Effective managers scan or search the environment for potential problems and targets of opportunity. Scanning activities include market and product research, long-range planning, and quality assessment. The development of management information systems may be essential for effective scanning. In large HCOs scanning activities are usually performed by special units of marketing, quality assessment, development, and planning. In smaller organizations managers may scan the environment themselves or with the assistance of subordinates or colleagues. Information about what similar organizations and managers do is available from journals, books, newsletters, and advertisements. Managers attend continuing education and trade association meetings where colleagues and experts discuss organizational and managerial opportunities and problems. Managers visit similar organizations to learn at firsthand about possible ways to improve effectiveness and efficiency. Openness to such visits is characteristic of public and voluntary HCOs.

Negotiating the Political Terrain. Effective managers maintain trust and build alliances with groups and individuals. A positive political climate contributes to effective decision making and implementation. New managers must find out "who is doing what to whom" in their organization; or, put another way, "What is the ball park in which I am playing, who are the players, and what are the rules?" Managers learn the informal organizational power structure by reading and listening. The operative rules are not always easy to ascertain. They vary by organizational setting, and they depend on the issue being discussed. Decision makers involved in establishing a management information system are different from those who decide to establish a renal dialysis unit.

Activities the manager undertakes in this set of roles include public relations, lobbying, labor negotiations, influencing decisions made by governing boards and medical staffs, arbitrating between internal units and departments, and negotiating with other organizations.

Generating and Allocating Resources. Effective managers spend a great deal of time analyzing organizational efficiency and finding ways to increase revenues and decrease expenses. In doing this, managers must consider past performance in this organization, present performance in like organizations, and industry standards.

Effective managers attempt to improve financial performance, for example, by making decisions about buying procedures, efficient securing of long-term and working capital, effective maintenance of buildings and equipment, appropriate price changes, and new construction. Effective managers attempt to understand whatever special circumstances may influence preferences among alternative objectives and strategies, and they listen closely to explanations and analysis by subordinates and clinicians.

Effective managers continually make decisions about generating and using resources. This occurs as part of the budgetary process and in response to emergency or extraordinary requests. Less tangible resources, such as staff time, must also be allocated, as must resources that may be less amenable to negotiation, such as space.

Tasks

Another way of looking at what managers do is in terms of the tasks or activities they perform, such as recruiting professionals and determining buying procedures. Managerial tasks can be grouped and analyzed as episodes of work, which can be examined in relation to organizational objectives, outcomes achieved, and resource costs involved. An example of what a hospital CEO does on a particular day is shown in Table 16.3 (Kovner, 1988).

As shown in Table 16.3, managers perform a great quantity of work and must continue beyond customary working hours. Their jobs are characterized by brevity of interactions with others, variety, and fragmentation. They favor verbal over written contact. Scheduled meetings consume more of managers' time than any other activity (Hales, 1986).

Skills and Experience

What are the skills and experience needed to obtain and perform managerial jobs in HCOs? Managers use communication and analytical skills in their work. Communication skills include reading, writing, speaking, and listening. Analytical skills include judging and deciding.

Communication Skills. Managers spend more time communicating than they spend deciding. In understanding what managers do, communication skills are probably underemphasized relative to analytic skills. As Urmy indicates,

> Hospital administration is not about sitting in your office with a calculator.... About ten percent of the job is pushing paper, bureaucratic work.... Although I may have gone to six meetings and put in a ten-hour day, sometimes I feel I didn't get anything done.... The primary function of a hospital administrator is to provide integration and coordination within the hospital.... This means meeting and talking with people. [Kovner, 1984, pp. 193–195]

Although communicating and deciding can take place simultaneously, lengthy communication often takes place before decisions are made and while they are being implemented.

Managers receive and send out a great deal of written material. Some managers compensate for limited reading and writing capability by doing most of their work in person or by phone. Reading, of course, includes analyzing numbers as well as concepts or service plans. Being able to interpret numbers critically is an important skill for health services managers.

Reading and writing skills can be learned. Managers should have learned them

TABLE 16.3   Episodes and Activities for Chief Executive Officer (CEO) T. Grover on Monday (12.25 hours)

Episodes and Activities	Time Spent
1. CEO is informed by Chief Operating Officer (COO) of phone threat to V.P. for Human Resources.	Brief (less than 10 min)
2. CEO is informed by COO that applicant has accepted offer as new Chief of Genetics.	Brief
3. CEO is informed by COO of office space mix-up involving physician whom the hospital is attempting to terminate.	Brief
4. CEO is informed by clinical chief about perceived ineffective behavior of another clinical chief.	Brief
5. CEO responds that he will meet state surveyors after being informed by COO of preparation underway for the state Health Department Inspection Survey.	Brief
6. CEO requests information from COO concerning drop in census.	Brief
7. CEO informs COO about the progress in planning hospital budget reductions.	Brief
8. CEO informs COO regarding implementation of changes in the hospital's fringe benefit plan.	Brief
9. CEO informs COO about MRI (magnetic resonance imaging) lease.	Brief
10. CEO informs COO about progress on a second site construction budget.	Brief
11. CEO is informed by COO about cost/productivity information that may be available for each hospital cost center.	Brief
12. CEO informs COO re continuation of captive malpractice insurance company involving other hospitals as well.	Brief
13. CEO informs COO re arrangements for delayed payments to pension fund.	Brief
14. CEO informs COO that he will review Executive Committee meeting later with Chief Financial Officer (CFO).	Brief
15. CEO informs other hospital CEO and consultant of merger and is informed by them: he requests and is asked for further information.	Very long (more than 1 hr)
16. CEO requests CFO obtain information regarding obtaining increased state reimbursement after CEO informs re progress in rate adjustment by the state.	Brief

(continued)

TABLE 16.3 *Continued*

Episodes and Activities	Time Spent
17. CEO requests from COO of second site the channeling of a donation through the hospital development program in response to being informed of such a donation.	Brief
18. CEO is informed by the COO about awards ceremony at second site.	Brief
19. CEO responds to trade association secretary that he can't attend a meeting after being informed about proposed state malpractice insurance rates and legislation.	Brief
20. CEO responds to secretary of medical disease organization affirmatively to requested use of his name to sponsor charitable luncheon for another organization.	Brief
21. CEO tells secretary that he cannot attend a medical school consortium meeting.	Brief
22. CEO responds to CEO of other hospital with his preferences after being informed of options in reorganizing state payment for uncompensated care.	Brief
23. CEO is informed by VP of Medical Affairs regarding planned dismissal of a physician.	Brief
24. CEO is informed by Assistant Administrator re implementation of hospital's quality assurance program.	Brief

as part of an elementary and high school education, but unfortunately some have not. Many colleges and graduate schools have instituted special remedial writing courses and workshops. Speed reading courses are widely available as well.

Listening and speaking effectively are even more important for managers than skill in reading and writing. Many managers are not even aware that listening and speaking skills (other than public speaking) can be learned. However, managers can learn to make focused yet personal phone calls. They can learn to conduct meetings that accomplish goals yet make attendees feel that their points of view have been listened to and their feelings have been adequately taken into account.

Analytical Skills. Perhaps more clearly identifiable than communications skills are the analytical skills of judging and deciding. Brown (1966) has defined judgement as "knowledge ripened by experience." Many managers feel that skill in judging and deciding can come only from experience, that it cannot be taught in school. Others argue that by analyzing and responding to managerial situations such as structured cases or simulations, with students taking parts or playing roles of different participants, judgmental and decisional skills can be assessed and improved.

Before managers can judge or decide, they must, of course, be able to define a problem, gather data, structure alternatives, and calculate benefits and costs for each alternative. Each step of this problem-solving approach involves judging and deciding. For example, how valid is the manager's definition of the problem relative to that of key clinical chiefs? How much time should the manager spend gathering what data?

Computational skills are also required—for example, in making decisions regarding appropriate scheduling of patients for appointments, discounting the value of money over time to assess the true cost of capital financing, or pricing services to different payers so that revenues can be maximized.

Experience. Like other professions, skill as a manager involves learning through practice and being coached by others on how to avoid mistakes and achieve better outcomes. Participating in meetings and writing memos can be learned by self-analysis and feedback from peers, superiors, and subordinates. Experience also can be gained as a student in reading, listening, writing, computing, and interpreting data or in working as a member of a team doing a project for a local HCO.

Persona

The effectiveness of managers is determined as much by who they are and how they manage as by what they do. Managers are trusted, at least in part, based on how they are perceived by others. Managers are likely to think that how they manage—rather than race, sex, age, or beliefs—affects how others view their contribution. However, workers tend to feel more comfortable with, and more trusting of, persons whom they see as similar to themselves.

Superiors, subordinates, and peers sometimes react to managers primarily in terms of the question "Is the manager one of us or is he part of some outside group whom we dislike or fear?" The group practice administrator in a rural community in west Texas may have great difficulty gaining the trust of her board of directors if she is well educated and from New York City. Or a west Texas graduate of a small religious school will have a similarly hard time gaining the confidence of the medical and administrative staff in a public hospital in New York City serving Hispanics and blacks.

People trust one another partly because of what they think others believe. "If she believes in the same things that I do, perhaps it doesn't matter so much whether I like her. I can trust her because she is likely to do what I would do in a similar situation for her own reasons."

Registered nurses distrust managers when they see managers as being interested only in money, with little or no perceived commitment to providing high-quality patient care. Such distrust may or may not be justified, but it is usually dissipated only over time, as managers' actions indicate what their beliefs really are relevant to a particular work situation.

Educating Health Care Managers

How do people learn to be health care managers? Can health care management be taught? Is it a science, an art, or a craft? What can best be learned at school and on the job?

Graduate Programs. Graduate education is increasingly being required of persons seeking employment as health care managers. There are over 100 graduate programs in health care management in the United States today. Such programs may be called health care or medical care administration, health planning and policy, hospital administration, nursing home administration, medical group practice management, and public health administration. Many graduate programs are members of the Association of University Programs in Health Administration (AUPHA), headquartered in Washington, D.C. Of the 67 AUPHA American and Canadian members in 1992, 20 graduate programs are housed in graduate schools of business management or public administration, 13 in schools of public health, and 34 in one or more of the following schools: business, allied health, community health, and medicine (AUPHA, 1991).

In the academic year 1991–1992, a total of 5,696 students enrolled in 59 AUPHA graduate programs; less than half were full-time. Of these students, 60.2% were women, and 12.3% were members of minority groups. In the same year 5,571 persons applied to the programs, and 48% were accepted. Master's degrees were awarded to 1,683 students (AUPHA, 1991).

As of 1992, 62 programs had been accredited by the Accrediting Commission on Education for Health Services Administration (ACEHSA). ACEHSA is sponsored by AUPHA, together with the American College of Healthcare Executive, the AHA, and the American Public Health Association. For accreditation, ACEHSA requires that the curriculum of a graduate program cover the following areas:

- Social-behavioral disciplines—economics, sociology, psychology, and political science.
- Determinants, of health, disease, and disability: the study of what health is, how it is measured, patterns and characteristics of illness, and interventions possible with a health care system.
- Elements of personal health systems and their interrelationships: evaluation, governance, financial structure, organization, function and structure, quality assessment, and social accountability.

- Management and administrative skills and their applications: organizational behavior, quantitative methods, financial management, information systems, law, strategic planning, and health regulation.

In addition to curricular requirements for accreditation, ACEHSA sets criteria in the following areas: program eligibility, resources, objectives, faculty, students and alumni, research, community service, continuing education, and program evaluation.

Most graduate programs include an academic and a practice component, which may involve employment with or without pay in an HCO for a period of 3 to 12 months. Some programs do not require a practice component at all. As the supply of graduates increases in relation to demand, programs may extend the formal training period to 3 years, 1 year of which would be a residency.

Undergraduate Programs. Undergraduate programs in health care administration are a more recent development. As of 1990–1991, 32 undergraduate programs in the United States were members of AUPHA, with 684 graduates in that year (AUPHA, 1991).

Most of the undergraduate programs attempt to produce managers for intermediate-level positions in hospitals and for top-level positions in those health services organizations that have been found less attractive to graduates of the master's degree programs. The curriculum offered by the undergraduate programs is generally similar to that offered by graduate programs. Courses that are generally required include introduction to the health care field, economics, health law, administrative theory, personnel administration, financial management, health planning, medical sociology, quantitative methods, system analysis, and management of specific types of health care facilities.

Continuing Education. In addition to graduate and undergraduate programs, there is a great variety of continuing education programs in health services management. They are of various lengths and cover various subjects. Some continuing education programs are offered by the university programs themselves. Others are offered by centers of continuing education that are freestanding or that have been sponsored by professional associations or corporations that sell equipment and services to health services organizations. Still others are offered by the large HCOs themselves.

On the Job. Much of what managers learn about what works in an organization and about how they can best work with physicians and nurses is done on the job. This includes what managers say, how they write, how they look, and how they influence others. Superiors, subordinates, and peers can assist managers in teaching about an HCO.

Managerial Contribution to Effective Performance in HCOs

HCOs are seldom formally evaluated in terms of their own preset specified goals. Part of the reason is the difficulty of securing agreement among the various parties of interest as to what these goals are, what acceptable standards of performance are, and who should evaluate performance and by what methods. Yet the basic problem in public organizations, according to Drucker (1973), is not high cost but lack of effectiveness: "Only if targets are defined can resources be allocated to this attainment, priorities and deadlines be set, and somebody be held accountable for results."

Measuring Organizational Performance

One reason for attempting to specify effective or acceptable organizational performance is to focus attention on whose organization it is. If performance is acceptable to managers, physicians, and trustees, does it matter what anyone else thinks? If it does matter, what are others going to do if they find performance unacceptable?

Another reason for developing measures of organizational performance has to do with the distribution of organizational resources. In order to adjudicate claims on resources among claimants, questions may need to be raised about the organization's purposes. For example, "How is the HMO doing? How does what we do compare to what our competitors do? How does what we do compare with what our doctors, nurses, trustees, customers, and potential customers think we ought to be doing?"

Prior agreement about standards of performance facilitates agreement on performance evaluation. Otherwise, performance is not measurable in terms such as excellent, acceptable, and unacceptable. Statements such as "The hospital operated at a $100,000 surplus this year, one percent of the patients made formal complaints, and our turnover rate in nursing was 15 percent per year" are uncertain indicators of performance unless they can be related to agreed-upon standards and purposes. The standards of performance for which the organization and its managers are to be held accountable must be made clear in measurable terms and in advance. Of course, targets can be adjusted for fully explained reasons as circumstances change.

Putting Performance Requirements into Operation

Standards can be developed regarding performance requirements. Certain standards, such as financial ratios, are easier to quantify than others, such as commitment of physicians and nurses to organizational performance requirements. Yet commitment can be quantified in terms of turnover and absenteeism rates; unit costs per clinical service relative to industry standards; nurses' attitudes, as measured by surveys; and physician commitment measured by attendance at key committee meetings and contributions to fund-raising campaigns. Whether the effort and cost of putting such requirements into operation and then measuring performance is "worth it" is, of course, a separate and not a trivial question.

Griffith (1978) has argued that guidelines need to be developed for hospital performance in the face of national concern about rapidly increasing health care costs. Accordingly, there should be a few, well-understood measures of hospital care—uniformly available and designed to permit each community to compare itself to other, similar communities, its state, its region, and the nation as a whole.

Reasons for Not Specifying Objectives. One of the difficulties in measuring organizational performance is that, according to Perrow (1982), the concept of organizational goals as a major influence on organizational behavior is "only a convenient fiction," and much of what happens in organizations results from

"happenstance, accidents, misunderstanding, and even random, unmotivated behavior. . . . Programs are started for a variety of vague and conflicting reasons, with the help of a lot of trivial or even accidental events. . . . Decision makers do not look for optimal solutions, have trouble discovering what they want, and settle for the first acceptable solution that comes along, which is usually what the organization has been doing. That is, they settle so long as some important person or group doesn't want to change what the organization is doing and how the organization has been doing to it."

Goal specification may not be necessary to achieving acceptable performance results, at least not in the eyes of major contributors of resources. Specification costs may be high in relation to projected benefits. It may be easier to accommodate diverse interests if goals are not specified. Competing members of a coalition may rarely see conflict among organizational objectives until goals are specified, at which time they may be forced to recognize and deal with the conflict. It may be easier to shift organizational direction if the proposed change does not have to meet criteria that have been previously defined and agreed to. Finally, trustees, managers, and clinicians may choose not to specify goals in order to avoid accountability and to maximize discretion or authority.

Results of Not Specifying Goals. Not specifying or targeting organizational performance requirements may result in lower levels of performance than would otherwise occur. By not focusing on particular goals and levels of attainment, the organization may fail to perform satisfactorily. Strong members of a coalition may gain more power or resources at the expense of the weak than they would have if the goals of the weak had been considered formally by all participants

When performance requirements are not specified and opportunistic interests prevail, long-term survival of HCOs may be threatened, or short-term organizational crises may become more frequent and more severe. Without goal specification, it may become more difficult to make and implement policy decisions— that is, to the extent that there is disagreement regarding effective performance requirements among the controlling coalition.

Not specifying performance requirements favors retention of the present power structure. And as long as the organization can continue to obtain necessary and appropriate inputs and sell or dispose of adequate quantities of outputs, the status quo will tend to be perceived as a satisfactory level of goal attainment.

The environment that many HCOs will be facing in the 1990s is expected to be increasingly competitive and problematic. Hospitals are competing for patients with physicians on their own medical staffs. Attending physicians are in conflict with staff nurses about nurse functions. Nurses are in conflict with managers and trustees regarding pay and working conditions. In these circumstances goal specification may be increasingly perceived by effective HCOs as less costly than direct conflict over limited resources. Evidence of a trend toward goal specification may be found in the startling growth of investor-owned corporations, some of which have well-developed internal systems specifying performance requirements by unit or department.

Measuring Managerial Contribution

Managers disagree regarding how and whether they should be evaluated by whom, and it is indeed difficult to isolate managerial contribution to organizational performance, about which there is also disagreement. For example, despite substantial managerial contributions, an organization may be floundering because of a hostile environment or poor decisions by previous managers. Or the reverse situation may be occurring: despite little or ineffective managerial contribution, an organization may be growing rapidly or raising quality standards and performance because of lack of competitors or excellent management in the past and excellent physicians and nurses now.

Reasons for Evaluating Managers. Generally, health services managers are evaluated to avoid setting them apart from all other employees who are evaluated, to determine continued employment and terms of employment, to set prospectively agreed-upon managerial performance requirements and to assess how these requirements may be accomplished, and to force self-examination in regard to managerial performance and improvements that would enhance managerial performance. A manager may be evaluated relative to what he or she has accomplished previously or relative to what managers in like organizations contribute, assuming a correlation between managerial and organizational performance.

Evaluation is a way of communicating to managers how superiors feel about them and of learning from managers how they feel about superiors' assessments. This can serve as a basis for desired changes in behavior by managers, or it may stimulate superiors to make certain changes that would enable managers to perform as desired. The evaluation process can make both superiors and managers focus on the most important organizational objectives for the time period ahead and can stimulate efforts to generate additional resources necessary to attain goals. Evaluation of managers also serves as a standard for managerial evaluation of others in the organization.

Formal evaluation may not be necessary for a high level of managerial performance or for a high level of satisfaction with managerial contribution by superiors. Nor is formal evaluation of the manager a panacea for effectively adjudicating political conflict between board members and physicians. Formal evaluation can avoid misunderstandings about what constitutes satisfactory managerial performance. The process can facilitate specification of managerial performance requirements that are realistic yet responsive to organizational constraints and opportunities.

Current Issues

Some key issues in HCO management for the 1990s include the following: (1) What should managers do in HCOs? (2) Is too much money spent on managing HCOs? (3) How should managers be trained? (4) To what extent does management performance need to be improved?

Functions of HCO Managers

Should HCO managers basically support the work of more or less independent clinicians, or are managers responsible for integrating the HCO with its environment and coordinating work in the organization? What should be the relationship of line and staff managers in large HCOs? For example, to what extent should a local HMO manager be responsible for marketing relative to the marketing specialists in the HMO central headquarters? How should front-line managers best spend their time—attending internal meetings and writing memos or listening to customers and influencing legislation?

Assuming again that the health care sector is becoming increasingly competitive, with too much capacity relative to demand, there will be an increasing need for managers to be skilled in the production of care and the sale of services in order to gain market share in a competitive situation. This means being the low-cost producer or else providing a differentiated service for which customers are willing to pay higher prices.

If this is so, there will be an increasing requirement in HCOs to specify objectives with regard to cost, quality, and market share and for managers to spend more of their time in activities that contribute to attainment of these objectives. This means more time spent in listening to customers, determining their perceptions and preferences, and in developing production standards to assist clinicians and others in meeting standards.

Resources Spent on Management Functions

Is too much money spent in HCOs on management relative to provision of care? Do managers make too much money related to their contribution as compared with clinicians, technicians, and nonprofessional workers? How should managers be paid, and to what extent should pay be related to performance?

Himmelstein and Woolhandler (1991) estimated the total cost for health care administration in 1987 to be between $96.8 billion and $120.4 billion, 19.3 to 24.1% of all spending for health care. This represents an increase of approximately 37% since 1983. They divided expenditures into $25.3 billion for program administration and insurance, $39.3 billion for hospital administration, $6.4 billion for nursing home administration, and between $25.8 billion and $49.4 billion (depending on which of two methods was utilized) for physicians' overhead. They argue that the institution of a single-payer health care system like Canada's would generate substantial savings between $69.0 billion and $83.2 billion by eliminating the majority of the private health insurance industry, much of the hospital and nursing home bureaucracy, and some of the expenses of doctors' offices (Himmelstein & Woolhandler, 1991). Their critics can argue that, yes, the British system is cheaper; but no, that is not the kind of health care system that Americans want.

Proponents of paying managers more can argue that health care is increasingly a competitive sector of the economy as patients are increasingly being steered away from high-cost and low-quality HCOs and toward those of low cost and high quality. The management function may be generally responsible for keeping costs down and quality high in large complex organizations, and managers must be attracted to work in health care as opposed to other organizations.

In the United States payment to workers is largely determined by market forces. Markets, of course, are influenced by reimbursement policies of payers, subsidies to suppliers, and governmental licensing of providers. So what managers earn relative to orthopedic surgeons, pediatricians, nurses, x-ray technicians, nurse's aides, and accountants is determined by what HCOs must pay to hire the type of staff they require to perform in variably competitive local markets. Hospital and other HCO managers are not licensed; nursing home administrators are licensed in certain states. Whether earnings of health care managers are too high, too low, or just right relative to other workers may depend on their relative contribution to organizational performance as determined by the board of directors. Obviously, different health care workers will answer this question differently, depending on different interests and perceptions.

Training of HCO Managers

Should managers be trained in business schools, schools of public health, medical schools, schools of public administration, or schools of allied health professions? Should managers of hospitals or group practices be physicians, lay managers, or nurses with management training? What kind of management training should managers receive?

There are no simple answers to any of these questions because of the variability of HCOs and the jobs of managers within them. Trends in the industry are toward a greater supply of physicians to population (hence, more physicians interested in management) and increasing surveillance of physicians, increased competition among HCOs, fewer and larger HCOs, and better-trained HCO managers. Given the tremendous changes taking place in the industry, this means a greater need for management training for those already working in HCOs compared to those entering the HCO managerial labor market.

What the industry trends imply for management training is that more physicians will want and require management training. Such training need not be the same as that required for lay managers, particularly if the managerial jobs of physicians so trained consist largely in supervising and recruiting other physicians while continuing to practice.

Increased competition among HCOs has implications for management curriculum that include more emphasis on economics, marketing, and planning, information systems, and accounting and reimbursement, as well as on production of care that meets quality standards and is responsive to consumer preferences.

Increased size of HCOs implies increased standardization and specialization of work, including managerial work. Large HCOs will spend more on managerial training and have more in-house training programs for new managers to teach them about the values, policies, and skills required in these HCOs.

Managerial Performance

To what extent does managerial performance in HCOs need to be improved? Does the health care sector require more MBAs, and would business managers do a better job of running HCOs than do those who currently manage them? Should expectations be any different for managers of particular types of HCOs, such as public hospitals and health clinics?

Kovner (1986) reports in interviews with 29 HCO managers and educators the following views regarding effective health care management and the education of health care managers. Health care managers have difficulty responding appropriately to a new environment of competition and purchaser price pressure; they have difficulty managing changing power relationships between physicians and governing boards; they have a lack of knowledge regarding efficient production of services of adequate quality; and they have employers who make a low investment in continuing professional education and career development for managers.

Similar problems have confronted managers in other service industries facing rapid change, such as airlines and banks. Power relations problems require board leadership for effective responses. MBAs have a useful contribution to make to HCO management, particularly in the functional areas—marketing, finance, information systems, accounting—where expertise can be applied across sectors of the economy and the commitment of the functional specialist is to the function rather than to the sector. On the other hand, to develop successful agendas and networks in HCOs, managers require a knowledge of the health care sector that cannot be learned in business schools without specific health care programs. MBAs can learn on the job about the production of health care, quality assurance, health economics and reimbursement, and government regulations and medical politics, but they are not generally a good investment for HCOs short of scarce front-line management talent. Certainly, HCO managers require continuing training to cope with changing circumstances, and HCOs would probably benefit from devoting more resources to training managers relative to organizational objectives—rather than viewing such training as to be enjoyed by managers in vacation resorts as a fringe benefit of employment.

Two differences in managing public HCOs are legislative "ownership" of the programs and civil service regulations that constrain rather than facilitate organizational flexibility. To the extent that public HCOs provide services for which insurance does not pay to people who can not afford to pay either, they face less competitive pressure. Such services, particularly for low-income populations in large cities, include long-term psychiatric and nursing home care and acute care for substance abusers and AIDS patients. However, expectations need to be set in a similar way for public HCO managers as for managers of other types of HCOs. Managerial performance in public HCOs, as in other HCOs, needs to be improved; and this includes billing and collecting of revenues and even marketing of services as appropriate and certainly listening to customers and responding to their preferences.

References

Allison, R. F., & Dalston. J. W., Governance of University-Owned Teaching Hospitals." *Inquiry, 19* (Spring), 11, 1982.

American Hospital Association. *Guide for Preparation of Constitution and By Laws for General Hospitals.* Chicago: AHA, 1981.

Association of University Programs in Health Administration (AUPHA). *Annual Survey of Health Administration Programs.* Washington, DC: AUPHA, 1991.

Brown, R., *Judgment in Administration.* New York: McGraw-Hill, 1966.

Burling, T., Lentz, E., & Wilson, R., *The Give and Take in Hospitals.* New York: G. P. Putnam's Sons, 1956.

Dayton, K. N., "Corporate Governance: The Other Side of the Coin." *Harvard Business Review, 84* (Jan–Feb), 34, 1984.

Drucker, P. F., "Managing the Public Service Institution." *The Public Interest, 33,* 46, 1973.

Gray, B. (Ed.), *For Profit Enterprise in Health Care.* Washington, DC: Institute of Medicine, National Academy Press, 1986.

Griffith, J. R., "Measuring Hospital Performance." *Inquiry, 3,* 1978.

Hales, Colin P., What do Managers Do? A Critical Review of the Evidence, *Journal of Management Studies* 23(1): 88–115, 1986.

Himmelstein, D. U., & Woolhandler, S., "The Deteriorating Administrative Efficiency of the U.S. Health Care System." *New England Journal of Medicine, 324*(18):1253–1258, 1991.

The Hospital Research and Educational Trust. *The Changing Character of Hospital Governance.* Chicago: HRET, 1990.

Joint Commission on Accreditation of Healthcare Organizations. *Accreditation Manual for Hospitals.* Chicago: JCAHO, 1993.

Kovner, A. R., "Improving the Effectiveness of Hospital Governing Boards." *Frontiers of Health Services Management, 2* (August), 4, 1985.

Kovner, A. R., *Really Trying: A Career Guide for the Health Service Manager.* Ann Arbor, MI: Health Administration Press, 1984.

Kovner, A. R., "Reflections in Health Management Education." *Journal of Health Administration Education 4*(3) 359, 1986.

Kovner, A. R., *Really Managing*: The work of effective CEOs in large health organizations, Ann Arbor, MI: Health Administration Press, 1986.

Longest, B. B., *Management Practices for the Health Professional.* Reston, VA: Reston Publishing, 1980.

Mintzberg, H., *Power in and around Organizations.* Englewood Cliffs, NJ: Prentice-Hall, 1983.

Pelligrino, E. T., "The Changing Matrix of Clinical Decision-Making." In B. Georgopoulos (Ed.), *Organization Research in Health Institutions.* Ann Arbor, MI: Institute for Social Research, University of Michigan, 1972.

Perloff, E., "For the Trustee, Deepening Responsibilities." *Hospitals 44,* 84, 1970.

Perrow, C., "Disintegrating Social Sciences." *Phi Delta Kappa 63,* 684, 1982.

Peters, J. P., & Tseng, S., *Managing Strategic Change in Hospitals.* Chicago: American Hospital Publishing, 1983.

Pfeffer, J., "Size and Composition of Boards of Directors: The Organization and Its Environment." *Administrative Science Quarterly 17,* 219, 1972.

Ritvo, R. A., "Adaptation to Environmental Change: The Board's Role." *Hospital & Health Services Administration, 25* (Winter), 23, 1980.

Seay, J. D., & Vladeck, B. C., *Mission Matters.* New York: United Hospital Fund of New York, 1987.

Umbdenstock, R., *So You're on the Hospital Board* (2nd ed.) Chicago. American Hospital Publishing, 1983

Umbdenstock, R. J., "Refinement of Board's Role Required." *Health Progress,* 68(1) 47, 1987.

Underwood, J., "How to Serve on a Hospital Board." *Harvard Business Review, 47,* 73, 1969.

Utah County v. Intermountain Health Care Inc., S. Ct. Utah, No. 17699, Slip Op., June 26, 1985.

Witt, J., *Building a Better Hospital Board.* Ann Arbor, MI: American College of Health-care Executives, 1987.

17

Comparative Health Systems: A Policy Perspective

Victor G. Rodwin

Comparative analysis of health systems in industrially advanced nations has produced a large and growing literature that provides profiles of health care systems abroad.[1] This chapter begins with an overview of general issues in the comparative study of health care systems. Next it assesses some common problems of health policy in three countries: France, Canada, and Britain. Finally, it analyzes the U.S. health system from a comparative perspective and examines the uses of comparative analysis, for Americans, in learning from abroad.

Three stages may be distinguished in the evolution of comparative health systems research (Dumbaugh & Neuhauser, 1979). During the first stage, which dominated until the mid-1960s, and continues today, travelogues were written by physicians returning from overseas tours (Corson, 1948). During the second stage, health systems were described from a variety of perspectives—often with hopes of promoting health care reform.[2] During the third stage, there has been an attempt to make the study of comparative health systems into a kind of social sci-

[1]There is even a two-volume bibliographic manual with appropriate taxonomies and summaries of relevant research (Elling, 1980a). The references at the end of this chapter provide a good bibliography of this literature. Suggested readings on comparative health systems and policy appear at the end of this chapter.

[2]For examples of some classic books, see Douglas-Wilson and McLachlan (1974); Fry (1970); Raffel (1985); Roemer (1977, 1981, 1991); Saltman (1988); Victor and Ruth Sidel (1977); In addition, there are some excellent single country case studies: Andreopoulos (1975) on Canada; Gordon Forsyth (1966), Almont Lindsey (1962) on England; Gordon Hyde (1974) and Henry Siegerist (1947) on the Soviet Union; Richard Weinerman (1969) on Eastern Europe.

ence. The research has focused largely on explaining variation across health systems on the basis of received theories within such disciplines as anthropology, sociology, political science, and economics.[3]

The social science approach to comparative health systems has the inherent defect of its virtues. To achieve a rigorous study design, it has classified descriptive data, elaborated hypotheses, and tested them against available evidence. The focus has been largely on cross-sectional comparisons of health services utilization and expenditures, thus narrowing the scope of research questions and eroding the ideals shared by stage 2 scholars, who were more motivated by the pragmatic concerns of improving the delivery of medical care. Social scientists tend to display more interest in the theoretical concerns of their disciplines than in social change. Nevertheless, a number of excellent studies have been produced, and this has raised some conceptual and methodological issues.

Conceptual Issues

The concept of health system is clearly central. And yet there is no fully satisfactory definition of this concept, for it is difficult to agree both on the boundaries of the system and on a definition of health. Blum (1981) provides a visual model of health, suggesting that health care services are merely one input into health among three others—heredity, behavior and environment (See Figure 17.1). Weinerman (1971) defines the health system as "all of the activities of a society which are designed to protect or restore health, whether directed to the individual, the community, or the environment." Anderson (1972) has more concretely outlined the "boundaries of a relatively easily defined system with entry and exit points, hierarchies of personnel, types of patients"—in short, what he calls "the officially and professionally recognized 'helping' services regarding disease, disability and death" (p. 22).

Viewing the concept of health system at a macrosociological level, Field (1973) proposes the following formal definition: "that societal mechanism that transforms generalized resources . . . into specialized output in the form of health services." He adds that "the 'health system' of any society is that social mechanism that has arisen or been devised to deal with the incapacitating aspects of illness, trauma, and (to some degree) premature mortality . . . the five D's: death, disease, disability, discomfort, and dissatisfaction (pp. 768, 772).

---

[3]For a good example of how anthropologists approach the comparative study of health systems, see Leslie (1978). For a sociological perspective, see Anderson (1989), Elling (1980c), Field (1989) or Light and Schuller (1986). For an organization theory perspective, see Saltman and Van Otter (1992). For a political science approach, see Altenstetter (1978), Immergut (1992) and Leichter (1979, 1991). For an economic approach, see Hu (1976), Hurst (1992), McLachlan and Maynard (1982), and Schweitzer (1978). Also, for classic single country studies, see Eckstein (1959) and Klein (1983) on England, Wilsford (1991) on France, Stone (1980) on Germany, and Field (1967) on the former Soviet Union.

FIGURE 17.1   Inputs to Health

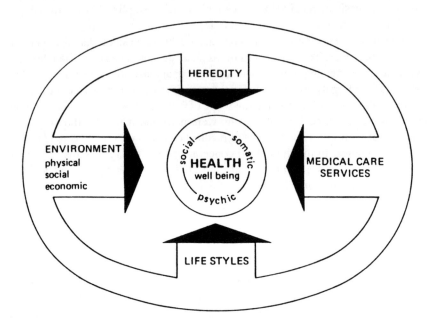

Source: Adapted from H. Blum, *Planning for Health* (2nd ed), New York: Human
Sciences Press, 1981, p. 3.

Another approach to the concept of health system is to define it implicitly by
postulating a casual model of it. Thus, drawing on Elling and Kerr's (1975) proposed framework for studying health systems, De Miguel (1975) outlines four
subsystem levels that influence health status: individual, institutional, societal, and
environmental. Such an approach allows one to analyze a health system by investigating the effects of a hierarchy of independent variables on the dependent variables, health status. It also raises questions about the most effective levels at which
to effect system change.

Methodological Issues

The fundamental methodological issue in comparative health systems research
involves devising a study design and selecting alternative systems that allow the
analyst to hold some variables constant while manipulating experimental ones. In
the area of health policy, for example, how does one evaluate the success of cost-

containment efforts in health systems characterized by diverse patterns of financing and provider reimbursement? Quasi-experimental research designs would suggest matching two health systems on all but a few policy-related factors. But "matching," let alone a real experiment, is rarely feasible in policy research.

One response to this difficulty has been to match health systems on at least some criteria (e.g., levels of health resources) and then to call for "in-depth studies of contrasting cases" (Elling & Kerr, 1975). Another response has been to use the language of natural experiment and view "most similar systems" as laboratories in which to assess the effects of alternative policy options at home (Marmor, Bridges, & Hoffman, 1978). A third response is to adopt a "modular approach" that examines systematically diverse components of health systems (Ellencweig, 1992).

Another methodological concern in the social science approach to comparative health systems research is whether the descriptive studies and data collected during stage 2 are actually comparable. If they are not, this casts great doubt on the utility of making international comparisons. If they are, qualifications must usually be made.

The most difficult methodological issues arise in evaluating health systems, for this involves specifying the relationship between the elements of a health system (inputs) and their impact on health (output). But how does one distinguish the impact of health services on health from the impacts of improvements in social services, income security, education, and transportation—not to mention the social and physical environment? This question raises the problem of devising indicators of health status. It also explains why, in his comparative study of the United States, Sweden, and England, Odin Anderson (1972) found it impossible to attribute differences in the usual health indices of morbidity and mortality to patterns of medical care organization in these countries. To evaluate health systems, it is necessary to agree on consistent definitions of health system inputs and to devise health status indicators to measure outputs.

Learning from Abroad

Although there is a large literature on the comparative analysis of health systems, there are rarely attempts to draw lessons from comparative experience. Comparative studies of health policy are sparse. Most often, they describe national experience in a range of policy areas; only rarely do they interpret, let alone evaluate, this experience. Exceptions to this general rule are of interest because they have contributed at least three ideas that have implications for learning from abroad.

First is the idea of evolutionary progress in health systems. Medical sociologists such as Field (1973) and Mechanic (1976) have argued that health systems in Western industrialized nations are evolving in similar directions. Drawing on Field's typology, consisting of five systems—the private health system, the pluralistic one, the national health insurance (NHI) system, the national health service (NHS), and the socialized health service—such views would suggest that the direction of change in modern societies is from the system of Type 1 to that of Type 5 (Table 17.1). Unlike Field and Mechanic, who are not convinced that such change necessarily implies "progress," Milton Roemer (1977) describes similar trends as a march toward a health ideal.

The second idea, the notion of public policy learning, is methodological in nature. It is highlighted in Glaser's studies of health policy in Western Europe and Canada. *Paying the Doctor* (1970) analyzes systems of physician remuneration. *Health Insurance Bargaining* (1978) explains how alternative administrative arrangements affect the process of bargaining between the medical profession and the state. *Paying the Hospital* (1987) describes systems of hospital reimbursement and assesses the implications for the United States. *Health Insurance in Practice* (1991) reviews a wide range of issues related to the financing and organization of national health insurance in cross national perspective. Each of these studies starts with the presumption that the United States has many problems and that the policies and experience of Western Europe and Canada shed light on and provide a useful range of solutions.

The third idea focuses on understanding either determinants of health policies or at least their effects. Leichter (1979), for example, analyzes the determinants of health policies in Britain, Germany, Japan, and the Soviet Union. Similarly, Altenstetter (1974) and Stone (1980) show how different structures and processes explain the differences in policy between the United States and West Germany; and Hollingsworth (1986) attempts to relate differences in structure and performance by comparing the United States and Britain. This approach views "most similar systems" as laboratories in which to assess the effects of alternative policy options at home (Teune, 1978). It is exemplified by Evans (1984) and Marmor and his colleagues (1978), who used this approach in their studies of Canada.

The idea of evolutionary progress in the development of health systems suggests that the United States can learn about future policy issues by studying nations whose systems are more advanced. Similarly, the idea that policy learning brings foreign solutions to bear on American problems is a variation on this theme. Finally, the idea of using comparative analysis to understand the determinants and effects of policies abroad can assist us in evaluating alternative policy options at home.

The ideas summarized above, indeed most of the literature in comparative health policy, often minimize or overlook the substantial problems of health systems abroad. An alternative, problem-oriented approach might be to reverse this emphasis. For example, another way to think about learning from abroad is to begin with the recognition that most countries, irrespective of their particular health system, face serious common problems with regard to the efficient and equitable allocation of scarce health care resources.

Economists, for example, emphasize the problem of inefficiency in the allocation of health care resources. They point out that cost containment should not be confused with allocative efficiency in the use of health care resources, and they study the possibilities of obtaining more value for the money spent on health care.

TABLE 17.1 The Evolution of Health Systems

Health System	Type 1: Private	Type 2: Pluralistic	Type 3: National health insurance	Type 4: National health service	Type 5: Socialized health service
General definition	Health care as item of personal consumption	Health care as predominantly a consumer good or service	Health care as an insured, guaranteed consumer good or service	Health care as a state-supported consumer good or service	Health care as a state-provided public service
Position of the physician	Solo entrepreneur	Solo entrepreneur and member of variety of groups, organizations	Solo entrepreneur and member of medical organizations	Solo entrepreneur and member of medical organizations	State employee and member of medical organizations
Role of professional associations	Powerful	Very strong	Strong	Fairly strong	Weak or non-existent
Ownership of facilities	Private	Private and public	Private and public	Mostly public	Entirely public
Economic transfers	Direct	Direct and indirect	Mostly indirect	Indirect	Entirely indirect
Prototypes	U.S., Western Europe, Russia in 19th century	U.S. in 20th century	Sweden, France, Canada, Japan in 20th century	Great Britain in 20th century	Soviet Union in 20th century

Sources: V. G. Rodwin. *The Health Planning Predicament: France, Quebec, England, and the United States.* Berkeley: University of California Press, 1984, p. 245. Adapted from: M. G. Field. *Comparative Health Systems: Differentiation and Convergence,* Final Report under Grant No. HS-00272, Rockville, MD: National Center for Health Services Research, 1978.

This applies not only with regard to improving health status, but also with respect to altering input mixes in the provision of health services: taking advantage of cost-effective treatment settings (e.g., ambulatory surgery) and personnel (e.g., nurse practitioners).

Public health and medical care analysts criticize the lack of continuity of care between primary, secondary, and tertiary levels. Although health planners have called for redistributing resources away from hospitals to community-based ambulatory care services and public health programs, the allocation of resources within health regions has been notoriously biased in the favor of more costly technology based medical care at the apex of the regional hierarchy (Fox, 1986; Rodwin, 1984). The consequence of this allocational pattern has been to weaken institutional capability for delivering primary care services. This has exacerbated the separation between primary, secondary, and tertiary levels of care, thus making it difficult for providers to assure that the right patient receives the right kind of care, in the right place, and for the right reason.

Consumers have noted the inflexibility of bureaucratic decision-making procedures and the absence of opportunities for exercising for what Hirschman (1970) calls "voice" in most health care organizations. Indeed, the problem of control and how it should be shared among consumers, providers, managers, and payers is at the center of most criticisms leveled against the current structure of health in Western industrialized nations. In all of these systems, decisions about what medical services to provide, how and where they should be provided, by whom, and how often are separated from the responsibility for financing medical care.

Resource Allocation Problems: France, Canada, and Britain

Drawing on the problem-oriented approach presented above, this section assesses common problems with regard to the efficient and equitable allocation of scarce health care resources in France, Canada, and Britain. Outside the United States there are two principal methods of health care financing: compulsory insurance and general taxation. France is an example of an employment-based national health insurance (NHI) system financed by compulsory payroll taxes on employers and employees. Canada and Britain both rely on general taxation. But whereas Canada uses federal and provincial general tax revenues to finance a highly decentralized NHI system, Britain relies overwhelmingly on central government funds to finance a national health service (NHS).

France

The French health system combines NHI with fee-for-service private practice in the ambulatory care sector and a mixed hospital care sector of which two-thirds of all acute beds are in the public sector and one-third are in the private sector. Physicians in the ambulatory sector and in private hospitals (known as *cliniques*) are reimbursed on the basis of a negotiated fee schedule. Roughly 30% of all physicians have chosen to engage in extra billing beyond the negotiated fees as payment in full (Rodwin & Sandier, 1993). And physicians based in public hospitals are reimbursed on a part-time or full-time salaried basis. *Cliniques* are reimbursed on the basis of a negotiated per diem fee. Public hospitals used to be reimbursed on a retrospective, cost-based, per diem fee, but they have received prospectively set "global" budgets since 1984.

There are several problems in this system. From a public health point of view, there is inadequate communication between full-time salaried physicians in public hospitals and solo-practice physicians working in the community. Although general practitioners in the fee-for-service sector have informal referral networks to specialists and public hospitals, there are no formal institutional relationships that assure continuity of medical care, disease prevention and health promotion services, post-hospital follow-up care, and more generally systematic linkages and referral patterns between primary-, secondary-, and tertiary-level services.

From the point of view of economic efficiency criteria, there are additional problems in the French health care system. On the demand side, two factors encourage consumers to increase their use of medical care services: the uncertainty about the results of treatment and the presence of insurance coverage. To reduce the risk of misdiagnosis or improper therapy, physicians are always tempted to order more diagnostic tests. Since NHI covers most of the cost, there is no incentive—neither for the physician nor for the patient—to balance marginal changes in risk with marginal increases in costs. This results in excessive medical care utilization.

On the supply side, fee-for-service reimbursement of physicians provides incentives for them to increase their volume of services so as to raise their income. Likewise, per diem reimbursement of *cliniques* and hospitals creates incentives to increase patient lengths of stay. The recent imposition of global budgets in France has eliminated this problem but the budgets represent a blunt policy tool—one that tends to support the existing allocation of resources within the hospital sector and, possibly, to jeopardize the quality of hospital care. It is relatively easy for a hospital to receive an annual budget to maintain its ongoing activities but extremely difficult to receive additional compensation for higher service levels, institutional innovation, or improvements in the quality of care. Even with prospective budgets, hospitals naturally seek to maximize the level of their annual allocations and to resist budget cutbacks.

In summary, under French NHI, providers have no financial incentives to achieve savings while holding quality constant or even improving it. Nor are there incentives—in public hospitals, for example—to increase service activity in exchange for more income. Consumers have few incentives, other than minimal co-payments, to be economical in their use of medical care. And there are no incentives to move the French system away from hospital-centered services toward new organizational modalities.

Canada

Under Canadian NHI, although coverage for drugs is far less than in France, there are no co-payments; there is first-dollar coverage for hospital and medical services. Physicians in ambulatory care are paid predominantly on a fee-for-service basis, according to fee schedules negotiated between physicians' associations and provincial governments. In contrast to France, physicians in hospitals are most often paid on a fee-for-service basis, as in the United States.

There are few private, for-profit hospitals in Canada such as French *cliniques* and American proprietary or investor-owned institutions. Most acute-care hospitals in Canada are private, nonprofit institutions. But their operating expenditures are financed through the NHI system, and most of their capital expenditures are financed by the provincial governments. In the United States, Canada's health system is often depicted as a model for NHI (Himmelstein & Woolhandler, 1989). Its financing, through a complex shared federal and provincial tax revenue formula, is more progressive than the European NHI systems financed on the basis of payroll taxes. Canada's levels of health status are high by international standards. And it has achieved notable success in controlling the growth of health care costs. What, then, are the problems in this system?

From the point of view of health care providers, there is, above all, a crisis of underfinancing. Physicians complain about low fee levels. Hospital administrators complain about draconian control of their budgets. And other health care professionals note that the combination of a physician "surplus" and excessive reliance on physicians prevents an expansion of their roles. Although Evans (1987) contends that Canadian cost-control policies cannot be shown to have jeopardized the quality of care, providers and administrators, alike, claim that there has been deterioration since the imposition of restrictive prospective budgets.

Leaving aside the issue of quality, the same issues discussed in the context of France are present in Canada with respect to economic efficiency. Neither the hospital physician nor the patient has an incentive to be economical in the use of health care resources. On the demand side, because patients benefit from what is perceived as "free" tax-financed first-dollar coverage, they have no incentive to choose cost-effective forms of care. For example, in the case of a demand for urgent care, there is no incentive for a patient to use community health centers rather than rush directly to the emergency room.

On the supply side, physicians lack incentives to make efficient use of hospitals, which are essentially a free good at their disposal. There are no incentives for altering input mixes to affect practice style. Nor are there incentives for providers to evaluate service levels and the kinds of therapy performed in relation to improving health status. It could be argued that these problems are common to all health systems, but they are especially acute in a system characterized by a bilateral monopoly that tends to support the status quo. On the one hand, providers organized in strong associations have strong monopoly power, which they use to defend their legitimate interests; on the other, the monopoly power of sole-source financing (NHI) keeps provider interests in check at the cost of not intervening in the organizational practice of medicine.

Stoddart (1984) has characterized the problems of the Canadian health system as "financing without organization." In his view, Canadian provinces "adopted a 'pay the bills' philosophy, in which decisions about service provision—which services, in what amounts, produced how, by whom, and where—were viewed as the legitimate domain of physicians and hospital administrators" (p. 3). The reason for this policy is that provincial governments were concerned about maintaining a good relationship with providers. This concern has not avoided tough negotiations and periodic confrontations. But there has been no effort to devise new forms of medical-care practice, for example, health maintenance organizations (HMOs) or new institutions to handle the long-term care for the elderly. The side effect of Canadian NHI has been to support the separation of hospital and ambulatory care and to reinforce traditional organizational structures.

As in France or the United States, there are, in essence, two strategies for managing the Canadian health system and making adjustments. The first involves greater regulation on the supply side: even stronger controls on hospital spending, more rationing of medical technology, more hospital closures and mergers, and eventual prohibition of extra billing. The second involves increased reliance on market forces on the demand side: various forms of user charges such as co-payments and deductibles now advocated as a form of privatization. Neither strategy is likely to succeed on its own. The former will control health care expenditures in the short run, but it fails to affect practice styles. Its effectiveness runs the risk of exacerbating confrontations between providers and the state and jeopardizing health care needs. The latter deals with only part of the problem—the demand side—and neglects the issue of supply side inefficiency. It provides no mechanism by which consumer decisions can generate signals to providers to adopt efficient practice styles. Moreover, it is likely to raise the level of total (public and private) expenditures.

Britain

There are many models of an NHS in Europe, ranging from decentralized systems in Sweden, Norway, Finland, and Denmark to more centralized systems in Spain, Greece, Portugal, and Italy. Because the British NHS is one of the oldest and most thoroughly studied models, it stands as an exemplar. It is financed almost entirely through general revenue taxation and is accountable directly to the

Department of Health and Social Security (DHSS) and Parliament. Access to health services is free of charge to all British subjects and to all legal residents. But despite the universal entitlement, Britons spend only 5.8% of their gross domestic product (GDP) on health care—one-half of what Americans spend as a percentage of their GDP.

Although the NHS is cherished by most Britons, there are, nevertheless, some serious problems concerning both the equity and efficiency of resource allocation in the health sector. With regard to equity, in 1976, the Resource Allocation Working Party (RAWP) developed a formula for the allocation of NHS funds between regions (DHSS, 1976). The formula represents one of the most far-reaching attempts to allocate health care funds because it incorporates regional differences in measures of health status. Slow progress is now being made in redistributing the aggregate NHS budget along the lines of RAWP, but substantial inequities still remain, from the point of view of both spatial distribution and social class (Townsend & Davidson, 1982).

With regard to efficiency, the problems are even more severe because NHS resources are extremely scarce by international standards. Because there is less slack, the marginal costs of inefficiency are higher than in Western Europe or the United States. And because the NHS faces the same demands as other systems to make available new technology and to care for an increasingly aged population, British policy-makers recognize that they must pursue innovations that improve efficiency. But there are numerous institutional obstacles in the way.

The tripartite structure of the NHS is, itself, a major source of inefficiency:

1. Regional Health Authorities (RHAs) are responsible for allocating budgets to hospitals in their regions. Hospital-based "consultants" are paid on a salaried basis, with distinguished clinicians receiving "merit awards," and all consultants have the right to see a limited number of private, fee-paying patients in "pay beds."
2. Outside the RHA budget are Family Practitioner Committees (FPCs) responsible for remunerating general practitioners (GPs), ophthalmologists, dentists, and pharmacists. The GPs are reimbursed on a capitation basis, with additional remuneration coming from special "practice allowances" and fee-for-service payment for specific services (e.g., night visits and immunizations).
3. Separate from both the RHAs and the FPCs are the local authorities (LAs), which are responsible for the provision of social services, public health services, and certain community nursing services.

Such an institutional framework creates perverse incentives to shift borderline patients from GPs to hospital consultants, to the community, and back to the hospital. GPs, for example, have no incentive to minimize costs and can impose costs on RHAs by referring patients to hospital consultants or for diagnostic services.

NHS managers can shift costs from the NHS to social security by sending elderly hospitalized patients to private nursing homes. And consultants can shift costs back onto the patient by keeping long waiting lists, thereby increasing demand for their private services. As in France and Canada, neither the patient nor the physician, in Britain, bears the cost of the decisions they make; it is the taxpayer who pays the bill.

Four recent strategies, all of them inadequate, have attempted to deal with this problem. The first came promptly with the arrival of the Thatcher government. After cautious attempts to denationalize the NHS by promoting a shift toward NHI and privatization, the conservative government backed off when they realized that such an approach would not merely provoke strong political opposition but also would increase public expenditure and therefore conflict with their budgetary objectives (McLachlan & Maynard, 1982). Instead, the strategy was narrowed in favor of encouraging competition and market incentives in limited areas. To begin with, the government allowed a slight increase in private beds in NHS hospitals. In addition, it introduced tax incentives to encourage the purchase of private health insurance and the growth of charitable contributions. Also, the government encouraged local authorities to raise money through the sale of surplus property and to contract out to the private sector such services as laundry, cleaning, and catering.

The second response was the Griffiths Report, which resulted in yet another reorganization in the long history of administrative reform within the NHS. Roy Griffiths, the former director of a large English department store chain, introduced the concept of a general manager at the department (DHSS), regional, district, and unit levels. This manager was presumably responsible for the efficient use of the budget at each level of the NHS. The problem, however, is that the tripartite structure of the system remained unchanged; and the general managers had very little information about least-cost strategies (across the tripartite structure) for generating improvements in health status.

The third response to the problem of improving efficiency was to reduce the drug bill (Maynard, 1986). Since April, 1985, the government limited the list of reimbursable drugs and reduced the pharmaceutical industry's rate of return. These measures helped contain the costs of the only open-ended budget within the NHS, but there is no evidence that they had any impact on the efficiency of health care expenditures.

Finally, the fourth and most recent reform for improving efficiency was announced in a government White Paper, *Working for Patients* (1989) passed in 1990 (The National Health Service and Community Care Act) and implemented on April 1, 1991. The White Paper proposed a range of significant changes, all of which attempt to create internal markets, within the public sector, by giving providers incentives to treat more patients and having "money follow patients." On the demand side, the government proposed that instead of operating as monopoly suppliers of services, district health authorities be required to purchase services for the patients they serve. On the supply side, the government proposed that some of the larger NHS hospitals be transformed into independent self-governing NHS trusts. It is too early, still, to evaluate these reforms. But they have already had far-reaching repercussions on reformers in national health service systems in Europe and the Newly Independent States.

The U.S. Health System: A Comparative Perspective

How does the United States health care system measure up in comparison to health sector problems in France, Canada, and Great Britain? To answer this question, we will review the ways in which the U.S. health system differs from and resembles that of other Western industrialized nations. Let us examine this issue from the vantage point of three characteristics that typically distinguish the United States from Western Europe and Canada: (1) American values and popular opinion, (2) the structure of health care financing and organization, and (3) policy responses to health sector problems.

American Values and Popular Opinion. The prevailing image of American values and popular opinion is that of nineteenth-century liberalism, which has colored American perceptions of equity, of the proper role of government, and of citizenship. These perceptions represent a range of American values and popular opinions that distinguish the United States from Western Europe and Canada.

American attitudes about equity with regard to health care were formed in the nineteenth century as the country became populated by immigrant populations in urban centers. During this period the concept of "truly needy" emerged (Rosner, 1982). Many Americans developed a sense of responsibility to come to their aid, but there were also harsher attitudes inspired by social Darwinist notions that distinguished between the "truly needy" and the "undeserving" or "unworthy" poor. Whereas in Western Europe broadly based socialist parties viewed poverty as an outcome of the economic system, in the United States there was an inclination to regard poverty as an individual problem. Hence the greater attention to *equality of opportunity* in the United States as compared with *equality of result* in the more left-leaning European social democracies.

As far as the proper role of government is concerned, in contrast to Western Europe and Canada, the United States has a long history of anti-government attitudes. The suspicion about excessive governmental authority and the attachment to individual liberties is a pervasive American value.

American perceptions of citizenship also present a striking contrast to Western European perceptions. In the United States individualistic values, on the other hand, and social and heterogeneity, on the other hand, have resulted in more "fractionalized understandings of citizenship" (Klass, 1985). In Western Europe and Canada, the understandings of citizenship are grounded in notions of solidarity and universal entitlements. The difference is that Western Europe and Canada have largely succeeded in covering all of their citizens under some form of health insurance; the United States has not.

There is a general aversion among Americans to universal entitlements. As Reinhardt (1985) has observed, when Americans face a trade-off between establishing tax-financed entitlements and leaving the uninsured on their own, they prefer to do the latter. It would be misleading, however, to draw any conclusions about how generous Americans are or how much social welfare they provide based only on the image of liberalism outlined above. In contrast to Western Europe and Canada, Americans prefer to promote redistribution policies through local assistance and indirect subsidies to the voluntary sector via tax exemptions.

Clearly, in comparison to Western Europe and Canada, there are important differences in the United States with regard to values and popular opinion. But how much of a difference do these differences make?

The Structure of Health Care Financing and Organization. The prevailing image of the American health system is one of a privately financed, privately organized system with multiple payers. These characteristics derive, in large part, from the absence of a publicly mandated NHI program. In comparison with Western European nations, Japan and Canada, the United States is last with respect to the public share of total health expenditures (Table 17.2). Although the United

TABLE 17.2   Sources of Finance for Health Care Expenditures: The Mix Between Public and Private in 1988–1989 as a Percentage of Total

	Public	Private
Australia	64.9	35.1
Canada[a]	73.5	26.5
France	68.2	31.8
Italy	68.2	31.8
Japan[d]	74.5	25.5
Netherlands[b]	75.8	24.2
Sweden	90.1	9.9
Switzerland	68.6	31.4
United Kingdom	84.7	15.3
West Germany	72.0	28.0
United States[c]	44.0	56.0

Source: Organization for Economic Cooperation and Development: Health Data File, 1993.
[a]1987
[b]1981
[c]1991
[d]1986

States has the highest per capita health care expenditures—public and private combined (see Table 17.3)—and spends the highest percentage of its GDP on health care (Table 17.4), it retains the lowest share of public expenditure as a percentage of total health expenditures (Table 17.4). Likewise, in comparing public health expenditures for the elderly as a percentage of gross national product (GNP) the United States spends the least (Table 17.5).

The organization of health care in the United States is noted for being on the private end of the public-private spectrum. In comparison with Western Europe, the United States has one of the smallest public hospital sectors. In the organization of ambulatory care, American private fee-for-service practice corresponds to the norm, at least in comparison to NHI systems. However, the absence of an NHI program in the United States has resulted in a system of multiple payers and has encouraged a more pluralistic pattern of medical care organization and more innovative forms of medical practice—for example, multispecialty group practices, HMOs, ambulatory surgery centers, and preferred provider organizations (PPOs).

The United States is also different, in comparison to Canada and Western Europe, with regard to the ways in which health resources are used. For example,

TABLE 17.3   Total Health Care Expenditures Per Capita 1988–1990 (in $US Purchasing Power Parities-PPP)

Country	$US (PPP)
United States[a]	2826
Australia	1321
Belgium[b]	926
Canada[a]	1847
Denmark	930
France	1609
Germany	1368
Greece	343
Italy	1172
Japan[b]	792
Spain[c]	504
Sweden	1174
Switzerland	1496
The Netherlands[d]	724
United Kingdom	931

Source: OECD Health Data, 1993.
[a]1991
[b]1986
[c]1987
[d]1991

TABLE 17.4 Health Care Expenditures, 1990

Country	Public health expenditures as % of total health expenditure	%Total expenditures on health in GDP
Australia	68.0	7.4[a]
Austria	67.1	7.9
Belgium	88.9	7.5[b]
Canada	72.2	9.7
Denmark	82.8	6.3[a]
Finland	81.0	7.2[a]
France	74.4	9.3
Germany	71.6	8.6[c]
Ireland	79.8	7.1[d]
Iceland	86.9	8.1
Italy	77.6	7.3
Japan	71.9	6.8[b]
Luxembourg	91.9	6.8[e]
Netherlands	71.3	7.7[f]
New Zealand	81.7	7.0
Norway	95.3	6.9
Sweden	79.8	7.3[c]
Switzerland	68.3	7.7
United Kingdom	83.5	5.8
United States	42.2	13.1

Source: OECD Health Data, 1993.
GDP = gross domestic product
[a]1988
[b]1986
[c]1989
[d]1991
[e]1987
[f]1981

the United States has fewer hospital beds per thousand population than any Western European country or Canada (Table 17.6). The United States also has the lowest use of inpatient care (hospital bed/days per capita) (Table 17.6). These data should not necessarily lead one to the conclusion that the United States is less prone to institutionalize patients than Western Europe and Canada, where a large portion of long-term care for the elderly is provided in hospitals.

These are ways in which the American health care system is different from that of Western Europe and Canada. But there are also some noteworthy points of similarity. For example, most health systems in industrially advanced nations are cen-

TABLE 17.5   **Public Expenditures for Health
Care of the Elderly, 1980**

Country	Public Expenditures as Percentage of GNP
United States	3.9
Canada	5.8
Denmark	6.4
France	6.1
Germany	6.2
Netherlands	6.5
Norway	5.8
Sweden	8.9
Switzerland	4.5
United Kingdom	5.2

Source: Adapted from U.S. Senate, Special Committee on Aging. "Long-Term Care in Western Europe and Canada: Implications for the United States," Washington, DC: U.S. Government Printing Office, 1984.

GNP = gross national product

tered around the hospital. They allocate roughly one-half of total health care expenditures to the hospital sector. The United States corresponds to the norm in this regard (Table 17.7).

There is also a high degree of similarity among the United States, Canada, and Western Europe in the broad structure of health care financing and provider reimbursement (Figure 17.2). From the point of view of both consumers and providers, the essential feature of modern health care systems is the central role of third-party payment, by either government or health insurers. On the financing end, all health systems are supported either by general revenue taxes or by payroll taxes. On the payment end, the magnitude of third-party payment dwarfs that of out-of-pocket payment by consumers.

For the consumer, what matters with regard to health care financing is not the relative public and private mix but rather the relative portion of *direct* versus *indirect* third-party payment. To emphasize the large private portion of health care financing in the United States is misleading; for the more critical factor is that public and private health insurance are both forms of third-party payment. This amounted to 73.1% of national health expenditures in 1990 leaving consumers with direct out-of-pocket contributions equal to 23.3% of total health expenditures (Levit et al., 1991). The most recent comparative analysis of consumers' out-of-pocket contributions to total health expenditures is based on 1975 data (Max-

TABLE 17.6   Hospital Beds and Use of Inpatient Care, 1990–1991

OECD Countries	No. of Beds per 1000[a]	Hospital Bed-Days (Per Person per Year)[e]
Australia	9.8[b]	2.8
Austria	9.7	3.0
Belgium	9.8[b]	2.6
Canada	6.7[c]	2.0
Denmark	5.7	1.7
Finland	12.5	4.0
France	9.7	2.8
Germany	10.4	3.3
Iceland	16.7[b]	5.0
Italy	7.2[b]	1.8
Japan	15.8	4.0
Luxemburg	11.8	3.7
Netherlands	11.4[d]	3.7
New Zealand	8.7[b]	2.0
Norway	14.5[b]	5.0
Sweden	12.4	3.5
Switzerland	9.5[b]	3.9
United Kingdom	6.4[b]	2.0
United States	4.7	1.2[f]

Source: OECD Health Data, 1993.
*This figure includes beds for all hospitals registered with the American Hospital Association.
[a]For 1990 unless otherwise indicated
[b]1989
[c]1987
[d]1991
[e]For 1991 unless otherwise indicated
[f] For 1990

well, 1981). Once again, the United States is different (Figure 17.3). It has the highest share of direct out-of-pocket contributions by consumers. But even under French NHI, consumers contribute roughly 16% of total health expenditures in the form of out-of-pocket payments. The difference is not as large as the image of private financing system would suggest.

The image of a private organizational structure in American health care is well founded. But that view, too, is incomplete. In spite of its *relatively* small size, there is an important role for the public sector in the United States—both in ambulatory services for the noninstitutionalized patient and in the provision of hospital services.

TABLE 17.7   Components of Health Spending, 1990–1991 (Percentage of Total Health Spending)

Country	Inpatient	Ambulatory	Pharmaceutical	Other
Australia	49.1	25.5	8.8	16.6
Belgium	33.9	39.8	14.9	11.4
Canada	49.1	22.1	13.8	15.0
Finland	44.9	34.5	9.9	10.7
France	43.8	28.3	16.8	11.1
Germany	36.6	28.0	21.3	14.1
Italy	46.7	27.3	18.4	7.6
Japan	31.1[a]	40.8	17.3	10.8
Luxembourg[b]	37.7	52.1	15.3	?
Netherlands[c]	54.4	36.8	9.9	?
New Zealand	56.6	16.5	12.7	14.2
Norway	70.4	23.3	10.4	?
United States	46.1	29.9	8.1	15.6

Source: OECD Health Data, 1993.
[a]1989
[b]1987
[c]1988

With regard to ambulatory care, there is a maze of special federal programs and a network of local government services largely for the poor. The services are provided either in county or municipal hospital emergency rooms, in local health departments, or in neighborhood health centers. As for hospitals, more than 30% of all acute-care institutions are owned and operated by governments. This includes the federal Veterans Administration hospitals and marine and military hospitals, as well as state, county, and municipal hospitals. Although Medicare and Medicaid were intended to bring the poor into "mainstream medicine," (i.e., into the private sector), local public hospitals continue largely to serve the poor. These hospitals are a major source of care not only for Medicaid beneficiaries but also for more than half of the poverty population who do not meet Medicaid eligibility levels and consequently often do not have access to private physicians or voluntary hospitals.

To sum up, there are distinctive characteristics of health care financing and organization in the United States, but there are also striking points of similarity when compared with Western Europe and Canada. The distinctive characteristics include the absence of an NHI program, preferences for institutional flexibility, and innovative forms of medical care organization. The points of similarity—the coexistence of both public and private provision and third-party payment—are structural features of the American health system as well as those of most other health systems.

FIGURE 17.2 Health Care Financing and Provider Reimbursement

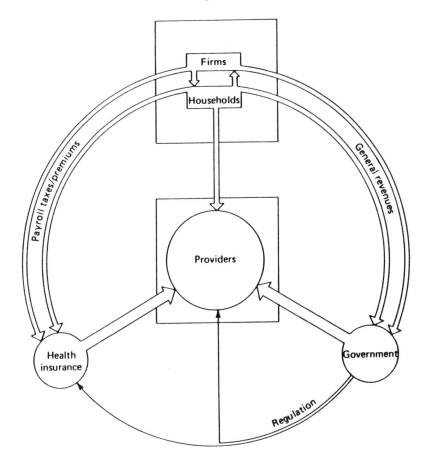

Policy Responses to Health Sector Problems. Abel-Smith (1985) argues that there is a growing divergence between Western European and American policy responses to the problem of containing health care costs. He suggests that Western Europe continues to rely on regulation, whereas the United States seeks to promote competition and greater reliance on market forces. Abel-Smith points to three examples of these unique American policy responses to health sector problems: (1) the growth of deductibles, co-payments, and other cost-sharing mechanisms; (2) the trend toward making those who benefit from insurance actually pay the whole cost—this implies, for example, reducing tax reductions and thus providing incentives for employers and employees to shop more prudently for insurance coverage; and (3) the growth of competitive bidding as a mechanism of forcing competition between alternative providers.

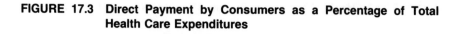

FIGURE 17.3 Direct Payment by Consumers as a Percentage of Total Health Care Expenditures

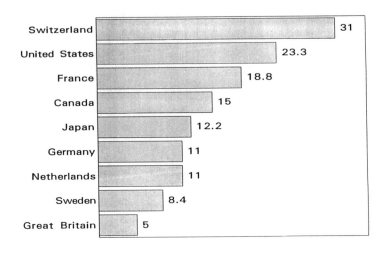

Sources: Germany, Great Britain and The Netherlands: *The Reform of Health Systems*, Paris: OECD, 1993. Canada: *Canada's Health System*, New York, Falkner and Gray, 1993. United States: *Health United States, 1991*. France: *ECO-SANTE, version 3*, Paris: CREDES, 1991. Japan: Rodwin, V. et al., *Japan's Universal and Affordable Health System: Lessons for the United States*, New York: Japan Society, 1994. Sweden: Appleby, J., *Financing Health Care In the 1990's* p. 12, Open University Press, 1992. Switzerland: Frei, A., & Hill, S., *Le Système Suisse de Santé*, 1992, Ed. Krebs SA, Bâle.

There are some insights behind this caricature of the American policy response to health sector problems. But there is probably more regulation in the eastern states with "all-payer systems" (e.g., New York, New Jersey, and Maryland) than in Western Europe. Even in well-known "pockets of competition" (e.g., California, Arizona, and Minnesota) regulation is essential, if only to enforce the rules of competitive game. The Prospective Payment System (PPS) for Medicare provides a good illustration. Although one of its effects was to intensify competition between hospitals, the use of diagnosis-related groups (DRGs) for hospital reimbursement was actually a highly regulatory strategy of centralized price controls—one that falls well within Western Europe policy traditions.

In regulating physician activities, American policy has not backed off. Rather, since the creation of Peer Review Organizations (PROs) under PPS, the regulation of physician behavior in the United States is surely stronger than any emerging European equivalent, including the French and Canadian systems of medical profiles, which are among the most developed outside of the United States (Rodwin, 1989a).

Three characteristics distinguish American policy responses from those of Western Europe and Canada:

1. The United States has long been concerned about the dangers of monopoly power and has pursued (until the recent wave of mergers both inside and outside of the health sector) a strong antitrust policy. A notable case in point is recent Federal Trade Commission measures to curb the monopoly powers of physicians and hospitals and to eliminate restraints on trade in health care by allowing advertising.[4] In the United States structural interests are not formally sanctioned and accepted as institutionalized counterparts for purposes of negotiating with the government. Instead, the more typical response of American health policy is to advocate proposals to fragment powerful groups that are presumed, as a consequence, to compete with one another.

2. Following directly from the first characteristic of the American policy response is the absence, in the United States, of institutional structures for negotiating between major groups of health care providers and the government or an NHI board of directors, or both. In contrast to the adversarial American approach, which attempts to fragment both the medical profession and the hospital associations—a strategy of "divide and conquer"—the Western European and Canadian response consolidates the organization of provider groups and confronts them with countervailing organizations.

   This important difference acts as a severe constraint, in the United States, on the possibilities of negotiating a national fee schedule for physicians or a uniform hospital payment system for *all* payers and hospitals. The constraint, however, has made it possible for individual payers (e.g., Medicare, Medicaid, and certain private insurance companies) to strike harder bargains with smaller groups and to foster competition and new organizational arrangements for medical care.

3. In contrast to Western European and Canadian strategies of comprehensive health care reform and strong centralized regulation, American strategies (with the exception of PPS for Medicare) are characterized by far greater decentralization and by more persistent social experimentation. Although major policy initiatives have usually come from the federal level and a range of government programs at the county and municipal levels, when compared to unitary European states (e.g., France), American federalism provides a striking contrast. But even in comparison to other federal states, such as Canada and Germany, the United States is still characterized by more decentralization and experimentation in the policy making process.

---

[4]This change of policy was prompted by the 1977 U.S. Supreme Court decision in *Bates v. State Bar of Arizona*, 433 U.S. 350 (1977) allowing health care professionals to engage in advertising.

These three characteristics of American policy responses to health sector problems highlight the ways in which the United States is different from Western Europe and Canada. But if one compares the evolution of American health policy over the past four decades with that of Western Europe and Canada, there are also points of similarity.

For example, Brown (1985) identifies four American policy responses to health sector problems: (1) the subsidy strategy—government grants on the supply side; (2) the financing strategy—third-party financing on the demand side; (3) the reorganization strategy—government inducements to promote new organizations for delivering medical care; and (4) the regulatory strategy—government attempts to influence the "use, price and quality of services, and the size, location, and equipment of facilities." Three of the four categories—subsidy, financing, and regulatory—are equally good descriptors of the Western Europe and Canadian policy response to their health sector problems.

In the 1950s and 1960s, during the expansion phase of health care systems, there was extraordinary convergence among Western industrialized nations around both the subsidy and financing strategies (De Kervasdoué, Kimberly, & Rodwin, 1984). In the mid-1970s and 1980s, during the containment phase, there was also convergence around the regulatory and reorganization strategies. Although one can point to examples of the reorganization strategy in all countries, Canada (particularly Quebec) and Western Europe have focused more on administrative reorganizations in the public sector, whereas the United States has encouraged reorganization in the private sector at the level of the delivery system. This is perhaps the most notable aspect of the American health policy response to health sector problems.

The Uses of Comparative Analysis in Learning from Abroad

Given the ways in which the health sector in the United States resembles that of Western Europe and Canada and the ways in which it is exceptional, what inferences can one draw about the usefulness of comparative analysis for purposes of learning from abroad? If the United States is truly exceptional in the health sector, then one can argue that there is little to learn from Western Europe and Canada. Countries often rely on this "assumption of uniqueness" to reject ideas from abroad (Stone, 1981). To the extent that the United States is unexceptional, however, a case can be made for drawing lessons from comparative experience.

For example, there is a widely shared belief among American policymakers that a national program providing for universal entitlement to health care in the United States would result in runaway costs. In response to this presumption, nations that entitle all of their residents to a high level of medical care, while spending less on administration and on medical care than does the United States, are often held up as models. The Canadian health system is the most celebrated example. French NHI, a prototype of Western European continental health systems, is another case in point. Britain's NHS, although typically considered a "painful prescription" for the United States (Aaron & Schwartz, 1984), nevertheless assures first-dollar coverage for basic health services to its entire population and, as we have seen, spends less than half as much money, per capita, as the United States (Table 17.3).

All of these countries have produced some of the leading physicians and hospitals in the world. Judging by various measures of health status, they are in the same league as, or better than, the United States (Table 17.8). In Britain, *life expectancy at 60*—when medical care may have an important impact—is lower than in the United States. But in the United States over 15% of the population remains uninsured for health care services while spending, as a percentage GDP, surpasses that of all industrially advanced nations (Table 17.4).

Should we adopt the Western European or Canadian models of health care financing and organization? Or should we maintain our present system and recognize that it is a manifestation of American exceptionalism, that is of the ways in which the United States is fundamentally different from Western Europe and Canada? Both of these responses are probably inappropriate. The second response—that comparative analysis is not useful—insulates us from the experience of other nations. It smacks of ethnocentrism, makes us conservative, and thereby supports the status quo in the United States. The first response—that we should adopt the West European or Canadian model—relies too heavily on the experience of those nations. It is misleading because, as we have seen, there are serious limitations in the Western European and Canadian health systems. Moreover, many of the present institutional arrangements of health care delivery in the United States are superior to those abroad.

The proliferation of medical technology combined with an aging demographic structure are trends common to all modern health care systems and have contributed to rising health care costs. Policymakers have responded largely by implementing systems with increasing control over expenditures on doctors' services as well as hospital budgets. Virtually no one in Canada or Western Europe views the American system as a model to emulate. Even under the government of Prime Minister Thatcher there is no significant challenge to the principle of an NHS in Britain (Klein, 1985; *Working for Patients*, 1989). Nor is there any question about eliminating NHI in such countries as France, Canada, Germany, Belgium, or the Netherlands.

Despite these attitudes, one striking aspect about how some common problems are currently being dealt with abroad is the extent to which a number of fashionable American themes have drifted north to Canada and across the Atlantic to Western Europe. In the context of the problems we identified earlier—inefficiency in the allocation of health care resources, lack of continuity between levels of care, and the absence of consumer "voice" in most health care organizations—the concept of an HMO, in combination with elements of market competition, has a certain appeal.

TABLE 17.8   Health Care Expenditures and Health Status (1990)

| Country | Health Expenditures (1984) as % of GDP | Life Expectancy | | | | Infant mortality Per 1000 live births (1990) |
| | | At Birth | | At Age 60 | | |
		Males	Females	Males	Females	
Britain[a]	5.8	73.8	78.5	17.5	21.8	7.9
Canada	9.7[b]	73.8	80.4	18.9	23.7	6.8
France	9.3	72.7	81.1	18.8	24.0[c]	7.2
Japan	6.3	75.9	81.9	20.0	24.4	4.6
United States	13.2[b]	72.0	78.8	18.6[c]	22.7[c]	9.1

Source: OECD Health Data, 1993.

[a] All data are for the United Kingdom

[b] 1991

[c] 1989

Since an HMO is, by definition, both an insurer and a provider of health services, it establishes a link between the financing and provision of health services. Because it is financed on the basis of prepaid capitation payments, its managers have an explicit budget as well as a clearly defined clientele. Moreover, since an HMO is responsible—on a contractual basis—for providing a broad range of primary-, secondary-, and tertiary-level services to its enrolled population, it has powerful incentives to provide these services in a cost-effective manner while simultaneously maintaining quality to minimize the risk of disenrollment.

The idea of introducing HMOs or similar kinds of health care organizations into national systems that provide universal entitlement to health care resembles in many ways the American experience of encouraging Medicare beneficiaries to enroll in federally qualified HMOs or competing medical plans (CMPs). The idea usually involves two reforms. It spurs policymakers to combine regulatory controls with competition on the supply side, and it encourages them to design market incentives for both providers and consumers of health care.

To the extent that the insertion of HMOs into NHI or NHS systems represents an American "solution" to *foreign* problems, it may provide a way in which Canada and Western Europe could learn from the United States (Rodwin, 1989b). It may also, paradoxically, have more practical implications for the United States than simply transposing a European NHI or NHS system into the American context. For example, the insertion of HMOs into NHI or NHS systems might provide insights on how to implement President Clinton's Health Reform Plan for the United States.

Just how policy learning occurs as a result of studying health care systems abroad is not thoroughly understood (Rodwin & Brecher, 1992). But there is no doubt that more policy research in the field of comparative health systems could potentially be helpful in learning from abroad.

Acknowledgements

I wish to thank Lyyn Kawasaki for assistance in updating the tables in this chapter.

References

Aaron, H. & Schwartz, W., *The Painful Prescription: Rationing Hospital Care.* Washington, DC: Brookings Institution, 1984.

Abel-Smith, B., "Who Is the Odd Man Out?" The Experiences of Western Europe in Containing the Costs of Health Care." *Milbank Memorial Fund Quarterly: Health and Society*, *63*(1), 1985.

Altenstetter, C., *Health Policy-Making and Administration in West Germany and the United States.* Beverly Hills, CA: Sage Publications, 1974.

Altenstetter, C., *Changing National-Subnational Relations in Health: Opportunities and Constraints*. DHEW Publication No. 6, NIH 78-182. Washington, DC: Government Printing Office, 1978.

Andreopoulos, S. (Ed.), *National Health Insurance: Can We Learn from Canada?* New York: Wiley, 1975.

Anderson, O., *Health Care: Can There Be Equity? The United States, Sweden, and England*. New York: Wiley, 1972.

Anderson, O., *The Health Services Continuum in Democratic States*. Ann Arbor: Health Administration Press, 1989.

Blum, H., *Planning for Health*. New York: Human Sciences Press, 1981.

Brown, L., *Health Policy in the American Welfare State*. Paper prepared for the Ford Foundation Project on the Future of the Welfare State, 1985.

Corson, J., *Loiterings in Europe*. New York: Harper, 1948.

De Kervasdoué, J., Kimberly, J. & Rodwin, V. (Eds.), *The End of an Illusion: The Future of Health Policy in Western Industrialized Nations*. Berkeley, CA: University of California Press, 1984.

De Miguel, J., "A Framework for the Study of National Health Systems." *Inquiry, 12*(10), 1975.

DHHS, *Sharing Resources for Health in England Report of the Resource Allocation Working Party*. London: Her Majesty's Stationary Office, 1976.

Douglas-Wilson, I., & McLachlan, G. (Eds.), *Health Service Prospects: An International Survey*. London: Nuffield Provincial Hospitals Trust, 1974.

Dumbaugh, K., & Neuhauser, D., "International Comparisons of Health Services: Where Are We?" *Social Science and Medicine*, 13B (221), 1979.

Eckstein, H., *The English National Health Services: Its Origins, Structure, and Achievements*. Cambridge, Harvard University Press, 1959.

Ellencweig, A., *Analysing Health Systems: A Modular Approach*. New York: Oxford University Press, 1992.

Elling, R., *Cross-National Study of Health Systems: Countries, World Regions and Special Problems*. Detroit, MI: Gale Research Co., 1980a.

Elling, R., *Cross-National Study of Health Systems: Political Economics and Health Care*. New Brunswick, NJ: Transactions Books, 1980b.

Elling, R., *Cross-National Study of Health Systems: Concepts, Methods and Data Sources*. Detroit, MI: Gale Research Co., 1980c.

Elling, R., & Kerr, H., "Selection of Contrasting National Health Systems for In-depth Study," *Inquiry* (Suppl. *12*), 2, 1975.

Evans, R., *Strained Mercy: The Economics of Canadian Health Care*. Toronto: Butterworths, 1984.

Evans, R., "Holding the Line: The Canadian Experience with Global Budgeting." In M. Berthod-Wurmser, V. Rodwin, et al. (Eds.), *Système de santé, pouvoirs publics et financeurs: qui controle quoi?*. Paris: Documentation Française, 1987.

Field, M., *Soviet Socialized Medicine*. New York, Free Press, 1967.

Field, M., "The Concept of Health Systems' at the Macrosociological Level." *Social Science and Medicine*, 7 (October), 1973.

Field, M., *Success and Crisis in National Health Systems: A Comparative Approach*. New York: Routledge, 1989.

Forsyth, G., *Doctors and State Medicine: A Study of the British Health Service*. London: Pitman Medical, 1966.

Fox, D., *Health Policies, Health Politics*. Princeton, NJ: Princeton University Press, 1986.

Fry, J., *Medicine in Three Societies-Comparison of Medical Care in the USSR, USA, and UK*. New York: Elsevier, 1970.

Glaser, W., *Paying the Doctor: Systems of Remuneration and Their Effects*. Baltimore: Johns Hopkins University Press, 1970.

Glaser, W., *Health Insurance Bargaining: Foreign Lessons for Americans*. New York: Gardner Press, 1978.

Glaser, W., *Paying the Hospital*. San Francisco: Jossey-Bass, 1987.

Glaser, W., *Health Insurance in Practice: International Variations in Financing, Benefits, and Problems*. San Francisco: Jossey-Bass, 1991.

Himmelstein, D., & Woolhandler, S., et al., "A National Health Program for the United States: A Physicians' Proposal." *New England Journal of Medicine, 320*(2), January 12, 1989.

Hirschman, A., *Exit, Voice and Loyalty*. Cambridge, MA: Harvard University Press, 1970.

Hollingsworth, J., *A Political Economy of Medicine: Great Britain and the United States*. Baltimore: The Johns Hopkins University Press, 1986.

Hu, T., *International Health Costs and Expenditures*, DHEW Pub. no. 78-184. Washington, DC: U.S. Government Printing Office, 1976.

Hurst, J., *The Reform of Health Care: A Comparative Analysis of Seven OECD Countries*. Paris: OECD, 1992.

Hyde, G., *The Soviet Health Service: A Historical and Comparative Study*. London: Lawrence and Wilshardt, 1974.

Immergut, E., *Health Politics: Interests and Institutions in Western Europe*. Cambridge University Press, 1992.

Klass, G., "Explaining America and the Welfare State: An Alternative Theory." *Health Affairs, 4* (Spring), 41, 1985.

Klein, R., *The Politics of the NHS*. London: Pitman Medical, 1983.

Klein, R., "Why Britains's Conservatives Support a Socialist Health Care System." *Health Affairs, 4* (Spring), 41, 1985.

Leichter, H. M., *A Comparative Approach to Policy Analysis: Health Care Policy in Four Nations*. Cambridge: Cambridge University Press, 1979.

Leichter, H., *Free To Be Foolish: Politics and Health Promotion in the United States and Great Britain*. Princeton, NJ: Princeton University Press, 1991.

Leslie, C. (Ed.), "Theoretical Foundations for the Comparative Study of Medical Systems." *Social Science and Medicine*, 12, Special Issue, 1978.

Levit, K. et al., "National Health Expenditures, 1990." *Health Care Financing Review*, Fall, p. 52, 1991.

Light, D., & Schuller, A. (Eds.), *Political Values and Health Care: The German Experience*. Cambridge, MIT Press, 1986.

Lindsey, A., *Socialized Medicine in England and Wales*. Chapel Hill: University of North Carolina Press, 1962.

Maxwell, R., *Health and Wealth*. Lexington, MA: Lexington Books, D.C. Heath and Co., 1981.

Marmor, T., Bridges, A., & Hoffman, W., "Comparative Politics and Health Policies: Notes on Benefits, Costs, Limits." In D. Ashford (Ed.), *Comparing Public Policies*. Beverly Hills: Sage Publications, 1978.

Maynard, A., *Annual Report on the National Health Service*. New York: Center for Health Economics, 1986.

McLachlan, G. & Maynard, A. (Eds.), *The Public/Private Mix for Health: The Relevance and Effects of Change*. London: Nuffield Provincial Hospitals Trust, 1982.

Mechanic, D., "The Comparative Study of Health Care Delivery Systems." In *The Growth of Bureaucratic Medicine: An Inquiry into the Dynamics of Patient Behavior and the Organization of Medical Care* (Ch. 2). New York: Wiley, 1976.

Raffel, M. (Ed.), *Comparative Health Systems*. Pennsylvania: The Pennsylvania State University Press, 1985.

Reinhardt, U., "Hard Choices in Health Care: A Matter of Ethics." In L. Etheredge et al. (Eds.) *Health Care: How to Improve it and Pay for It*. Washington, DC: Center for National Policy, 1985.

Rodwin, V., "The Marriage of National Health Insurance and La Medecine Liberale in France: A Costly Union." *Milbank Memorial Fund Quarterly: Health and Society*, 59, (Winter), 16, 1981.

Rodwin, V., *The Health Planning Predicament: France, Quebec, England, and the United States*. Berkely, CA: University of California Press, 1984.

Rodwin, V., "Physician Payment Reform: Lessons from Abroad." *Health Affairs*, (9)1, Winter, 1989a.

Rodwin, V., "New Ideas for Health Policy in France, Canada, and Britain." In Field, M. (Ed.). *Success and Crisis in National Health Systems: A Comparative Approach*. New York: Routledge, 1989b.

Rodwin, V., & Brecher, C., "Comparative Analysis and Mutual Learning." In Rodwin et al., *Public Hospital Systems in New York and Paris*. New York: New York University Press, 1992.

Rodwin, V., & Sandier, S., "Health Care under French National Health Insurance: A Public-Private Mix, Low Prices and High Volumes". *Health Affairs*, Fall, 1993.

Roemer, M., *Comparative National Policies Health Care*. New York: Marcel Dekker, 1977.

Roemer, M., & Roemer, R., *Health Care Systems and Comparative Manpower Policies*. New York: Marcel Dekker, 1981.

Roemer, M., *National Health Systems of the World*. (Vol. 1 and 2). New York: Oxford, 1991.

Rosner, D., "Health Care for the 'Truly Needy': Nineteenth-Century Origins of the Concept." *Milbank Memorial Fund Quarterly: Health and Society*, 60 (Summer), 355, 1982.

Saltman, R. (Ed.), *The International Handbook of Health Care Systems*. New York: Greenwood Press, 1988.

Saltman, R., & Von Otter, C., *Planned Markets and Public Competition: Strategic Reform in Northern European Health Systems*. Philadelphia, Open University Press, 1992.

Schweitzer, S., *Policies for the Containment of Health Care Costs and Expenditures*, DHEW Publication No. 78-184. Washington, DC: U.S. Government Printing Office, 1978.

Sidel, V., & Sidel, R., *A Healthy State: An International Perspective on the Crisis in the United States Medical Care*. New York: Pantheon, 1977.

Siegerist, H., *Medicine & Health in the Soviet Union*. New York: Citadel Press, 1947.

Stoddart, D., *Rationalizing the Health Care System*. Paper presented at the Ontario Council Conference, Toronto, May 14–15, 1984.

Stone, D., *The Limits of Professional Power*. University of Chicago Press, 1980.

Stone, D., "Drawing Lessons from Comparative Health Research." In R. A. Straetz, M. Lieberman, & A. Sardell (Eds.), *Critical Issues in Health Policy*. Lexington, MA: D.C. Heath and Co., pp. 135–148, 1981.

Teune, H., "The Logic of Comparative Policy Analysis." In D. Ashford (Ed.), *Comparing Public Policies*. Beverly Hills: Sage Publications, 1978.

Townsend, P., & Davidson, N. (Eds.), *Inequalities in Health: The Black Report*. London: Penguin, 1982.

Weinerman, R., & Weinerman, J., *Social Medicine in Eastern Europe: Organization of Health Services and the Education of Medical Personnel in Czechoslovakia, Hungary, and Poland*. Cambridge, Harvard University Press, 1969.

Weinerman, R., "Research on Comparative Health Systems." *Medical Care*, (9)3, 1971.

Wilsford, D., *Doctors and the State: The Politics of Health Care in France and the United States*. Durham: Duke University Press, 1991.

Working for Patients. London: Her Majesty's Stationery Office, 1989.

Suggested Readings on Comparative Health Systems and Policy

Anderson, O., *The Health Services Continuum in Democratic States*. Ann Arbor: Health Administration Press, 1989.

Ellencweig, A., *Analysing Health Systems: A Modular Approach*. New York: Oxford University Press, 1992.

Field, M. (Ed.), *Success & Crisis in National Health Systems*. New York: Routledge, 1989.

Graig, L., *Health of Nations: An International Perspective on U.S. Health Care Reform*. Washington, DC: CQ Press, 1993.

Glaser, W., *Health Insurance in Practice*. San Francisco: Jossey Bass, 1991.

Health Affairs, Special Issue: *Pursuit of Health Systems Reform*, (10)3, Fall, 1991.

Hurst, J., *The Reform of Health Care: A Comparative Analysis of Seven OECD Countries*. Paris: OECD, 1992.

Journal of Health Policy, Politics and Law. Special Issue on Comparative Health Policy, (17)4, Winter 1992.

OECD, *Health Care Systems in Transition: The Search for Efficiency*. Paris: OECD, 1990.

OECD Health Systems: Facts and Trends (1960–1991). Paris, OECD, 1993.

OECD Health Systems: The Socioeconomic Environment (Statistical References). Paris, OECD, 1993.

Payer, L., *Medicine and Culture: Varieties of Treatment in the United States, England, West Germany and France*. Salt Lake City, Utah: Henry Holt and Co., Inc., 1988.

Raffel, M. W. (Ed.), *Comparative Health Systems*. Pennsylvania: The Pennsylvania State University Press, 1985.

Saltman, R. (Ed.), *The International Handbook of Health Care Systems*. New York: Greenwood Press, 1988.

18

Health Care Ethics

Dena J. Seiden

Overview

This chapter will cover the historical development of the field of bioethics, the various methodologies used in bioethics, the more important ethical principles and issues, and major topics of current interest in health care ethics. It will provide considerable detail about all these topics, but will not attempt an exhaustive discussion of each issue. It will occasionally discuss actual cases that are of importance in the development of biomedical ethics, but it will not use a case-study approach. Rather, the point is to give the reader an idea of the impetus for the rise of the field, and of the current concerns in the field.

Introduction

The discipline of health care ethics, sometimes known as bioethics or medical ethics, is a relatively recent development, with its beginnings in the late 1960s and early 1970s. Though there was interest among both health care professionals and ethicists in the topic before that time, there was not a recognized group of scholars, practitioners, or a literature that supported that interest. The change to the present time is startling for both intensity and depth. Medical ethical questions appear on the front pages of newspapers and on the evening news with regularity. Bioethical journals have become fixtures (*Hastings Center Report, Journal of Medical Ethics*, etc.), and the standard medical journals routinely carry articles on moral questions in virtually every issue (particularly see *The New England Journal of Medicine* and *The Journal of the American Medical Association*). Degree-granting programs in the field have been established, and a national society for bioethical consultants has been formed, meeting for the first time in

1986. New professional organizations are being formed that are considering credentialing for the field. Despite this explosion of public, professional, and academic interest, health care institutions have been slow to hire ethicists as staff, preferring often a few ethics seminars through the year, or the establishment of an ethics committee, which is made up of professionals with fine intentions and little ethical training. As formal ethics teaching increasingly becomes part of the credentialing process for institutions, graduate school education, and residency training programs, it will be interesting to observe how the discipline and its practitioners are absorbed into the mainstream of institutional life.

Development of Health Care Ethics

Reason for Development

The quickening of interest in medical ethics as a concept began after World War II, and the acknowledgment of the complicity of the German medical profession in the death camp exterminations and in medical and scientific "experiments" upon prisoners, which were thought to be beyond any reasonable bounds of moral constraint, (see Alexander, 1949; Declaration of Geneva International Medical Agreements, 1949; Declaration of Helsinki Medical Agreements, 1964). There was general agreement among the world's medical associations that the profession had been corrupted, and strong national and international rules were needed to apply to the canons of scientific and medical experimentation on human beings, and also on how the profession should conduct itself, despite political pressure.

Once these agreements and canons were in place, however, little more followed in the establishment of a discipline of health care ethics. But the seeds for such a development were sown in the 1950s and 1960s, due to several factors. The first, seemingly nonmoral, was the rise and speed of innovation in medical technology, initially greeted as an unmitigated blessing, and then looked upon somewhat as a sorcerer's apprentice type of problem. That is, the ability to prolong life through use of respirators, dialysis, artificial nutrition, and hydration, etc., though often dramatically effective, frequently resulted in prolonging a vegetative existence, which many people questioned as meaningful.

The second, derived from the earlier concerns with World War II medical atrocities, but more truly generated by the preoccupation in the 1960s with individual rights and individual autonomy, was the ideal of patient autonomy, as opposed to the traditional beneficence model of the medical profession. The beneficence ideal has been dominant since at least the Hippocratic oath, with its statement, "the regimen I adopt shall be for the benefit of my patients according to my ability and judgment," (Hippocratic oath, Temkin & Temkin, 1967), in which the physician makes decisions without benefit of discussion and/or direction by the patient. The move toward patient autonomy directly challenged that posture, insisting that the patient be at least a co-partner in all decision making. Some ethicists in fact believe that the patient should be the sole decision maker.

Notwithstanding the degree of autonomy desired, the ideal of individual autonomy became the basis for concrete health care policies, such as the Patient Bill of Rights, (American Hospital Association, 1972), and a building block of health care ethics for such ideas as informed consent and the right to refuse treatment, of which more below. The ideal was given greater emphasis when startling incidents of patient mistreatment in the United States began to be revealed. Key among these were:

1. The Army's use of lysergic diethylamide acid (LSD) on unsuspecting volunteers during the 1950s and 1960s. Many of these servicemen suffered psychotic episodes and permanent psychiatric damage.
2. The Tuskegee syphilis experiments on black men in Alabama, which began in the 1930s and continued through the 1960s. The control group of black men were not treated for their disease, even when penicillin became available during the 1940s, and as a result many went blind, were institutionalized and/or died. These men were never given the option of treatment, for fear it would make the experiment less scientifically useful.
3. The Willowbrook hepatitis experiments on retarded children and adults in Staten Island, N.Y. Physicians and researchers at the institution injected the patients with a mild form of hepatitis, so as to have a controlled population experiment, in an effort to discover a vaccine for the disease. The patients were not informed nor given the right to refuse the inoculation. Parents who wanted their children placed at Willowbrook were told admission was conditional upon their agreement to the inoculation. In consequence, this already sick population was given an additional sickness without consent and without therapeutic benefit to the patient.

These examples of medical arrogance and abrogation of individual rights gained widespread attention and underscored the need for patient autonomy and for the introduction in a formal way of medical ethics into the profession.

Finally, specific topics such as abortion, euthanasia, and the special problems of keeping alive multiply handicapped newborn infants fueled public and professional debate about when life begins and ends. These questions also led to great debate about the "sanctity" of life, as opposed to the "quality" of life. These ultimate questions have formed the central topics in current health care ethics.

Historical Development of the Field

Medical ethics began as a subset of the disciplines of ethics and philosophy, and to a lesser extent, that of the law. Given the issues and pressures described above, it has become a discipline of its own. Important ethicists such as Paul Ramsey and Joseph Fletcher began devoting time to medical ethics (Fletcher, 1960, 1966, 1979; Ramsey, 1971), among their other ethical concerns in the 1950s and 1960s. By the 1970s, thinkers such as James Childress, Tom Beauchamp, Daniel Callahan, Albert Jonsen, (Beauchamp & Childress, 1983; Callahan, 1987; Childress, 1970, 1983; Jonsen & Garland, 1976) and many others began to devote their full-time efforts to ethical problems in health care. At the present time, there are hundreds of ethicists working in health care. In addition, it is estimated by the American Hospital Association that 80% of acute-care hospitals with more than 100 beds have some form of an ethics committee.

That last fact highlights the movement of medical ethics out of academic centers and into the health care industry. As noted before, to date a great deal of this is more well-meant words than specific policies or case decisions. Yet, there is a discernible movement into institutions, particularly nonprofit multi-hospital institutions, such as the Sisters of Mercy and Kaiser Permanente Health Plan. The for-profit hospitals have largely resisted this trend.

Methodology

There are a number of methods used in analyzing medical problems from a moral perspective. One is to bring established ethical traditions and schools of thought to bear on current medical dilemmas and situations. These traditions and philosophical currents are generally both secular and religious, with religion coming from the Judeo-Christian tradition, at least in the West. A second is to examine cases or health care problems and policies, and examine them against ethical standards, learning general ethical principles from the cross-fire of discussion. A recent influential book has identified this as *casuistry*, a term that means applying general rules of morality to particular instances in which circumstances alter cases or where duties conflict (Jonsen & Toulmin, 1988). A third method is to focus on health care ethical issues only, foregoing any attempt to learn the general ethical principles that have been collected over the last several millenia. A fourth method is to focus only on patient care cases or health care policies, assuming that the values generated in discussion will provide a sufficient ethical framework in which to judge the correct values of the dilemma. One ethicist has called this "practice become values" (Shinn, 1983).

Clearly, there are strengths and weaknesses in all these methods. In the first, there is the difficulty of and resistance to learning basic philosophical tenets of the Western world. This is true for working health care professionals, whose training has tended to be in the sciences, as opposed to the humanities. It is true also for those in professional graduate schools and residency training programs, who tend toward either fiscal programs or experiential medical learning. It requires work on the part of both teacher and student to adapt such essentially different disciplines to forge a rigorous, thoughtful, hybrid discipline, which combines such different needs as pure thought and immediate action. Ethics in a medical setting could easily become an abstract contemplation of humanity's existential dilemmas, which would almost immediately alienate health care providers. Or it could become a second-rate litany of catch phrases, for example, informed consent, patient autonomy, whose implications have not been fully explored, and so lose the interest and respect of academics and most intelligent people who have pondered these questions. The challenge is to keep both immediacy and ultimate meanings in the hybrid new discipline.

Ethical Principles and Issues Principles

The Deontological Principle. This principle represents an ethical pole, an absolutist ethic which exists both as a principle in itself, and also, in present times, as an extreme of ethical thought, against which other ethics can be measured.

The word "deontological" comes from the Greek "deon" or duty. It is an ethic that relies on duty, on law, on rules that are based on *a priori* agreement on essential facts.

Deontological thought focuses on the "right," which is different from "rights," of what is "good." The right is what one *ought* to do, and never deviate from. Ought is the key word here. If one follows the ought, without exception, the most moral decision will be reached. Importantly, within this ethic, one doesn't plan for consequences. Consequences are seen as truly unforeseeable. Life has too many permutations to allow for even a pretense of accurate prediction. Thus, one goes by the rules, the ought, the law. (Note the small "l" in law. We are talking about universal law, not categorical e.g., civil, criminal law).

Overall, this is a highly individualistic ethic. The individual is the end of all action. In the words of Immanuel Kant, an eighteenth-century German philosopher and perhaps the foremost exponent of this ethic, (Kant, 1949), each individual is in himself the end of action and never the means. Here we see how well this ethic can be applied to clinical medicine. As in clinical medicine, all efforts go to the individual, as there is no higher goal, and no other goal for that moment in time. To do else would be to denigrate the close to sacred meaning of the individual. Moreover, as in clinical ethics, one goes by the ought and the rules. Medicine's oughts are its protocols for diseases and procedures. Deontological oughts are, as stated before, the *a priori* laws, which are reached partially through reason.

The final point to keep in mind with this ethic is how firmly it is grounded in reason. It is reason, not emotion, that governs. There are many reasons for this, for instance, reason is thought of as more reliable than emotion. But the underlying point in favor of reason is that only men and women are capable of reason, on all the earth, and it is this faculty, reason, which allows the free use of will, allowing us to choose between good and evil. Reason and free will are inextricable in this ethic.

The Utilitarian (Teleological) Principle. This principle represents the other ethical pole, the furthest opposite from the individualistic, deontological ethic. Originally called teleological, (from the Greek, "telos" or end), in current parlance, it has become, to all intents and purposes synonymous with utilitarianism. By definition, it is an end-oriented ethic, with the end of human thought and action being human happiness. But it focuses on the mass happiness, as in utilitarian's most famous maxim, "the greatest good for the greatest number," as stated by J. S. Mill, (Mill, 1962). In this ethic, concern is for the group, the mass, the society as a whole or sometimes, even the world.

Clearly, if concern is with the end point of thought and action for any group, this is an ethic that expects to be able to predict for consequences. Different utilitarians approach this in various ways, but all assume that reason (again a dominant theme in an ethical school of thought), can allow calculation on the part of some that will be beneficial for the many, or at best, calculation for the many that will be beneficial for the many.

Happiness itself was not conceptualized as a vulgar fleeting pleasure, a charge which has undeservedly earned utilitarian ethicists the charge of being listed as hedonists. Happiness can consist of many components, such as quiet contentment, intellectual pursuits, even health itself, important in bringing this ethic back to health care. Health for utilitarians is thought of as a basic good, necessary for happiness.

At least one prominent utilitarian, Joseph Fletcher (1966) noted that this ethic depends on either a majority view of what is "the (ultimate) good," or at least an individual's view of what is the supreme good. (Remember here that "good" is different from "right," in that it finds its end in maximizing happiness. The deontologist will follow reason, the rule and the right and not trust to happiness as too chimerical). Fletcher notes that this leads at some point to a clash of overriding principles and that finally one principle must be defined as the supreme good in this ethic. Fletcher himself votes for love, in the disinterested, nonself-regarding variety (Fletcher,1966), but his underlying point holds, no matter what principle is used. The "good" must be defined. In a markedly pluralistic society, such as our own, this is extremely difficult, if not impossible. Consider, for instance, the debate of the last twenty years over abortion, as to what is best for the society as a whole. The difficulty of defining the good becomes readily apparent. This is a major flaw in the utilitarian stance. While a majority, perhaps even a temporary majority, may define the good, that leaves enormous room for a minority to feel that some very bad things are happening to them and to their society. Their happiness is not being maximized, by their standards.

An example of how this could apply in health care would be a decision that a high-technology procedure, such as liver transplants, does not maximize the health and/or happiness of the majority of the population, and that therefore such procedures should not be covered by insurance in this country. Rather, the same amount of money that would go for transplants should be used to provide a baseline "floor" of medical care for all Americans, so that access for some definition of basic care could be achieved. This might well maximize the health and/or happiness of a majority. It would, however, leave those in need of transplants with an alternative of either dying or raising the funds for transplant by their own means, now estimated at from $120,000 to $140,000. Their happiness would be at risk. This example could be used in any number of other high-technology applications, for example, in vitro fertilization, which can benefit a small number of infertile women at considerable cost, (and some risk). Could the money be better used to foster adoptions of "problem children" considered unadoptable, or going further, adoption of orphaned children from other countries, who live in dire straits? How would one ethically balance the greater happiness here. Obviously, these are complex, multifaceted issues, and the utilitarian solution, as well as the deontological solution may simply not work in such complexity.

Other Ethical Schools of Thought. The Ethics of the Fitting: H. Richard Niebuhr, a twentieth-century ethicist, is one of many ethicists who have tried to find a median point between the "right" and the "good." In his 1962 book, *"The Responsible Self,"* (Niebuhr, 1963), he posited a four-point system for ethical decision making, aimed at the "fitting" ethical move. The ethical decision maker (1) must first be able to respond, then (2) must make an interpretation of the issues at stake, in terms of "what is being done to me, to us, to them," *not* what is my "law/right" or my "ultimate end," leading to (3) accountability, or taking into account the reactions of others, making the community's reactions part of the individual's decision. All this leads to (4) social solidarity, when the decision is implemented, not as a completely final act, but rather becomes part of a continuing discourse or interaction within the relevant community.

There are some major problems with this valiant attempt to get past the problem of totally opposed ethical opposites. One problem is that with all the discussion, interaction and taking into account of the community's values, the decision reached may merely be one of the common denominator. The decision may then be one with which no one is fully morally comfortable, but with which all are somewhat quieted. Another even more potentially dangerous problem is that the values involved are derived from the community's values. If those values are distorted, there is no absolute corrective. This points to the reverse of the problem of having the absolutist values of either the deontological or teleological school. If there are no absolutes, no higher authority, law, or value system to which to appeal, then morals can become an infinite regression, without any ending or beginning moral point. Some philosophers have attempted to deal with this by proposing an ethics of virtues (MacIntyre, 1984).

Max Weber—Supplements, not Contrasts. Max Weber, a sociologist and political scientist of the early twentieth century, was interested in ethical systems as well. In his treatise, "Politics As A Vocation," (Weber, 1958), he wrote at length on the ethics of decision making and the need to take responsibility for the consequences of one's action. Weber called this "the ethics of responsibility" and was strong in support of this modality. He was highly condemnatory of what he called "the ethics of ultimate ends" condemning them as "political idiocy," and for being responsible for most of the bloody events then taking place in his native land, Germany.

In his criteria for ethical decision making, Weber relied on three characteristics: passion; (somewhat contradictorily), an ability to abstract and to distance oneself from the problem; and a sense of responsibility. One cursory glance at his praise of the ethics of responsibility would seem to exclude "passion" as a desirable quality. But Weber stated that decisions are made "not with the head alone, but also with the heart." And for Weber, passion and the emotions are linked to the despised "ethics of ultimate ends," Weber had to come to an understanding and a synthesis of the place of both passion and of absolutes.

Weber did this by postulating that the ethical, mature decision maker, must continue with the ethics of responsibility or being responsible for the consequences of one's actions, for as long as humanly possible. To do otherwise is to "intoxicate" oneself with "romantic sensations." Yet, even following along this path of reason and responsibility, one reaches a point where one says "Here I stand; I can do no other . . . and every one of us who is not spiritually dead must realize the possibility of finding himself (sic) at some time in the position. In so far as this is true, an ethic of ultimate ends and an ethic of responsibility are not absolute contrasts but rather supplements, which only in unison constitute a genuine human being."

Weber then admitted the necessity for some moral absolutes, but only as a last resort and only when the absolute comes from the totality of the person. This ethic also has serious problems. By Weber's very definition of wringing the absolute out of oneself, he acknowledges that (a) it will be somewhat different for each person, and (b) an absolute will call forth the strongest and potentially most dangerous, irrational behavior from human beings. That is of course, why he insists that the ethics of responsibility and the ethics of ultimate ends be supplements, not contrasts. Yet, by admitting that it is for an absolute principle that people will stand fast, and not for a relative principle, he concedes the problem.

Absolutes in ethics and morality are exceedingly dangerous, as they lead to nonnegotiable positions, and to bitter and sometimes violent argument. Yet, the alternative is a relativism that allows for no moral standing point, no appeal to an intrinsic or extrinsic higher authority, for which the moral dilemma is truly crucial and outside conventional morality. Weber's notion of supplements is useful, as a possible way to escape these dangers, at least for a good deal of the time and for a good many situations.

The Doctrine of Double Effect

This doctrine was developed over centuries by Catholic theologians, in an effort to make canon law more amenable to actual human predicaments. For instance, under this doctrine the removal of a cancerous uterus of a pregnant woman might be justified, notwithstanding the Catholic opposition to abortion.

The doctrine of double effect attempts to justify certain actions that produce indirectly certain evil consequences, but it does this only after four basic principles have been justified.

1. The action, by itself and independently of its effect, must not be morally evil;
2. The evil effect must not be a means to producing the good effect;
3. The evil effect is sincerely not intended, but merely tolerated;
4. There is a proportionate reason for performing the action, in spite of its evil consequences.

This ethical system may be understood best in one of its classical illustrations. The case, which dates back many centuries is this:

> A woman, nine months pregnant, has had an extremely difficult pregnancy. She wants very much to bring her child to term. She has been warned by the local physician not to exert herself. If she exerts herself, there is a real chance that she will lose the child she is carrying. She lives in a house on the river, and at the moment of moral decision is sunning herself by the river.
>
> Suddenly, she hears the cries of a child, drowning in the river and screaming for help. There is no one else around. The *moral* question is can she run to help the drowning child? The point is not whether she wants to, but whether, given the Catholic emphasis on protection of fetal life, can she run as a moral act.

Here is where the sophistication and precision of the doctrine of double effect can be shown. Going back to the first principle, the action, which is defined as *running* is not "morally evil." For the second principle, the evil effect, the possible loss of the child in utero, is not the *means* of producing the good effect, the saving of the drowning child. Running is the means. In the third principle, the evil effect is clearly not intended as the woman wants her child. For the fourth principle, there is of course a proportionate reason for performing the act, and that is the attempt to save the drowning child. The key principle and action in the above scenario, however, is the isolation of the evil effect from being the *means* of saving the drowning child. In using this kind of logic, formally called casuistry, defined earlier in this chapter, secular and religious ethicists are able to respond to particular human situations while still holding to firm general principles.

The above certainly does not represent an endorsement of this method as a sure means of solving ethical dilemmas. Rather, it can be used to identify what is the moral dilemma, which is the first step in attempting to solve the problem. Perhaps, if there is a method being advocated among all of the above methods, it is the use of supplements, not contrasts, between absolutes and relativities.

Health Care Ethical Issues

Autonomy

Currently, the most important issue within health care ethics is that of individual autonomy. What this has come to mean is that the patient is the chief decision maker in all situations, regarding her/his medical care. The provider, be it physician, nurse or other professional, may and should provide information as to the risks, benefits and alternatives to a course of treatment, a procedure and/or a medication. But, according to the theory of autonomy, the patient makes the decision, up to and including the rejection of all forms of treatment, including life-saving treatment. The professional must abide by the patient's wishes.

As explained in the section above on the development of medical ethics, this was an almost inevitable course for ethicists to follow. Both the fears and realities of medical excesses lead to a strong doctrine of individual autonomy. Certainly, also the political climate of the 1960s and 1970s, with its emphasis on maximized individual rights, would also lead in such a direction. Further, a reaction against professional beneficence (see section below) for a variety of reasons—e.g., the malpractice problem, excessive physician and hospital fees during the financially expansive Medicaid and Medicare years, fears of technology being used both for its own sake without thought of what it might and might not do for the patient, and simply to make money for those supplying it— all lead to individual patient autonomy as *the* central medical ethical principle. For good discussions of these ideas, Gerald Dworkin, George Annas, and Ruth Macklin have done superb work (Annas, 1984; Dworkin, 1978, 1983; Macklin, 1986, 1987).

Most theories of individual patient autonomy are grounded in the work of Immanuel Kant (discussed above) and his notion of each individual as endowed with reason and free will, and therefore, unique in the universe. Each human being is a creature making choices for her or himself. Further, this theory holds that it diminishes the individual to have others make choices for him, as this is, in effect, an insult to her or his reason and unique individuality.

However, there are limits to the position of full professional autonomy, both in reality and in theory. In reality, the patient is dependent on the health care professional for information, and no matter how scrupulous the professional, it is difficult to keep professional biases out of the discussion. In addition, the professional knows a great deal more of the medical and scientific facts regarding the patient's situation, simply by virtue of years of study of the subject, which the patient has not had. Also, in reality, the patient may sometimes reject being given the option of choice, through fear, denial, indecision, etc., and the cliche, "Do whatever you think is best, Doc," is far from being history.

In terms of both reality and theory, there is a clearer limit on patient autonomy in asking for treatment than in rejecting treatment. Autonomy has been held to be grounded in *the right of privacy* in a number of legal decisions, notably in Roe versus Wade, (1973), the landmark abortion decision. It has been held to be the basis for rejection of treatment in a number of the so-called, "right-to-die" cases, beginning with the Karen Anne Quinlan case in 1976, and continuing with the major cases in the field, e.g., In Eichner (1981), In re Storar (1981), In re Spring (1980), Brophy vs. Mount Sinai Hospital (1986). In these and many like cases, the individual's right *not* to be treated has been based on privacy, or the freedom to do what one wants with his or her own body. Given the highly individualistic nature of American political, economic, social and legal thought, it is natural to have reached this point. But does individual patient autonomy include the right to demand treatment, particularly treatment that may be useless to the individual?

A relatively benign example is the patient who demands antibiotics for a viral infection. In fact, antibiotics will not attack a viral infection, only a bacterial infection. Yet, many patients have become so accustomed to getting a "shot" for the "flu" that anything less seems like shoddy care. Clearly, the right to demand this kind of useless treatment cannot be grounded in privacy. Can it and should it be grounded in some other notion of autonomy? (For a discussion of these and similar questions, see Brett and McCollough, 1986.)

A less benign example, and one anchored in theory as well, is that complete patient autonomy may lead to a major consumption of resources by one individual, or group of individuals, to the enormous detriment of the community as a whole. A few examples will make the point. A terminally ill patient may demand a large quantity of blood transfusions, which will minimally prolong his life. Yet, the hospital or the region may be so short of blood, which is now often the case, that to transfuse that individual at that rate may make it impossible to care for motor vehicle accident cases, or other types of trauma cases where transfusion is key. A patient or her or his family may demand that the patient remain in a critical care unit, long after some definable clinical benefit can be achieved by the stay, because they "want everything to be done" or because of fear or guilt or a host of other reasons. Yet, the bed may be desperately needed for a patient who can clinically benefit from the stay in a critical care unit. Finally, the transfer of medical resources to the elderly population through the Medicare program, and the recently passed catastrophic care bill, in an era of deliberate cost-containment have begun to raise serious questions about whether the remaining resources can adequately meet the needs of all other Americans. Some recent journal issues and books have begun to deal with this question (*The Journal of Medicine and Philosophy, 13*,[1]; Daniels, 1988a, 1988b), as well as various governmental leaders and the popular press.

The basic question is relation to autonomy, which arises from this, is how much can any person, elderly or not, demand in having their requests for aggressive, maximal treatment honored? This question particularly holds when the patient is terminal, but it may apply in other situations as well, when allocation of scarce resources is a serious problem. One author has gone so far as to suggest that as an incentive, if people didn't use their benefits themselves, they could transfer them to others (Hartwig, 1988). This is a very new idea, which remains to be explored for moral and administrative problems. (For a general discussion about the limits of autonomy, and age as a criteria, see Callahan, 1984, 1987a, 1989.)

Professional Beneficence

The doctrine of professional beneficence is deeply embedded in medical history. It is part of the Hippocratic Oath. The Oath states on part, "The regimen I adopt shall be for the benefit of my patients according to *my* (emphasis added) ability and judgment, and not for their hurt or for any wrong." Note that the patient has no say in the regimen adopted. The physician decides alone.

The roots of professional beneficence, sometimes less flatteringly called paternalism, lie very deep in medical history. The healing function and the priestly function have been combined in many societies, including our own. In biblical times, holy men were thought to be able to heal the sick by virtue of their ties to God. Jesus Christ healed by the laying on of hands, or in a more startling example, by having a hemorrhaging woman, unbeknownst to Him, touch the hem of His garments. In the Middle Ages, monks and priests practiced the art of healing as part of their role in keeping learning and knowledge alive, but also, in part, in imitation of the example of Christ. Nuns nursed the sick in hospitals and elsewhere.

In many other cultures, in the past and continuing to the present, the healer was the local religious person, whose power derived from the deity of the culture. Often the healing ritual and the priestly ritual would be combined. It is certainly worth noting that in the Hippocratic Oath, quoted above, the opening appeal, by the Greek writers of the fourth century B.C. is to "Apollo *Physician* (emphasis added) and Asclepias and Hygieia and Panaceia and the gods and goddesses, making them my witnesses, that I will fulfill according to my ability and judgment this oath and covenant." Again, there is the tie of the art of medicine to the reigning deities, to the extent of noting that one of the most powerful gods is himself a physician.

Given this background, the power of professional beneficence and/or paternalism is quite logical in the practice of medicine. Does not healing come from the highest authority, the most powerful Father of them all, at least for many people in the world? The switch into medical paternalism is an easy one to make emotionally and psychologically.

Moreover, as noted in the section on informed consent, there is an internal logic to it. The physician and nurse do indeed know a great deal more medically and scientifically than the patient, and their *medical* judgment is certainly more informed. In fact, leaving consideration of the basis of the doctrine to go to consideration of its central place in the twentieth century is instructive. As medicine has learned more, and become so specialized that physicians from different specialties cannot claim much knowledge of the other's specialty, the reason for beneficence/paternalism appeared even clearer. Physicians seemed to be extraordinary people, who knew and could do extraordinary things, perhaps even cheat death itself. For ordinary patients to enter into a dialogue with people of such knowledge and skill seemed foolish.

Of course, as the section on autonomy tried to make clear, this was not the case. The physician knows the medical facts. She or he may empathize greatly with the patient's plight and feelings, but it is the patient's body and mind that is at stake, and thus the patient has the right to decide what to do, after listening (hopefully) to sound advice. Moreover, as the most cursory reading of history shows, investing unchecked power in any group leads to abuse of power. Despite their long-standing ethical codes and traditions, this is as true of the medical profession as of any other profession.

Professional Autonomy

Given the struggle between individual patient autonomy and professional beneficence, what balance can be achieved? Many ethicists, including this one, think that the answer lies in professional autonomy. In a sense, this is giving to the health care professional the same dignity and respect accorded to the patient. It takes into account that the health care professional has striven to master a body of knowledge which allows for informed, discrete judgments. It also allows for the fact of the health care professional as a human being, with feelings, beliefs, and values, not a technician who performs at the behest of patient, science, or employer.

One notable example of where this has occurred is in the abortion situation. There are health care professionals who have strong beliefs against abortion. Most hospitals have recognized this, and not assigned such staff to areas where they would be dealing with abortions.

Equally compelling are cases in which the patient will be allowed to die being taken off life-sustaining technological equipment. Some physicians and nurses feel very strongly that this is either tantamount to murder or against all medical ethics or both. Some feel, perhaps more strongly than the patients own family, that this is the only possible course to end pointless and intractable suffering. In the first case, can medical staff be forced to terminate treatment? Clearly not, as to do so would be to negate their individual moral worth. Such professionals should be transferred off these cases and professionals who are in agreement with the beliefs and wishes of the patients and families can take over in each case. This option should never be used as a subterfuge to allow health care professionals to abandon patients whom they do not wish to treat. The clearest current example of this is the way a few clinicians have declared that they will not treat AIDS patients because of fear of infection for themselves and their families, or sometimes because of their dislike of the life styles of AIDS patients.

In the second case of professional-patient value differences, can medical staff override family wishes, in a commendable desire to end suffering? This is the subject of increasing debate. What becomes of professional responsibility, autonomy and standards when a family requests, for example, the continuation of aggressive treatment for an irreversibly comatose patient? In another example, should a patient be offered the prospect of cardiac resuscitation if professional opinion is that such treatment would inevitably have the patient in a worsened medical state than before, with an even more dismal prognosis. The debate over what has come to be called "futile" treatment is vigorous on both sides, and is far from conclusion. The debate clearly involves varying conceptions for professional autonomy. Almost inevitably, it has also become tied to a debate on resource allocation, which alarms some observers while seeming rational to others (Tomlinson & Brody, 1990; Blackhall, 1987; Younger, 1988; Truog, 1992; Veatch & Spicer, 1981, 1992).

While some ethicists feel professional autonomy may be a way to bring back the discredited notion of professional beneficence, many others feel that this may be a means of humanizing medicine. Health care professional training now focuses overwhelmingly on technology. By acknowledging that professionals have determining beliefs and values, and making sure that the arena is open for them to act on those beliefs and values, the practice of medicine may become more cooperative, less adversarial, and more humane. The patient or surrogate still decides, within the bounds of reason, what is done with her or his mind and body. But the professional does not have to slavishly follow this dictate. In this view, the practice of health care also contains its own inherent values.

Societal Risk and Benefit

Medical ethics has tended to emulate medicine itself, in that the ethics have had an individualistic flavor, as has medicine. A great deal of this arises from the focus on individual autonomy, as discussed above. A less-noticed reason for the emphasis on individualism is that working ethicists outside of think-tanks or academia, work on cases much the way medical staff do. That is to say, both groups focus intensely on one patient at a time. Even those ethicists outside the institutional maelstrom tend to comment on specific cases involving specific individuals. To date, there are no public health ethicists, that is, ethicists whose concern is the health of large groups of people and/or whole societies.

There has been a change in this tendency within the last few years, as cost-containment has become a major theme in health care. Once resources are acknowledged as scarce, it forces consideration as to how these newly scarce resources may best be used to benefit society as a whole. It also raises the converse question. What is the risk to society of failing to use these resources appropriately, or using resources disproportionately for particular groups at the expense of other groups? (See Churchill & Davis, Callahan, Maguire, Zoloth-Dorfman.)

Other changes in the health care field have also forced reappraisal as to the good of society. The AIDS epidemic is key in this respect. Both the health professions and society as a whole are struggling to find the balance between protection of the AIDS-infected individual and the ability of society to have enough information to protect against the further spread of the disease. This has involved a reappraisal as to the limits and benefits of confidentiality, as well as consideration of the protection of individuals against bigotry and discrimination.

The aging of the American population has also forced reconsideration of the use of resources. Medicare expenditures have continued to rise, despite sustained efforts to control the increases and specific, heavy cuts in the Medicare budget. Nursing home care for the elderly consumes a large proportion of the Medicaid budget, originally intended for care for the poor. Numerous demographic studies show that the need for long-term care for the elderly will increase sharply as the baby boom generation of the 1940s and 1950s ages, and various proposals have been advanced to deal with the problem. They range from making long-term care a Medicare benefit to a tax increase for the population as a whole to support this service. While the need for long-term care for the elderly is a reality, the increasing allocation of resources to the health needs of the elderly can easily cut very deeply into the funds left for care for the remainder of the population, unless the society is willing to accept a substantial increase in the amount of national resources going into health care as a whole. It is unclear whether society is willing to do so, or what society wants to do about long-term care as a unique problem. Polls and studies are conflicting.

A classic example of difficulty in allocation of scarce resources has arisen in organ transplantation. There are far fewer potential donors for organs, (livers, kidneys, hearts, etc.) than there are recipients. This is a problem in itself, but it is further complicated by the fact that many foreign nationals come to the United States for transplants because this country is using this technology so much more than any other. There is thus a debate on whether and/or how many foreign nationals should be put on the waiting list for organs, instead of American citizens. Beyond this problem, and certainly more important than this problem, is how to justly allocate these scarce organs among those whose lives depend on the transplant. All too often, intense media publicity by distraught patients or their families has resulted in a patient being jumped from a low place on the waiting list to a top place, leaving those who have been waiting to wait still longer. This "jumping the list" has been fairly criticized as unjust. The current proposal is to have a national consortium, privately run, to deal with the allocation.

Beyond even this question is the ethically and politically difficult question of whether this country should be doing transplants at the rather rapid rate that it is, compared to other countries. Organ transplantation is extremely costly, and benefits a relatively small number of patients, albeit very sick patients. Many ethicists and health care professionals argue that this money could be far better spent on basic public health services, preventive care, and health education. They further argue that such activities would diminish the need for organ transplantation as people learned better nutrition, more useful exercise, or less-damaging health habits such as stopping smoking, drinking alcoholic beverages to excess, or the abuse of drugs. Those in favor of organ transplantation point to the enormous need currently present in these very sick patients, who will surely die without the transplantation.

All of the above are examples of the vexing nature of consideration of balancing risk and benefits to the society as a whole, while still considering the individual as an enormously important end point in him or herself. Health care reform, proposed by the Clinton administration, has not explicitly addressed societal risk and benefit, or who gets what and how. Underneath the goals of universal coverage and cost-containment, the issues of commensurate benefit with finite resource remain open questions.

Meaning of Institutional Integrity and Survival

This chapter is concerned with the very great pressures on health care institutions and health care professionals to provide optimal care while limiting the cost of that care. It is very much an open question as to whether this can in fact be done, (Shortell & Hughes, 1988; Feldstein et al., 1988; Schramm & Gabel, 1988, McCarthy, 1988). It is difficult, in life, to have it all. However, such are the signals being given by patients, the government, insurers, and businesses to American health care, with the declared goal of universal coverage and lowered cost.

Under the pressures, there is a strong incentive for hospitals, or other health care institutions such as HMOs and health care professionals to cut corners in a variety of ways. Hospitals may cut back on less visible but needed staff in an effort to hold down costs. Physicians in a fee-for-service practice may turn a treatment or a procedure that can be accomplished in one visit into several, at risk and difficulty to the patient. HMOs may provide patients with fewer referrals to specialists or hold off on patient hospitalizations past the point of patient safety. Currently, with the emphasis on both "managed care" and "managed competition," the threat is more in this direction. Physicians who have promised an insurer, employer, or the proposed health provider insurance cooperatives that they will deliver care at a set prime per month per patient may simply not deliver care. This can be accomplished in a variety of ways. An HMO can make the wait for an appointment so long that the patient will become discouraged, or go elsewhere, paying out-of-pocket costs to a private provider. Or staff can minimize the difficulty a patient is having, incorrectly deflecting(?) care. Or the patient is given a greatly shortened visit in which little is discussed or diagnosed. Under the proposed "managed competition" scenario, this may become endemic. Controls against such practice have not been proposed by the government authorities advocating them, other than economic market forces of supply and demand, which have not worked well in health care to date.

Clearly, if an institution or a single health care professional does not survive professionally, no care at all will be given. This is almost always the reason given when care becomes shoddy and/or dangerous. The reasoning is that some care is better than no care at all. This is true to a degree. At some point, however, the integrity of the institution or individual is so compromised that the care given is worse than no care, because it prevents the patient from using an alternate source or even understanding that an alternative is available. This may be at the heart of the ethical dilemma for health care as both an industry and a profession in the immediate future. There is no fixed point where any ethicist or in fact, any person, can say that the balance has tipped irretrievably. But it can and has, as in some notable scandals, and the danger must be taken seriously. For example, a managed competition scenario that relies on market forces to direct allocation has moral implications for institutions, such as the temptation to limit quantity or quality of care in order to preserve competitive prices for those who would purchase insurance.

The Two-Tier System of Health Care

The two-tier system of health care refers to the general fact that the lower classes receive a lesser level of care than the middle and upper classes. It also refers to the fact that, by and large, the poor are treated in physically different settings than the well-to-do. The poor are treated in public hospitals, and to a large extent in ward-like settings of private hospitals, while the well-to-do are treated in private hospitals, in more pleasant, small room settings. The more serious problem is seen as the first one, since it means that the lower classes are treated by less experienced staff in overcrowded and generally understaffed settings. Though a substantial number of poor people have had health insurance (such as Medicaid) since 1965, this has not substantially changed the situation. In part, this is due to the fact that Medicaid is—of all insurance plans—the one that reimburses the least well, so hospitals and physicians claim that they cannot afford to treat these patients, or to treat them as well as patients with better forms of insurance. But in part the phenomena seems to be due to such well-known factors as the social stigma of poverty, racism, and the lesser amount of political power of the poor.

In a real sense, the two-tier system is almost a passe issue. What is evolving now is a multi-tier system, as different types of health maintenance organizations, preferred provider organizations, employer self-insured managed care plans, and the like press workers into a variety of less well insured medical programs. A middle-class patient may be covered by insurance that either doesn't cover the illness with which he or she presents, or which insufficiently covers that illness. Since the majority of even middle-class people cannot pay for the cost (or even part of the cost) of a serious illness, the institution or physician judges this type of patient to be a poor financial risk, and some tend to act in ways that are not to the medical benefit of the patient. They may refuse care, attempt to transfer the patient, or skimp on care for this type of patient, following the financial incentives. This sort of problem was traditional for the poor in the old two-tier system. What is new is the beginning of its extension to the working middle classes.

The ethical dimensions of this phenomena are clear. The ethical issue is justice, or less dramatically put, the just and fair allocation of health resources in terms of manpower, technology, and access. The allocation has been traditionally done on the random factor of class and race. The injustice will be further deepened by the multi-level system now going into place, driven by the pressures of cost-containment. Some philosophers from the egalitarian school have advocated a theoretical "veil of ignorance" behind which no one would know his or her advantages or disadvantages, as a means of combating the injustices of this system (Rawls, 1971). Others from the libertarian school have accepted the system as "unfortunate but not unfair," and part of the price for preserving our pluralistic society (Engelhardt, 1984).

Within the healthcare professions, there has been a long-standing tendency to descry the problem, but there has also been a lack of sustained effort to change the system. Within ethical circles, with the major exception of the libertarian stance noted above, the same tendency to deplore the system has consistently appeared. There have been a number of proposals put forth to change the system, ranging from a National Health Service to a free-market competitive system where all would be given "vouchers" to purchase the best health care they could find. But as noted, the system has remained, and is in fact, expanding to the middle class. A solution proposed by some physicians, ethicists, and health care theorists is a move toward the so-called "Canadian" system, which provides universal coverage under a single insurer—the government. While this would provide difficulties of its own such as the unemployment of those currently involved in processing the paperwork of the current system, as well as charges of undue government involvement in the private sector, it would improve access to care for the uninsured and diminish some of the harsher effects of multi-plan insurance.

Major Topics in Health Care Ethics

To this point, we have discussed general ethical principles as they apply specifically to health care. But the field of bioethics has spawned a number of topics that are intrinsic to health and have become key in understanding and appropriating the body of knowledge in the field. What follows will be a summary of such issues, including how they relate to the larger ethical principles discussed above.

Informed Consent

This is currently seen as a central issue in bioethics. It rests on the general principle of individual autonomy, and means that with a patient who has some capacity to understand the information being given, that no treatment, procedure, or medication can be given or done without the consent of the patient. Moreover, such consent must be in writing, or if the patient is not capable of that, such consent must be fully documented in the patient's medical record.

These statements may appear self-evident to a reader in the late 1980s, but twenty years ago they were hardly thought of, and almost never put into practice. Patients were (sometimes) told what would happen to them, and would often be told that this was to be done based on sound medical judgement, and there the matter generally ended (see Professional Beneficence above). That this state of affairs should have existed is particularly unsettling as no less a personage than Justice Benjamin Cardozo, later to be on the United States Supreme Court, had upheld the principle of informed consent in 1914. The decision was *Schloendorff versus Society of New York Hospital,* (211 N.Y. 125, 127, 129; 1914). It read, in part, that "every human being of adult years and sound mind has a right to determine what shall be done with his own body; and a surgeon who performs an operation without his patient's consent commits an assault, for which he is liable in damages . . . This is true except in cases of emergency where the patient is unconscious and where it is necessary to operate before consent can be obtained."

The *Schloendorff* ruling could have been, narrowly, held to apply to only surgery and surgical procedures. Yet, even this was not done. It would be fifty years before the next two major court rulings would clarify the meaning, necessity, and force behind informed consent.

The first, *Cobbs versus Grant,* S.F. 22887, Supreme Court of the State of California, 1972, was a response to the then current practice of defining what constituted informed consent by what everyone else practicing in a particular medical community did, rather than a universal obligation. *Cobbs v. Grant* said, in part, that the necessity of obtaining informed consent prior to diagnosis and treatment of disease is not governed by ". . . the standard of practice in the community; rather it is the duty imposed by law."

The second, *Canterbury versus Spence,* 464 Federal Reporter, 1972, dealt with standards of disclosure. Again, this had been something of a "standard practice" problem, in that physicians and the courts had used standard practice in a particular community as a sound rule for what could be disclosed. In addition, individual physicians had used, as an indicator, what *they* thought patients wanted to hear and were emotionally capable of hearing. *Canterbury v. Spence* changed to the ideal of the "reasonable person," who is defined as a composite or ideal of reasonable persons in society. The individual patient is not in question. Rather, the information, the patient must be given is what the reasonable person would want to know.

The temper of the times plus the universal claims of the decisions combined to make them much more acceptable than Justice Cardozo's decision in 1914. The idea of informed consent as a necessity in the clinician/patient or institution/patient relationship began to take hold. The difference between *simple* consent and *informed* consent became both clearer and more inflexible. Simple consent is a process where the patient is told what someone else thinks she or he can or wants to comprehend, and what the particular community, which may well be the medical community, believes the patient should know. The patient can then consent or refuse to consent, but refusal carries little weight, if there is a good "medical" reason on the other side. Informed consent turns that situation on its head. The patient is *informed* by a clinician telling all a "reasonable" person would want to know, stating it in comprehensible, not obscure medical language, and stating it out of a universally recognized obligation. Moreover, if a competent patient refuses, in a nonemergency situation, that refusal carries over the clinician's wishes.

All this derives from the autonomy principle, though most ethicists would also argue that it derives somewhat from the principle of justice. The mechanics of informed consent require that this consent arises from the clinician/patient or institution/patient relationship, and presupposes reciprocity. Philosophically, ethically and legally the person performing the procedure, or prescribing the medication or undertaking the treatment should obtain the consent. This should not be delegated to some lower level of staff. All this should be done in an absence of coercion, such as threats of abandonment, or undue influence. It should be done in the patient's own language, and should be understandable to the patient. This last point is more difficult than it sounds theoretically and practically. On the practical level, clinicians all too easily slip into "medicalese," and the patient is often embarrassed to say that she or he does not understand what was said. On the theoretical level, there are a number of quite depressing studies, (Cassileth et al., 1980), which show that the simplest, most understandable professionals attempting to give information to their patients in an effort to obtain consent are wildly misunderstood by their patients. Many patients, even after being told the contrary several times, stated that they believed that they had to sign the form, and a substantial number said they didn't know or even care what it was that they were signing. This is disconcerting. Nonetheless, the ideal and hope is to communicate the risk, benefits, and alternatives of what is being undertaken.

There are, of course, exceptions to the principle. One has already been discussed. The exceptions are:

1. Incapacity. The patient is not capable, mentally, of understanding the conversation. This can be temporary or permanent. Obvious examples are patients

who are severely mentally retarded, who arrive or slide into a comatose state, or who are minors (Curran & Beecher, 1969; Ramsey, 1971).

It is essential to note that even within this, efforts should be made to communicate with the patient. An adolescent or even preadolescent minor child, for instance, may well be able to comprehend the situation, and may have very strong feelings and beliefs about his or her care. Physicians, lawyers, and ethicists all disagree about what age it is appropriate to begin involving children in their care, but there are few who would deny minors some say in their treatment.

Further, the mentally retarded or mentally ill may have degrees of capacities to understand their condition, and be able to make decisions about much of their care. This section deliberately did not use the word "competence" as a condition that would constitute an exception to informed consent. Competence/incompetence is a legal term, and we are attempting to deal in matters of ethics, and not the law. We therefore deal with the terms *capacity* and *incapacity*. Within some levels of incapacity, a patient may still have the *capacity* to make decisions on other matters as grave as surgery or chemotherapy for life-threatening conditions. The courts are currently attempting to decide if a mentally ill patient can refuse medication that might alleviate their disease, or the symptoms of their disease. The ethical community is divided on this question, but tends toward allowing participation in decision making on this subject (Dworkin, 1983).

Finally, the patient who arrives in a stupor or becomes comatose may well improve and become lucid. At this point, it is incumbent on the clinician or institution to advise the patient of risks, benefits, and alternatives, and ask for consent, regardless of what may have gone before.

2. Emergency treatment. In these cases, ethics, the law, physicians, and common sense agree. When a patient presents in an emergency, life-threatening situation, and is not capable at that moment, due to pain, or unconsciousness, of giving consent, the clinician may treat in the absence of consent. In fact, major operations may be performed with a lack of consent, if this is what is needed to save the patient's life. There are some in the above communities who will go further and say that even if a patient refuses consent after presenting in an emergency, life-threatening situation, the clinician may still treat. They base this on the terror, confusion, and misapprehension that often attend the fact of suddenly being about to die.

Where one stands on consent within the context of a life-threatening emergency depends in part on how strongly one believes in the autonomy principle, and how strongly one believes in the beneficence principle. Beyond this, it is still somewhat subjective. If a patient is clearly so terrified of illness and death that communication is impossible, it may be ethically permissible to treat. However, if there is time, strong attempts should be made to communicate. The point in all this is that if the clinician hesitates until the situation clarifies and the patient is able to give consent, it may well be too late to save the life of the patient. There are times when a second's hesitation has the potential to be fatal. This exception is meant to deal with that situation.

3. Waiver. This exception is meant to apply to those patients who refuse to make a choice about the type of care they want, or whether they want care at all. Colloquially put, this is the patient who says, "Whatever you say is fine, doc." There are a number of reasons why patients do this, among them: fear, denial, life-long training to regard physicians as omniscient, indecision, etc. If a patient indicates nonaction along these lines, the patient's delegation of authority or waiver should be carefully documented in the patient's medical record. After recovery, some patients may deny that this was ever their stance.

4. Therapeutic privilege. This exception means that in the judgement of the clinician, the patient is too sick to be able to hear the diagnosis, prognosis, risks, etc. It generally also means that in the judgement of the clinician the patient's condition will worsen if such is discussed with the patient. This position is increasingly frowned upon by ethicists as a means of bringing the discredited professional beneficence doctrine back in the door.

A variation of it, has however, been brought back via the 1988 New York State Do Not Resuscitate law, (State of N.Y. Public Health Law, 4/1/88). This law allows a physician to write a Do Not Resuscitate order (DNR) if the attending physician determines that, to a reasonable degree of medical certainty, the adult with capacity would suffer immediate and severe injury from a discussion of CPR, (cardio-pulmonary resuscitation)." The attending physician may then write a DNR order after getting a concurring opinion from a second physician, and also ascertaining the patient's wishes to the extent possible without having the discussion! Presumably, this is to be done by discussion with family, review of the patient's lifestyle for clues for beliefs on the issue of resuscitation. Again presumably, the physician objectively weighs the benefits and burdens to the patient, this last, of course, not being the patient's wishes, but the physician's best thinking on the subject. The problems that arise by ascertaining the patient's wishes without discussion become enormous when there is no family to consult, there is a divided family, or when the patient is new to the physician and previous lifestyle is unclear or unknown. Then, the physician can only rely on objective benefits and burdens, which have nothing to do with patient beliefs or wishes. It is these kind of situations that makes the use of therapeutic privilege such a dubious tool, at least for ethicists.

There are in fact, some rare cases where the patient cannot bear to have any discussion or even hear the name of the disease she or he has. It was for these circumstances that the concept of therapeutic privilege was brought forth. However, most patients are generally extremely glad to have someone finally tell them what is going on. They may be sad, grieving, or even distraught, but they are somewhat back in control, and can plan for how they want to lead the lives that are left to them.

Do Not Resuscitate Orders

The above discussion leads us to the topic of cardio-pulmonary resuscitation, and ethical concerns about its use. Simply put, cardio-pulmonary resuscitation is the welter of mechanical interventions that physicians, nurses, and technical medical personnel initiate when a patient's heart stops beating. This is probably the best-known and most-debated technology in public discussion.

There has been a medical tendency to automatically resuscitate a patient when his or her heart stops, regardless of the condition of that patient. The patient may have been in intractable pain and suffering, or have expressed a wish to die, given the miserable quality of life available, or the physicians may know that resuscitation may "bring back" (from the dead) the patient in an even worse condition than he or she was in formerly. Yet, all medical training has been aimed at the preservation of life, and despite all the above, the patient would be resuscitated (or to use the slang "coded," for code blue or code zero, as notifying the relevant staff that a patient's heart has stopped is called in many hospitals).

, The reaction against this practice has been very strong among the public, and the shift has gradually come within the medical profession itself. In recent years, a substantial number of physicians have felt a repugnance at attempting CPR on a patient for whom they have no reasonable expectations. However, even these physicians have been reluctant to write a DNR order, or even communicate such an order to other personnel such as house staff and nurses, for fear of medical malpractice litigation against them. Until quite recently, most states have had neither legislation nor statute that would prevent such physicians from being sued for murder, assisted suicide, or the like. Some physicians in some hospitals have resorted to such methods as erasable blackboards to indicate which patients should not be resuscitated, or used multi-colored dots on the patient's medical record for the same purpose. This is not only ludicrous, but can lead to mistakes, for example, the dots might fall off. The same mistakes can happen with whispered verbal orders. A house officer, going off duty, could inform the next shift that the *wrong* person was not to be resuscitated.

Some other ways around physicians and nurses fear of failing to resuscitate have been the "slow code" and the "show code." Since CPR depends on speed, if the "code" team takes its time getting to the area of a person in cardiac arrest whom nobody wants to resuscitate, the patient may well be past the point of no return by the time the team arrives. A "show code" is quite literally a show put on for the patient's relatives, so that they will think that all possible is being done for their loved one, while in reality, nothing of any significance is happening.

As mentioned, public repugnance against this charade, as well as the actual practice of resuscitating hopelessly ill patients, began to build up in the late 1970s with the Karen Anne Quinlan case, though in reality, that was a different type of case. However, it brutally served to make the point that technology could "keep alive" those who would prefer not to live in such conditions. It also became known, though more in the medical community, than in the community at large, that the statistics on patients who were able to leave the hospital, ever, after receiving CPR were very dim (Bedell et al., 1984; Tomlinson & Brody, 1990; Blackhall, 1987).

It could be said that by the late 1980s, public consensus had switched away from CPR to DNR. This can be measured by the passage of a number of state laws designed to declare someone who is brain-dead legally dead: the California Natural Death Act, 1976; the California Durable Power of Attorney Act, 1985; the New York State DNR law, see above (despite its peculiarity), and by the report of the *President's Commission for the Study of Ethical Problems in Medicine and Biomedical and Behavioral Research*. These kinds of documents embody what has come to be the conventional wisdom, at least in this area of health care. That is, that the technology to "stop" death far outstripped our capacity to use it rationally, and that there are many people who would prefer to die than live in states of dependency, pain, and disease. Furthermore, that at least as far as resuscitation is concerned, such people have the right not to be resuscitated and to be allowed to die. Furthermore, that this principle rests firmly on autonomy, privacy, and free-will, which are governing principles not simply in medical ethics, or even ethics, per se, but in the political system of the country. With the exception of a few groups such as some "Right-to-Life" believers, Orthodox Jews, and some native Americans, this would seem to be the prevailing view of the public, who in this case may have been said to have pulled along the medical profession. Many physicians and some ethicists in the last few years have questioned whether CPR should even be offered to certain classes of patients, such as the permanently comatose or the severely demented.

Foregoing Life-Sustaining Systems

Just as a discussion of informed consent lead us to a discussion of Do Not Resuscitate orders, so does a discussion of DNRs lead us to contemplate the use of other life-sustaining technology as an ethical problem. Some of this technology goes back more than forty years, such as the use of antibiotics to treat infections. Some is relatively new, such as the use of hyperalimentation or total parenteral nutrition (TPN) to feed patients who can no longer absorb sufficient nutrients to survive. The list of life-sustaining technologies includes, but is not limited to: antibiotics, artificial nutrition and hydration, dialysis, drugs, surgery, cancer chemotherapy, ventilation, the insertion and changing of catheters and other "lines," and transplants. The same questions apply here as do those in a discussion of DNR orders. Is life itself sacred and to be maintained at all costs, as the ultimate good? Or is quality of life to be taken seriously, despite its subjective nature? When a certain quality of life can no longer be maintained, which may differ enormously from person to person and group to group, does the considerable array of current technology *have* to be used to forestall death, or perhaps merely prolong the dying process? What indices, if any, can be used for quality of life and its converse, futile treatment, to universalize these questions, rather than leave them so subjective that practice may vary in hospitals a mile from each other?

One source many students may think of as unlikely has spoken on some of these questions. In 1957, Roman Catholic Pope Pius XII, speaking to a group of anesthesiologists said that "extraordinary" means do not have to be used to keep alive those who are surely dying (*The Pope Speaks*, 1958). Reiterating and clarifying this in 1980, Pope John Paul II spoke of the "benefits and burdens" of treatment, and stated that when the burdens have outweighed the benefits to the individual patient, that treatment is no longer obligatory and may cease. This weighing of benefits and burdens is not only a Catholic mode of ethical thinking, but a general ethical method. The change that many modern ethicists might ring on it though, is that when the patient's condition is extraordinary, all treatment is extraordinary. In such an extreme condition, there is no ordinary treatment.

Consider the case of a patient who has survived a severe heart attack and a stroke, but is now in a persistent vegetative state. The patient develops a pneumonia that could be treated by antibiotics. Antibiotics, in the modern world, fall under the rubric of ordinary treatment. But the patient has lost all higher brain functions, and cannot relate to himself or to others. The point of life, beyond biological life, has arguably been lost. The patient's condition is thus extraordinary, and so the treatment is also extraordinary. The concept of what is "ordinary" changes as the patient's condition changes.

There is not as yet a clear consensus from the society in general or from the health care professions as to the issue of the sanctity of life versus the quality of life in cases of foregoing life-sustaining treatment. Most health care ethicists feel strongly that the quality issue is the dominant issue, but even among this group, there are various beliefs as to the definitions of quality. Some feel that it is consciousness, and/or the ability to reason (Augustine, 1963, 1984; Fletcher, 1979). Some believe, as noted above, that quality of life lies in the ability to relate to oneself and to others. Those who believe in God, add a third relationship, the ability to relate to God (McCormack, 1974). Some believe that quality is found in the ability to derive some meaning and happiness from life, by the sick individual's own definition.

There are some in the medical profession and in the public at large who point to some of the dreadful historical consequences of making decisions on the qualities of lives lived, as happened with the Nazis. These people hold that the sanctity of life is the central point, and that to do anything other than maximally preserve life is to make a pact with the devil. The phrase "playing God with people's lives" is often heard in this context.

The fallacy in the "playing God with people's lives" theory is that the practice of medicine has always involved rigorous, sometimes brutal interventions in people's lives. From the beginning of the practice of medicine strong drugs were used to halt disease. Harsh practices such as "bleeding" the patient and surgery, certainly including amputations without benefit of anesthesia, were carried out. These drugs, practices, and procedures often killed the patient. Their purpose, though, was to cure disease and prolong life, and so they were generally accepted. But the usual understanding of "playing God" is direct intervention in people's lives (and in the case of health care, intervention in their disease process), and withholding or withdrawing treatment continues in this line. It doesn't alter the overall thrust of medicine, rather, it acknowledges the limits of technology, which have always been present (as in the examples above). Withholding or withdrawing treatment intervenes to end suffering, or put more correctly, allows the illness to claim what it has already claimed, that is, the patient's meaningful life, as the patient or family would understand it.

There are a fair number of signals that this view is becoming a consensus view in the health care professions and in the larger community as well. Many recent court decisions in differing states (Conroy, 1985; Jobes, 1987; Delio, 1987; Brophy, 1986) have held that withdrawing life-sustaining treatment is in the best interests of the patient. In all of these cases, the patient has been unable to express his or her own wishes at the time. Still, the courts have found for withdrawing treatment. In the only such case to reach to United States Supreme Court, the Court found the right to die in the 14th Amendment to the Constitution. The Court also held that artificial feeding is similar to therapies such as respirators and hemodialysis. However, the Court did not find a compelling federal interest in determining standards for treatment withdrawal and left this decision to the "laboratory of the states" (Cruzan, 1990). In the case of a conscious patient who can state wishes and desires, the courts have shown unanimity that such a patient can have a request for cessation of treatment honored, even including a stated wish to die due to deeply distressing circumstances (Bouvia, 1986). In another setting, the American Medical Association's Council on Judicial and Ethical Affairs, in 1986, allowed the cessation of feeding a patient by artificial means, when to do so would simply prolong the dying process. There has been little direct polling on these issues, but those health care organizations that have done so have found a considerable willingness to forego treatment by their patients, when the case is hopeless.

The distinction between withholding and withdrawing treatment is often made by many professionals. In fact, ethically, there is no difference between not starting a treatment, or stopping one that has already begun. The principle, as above, is whether the treatment will be or has been of benefit or burden to the patient. However, there is a clear emotional difference between not starting a treatment and stopping a treatment. In stopping a treatment, the professional also breaks the emotional bond with the patient, and this is difficult to do. Family members often feel the same way. However, unless one is permitted to stop a treatment, in reality, one could never start a treatment, for fear that it would continue pointlessly, after all hope for recovery had been lost.

The other emotional sticking point seems to surround the difficulty in feeding or not feeding a patient by artificial means. What appears to be at stake here is the symbolic value of eating and drinking in everyday life. A common theme here is "I can't stop feeding the patient, because that's a natural part of life." There is also a fear that the patient will suffer hunger and thirst. As to the former complaint, the idea of the natural act, it is again important to remember that it is the patient's condition that matters, not the type of treatment. If the patient is being maintained in a hopeless situation by artificial feeding, that can well be considered neither natural nor ordinary. As for the second problem, the fear of hunger and thirst, if the patient shows any sign of either, the patient should be fed and hydrated, (with consent, of course). However, patients in a persistent vegetative state or permanent loss of consciousness do not experience these sensations. For the sake of patient dignity, and also the feelings of family and staff, the patient's mouth can be kept moistened, after artificial hydration has been withdrawn. There is still considerable disagreement on the topic of artificial nutrition and hydration.

This is a lengthy topic and this section has only touched on some major issues. Many institutions have worked out elaborate protocols for different levels of care for different types of patients, such as general nursing care for those in a persistent vegetative state. Students are referred to several articles for further exploration of this subject (Wanzer et al., 1984; Meisel et al., 1986).

A relatively new development in this area has been the topic of physician-assisted suicides, in which a physician supplies the patient with the means to end his or her own life. Several states have had voter initiatives to enact legislation legalizing this practice (e.g., California and the state of Washington). Laws contesting this practice are being discussed as unconstitutional. Though the publicized cases have attracted enormous media attention, there is little professional or societal consensus on assisted suicide in this country.

Newborns with Multiple Handicaps

The previous discussion of foregoing life-sustaining treatment leads to an extension of an ethical question. The question is when, if ever, should a child born with multiple anomalies, be allowed to die, rather than treated. While the issue contains many of the same ethical points of that for a discussion of foregoing life-sustaining treatment for adults, it differs in the following ways. One, the infant can never express wishes, and the decision makers cannot be guided by previous wishes. Two, the infant is at the beginning of life, and has had no experience of life. It is emotionally more difficult to terminate life in these circumstances. Three, diagnosis and prognosis are often less clear than with adult patients, and this creates a hesitation to make any irrevocable moves. Four, the tests of quality for an adult, whether they be rationality or ability to relate simply do not apply. Perhaps the only tests of quality that can apply are estimates of the potential for consciousness and relationship, and more surely, whether the infant appears to be enjoying, or finding pleasure in her or his babyhood.

The questions came to the fore with some highly publicized cases in the early 1980s. In the first, a child with Down's syndrome and an esophageal fistula was not treated for the fistula, which is easily corrected by surgery. His parents made the decision not to treat on the basis of his Down's syndrome, and the obstetrician concurred. The local district attorney sued, but the child died before the case could be heard. This case, the Baby Doe case, created a sensation, and the federal government responded with regulations that demanded the aggressive treatment of *every* infant born, regardless of handicap. The government created severe penalties for noncompliance and a new federal office, nicknamed the "Baby Doe squad," which was staffed around the clock to monitor such cases and receive complaints. The American Academy of Pediatrics, and later, the American Medical Association successfully sued in federal court to rescind these regulations. Less stringent regulations are presently in effect that attempt to leave the bulk of the decision making with the parents and attending physicians(s), (Public Law 98-457, 1984).

While the double suit was continuing, the second of the well-publicized cases arose. This was a spina bifida infant, with hydrencephaly, whose parents, in consultation with physicians and clergy decided against proposed treatment for the condition. A local right-to-life lawyer sued on behalf of the child (Court of Appeals, 2d, No. 679, 2/23/84). The federal government then intervened, though unsuccessfully. The Supreme Court ruled against the government on the narrow ground of medical record confidentiality, leaving open the larger question of what parties may make what kinds of decisions for minor children and infants, (*Bowen vs. AHA*, 6/9/86). The case, named the Baby Jane Doe case, ended somewhat inconclusively. The parents eventually allowed some treatment, and the child surprisingly, spontaneously made some improvement. Baby Jane Doe eventually left the hospital to live with her parents.

The only area of consensus within the issues involving treatment of newborns with multiple anomalies is possibly that of anencephalic infants. The fact that there are no documented survivors for this condition, and that the infants normally die within a few days to a month, has lead to an understanding that anencephalic infants will not be placed on respirators. Yet, even this virtual unanimity has been displaced by a new issue. Brain tissue of anencephalic infants can be transplanted into adult patients ill with Parkinson's disease. One consequence is a policy of placing the infants on respirators until their tissue can be used. Another consequence is that mothers who are diagnosed as carrying such infants in utero are choosing to carry such children to term, to "redeem" their pregnancy. Another issue involving anencephalic infants is similar—the use of their organs for transplantation into otherwise viable infants. The ethical question is to what degree, if any, may anencephalic infants be used as organ donors, if there is no benefit to them by being kept alive until transplant is possible. There is little agreement here. The traditional touchstone suggested by Paul Ramsey (1971) has been that all research and treatment of a child must benefit that child. In the face of this traditional claim, the problem of anencephalic infants as donors to adults or children remains an ethical conundrum.

The issues involved in the cases of infants born with multiple anomalies have proved so difficult ethically and emotionally that at the present time, most are being decided on a case-by-case basis. There is no agreement on who, among the various parties (parents, physicians, the State, the infant, the adult in potentia), should make the decisions, and no agreement on what method the parties should use for their decision making. There is very little agreement on how long to wait before questions on diagnosis and prognosis become clear, except a tentative accord to immediately resuscitate infants born without the ability to breathe on their own, until consultation with parents can take place. There is some belief that Down's syndrome and other indications of mental retardation are in themselves insufficient reason not to treat. However, that perception is somewhat mitigated by the abortion issue (see below). For the student who wishes to pursue these issues further, see referenced articles by Shaw, 1973; Duff & Campbell, 1973; Lantos, 1987.

Perhaps, the most difficult and exciting issue is that the threshold of what defines a salvageable infant is constantly being thrust backward. A child with a birthweight of 750 grams or even lower is now considered a salvageable child, as is an infant born at 20 weeks. Some argue that any child with a "gasp" at birth can be considered salvageable. Given that the technology is changing and improving at almost miraculous speed, the challenge is to arrive at an ethic that can rationalize care. The principle of benefit and burden is applicable in this area, but understanding of what is technologically possible for various diseases, birthweights and gestational ages, and understanding long-term prognoses will be key before further progress can be made ("Imperiled Newborns" December, 1987).

One useful addition may be the infant care review committees that the revised federal regulations suggested, and that 80% of American hospitals have now established. These are, in effect, ethics committees for decisions on infants, hopefully containing a broad spectrum of views and varying types of members. The committees mainly review issues on a case-by-case basis, but the combined experience of these committees may provide a framework for deciding the pressing moral issues on a policy basis.

Abortion

The question of legalization of abortion was to a degree settled legally by the Supreme Court decision in *Roe versus Wade* in 1973. The decision, in brief, held that abortion was solely in the province of the mother-to-be for the first trimester, and was a matter for consultation between the mother-to-be and her physician until the end of the second trimester. Abortion was not permitted through the third trimester, on the usual grounds of the interest of the State in the preservation of life, and with the usual exceptions, such as abortion to save the life of the mother. The ground on which the Court made its decision was viability, that is, whether the child could survive outside the body of the mother at a given point. In 1973, six months was not an unreasonable time to set for viability. The moral and legal reasoning was based on the doctrine of privacy, in this case, that the decision of the woman on what to do with her body was a question of her privacy. A number of ethicists believe that autonomy would have been a stronger moral reason than privacy, which has traditionally fallen in many areas when challenged by the rights of others.

The question of viability has been sharply altered, as seen in the above discussion on salvageable infants. As mentioned, it is now possible, with enormous effort and great expenditure, to salvage infants at 20 weeks, which is, of course, the cut-off point in *Roe vs. Wade*. The development of fetal surgery, which allows the correction of some congenital defects in utero, also challenges the point of viability, as these procedures may allow the possibility of a healthy infant at an age when abortion is still permissible. Finally, the developing doctrine of *fetal rights*, a prolonged discussion of which is beyond the scope of this chapter, has raised difficult questions of what rights the fetus may have in utero, (Murray, 1987; Robertson & Schulman, 1987). Some examples of this doctrine are the right of a fetus to a mother who refrains from unhealthy behavior, or even the right-to-be born and not be aborted if the mother has declared her earlier intention of bringing the child to term. All these developments since 1973 have called into question, for some, the very basis of the thinking in *Roe vs. Wade*. Strong proponents of the theory that a woman has the sole right to control what is in her body largely remain highly supportive of *Roe vs. Wade*.

It is important to remember, however, that while the Supreme Court decision settled the legal questions on abortion, the political and ethical questions were not settled. Those who opposed the decision, for religious and other reasons, opposed it from the date it was issued. They have continued to oppose the decision legally, with legislative campaigns to overturn it by Constitutional amendment, by marches, petitions, and publicity. They have sometimes opposed it by illegal means, such as the bombing of abortion clinics and the murder and attempted murder of physicians who perform abortions. This is certainly not meant to link all the opponents of legalized abortion together in one camp, including those who use violent means. Rather, it is to reinforce how strongly this decision was opposed by large segments of the population, even at the moment when the Court's definition of viability made medical sense. Many of those who oppose legalized abortion see the procedure as legalized murder. They believe that either an embryo becomes human at the moment of conception, or perhaps at the moment of individuation. Some will extend this to the moment of "quickening" or the fetus' first movements in the uterus. But to its opponents, abortion is the taking of human life.

To its proponents, the issue is intrinsic to women's rights. They point to the long and bloody history of illegal abortion, in which many women, who felt unable to bring their child to term, died in unsanitary and brutal procedures. They point out that many more suffered irreparable harm to their health from such procedures. They believe that this situation was allowed to continue because the value of women was historically low, and because it allowed men to control the reproductive process. For these advocates, abortion is central to women's gaining control of the reproductive process, and with it, control of their own lives from male rule. They go further, to point out that our society continues to value neither women nor children, in their view, by the lack of support for universal child health care, and by lack of focus on the particular needs of children in the society. For this view (Harrison, 1983), the anti-abortion position is a sham, as it is not children's lives that are at stake, but rather power in the society.

Obviously, such diametrically opposed views have had difficulty finding any meeting ground, or in the ethical parlance we have used, any balance. Each side has won some political victories. The anti-abortion people won a Supreme Court ruling that Medicaid funds could not be used to pay for abortions, but many states have funded abortions for poor women from their tax funds. The pro-abortion forces have fought back several strong challenges to the overall ruling in the legislature.

As there is no moral consensus within the nation on when life begins, or what the meaning of that life is in utero, so there can yet be no consensus on abortion as an ethical and political problem. There is no clearer case in health care of how personal morality affects health care decisions. One's perceptions and beliefs on the very meaning of life, and the place of women and children in the society, have determined and will continue to determine how this issue is handled by American society. There may well be further Supreme Court decisions changing and/or clarifying *Roe vs. Wade,* beyond the 1989 *Webster versus Missouri Reproductive Health Services,* that allowed states to ban abortions by public employees in public institutions. The upholding of a Pennsylvania case added new levels of allowable restrictions, for example. Recent additions to the Supreme Court make for unpredictability on this issue. (For further references see Noonan, 1970; Thomson, 1971; Warren, 1973.)

Confidentiality

The ideal of confidentiality is one that is deeply held in the practice of medicine. Once again, this is a precept that is found in the Hippocratic oath. "Whatever things I see or hear concerning the life of men, in my attendance on the sick or even apart therefrom, which ought not to be noised abroad, I will keep silence thereon, counting such things to be as sacred secrets." An influential volume published at the beginning of the nineteenth century, Thomas Percival's *Medical Ethics* (Percival, 1927), orders that "professional visits should be used with discretion and with the most scrupulous regard to fidelity and honour." The American Medical Association, in 1980, stated that "a physician shall safeguard patient confidences within the constraints of the law AMA, 1980," (1984). The American College of Physicians goes further in saying that a physician may break the law to protect her or his patient, if prepared to accept the consequences of such behavior (ACP, Ethics Manual, 1984).

The ethics on which all this rests are again autonomy, privacy, and the protection of the individual. Interestingly, there is another ethic at work in protecting confidentiality, and that is utilitarian. The premise is that if patients cease to trust their physicians, they will not go for treatment, and that the society as a whole would be harmed by such behavior, for example, an outbreak of epidemics or untreated mental illness.

Clearly, all health care professionals by the very nature of their work, hear and see things that patients would not wish publicly known, such as sexually transmitted diseases or genetic chronic diseases. Until fairly recently, the standard of confidentiality has remained strong in the health care community, though tested by such problems as teenage drug use. (For example, does the treating pediatrician tell the parents of a teenager's drug use, over the patient's objections?) But the question began to become more pointed over the use of confidentiality in the case of mentally ill, violence-prone patients, and has now become a national debate, with the rise of the AIDS epidemic.

The issue of confidentiality regarding violent, mentally ill patients came to a turning point with the Tarasoff case, (*Tarasoff v. University of California*, 1976). Prosenjit Poddar killed Tatiana Tarasoff on October 27, 1969. They were both students at the University of California at Berkeley, and Mr. Poddar had been seeing a campus psychologist over the issue of his unrequited loved for Ms. Tarasoff. After nine or ten sessions, Mr. Poddar confided that he had purchased a gun, and intended to use it against a woman who could be readily identified as Ms. Tarasoff. The psychologist, Dr. Moore, asked the campus police to detain Mr. Poddar, which they did. They found him rational and warned him to stay away from Ms. Tarasoff. Dr. Moore consulted with his superior, Dr. Powelson, director of the Department of Psychiatry, who ordered that all records of the case be destroyed, and that Poddar *not* be placed in a treatment and evaluation facility. Mr. Poddar then killed Ms. Tarasoff, after ingratiating himself with her brother in order to find out when she was returning from a summer vacation.

Ms. Tarasoff's parents sued Dr. Moore, Dr. Powelson, and the Regents of the University of California, who was ultimately responsible for all services at the University. Their belief was that they and Ms. Tarasoff's brother, as the people most directly concerned with Ms. Tarasoff's welfare, should have been warned. In a hotly disputed and narrowly split decision, they won their case. In a sentence that became famous, the majority opinion held that "The protective privilege ends where the public peril begins." The opinion stated that the therapist "owes a legal duty not only to his patient, but also to this patient's would-be victim" and that "professional inaccuracy in predicting violence cannot negate the therapist's duty to protect the threatened victim." The majority did not state, however, who they felt should have been warned by Dr. Moore or Dr. Powelson. The dissenting opinion held that the majority opinion would destroy the practice of psychiatry, because without strict confidentiality those needing assistance would be deterred from doing so. Further, that patients who are in treatment would no longer confide in their therapists, should it became known that their thoughts might be told to others. The minority held that the majority had not only invaded individual rights, but also increased the possibility of civil commitment as the likely alternative when a third-party is warned of impending danger.

The Tarasoff decision has been used by both sides in the dispute over whether to warn the sexual and/or drug using contacts of Human Immunodeficiency Virus (HIV) positive patients, (the AIDS virus), that they are in danger of contracting the virus from their contacts. Most HIV positive patients are in fact cooperative in warning contacts whom they know. Some, however, refuse to do so, putting these contacts at great risk. The sentence from "Tarasoff," "The protective privilege ends where the public peril begins" is often used by advocates of breaking confidentiality to warn contacts over the objections of the patient. These advocates argue that the public peril is clear, and that the individuals are at risk of their lives. Moreover, since unknowing individuals may spread disease to others, whereas, if they knew of their danger, they might take protective measures or abstain from sex or drugs, that keeping silent means an intolerable risk to the whole of society, by means of a fatal illness for which there is no cure. These people are making an essentially utilitarian argument from "the greatest good for the greatest number." Those who favor keeping confidentiality in all circumstances take issue as to whether the utilitarians are correct in their premises much less their ethics. Echoing the minority opinion in "Tarasoff," they claim that if those who are HIV positive know that their physicians will inform their contacts, that they will go underground and never receive either counseling or treatment. Thus, the epidemic will spread more rapidly. This premise remains unproven. It is interesting to note that with regard to "Tarasoff" a study published 10 years after the final decision found that there had been no diminution in the practice of psychiatry as a result of the decision (Mills, Sullivan & Eth, 1987). However, the very real cases of discrimination against HIV positive people, wherein they have lost jobs, homes, and insurance due to their health status gives credence to the possibility of these people hiding their status from the health care system.

The other argument that advocates of absolute confidentiality make also mirrors that of the minority Tarasoff opinion. That is, that privacy is a right, based on individual autonomy (Walters, 1974). Therefore, no one, including health care professionals, has the right to violate it. This is harking back to deontology as an ethical touchstone. The new and allied problem of drug-resistant tuberculosis in immuno-compromised patients has added further controversy to the debate. The disease is far more communicable then AIDS, and needs strict compliance with a treatment regimen from those infected. Discussion has ranged from warnings to civil and criminal sanctions, including quarantine in a variety of forms.

The medical, legal, and bioethical professions are actively debating these issues, and that several state legislatures have also become involved. Yet, there is not yet a societal and a professional consensus on this issue. Such agreement as exists appears to be taking shape as the right (not the obligation) to warn *known* others, if their contacts refuse to do so. New York State is among several states that has put forward legislation that would free physicians from liability should they warn known contacts. However, there is no move afoot to attempt to track down fleeting or anonymous contacts, and attempt to warn them of danger. This has been the standard means of treating sexually transmitted diseases in the United States in the twentieth century, so it is possible that the position taken eventually includes this traditional public health function as well. As the epidemic progresses, it will put confidentiality, among many other principles, under severe strain.

Allocation of Scarce Resources

The problem of the allocation of scarce resources is a new topic in American health care. The problem itself is not new, as resources are by definition finite. But the topic itself has not been under discussion in American health care, for two reasons. The first reason is that Americans have historically rationed health care by level of socioeconomic status, (see the section on the two-tier system above). The second reason is that, other than using income as a measure, the United States has not rationed or even allocated care by planning. Those attempts which have been tried, as for instance in the Health Systems Agencies (HSAs) of the 1970s have failed for a variety of reasons beyond the scope of this chapter. (The HSAs were health planning agencies, established by Congress, to coordinate health care within states, cities and localities.) When faced with a rationing or allocation problem beyond income, the American health care system has expanded. This has been possible because the overall economy has been expanding, because the public wanted increased access and technology, and because various interested groups mobilized successfully to continue the expansion, for example, the elderly and those in need of renal dialysis.

As noted previously, in the 1980s, the situation changed. The economy found itself under pressure from other countries such as West Germany and Japan, whose prices were more competitive than American prices. American business claims that at least in part, this is due to the huge costs of health care benefits to workers, dependents, and retirees. Therefore, American business began strong efforts to contract their portion of the health care budget. In addition, the federal government claimed, at the beginning of the 1980s, that the Medicare trust fund would soon be depleted (Office of the Actuary,1984), and in response, also began efforts

to contract the costs of their share of the health care budget. The insurance industry claimed that it was experiencing heavy losses from the health care section of
its business, and also began contraction. Resource allocation thus began to appear
as a debateable topic, under the pressure of all these cost-containment efforts, with
the specific fear that quality of care would suffer as funds diminished.

Moreover, health care inflation continued to be at least double that of the general inflation rate throughout the 1980s. And the proportion of the Gross National
Product that is consumed by health care services rose to around 14% in 1992,
compared with around 6.5% in 1977. Though a variety of polls indicate that the
American people are willing to pay that and more for optimal health care for themselves and their neighbors, the triad of business, insurance industry, and federal
government views these numbers with alarm and dismay. The issue became greatly
politicized in the 1990s, affecting various Senate campaigns, and the 1992 Presidential campaign.

The debate on allocation of resources has also been heightened by the advent
of managed care, itself partly an outgrowth of cost-containment efforts. In health
maintenance organizations, and to a lesser extent in preferred provider organizations, the budget is fixed, generally on a yearly basis. Therefore, expensive treatments for a few patients, or a group of patients with a particular disease, can mean
that the organization may have to cut back on routine care for the remainder of its
members/patients. Setting aside the problem of financial incentives for under-
treatment, with which some charge the managed care organizations, expensive,
repeated treatments raise serious questions of resource allocation. This is a new
problem for the American health care system, accustomed as it is to third-party
billing in a fee-for-service setting and the consequent lack of a fixed budget
(Levinson, 1987; Reagan, 1987).

Finally, the finitude of resources has been dramatically demonstrated by the
questions inherent in organ transplantation, as noted above in the section on societal risk and benefit. The principle of justice has been the dominant ethical theme
in considerations of organ transplantation, both in questions of who gets transplanted, and what proportion of the national health care dollar will go to support
these services. But the consideration of justice is, in fact the principle theme in
the allocation of resources, tempered by compassion. Now that the allocation problem is moving into the open, it will be a sure test of a democratic society to determine how ethics can affect the political and economic processes of resource allocation. President Bill Clinton has made health care reform a priority, if not *the*
priority of his administration. However, little attention has been paid to resource
allocation and none to rationing. A few of these more egregious examples of overuse of treatment have been mentioned experientially. The guiding assumption
appears to be that the market forces of managed competition will guarantee equity
in resource allocation. Several in Congress, notably Fortney (Pete) Stark and Henry
Waxman have questioned the validity of this assumption.

Equity of Access

Any discussion of allocation of resources is based on the idea of equity of access. Without access to the health care system, it is not possible to receive care at all. Equity of access can be defined as all people having the right and ability to receive similar treatment for similar conditions. Some moral limitations on access are arguable, that is, the distinction between "basic" medical needs and "felt" medical needs. An example of a basic medical need could be asthma control programs for children. An example of a felt medical need could be cosmetic surgery, such as face-lifting. The distinction between basic needs and felt needs, however, is often more difficult to make. An example is infertility treatment. There are those, for instance, who believe that treatment for infertility is a basic medical need. There are those who believe it is only a felt medical need. There are those who believe that it is not a problem for health care, but rather a societal problem of the imbalance between infertile couples and children already available to adoption, or a problem of narcissism. When definition of need itself is controversial, it is more difficult to define equity of access. However, there are broad categories of need, such as primary, emergency, critical, and chronic care, which most ethicists agree demand equity of access.

There are any number of impediments to equity presently. Income problems have been discussed, as how the cost-containment efforts that have deepened the problems of socioeconomic status. The two-tier and now the multi-tier health care system has been explored, and this is one of the bases for inequity. But there are many other barriers as well. Approximately 38 million Americans are estimated to have no health care insurance of any type. Estimates on the number of Americans with drastically inadequate health care range from 18 million to 40 million. Though public facilities funded by tax monies are available to some of these people, it is these facilities that are overcrowded and understaffed. Rural areas and indeed some states may have no public facilities at all. A small number of uninsured people find their way into private hospitals, but decreasingly, as cost pressures cause "dumping" of these patients into such public facilities.

Another barrier is geographic. People in rural areas may be truly isolated from any facilities or physicians, as these areas are largely financially unattractive places in which to practice. People in urban slums may have difficulty in achieving access, for the same reasons. That is, many hospitals and physicians find that they cannot stay in business in these areas and depart for more financially rewarding locations.

In addition, in what is overall a deeply organized system, but what is for the individual often a fragmented, confusing system, it is difficult for a patient to find out what kind of care she or he needs, and then locate that care. In an era of heavy medical specialization, the lack of primary care may itself be a barrier to access. The information necessary to understand how to use the system is most easily possessed by those within the system. The individual patient, without the guide of a primary care practitioner may be unable to reach care, even if insured.

Equity of access is a key ethical problem, as it is almost impossible to discuss fair distribution, or indeed any distribution, without it (President's Commission, *Summing Up*, 1983). Here, too, the Clinton administration has made a major effort to assure access for all citizens, excluding illegal aliens, in its proposed plans. The political process will be deeply involved in a question, that is also a moral decision.

Adult Immunodeficiency Syndrome (AIDS)

The AIDS epidemic contains almost all current dilemmas in ethics within it. These detailed above, include such matters as confidentiality, resource allocation, and physician responsibility to patients. The epidemic can be seen ethically, in the words of Albert Camus, writing in *The Plague*, as coming for the "bane and enlightenment of men," the possible enlightenment being the focus the epidemic brings to vital moral questions.

AIDS is an infectious disease caused by a retrovirus, which is capable of replicating in the body, and causing the destruction of the body's immune system. Thus, the individual becomes prey to opportunistic infections, which it could otherwise protect against. The AIDS virus, Human Immunodeficiency Virus (HIV) is effectively transmitted by sexual contact between men, from men to women, and somewhat less effectively, from women to men. Transmission is also bloodborne, thus putting those who share syringes for intravenous drug use at risk. It also leaves at risk those who have been transfused with large amounts of blood, such as hemophiliacs, though since 1985, the blood banks have effectively cleaned their supplies of HIV. Perinatal transmission is also possible, from infected mothers to their infants in utero, during parturition, or during postpartum breast-feeding. Infection is also possible from accidental injuries, such as needle-sticks to healthcare workers during the course of caring for an HIV positive patient. Such cases have been few, however. There is reason to believe that a single inoculation of HIV is unlikely to transmit the virus. The single American case of transmission from an HIV-infected health care worker remains unclear as to mode of transmission. It is still believed that the most effective means of AIDS transmission is receptive anal intercourse with multiple partners.

AIDS is a fatal disease for which there is no cure nor vaccine. The pandemic contains most of the issues of health care ethics within it. The discussion of confidentiality touched on one such issue. The issue of mandatory versus voluntary screening for the HIV virus is a spin-off from that issue, though there is more involved than simply confidentiality. The issue, so far unresolved, is whether to institute a mandatory testing program for groups at high risk, such as homosexuals, bisexuals, and intravenous drug-abusers, or for groups the society might especially want to protect, such as expectant mothers, or to institute such testing for the entire society.

Those in favor of mandatory testing on any of the above levels give many reasons for their advocacy. They state the value of tracking the disease epidemiologically. They claim it will alert health care workers to take extra precautions to guard against risk of infection. They claim it will give either the government or various other institutions the opportunity to offer help to these individuals. They say it will alert those who unsuspectingly have the virus to change behavior patterns in ways that can protect others.

Those who oppose mandatory testing, particularly at the broad level of the whole of society, raise strong civil liberties objections to the concept. They point out that there are few guarantees in most states against discrimination against HIV-positive people and that individuals who tested positively could easily be subject to punitive action. Some take that thought a step further, in fearing that HIV-positive people or those with drug-resistant tuberculosis would be quarantined, and/or subject to criminal sanctions for transmission of the disease. They emphasize that so far, the disease has affected those people already at the margins of society, such as homosexuals, bisexuals and illegal drug users, and the concerns and protection of marginal peoples are historically quickly discarded. They also state that such a program would cost enormous amounts of money, yielding little in the way of hard results and a great deal in the way of false-positives. The lack of hard results would come about because the homosexual and bisexual communities largely already assume infection and have moved to take precautions, as evidenced by the falling rates of other sexually transmitted diseases in these groups. The false-positives are a problem because such incorrect knowledge could harm or destroy a person's life, before the misinformation became corrected.

Those opposed to mandatory testing often oppose it for particular groups as well, such as expectant mothers and patients about to undergo surgery. As to the former, once again, they believe testing to be a violation of individual autonomy and privacy and a dangerous invitation for future invasions. As to hospitalized patients awaiting surgery, they cite the Center for Disease Control (CDC) standards, which are, in essence, that every patient be treated as an AIDS patient, so that full precautions are taken on every patient (Bayer et al., 1986).

Other ethical issues which have been discussed in other contexts above are the use of life-prolonging technologies and the allocation of resources. The question of the use of life-prolonging technologies for an invariably fatal and degenerative disease, adds even more tension to the problem than it normally generates. This tension is coming from a variety of sides. There are a considerable number of AIDS patients who refuse technologies, such as respirators, from virtually the onset of the disease. This may produce tension with medical staff who believe that the patient could have months or even years of meaningful life, if the patient accepted technological help. On the other hand, there are patients who will request major interventions when all hope is gone, and there can be no clinical benefit received from the intervention. Many health care professionals find it difficult to deny such interventions, however, to young patients, the very sort of patient for whom they historically have used the most aggressive treatments. Another issue along these lines is the use of experimental and/or very expensive drugs for AIDS patients, or for patients who are HIV positive. Patients will often request these drugs before there is approval from the Food and Drug Administration and/or reason to believe that patients will benefit from the drugs. There is thus resistance to ordering such drugs for patients, yet patients will demand them as a last chance at life, however unrealistic this seems.

The ethical and emotional issues can become confused in this situation. For at least one ethical issue involved here is the allocation of resources, and there are a welter of emotions regarding HIV-positive patients that complicate the allocation issue. For instance, there are many in society who believe that the life style choices of homosexuals and illegal drug abusers have brought the punishment of AIDS upon its victims. Whether this is divinely inspired wrath, or a secular settling of scores, such people would not choose to allocate much in the way of treatment for AIDS patients. Yet, on the other side, there are also many in society who feel that AIDS is a horrendous additional burden for those already carrying the onus of bigotry, and that considerable resources should be apportioned to those afflicted. This problem will deepen in the years to come, as the epidemic increases, and the dollar amounts to pay for care increase as well.

Another ethical problem is the response of the health care community to the risk inherent in caring for AIDS patients. Presently, there are many thousands of health care workers who have accidentally exposed themselves to HIV, from needle-stick injuries, blood splashes, contact through open skin lesions, and the like. They are being followed by the CDC, and in the last major survey in 1989, only about 20 had become HIV positive. Yet, there is considerable fear and resentment in the medical community, from some, and a refusal to treat from a very small number of professionals.

There has been an extensive discussion of this question, and there is a clear professional consensus that the duty to treat must overcome all hesitation due to fear of infection. This stand has been embraced by the AMA, the American College of Physicians, and the American Hospital Association, among others. All have pointed to the long-standing tradition in medicine of caring for the sick at great personal risk. Many have also pointed out that freedom from risk of infection is a very new development in the history of medicine, and that professionals were routinely at risk until the development of antibiotics, which is as recent as the 1940s, (Zuger & Miles, 1987; Pellegrino, 1987).

This certainly does not exhaust the list of ethical problems that the AIDS epidemic has brought about. There is, for instance, the question of what role the health care professions should take to protect their patients, when society has not provided such protections, such as anti-discrimination laws. There is the problem of confidentiality and protection of HIV-positive health care workers, who are apt to be immediately dismissed from their jobs unless other policies are in place. Some have hospital privileges removed without benefit of hearing or evidence of likely transmission routes. There is the problem of finding some means of dealing with those, such as prostitutes, who have a better than average chance of being HIV positive, and who continue to practice their trade, as well as what to do with those who patronize them. For those interested in these areas, there are a number of good reference works on the AIDS epidemic dealing with the study of the ethical problems involved (Macklin, 1986; Gostin & Curran, 1986; Steinbock, 1986; Osborn, 1988; Steinbrook et al., 1986; "AIDS: The Responsibilities of Health Professionals: A Special Supplement," *Hastings Center Report*, 1988).

Ethics of Managers in Health Care

The health care administrator has been gaining power steadily through the last few decades, for reasons made clear in other chapters. This has been particularly true during the 1980s, due to funding changes, the physician surplus, the determination of government, business, and the insurance industry to curb health costs (making the administrator the point man in the effort), etc. The balance of power has shifted dramatically from the physician to the administrator/manager, and will continue to do so in the foreseeable future. This shift also entails a change in outlook. Clinicians tend to an individualistic ethic, centered on the patient they are caring for at that moment. Administrators tend to look at the institution's needs as a whole, by both training and inclination (Seiden, 1982, 1985).

Administrators were perhaps not well prepared for the power they would have thrust upon them, or which they would assume. But they have certainly not been prepared for the ethical responsibilities that power entails. Physicians, as has been shown many times in this chapter, have a tradition of ethics that extends back at least 2,500 years in the west, and at least 3,500 years in the east. Administrators/managers have been trained to think of budgets, staffing, reimbursements, development etc., with a conspicuous lack of moral tradition to center these activities. This is a considerable problem, as power without morality inevitably degenerates into abuse.

Administrative training programs infrequently include training in ethics. A reversal of this in the undergraduate and graduate schools seems an obvious place to begin educating administators-to-be to the moral implications of their work. But that strategy leaves unchanged the current generation of working administrators, and that is an unacceptable solution. The American College of Health Care Executives revised its Code of Ethics in 1987 to try to delineate the moral responsibilities of administrators. This is a beginning, but formulated codes from voluntary organizations cannot change thought processes geared to "the bottom line." In-service training on a continuing basis, substantial regional and local conferences on topics of interest such as resource allocation, and a serious literature on administrative ethics are all needs that should be fulfilled for the good of the health care professions and the patients that are its charge (Darr, 1984).

Further, since administrators/managers now have great power, they cannot follow ethical trends, but should rather take the lead in establishing policies and protocols in their institutions on ethical issues. To do this, they must involve all the constituencies involved with their institutions, such as physicians, nurses, ancillary personnel, patients, community members affected by their institutions, and so on. Once policies are in place, institutions can begin to act on individual cases within a given framework, and except in emergency cases, patients can find out an institution's stance on questions that concern them beforehand and act accordingly. For instance, if an individual with a terminal disease knows before entering a hospital that the staff is committed to the most aggressive measures for treatment, that patient can choose to enter that hospital or find another, in accordance with individual preferences.

In a time of fierce competitive pressures, when the impetus to cut corners is very great, administrators/managers must come to a new understanding of the moral implications of their role. A major role can be as an advocate for the community's health. It is not a difficult step to take that bias to a consideration on what best serves the community. This would give administrators a new, moral role that could protect against the inroads that cost-containment pressures may make on delivery of good care (Westbury, 1983).

This differs from the roles of both clinicians and patients. The patient is generally concerned with her or his health, and perhaps how that health or lack of it will affect family and friends. The clinician is similarly concerned, and also concerned with collegial relationships, referrals, consultants, and the various pressures of operating a practice or participating in a group practice or HMO (Veatch, 1981). The administrator/manager of necessity is concerned with the entire institution or program, and as just mentioned, it is an easy jump from that concern to acting as advocate for the health of the community. However, to do all this, administrators will have to seriously reassess their education, training, and career pressures, and begin to think in new ways.

Another issue that is much in the public mind is the amount of the health care dollar that is consumed by administrative tasks and administrators themselves. This has been variously estimated at 10 to 20% of each health dollar. There is concern that health care administration and salaries have diminished the primary purpose of health care, which is the well-being of the population. A somewhat allied concern is the extent of physician's incomes and whether physicians should have fees adjusted to diminish their share of the total. Physicians argue that their lengthy, expensive training and the costs of staying current with new medical practices necessitate high motivational incomes. Others believe that while different kinds of people might be drawn toward the practice of medicine, if given diminished financial rewards, the quality of care would not suffer.

These are matters that affect all health care professionals, and all society (*American Journal of Nursing,* 1977). In a very real sense, how we decide these issues will shape the type of civilization we become. If the moral implications of medicine are ignored, glossed over, or trampled upon, the civilization will be deeply harmed. Though medical ethics is a new discipline, it arose because the problems and the challenges were there. It will be instructive to see how all branches of the professions, in concert with the community, act to adapt ancient and modern theories to very new concerns. Health care administrators will be judged by more than the bottom line. They will be judged by health care reform initiatives in terms of the time-worn imperative of medicine: insuring the health of the individual and community to the maximum of their collective capacities.

References

"AIDS: The Responsibilities of Health Professionals" [Special supplement]. *Hastings Center Report, 18*(2), April/May 1988.

Alexander, L., "Medical Science under Dictatorship." *New England Journal of Medicine, 241*(2), 1949.

American College of Physicians. *Ethics Manual,* 1984.

American Hospital Association. *Patient Bill of Rights,* Chicago, 1972.

American Medical Association. *Proceedings of the Judicial Council.* Chicago: Author, 1980.

American Medical Association. *Proceedings of the Council on Judicial and Ethical Affairs.* Chicago: Author, 1986.

Annas, G., "Prisoner in the ICU: The Tragedy of William Bartling." *Hastings Center Report, 16*(4), December, 1984.

Annas, G., & Densberger, J., "Competence to Refuse Medical Treatment: Autonomy vs. Paternalism." *Toledo Law Review, 15*(561), 1984.

Bayer, R. et al., "HIV Antibody Screening: An Ethical Framework for Evaluating Proposed Programs." *Journal of the American Medical Association, 256*(13), 1986.

Beauchamp, T., & Childress, J., *Principles of Biomedical Ethics.* New York: Oxford University Press, 1983.

Bedell, S., & Delbanco, T., "Choices about Cardiopulmonary Resuscitation in the Hospital." *New England Journal of Medicine, 310*(17), 1984.

Blackhall, L., "Must We Always Use CPR?" *New England Journal of Medicine, 317*(10), 1987.

Bouvia v. Superior Court, 1986, 179 Cal. App. 3d 1127.

Brett, A. S., & McCullough, L. B., "When Patients Request Specific Interventions: Defining the Limits of the Physician's Obligations." *New England Journal of Medicine, 315*; 1347–1351), 1986.

Brophy, v. New England Sinai Hospital, 479 N.E. 2d 626 (Mass. 1986).

California Natural Death Act. California Hospital Association, December 1976.

Callahan, D., "Autonomy: A Moral Good, Not a Moral Obsession." *Hastings Center Report, 15*(1), April 1984.

Callahan, D., *Setting Limits: Medical Goals in an Aging Society*, New York: Simon and Schuster, 1987 (a).

Callahan, D., "Terminating Treatment: Age as a Standard." *Hastings Center Report 17*(5), Oct./Nov. 1987 (b).

Camus, A., *The Plague.* NY: Vintage Books, 1972, p. 287.

Canterbury v. Spence, 464 Federal Reporter, 1972.

Cassileth, B. et al., "Informed Consent—Why Are Its Goals Imperfectly Realized?" *New England Journal of Medicine, 302*(16), 1980.

Childress, J., "Who Shall Live When Not All Can Live." *Soundings, 43*(1), Winter 1970.

Cobbs v. Grant, S. F. 22887, Sup. Court, Calif., 1972.

Cruzan v. Director. Missouri Dept. of Health, 497, U.S. 261, 280, 1990.

Curran, W., & Beecher, H., "Experimentation in Children: A Reexamination of Legal Ethical Principles." *Journal of the American Medical Association, 10*(1), 1969.

Daniels, N., *Am I My Parent's Keeper?* New York: Oxford University Press, 1988a.

Daniels, N. (Ed.), "Justice Between Generations and Health Care for the Elderly" [Special issue]. *Journal of Medicine and Philosophy, 13*(1), February 1988 (b).

Darr, K., "Administrative Ethics and the Health Services Manager." *Hospital and Health Services Administration, 29*(2), 1984.

Davis, M., & Churchill, L., "Autonomy and the Common Weal." *Hastings Center Report, 21*(1), 1991.

Declaration of Geneva. Adopted by the General Assembly of The World Medical Association, Geneva, Switzerland, September 1948. Amended by the 22nd World Medical Assembly, Sydney, Australia, August 1968.

Declaration of Helsinki. Adopted by the 18th World Medical Assembly, Helsinki, Finland, 1964. Revised by the 29th World Medical Assembly, Tokyo, Japan, 1975.

Delio v. Westchester County Medical Center, N.Y. Sup. Ct. App. Div. 1987, 516 N.Y.S. 2d 677.

Duff, R., & Campbell, A. G. M., "Moral and Ethical Dilemmas in the Special Care Nursery." *New England Journal of Medicine, 289*(17), 1973.

Durable Power of Attorney for Health Care. California Civil Code Sections 2410-2443, January 1, 1985.

Dworkin, G., "Moral Autonomy." In H. Engelhardt, Jr., & D. Callahan, (Eds.), *Science and Sociality*, Hastings, NY: The Hastings Center, 1978.

Dworkin, G., "Autonomy and Informed Consent." *President's Commission for the Study of Ethical Problems in Medicine and Biomedical and Behavioral Research*, Appendix F, Washington, DC: Government Printing Office, 1983.

Engelhardt, H. T., "Shattuck Lecture: Allocating Scarce Medical Resources and the Availability of Organ Transplantation." *New England Journal of Medicine, 316* July 5, 1984.

"Ethics." *American Journal of Nursing*, Chicago: American College of Physicians, May 1977.

Feldstein, P. et al., "Private Cost Containment: The Effects of Utilization Review Programs on Health Care Use and Expenditures." *New England Journal of Medicine, 318*(20), 1988.

Fletcher, J., *Morals and Medicine.* Boston: Little, Brown, 1960.

Fletcher, J., *Situation Ethics: The New Morality.* Philadelphia: Westminster Press, 1966.

Fletcher, J., *Humanhood: Essays in Biomedical Ethics*. Buffalo, NY: Prometheus Books, 1979.

Francis, D., & Chin, J., "The Prevention of Acquired Immunodeficiency Syndrome in the United States." *Journal of the American Medical Association, 257*(10), 1987.

Gostin, L., & Curran, W., "The Limits of Compulsion in Controlling AIDS." *Hastings Center Report, 16*(6), December 1986.

Harrison, B., *Our Right to Choose*, New York: Beacon Press, 1983.

Hartwig, J., "Donating Your Health Care Benefits." *Hastings Center Report, 18*(2), April/May 1988.

Hirsch, D., & Enlow, R., "The Effects of the Acquired Immune Deficiency Syndrome on Gay Lifestyle and the Gay Individual." *Annals of the New York Academy of Science*, 1985.

"Imperiled Newborns" [Special issue]. *Hastings Center Report, 17*(6), December 1987.

In re Eichner (Brother Fox), Court of Appeals, 52 N.Y.S. 2d 266 (1981).

In re Quinlan, 70 N.J. 10, 355 A. 2d 647, cert. denied, 429 U.S. 922 (1976).

In re Spring, (Mass. 1980) 405 N.E.2d 115.

In re Storar, 420 N.E.2d 64 (NY 1981).

In the matter of Conroy, N.J. 1985, 486 A 2d 1209.

In the matter of Jobes, N.J. Supr. Court, No. A-108/109, 1987.

Jecker, N., "Knowing When to Stop: The Limits of Medicine." *Hastings Center Report*, May-June, 1991.

Jonsen, A., & Garland, M., *Ethics of Newborn Intensive Care*, San Francisco and Berkeley: University of California, 1976.

Jonsen, A., & Toulmin, S., *The Abuse of Casuistry*. University of California Press, 1988.

Kant, I., "Metaphysical Foundations of Morals." In C. J. Freidrich (Ed.), *The Philosophy of Kant*. New York: Modern Library, 1949.

Kass, L., "Regarding the End of Medicine and the Pursuit of Health." *The Public Interest, 40*, Summer 1975.

Lantos, J., "Baby Doe Five Years Later: Implications for Child Health." *New England Journal of Medicine, 317*(7), 1987.

Levinson, D., "Toward Full Disclosure of Referral Restrictions and Financial Incentives by Prepaid Health Plans." *New England Journal of Medicine, 817*(27), 1987.

MacIntyre, A., *After Virtue*, 2nd Edition. University of Notre Dame Press, 1984.

Macklin, R., "Predicting Dangerousness and the Public Health Response to AIDS." *Hastings Center Report, 16*(6), December 1986.

Macklin, R., *Mortal Choices: Bioethics in Today's World*. New York: Pantheon Books, 1987.

Maguire, D., "What's So Good About the Common Good?" From *A New American Justice*, Doubleday, 1980.

Matthews, G., & Neslund, V., "The Initial Impact of AIDS on Public Health Law in the United States—1986." *Journal of the American Medical Association, 257*(3), 1987.

McCarthy, C., "DRGs—Five Years Later." *New England Journal of Medicine, 318*(25), 1988.

McCormick, R., "To Save or Let Die." *Journal of the American Medical Association, 229*(2), 1974.

McKinlay, J., & McKinlay, S., "The Questionable Contribution of Medical Measures to the Decline of Mortality in the United States in the Twentieth Century." *Milbank Memorial Quarterly, 55*(4), 1977.

Meisel, A. et al., "Hospital Guidelines for Deciding about Life-Sustaining Treatment: Dealing with Health Limbo." *Critical Care Medicine, 14*(3), 1986.

Mill, S., "Utilitarianism." In A. Smullyan et al., (Eds.), *Introduction to Philosophy*. Belmont, CA: Wadsworth, 1962.

Mills, M. et al., "The Acquired Immunodeficiency Syndrome: Infection Control and Public Health Law." *New England Journal of Medicine, 314*(14), 1986.

Mills, M., Sullivan, G., & Eth, L., "Prohibiting Third Parties: A Decade After Tarasoff." *American Journal of Psychiatry, 144*(1), 1987.

Murray, T., "Moral Obligations to the Not-Yet-Born: The Fetus as Patient." *Clinics in Perinatology*, June 1987.

Niebuhr, H., *The Responsible Self: An Essay in Christian Moral Philosophy*. New York: Harper and Row, 1963.

Noonan, J., *The Morality of Abortion: Legal and Historical Perspectives*. Cambridge, MA: Harvard University Press, 1970.

Office of the Actuary. *1984 Annual Report of the Board of Trustees of the Federal Hospital Insurance Trust Fund*. Washington, DC: Health Care Financing Administration, 1984.

Osborn, J., "AIDS: Politics and Science." *New England Journal of Medicine, 318*(7), 1988.

Otis, Bowen v. American Hospital Association, et al., U.S. Supreme Court 106 S. Ct. 2101, No. 84-15-9, June 9, 1986.

Pellegrino, E., "Altruism, Self-Interest and Medical Ethics." *Journal of the American Medical Association, 258*(14), 1987.

Percival, T., *Medical Ethics* (C. D. Leake, Ed.). Baltimore: Williams and Wilkins, 1927.

Pope Pius Xll. "The Prolongation of Life." In *The Pope Speaks* (Vol. 4, pp. 393–398), 1958.

President's Commission for the Study of Ethical Problems in Medicine and Biomedical and Behavioral Research. *Summing Up*, Washington, DC: U.S. Government Printing Office, 1983.

Ramsey, P., *The Patient as Person*. New Haven, CT: Yale University Press, 1971.

Rawls, J., *A Theory of Justice*. Cambridge, MA: Harvard University Press, 1971.

Reagan, M., "Physicians as Gatekeepers." *New England Journal of Medicine, 817*(27), 1987.

Roe v Wade, 410 U.S. 113, 93 Supreme Court 705, 35 L.E.D. 2d 147, 1973.

Robertson, J. & Schulman, J., "Pregnancy and Prenatal Harm to Offspring: The Case of Mothers with PKU." *Hastings Center Report, 117*(4), Aug./Sept. 1987.

Saint Augustine. "On the Trinity." In J. Burnaby (Ed.), *Augustine: Later Works*. Philadelphia: Westminster Press, 1963.

Saint Augustine. *Confessions, Book 10*. New York: Penguin Books, 1984.

Schloendorff v. Society of New York Hospital, 211 N.Y. 125, 127, 129; 1914.

Schramm, C., & Gabel, J., "Prospective Payment: Some Retrospective Observations." *New England Journal of Medicine, 318*(25), 1988.

Seiden, D., "Ethics for Hospital Administrators." *Hospital and Health Services Administration, 28*(2), 1982.

Seiden, D., "Diminishing Resources, Critical Choices." *Commonweal, 112*(5), 1985.

Shaw, A., "Dilemmas of Informed Consent in Children." *New England Journal of Medicine. 289*(17), 1973.

Shinn, R., *Forced Options: Social Decisions for the 21st Century.* San Francisco: Harper and Row, 1983.

Shortell, S., & Hughes, E. F. X., "The Effects of Regulation, Competition and Ownership on Mortality Rates among Hospital Inpatients." *New England Journal of Medicine, 318*(17), 1988.

State of New York Public Health Law, Article 29-B, Statute 413-A, April 1, 1988.

Steinbock, B., "Patient vs. Public: Whose Right Is It Anyway." *Medical Ethics, 1*(5), December 1986.

Steinbrook, R. et al., "Preferences of Homosexual Men with AIDS for Life-Sustaining Treatment." *New England Journal of Medicine, 314*, 457–460, 1986.

Tarasoff v. Regents of the University of California, 17 Cal. 3d 425, 1976.

Temkin, O., & Temkin, C. L. (Eds.), *Ancient Medicine: Selected Papers of Ludwig Edelstein.* Baltimore: Johns Hopkins University Press, 1967.

Thomson, J. J., "A Defense of Abortion." *Philosophy and Public Affairs, 1*(1), 1971.

Tomlinson, T., & Brody, H., "Futility and the Ethics of Resuscitation." *Journal of the American Medical Association, 264*(10), 1990.

Truog, R., Brett, A., & Frader, J., "The Problem with Futility." *New England Journal of Medicine, 326*(12), 1992.

University Hospital, State of New York at Stony Brook, U.S. Court of Appeals of the Second Circuit, No. 679, February 23, 1984.

U.S. Child Abuse Protection and Treatment Amendments of 1984, Public Law 98-457.

Veatch, R., "Nursing Ethics, Physician Ethics and Medical Ethics." *Law, Medicine and Health Care*, October 1981.

Veatch, R., & Spicer, C., "Medically Futile Care: The Role of the Physician in Setting Limits." *American Journal of Law and Medicine, 18*(142), 1992

Walters, L., "The Principle of Medical Confidentiality," from Contemporary Issues in Bioethics," T. Beauchamp & L. Walters (Eds.), Encino, CA: Dickinson Publishing Co., 1978.

Wanzer, S. et al., "The Physician's Responsibility toward Hopelessly Ill Patients." *New England Journal of Medicine, 310*(15), 1984.

Warren, M. A., "On the Moral and Legal Status of Abortion." *The Monist, 57*(1), 1973.

Weber, M., "Politics as a Vocation." In H. H. Gerth & C. W. Mills (Eds.), *Max Weber: Essays in Sociology.* New York: Galaxy, 1958.

Wesbury, S., "Ethics and Hospital Decision Making." *Michigan Hospitals, 19*(4), 1983.

Youngner, S., "Who Defines Futility?" *Journal of the American Medical Association, 260*(8), 1988.

Zolorf-Dorfman, L., "First, Make Meaning: An Ethics of Encounter for Health Care Reform." *Tikkun, 8*(4), 1993.

Zuger, A., & Miles, S., "Physicians, AIDS and Occupational Risk." *Journal of the American Medical Association, 258*(14), 1987.

19

Futures

Anthony R. Kovner

Forecasting is an old art and a recent science. It has involved everything from Joseph's interpretation of the Pharaoh's dreams to econometric models and political scenarios. There are many methods for predicting the future. One is the extrapolation of a past trend. Cyclical trends such as consumer control of health care, are particularly amenable to this method. In the mid-1800s the health care consumer was dominant, but by the middle of the 20th century the physician had gained control. Since the 1970s, however, the consumer has begun to gain dominance again.

Another type of forecasting deals with predicting technological inventions that create breakthroughs and are followed by major developments. Such a breakthrough was the discovery of the microbial cause of disease; another, more recent breakthrough has been the discovery of the impact of environmental factors on disease causation. With this second type of forecast, a trend is likely to come slowly at first while the concept or idea develops and spreads, then the trend will gather momentum, moving into a phase where the development is exponential. Later the trend will flatten at a new level.

The Rand Corporation developed a forecasting technique called Delphi, in which large numbers of observers' opinions are polled and responded to, and projections are made with less bias than results from the predictions of individuals or small groups. Several Delphi studies have been done in health care, and it is perhaps instructive to review two such studies conducted in 1967 (Bender et al., 1967) and 1974 (McLaughlin & Sheldon, 1974). Table 19.1 presents certain projections taken from these studies. Some of the projections, such as widespread use of physician assistants, have been borne out in the 1980s. Others, such as "never" for a "second class" system for medical care in the "wake of a wave of health centers, clinics, and prepayment systems," have come to pass. Still others, such as "solo practice virtually disappeared except by doctors over 50 years of age has not taken place, as of 1993.

TABLE 19.1   Effects of Internal and External Forces on the Elements of the System

	Time Implemented
Technology	
Transmission of genetic information[a]	1980 ± 5 years
Electronic control of human behavior[a]	never
Chemical control of human behavior[a]	never
Use of computer for information storage and retrieval[a]	1978 + 10 years
Development of Mechanical Heart[a]	1988 + 5 to 10
Genetic control[b]	1990–1994
Computer record bank covering 80% of U.S. population[b]	1987
Government	
De facto federal control of psychiatric and medical facilities	1980–1994
Medical industry	1975–1984
12% GNP[b]	1994
20% GNP[b]	
Uniform geographic districts for political and public health education and all human service industries	Never
Physicians	
Few if any physicians in solo practice[a]	1993 ± 6 years
Solo practice virtually disappeared except in doctors over 50[b]	1981
Physicians undergo compulsory reexam[b]	1984
Other health practitioners	
Other health care systems workers in independent practice[a]	1993–1995
Widespread use of physicians assistants[b]	1975–1979
Organization	
Direct public participation in decision making with "real time" polling[b]	1985
A "second class" system for medical care in wake of a wave of health centers clinics and repayment systems[b]	Never
Broad community participation in all medical institutions[b]	1980–1989

[a]Bender et al. (1967)—90% probability

[b]McLaughlin and Sheldon (1974).

Samuel P. Martin and Anthony R. Kovner, Futures, in Kovner, Anthony R. & Samuel P. Martin (eds.) *Community Health & Medical Care*, New York: Arvine Stratton 1978, pp. 413–442, pp. 415

Vladeck (1987) noted that in 1982 experts were predicting that the trend toward increasing control of hospitals by national investor-owned corporations would reach a peak of 50 to 60% by the year 2000. Almost no one believes this in 1993, as the major national chains have closed or sold off almost one-third of their facilities, and several small hospital companies have lost great amounts of money or have gone into bankruptcy.

In a January 1985 study conducted for the Health Insurance Association of America, based on interviews with 40 "nationally recognized leaders in health care," Arthur D. Little and Company (1985) made the following predictions for the health care system in the mid-1990s:

- Health care will increasingly be perceived as an economic good subject to the influence of supply, demand, and price.
- Government and business purchasers of health care will intensify efforts to contain costs, which will dominate the health care agenda.
- The health system in 1995 will be highly competitive and, to some degree, regulated.
- Regulation is most likely at the state level, varying from state to state.
- Evaluation of cost-containment strategies will be aided by a major improvement in the availability of information on health care utilization, cost, and quality.
- Consumers will increasingly accept responsibility for their own health care.
- There will be more health services for the aged, increasing public pressure for protection against the costs of long-term care; a variety of emerging specialized services; a shift from inpatient to ambulatory care; and more care delivered in managed-care systems.
- A limited "safety net" will provide some guarantee of access to care.
- A "tiered" system of care will be recognized and accepted.
- Cost containment and overcapacity will combine to change the way hospitals function.
- The growing surplus of physicians amid pressure for cost containment will change the nature of physician practice (e.g., more physicians will be salaried, and the use of midlevel practitioners will be inhibited).
- Health maintenance organizations (HMOs) and other capitation arrangements will experience explosive growth.
- Negotiated provider contracts will be based on services and management efficiency rather than on price discounts.
- Cost increases will taper off.

Similar predictions for 1995 were made by 1,600 "national health care leaders and astute observers" in a study conducted by Arthur Andersen and Co. and the American College of Health Care Executives (1987):

- Growth in the elderly population will affect the health care system in 1995 more than any other issue.
- Adequate quality for all should drive health policy, but budgetary concerns will be the primary driving force behind federal health policy through 1995.
- A majority of all panelists believe there will not be a comprehensive national health policy by 1995.
- Health care's share of the gross national product (GNP) will exceed 12%.
- Rationing of health services will be the top medical ethics issue.
- Elderly consumers will exercise increased influence on U.S. health care policy.
- Ethical and legal issues surrounding AIDS will be addressed (61% of all respondents predict a cure for AIDS by 1995).
- Length of stay and admissions to hospitals will continue to decline.
- 700 of the nation's hospitals will close by 1995 (75-84 per year).
- Preferred provider organizations (PPOs), and HMOs will continue to grow.

In 1988, Amara and his co-workers, of the Institute for the Future, singled out trends most likely to change health care by the year 2000 by describing two different scenarios of "tough choices" and "health and wealth" depending on the amount of resources available to the health sector. Key driving forces included aging of the population, more sophisticated consumers, cost pressures from payers, pluralism and diversity of the system, new technologies, excess capacity, growth in health care expenditures, and government as a steering agent. Structural shifts from 1985 forward to the year 2000 were predicted to include growth of managed care, more salaried physicians with less autonomy, fewer hospital admissions and more ambulatory care, increased intensity of inpatient care, decline in medical school applicants, increasing concentration of medical research dollars, and a growth in the cost of health benefits administration and the net cost of insurance (Amara et al., 1988).

My own predictions as of early 1994, with rationales, for the next 5 years are as follows:

Prediction 1: There will be national health insurance.
Rationale: Americans' preferences for pluralism and diversity, plus distrust of government, will not overcome President Clinton's political priority extending universal health coverage to all Americans.

Prediction 2. Fewer larger groups of health care providers will compete for capped purchaser dollars in increasingly organized local markets.
Rationale: There are economies of scale in the marketing, production, and financing of health care. Certain organization can provide certain services better and cheaper than others and will be so perceived by increasingly sophisticated purchasers.

Prediction 3: Consumers will use less medical care per capita on an age-adjusted basis.

Rationale: Budgets will increasingly be limited, based on purchaser preferences, as validated by consumers and providers. More of each health-benefit dollar will be spent on cost-effective treatment and prevention. Less of each dollar will be spent on services that do not predictably improve health outcomes.

Prediction 4. Governmental regulation will increase regarding cost, quality, and access to health care.

Rationale: Access to care is a political issue for populations in rural areas and inner cities, as is the uneven quality of care in these areas. States face increased costs for Medicaid beneficiaries and state government employees. The federal government will supersede state government on these matters.

Prediction 5: The power of physicians to shape and benefit from decision making in health care will diminish.

Rationale: Managers, including clinician-managers, will have more power relative to practicing physicians and nurses. This will result from less per capita utilization of health services, more physicians per capita, and more pervasive standards regarding clinical process and outcome.

An oversimplified model of some of these predictions and relationships is shown in Figure 19.1.

Important factors that will influence the shape of health care in the future include population demographics, disease patterns, information systemization, and medical technology.

FIGURE 19.1   Forecasted Health Sector Pressures and Responses, 1988–1993

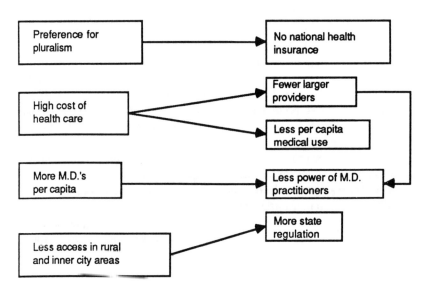

Demographics: Age and Income

By the year 2000 the percentage of persons over 75 years of age is expected to represent 50% of all persons 65 years and older. The percentage of the eldest elderly, those over 85 years is expected to increase from 10% of those over 65 years in 1990 to 24% in 2050. Already persons 65 and over account for more than 40% of inpatient days in general hospitals and more than 30% of all physician visits. At the same time there is a shrinking number and percentage of adolescents and young adults. It has been estimated that from 1985 to 2000 the number of persons between the ages of 18 and 24 in the United States will decrease by 14% while the number of persons 25 to 34 falls by 13%. The impact of these trends is expected to be increasing political pressure to provide national health insurance for long-term care and a shortage of younger health workers to provide care, especially on nights and weekends.

Another demographic trend is the increasing growth of a minority, low-income underclass population in large cities. This population has special health problems but has equally important other problems relating to jobs, education, and housing, all of which have received little national attention during the Reagan years. Per Arthur D. Little's prediction of a tiered system in 1985, different levels of services to consumers based on income is perhaps recognized and accepted in the United States, circa 1993.

Patient Preferences and Values

As Americans have become more educated, they have acquired higher expectations for health care and for the physician. When expectations are not met, there is great disenchantment. Physicians are sued frequently for their failure to cure. Patients want to know more about health care and to participate more fully in decisions regarding it, including the right to die.

The past 65 years have been characterized by a shift from the extended family to the nuclear family. Now, even the nuclear family is showing great strain. There is one divorce for every two marriages. Working mothers have become the norm rather than the exception, and many single parents, both male and female, are heading households. Mobility (20% of the population moves each year) also has contributed to the instability of the family and family neighborhood structure.

One impact of these trends has been to move more responsibility for health care away from the family and toward the educational system or employer. Schools are more responsible for student competency with regard to knowledge about health and health care, and more of them provide on-site services from nutrition to family planning. Employers provide health benefits ranging from health insurance, day care, and exercise classes to management of long-term care for workers' parents.

The Information Revolution

According to Griffith (1987), by the middle of the 21st century, patient care in hospitals will be highly computerized:

> [T]he doctor will guide an electronic system which suggests a plan of care for each patient based on analysis of both the patient's history and detailed data about specific treatment options. Forecasts of all patients' needs will be available to each patient service unit. Systems will optimize schedules, order supplies, and prompt completion of the original assignment and follow-up of any unexpected occurrence. Complete records will be available to establish expectations and monitor performance for the doctor and the nurse. [p. 330]

As of 1990 the processing ability of the computer has far exceeded its use in practice. The computer has had much wider acceptance in finance and billing for services than in patient care. But computers are being used increasingly in analyzing treatment in relation to outcome and in developing standards for diagnosis and treatment.

Near-term (3–5 yrs) directions for expanded computer capability are in areas of revenue control, budgeting and accounting control, clinical review, final product cost accounting and risk management (Griffith, 1987). Information systems can increasingly break down revenues by services rendered and by payer, employer, and insurance group. Expenses can be allocated increasingly to a larger number of cost centers, and flexible budgeting can be implemented for varying volumes of service.

Medical records are increasingly being automated, with larger and more detailed patient abstracts integrated with cost and revenue data. Many health care organizations (HCOs) have implemented quality of care review while the patient is currently undergoing treatment. Such review adds to the cost of care. For example, in 1988 the Lutheran Medical Center, a 550-bed hospital in New York City, had 20 staff members dedicated to quality assurance, at a cost of $650,000 per year.

Other near-term trends include movement toward final-product cost accounting, by which services for groups of patients requiring regular treatment can be budgeted at alternating levels of demand; and risk management, by which all untoward incidents can be aggregated and analyzed from incident reports.

New Technology

New technology in health care will be developed and increasingly assessed. Among examples of such technology and assessments are periodic findings of studies funded by the Agency for Health Care Policy and Research (AACPR) the Office of Technology Assessment. For example, findings released in 1987 on the efficiency and uses of fully automated blood pressure monitoring, cochlear (inner ear) implant devices for the deaf, and continuous positive airway pressure for treating obstructive sleep apnea in adults were as follows:

- Although safe and accurate, automated blood pressure monitoring's role in blood pressure measurement other than during sleep "has yet to be clearly differentiated" from that of the traditional manual method and of semiautomatic monitoring.
- Cochlear implant devices (surgically inserted special hearing devices) are "considered to be safe and to help patients by restoring auditory sensation and speech detection and by improving voice modulation."
- Continuous positive airway pressure (PAP) provides even levels of air pressure from a flow generator through the nose to counteract obstructed sleep apnea (OSA) in which a sleeping person's respiratory airflow stops for 10 seconds or more. PAP "appears to reduce signs and symptoms of OSA and in appropriately selected patients, may completely prevent upper airway obstruction during sleep."

These assessments were conducted relative to coverage under Medicare. The Health Care Financing Administration decides on whether new technologies are reimbursable based in large part on an assessment of safety and effectiveness. One of the weaknesses of diagnosis-related group (DRG) reimbursement under Medicare is the lack of responsiveness in rate changes to new technology, thereby discouraging its introduction.

The last 35 years have seen great advances in technology and the development of the belief that all problems can be solved by the engineering biological science approach. This approach was eminently successful with antibiotics for the acute infectious diseases and neuropharmacological agents for nervous disorders; but despite new diagnostic advances such as lasers and magnetic resonance imaging, technology has not yet been able to combat chronic diseases. Although confidence is being strained, it is still strong.

With regard to predictions of clinical advances, 23 experts were invited by *Medical World News* ("Tomorrow's Medicine", 1988) in 1976 to predict what two or three useful clinical advances in their specialty would become conventional medical practice within the next 25 years. Examples of the predictions are as follows:

Oncology

1. Enzyme or radioimmunoassay detection of people at high risk   1985
   of cancer
2. More careful screening of environment for carcinogens by   1990
   bacterial and mammalian cell systems
3. Interruption of carcinogenic process in high-risk individuals   2000

Bioengineering

1. Clinical use of implantable artificial bladder, heart, kidneys,   1990
   pancreas, and liver
2. Instrumentation for home use with information relayed by   1990
   telephone or telemetry to physician base for analysis with
   treatment prescribed by phone
3. Completely computerized general health care centers for   1990
   treatment of mass populations

Neurology

1. Nonnarcotic treatment of pain   1980
2. Prevention or treatment of multiple sclerosis, perhaps by   1990
   vaccine
3. Chemical treatment of malignant brain tumor   2000

Coile (1988) has made a more updated assessment for the 1990s, with the following forecasts, among others: biosensors will be implanted in the chronically
ill to provide a continuous stream of physiological data and alert caregivers if health
status falters; drug-dispensing pumps will provide more precise and self-regulating
drug therapy to diabetics and chronic-disease patients and will relieve problems
of overmedication and missed dosages; self-care robots will provide support in
daily living to the disabled; and many forms of cancer will yield to genetically
engineered drugs, blocking the damaging spread of defective cells by chemically
altering the cellular structure.

Politics of Health Care Costs

Blendon and Altman (1987) summarized the major themes drawn from 15 national opinion polls regarding health care costs. Conducted between 1981 and 1984,
the polls showed the following:

- Rising health care costs do not rank very high on a list of most important
  problems now facing the nation.
- Most Americans are concerned about their own, not business's or the gov-
  ernment's, health cost problem.
- People are happier with the status quo than one might think.
- Most Americans do not see themselves as having any responsibility for cre-
  ating the problem of health care costs.
- The view of practicing physicians are often more influential with the public

than the opinions of groups proposing change, such as government officials and business and labor leaders.

- Although the majority of Americans see the deficit as a major threat to the nation, they do not see cutting federal health outlays as the most desirable way to reduce it.

The above conclusions were challenged by the 1988 Harris poll referred to in Chapter 1. According to this survey, Americans were significantly less happy with their health care system than either the British or the Canadians are with theirs (Blendon, 1989). According to Blendon, Americans said "they want a fundamental break with their current health care policies and a much more central role played by the central government in remedying America's health problems." I believe that in the 1990s such a break will occur because of the increasing numbers of the uninsured.

American Culture

Consumerism, a force in the late 1960s, continues to grow. Government and business purchasers intervene on behalf of consumers and influence client–provider behavior. Increasingly purchasers of care are steering their beneficiaries by paying in full only for care given by providers who are preferred in terms of quality and price.

Income distribution in the United States has become more inequitable. Instead of increasing purchasing power of the poor, who have a greater need for health services, the next few years may see increased governmental activity in restricting choice of providers for beneficiaries of public programs. Higher income is associated with increased demand for care and hospitalization, often leading to overutilization of services. Affluence itself can influence disease patterns as a result of life-style.

After a period of 40 years of unbridled health care cost expansion, there has developed among purchasers a serious concern for cost and benefit. There is increasingly serious scrutiny of the cost of medical services. This is being accomplished through evaluation of the quality of health services and some control of ineffective utilization. There is strong demand to prove the effectiveness of hospitalization, laboratory tests, and medications.

Large corporations meet most of our needs, and this ethos has an impact on health care in three ways. First, hospitals and clinics are increasingly being organized and managed like large corporations. Second, health care has become a promising market for large and small corporations. Third, large corporations see health care costs for their employees as one of their largest and most rapidly increasing expenditures.

An example of what corporations are doing to control health care costs is General Motors's Informed Choice Plan, which went into effect in 1985. Workers were given a choice of three types of coverage: a traditional fee-for-service plan (with strict utilization controls), HMOs, and PPOs. In 1984, GM spent $2.35 billion on employee health benefits, and the objective of the new plan was to save the company money. In the first 9 months, enrollment in the managed-care plans increased significantly. HMO enrollment among GM employees and retirees rose from 70,000 to an estimated 123,000, and PPO enrollment—nonexistent before the contract—climbed to almost 75,000. Add in an estimated 330,000 dependents, and the total equals nearly 24% of those eligible for health insurance benefits.

Government has increasingly seen health care costs as something to be controlled for its beneficiaries and employees rather than for its own sake. And health care has increasingly been viewed as an economic good, access to which is available to poor people only on limited terms, that is, through Medicaid or through local charity; and over 35 million Americans lack adequate health insurance.

Effect of External Forces on the Elements of the Health Care System

The major forces described previously are producing significant changes in the health care industry. Rather than health care being the fiefdom of the physician, it is becoming the domain of the consumer and the corporation. A mature, sophisticated, technological society cannot accept on faith the physician's assurance of the effectiveness and quality of the care provided. When quality control of health care is so important to so many individuals, some wonder why government has not taken more responsibility in this area. A number of movements are afoot to assure quality control. Some are implemented in the name of quality and outcome measurements. Legislation for quality control has had the same history as legislation for payment systems. The legislative mandate is opposed with extreme vigor, but when it is passed, its force is diverted by the medical providers to their control and ultimately to their benefit. Efforts to control and assure quality of care will increase during the next 5 years.

Within the health care industry, as in all industries, there is a demand for freedom of information. Increased data availability in the doctor's office and in the hospital involving quality of care has created greater demand for disclosure, more openness and availability of the data. Most importantly, such availability can alter doctor and hospital behavior.

Government

Health care remains politicized. Politicians seek election or reelection based in part on their position on health issues, whether on universal health care coverage, treatment of AIDS patients, health care for the homeless, the amount of Medicare rate increases, or the quality of care in public hospitals.

Government participation in health care has changed. It used to consist of limited provision of services to the poor, services for government employees, administration of communicable disease programs, statistics compilation, licensing, and financing of research and construction. It now also consists of financing the bulk of health care for the elderly and the poor and extensive regulation of quality and cost in these programs. At the same time, governmental provision of direct care, at all levels, is diminishing.

Government initiatives in the early 1970s included stimulation of HMOs, Professional Standards Review Organizations (PSROs), certificate-of-need legislation, and research in health care delivery. This was accompanied by cutbacks in the ambitious direct service programs of the 1960s, such as neighborhood health and community mental health centers. More recently there have been attempts to control the increase in the governmental cost of the Medicare and Medicaid programs, to stabilize the basic research expenditures of the National Institutes of Health, and to slow hospital construction and the supply of physicians.

In 1978, Kovner and Martin predicted inaccurately that the next 3 to 5 years would see universal health coverage, the establishment of a national council for health services policy similar to the Council of Economic Advisors, and the establishment of a national center to evaluate medical procedures and tests equivalent to the Food and Drug Administration. We also stated that government attempts to directly proscribe the behavior of providers, such as PSROs; rate setting; and certificate-of-need legislation were bound to fail, as these created counterpressures to "beat the system" rather than altering basic incentives. This reaction on the part of health care providers would be similar to that of producers in other heavily regulated industries. The first response is frequently to enact regulation, and it is often counterproductive. Through political influence and campaign contributions, the regulated often become the regulators. Of course, we based our predictions on a rationality in public affairs that, we should have been aware, often belies reality.

No one in 1980 could predict the AIDS epidemic, which has had a major impact on the American population since 1982. In 1988 on any given day in New York City, for example, approximately 1,500 inpatient beds are occupied by patients with AIDS or AIDS-related illnesses. The already significant demands that AIDS places on the health care system will only increase in the next 5 to 10 years, perhaps substantially. The government has spent millions of dollars on AIDS research and services that do not yet meet the need or cure the disease.

Through DRG reimbursement of hospitals and RBRVS reimbursement of physicians the federal government did pursue an incentives policy that alters provider behavior not only by provision of rewards but also by changing cognitive patterns as to what is acceptable. I see increased governmental regulation in the area of quality of care such as that undertaken in New York State, where all hospitals must meet strict criteria in quality assurance programs, state investigations of quality are frequent, limitations on house staff working hours have been enacted, and proposals have been made for recredentialing physicians.

Unfortunately, improved planning and regulation in government is constrained, especially at the state and local level, by the lack of accountability for the performance of its own bureaucracy. The uneven quality of state government may result in increased federalizing of the regulatory system, either directly or indirectly, by means of incentives to reward or punish performance by state bureaucracies.

The federal government will continue to support medical and nursing research and some part of medical and nursing education. The health care industry will continue to meets its capital expenditures by long-term debt financing in the capital market. The debt is amortized over a long period by devoting a part of the service cost to capital debt. Local mechanisms to secure the loans and develop taxfree status for the bonding mechanism have become widespread.

Clinicians

Physicians are being challenged from inside and outside the health care system. The physician's place within the system has narrowed and moved toward the purely curing role of the technician, as other professionals encompass the care, cure, and support functions. Physicians are increasingly employed by large HCOs and supervised by physician-managers with special management training.

The 1970s witnessed an increasing attack on the authority of the physician: by the patient for a lack of responsiveness to personal and primary care needs, by the taxpayer for a lack of concern in controlling medical care costs, and by increasing numbers of other professionals regarding their remuneration and power relative to the physician.

The 1980s witnessed increasing competition between physicians and hospitals. Services that had been provided primarily in hospitals, such as ambulatory surgery and rehabilitation, were now provided by physicians on an outpatient, freestanding basis.

There is increasing skepticism concerning the efficiency of physicians and their capacity to allocate resources. They are being criticized for performing unnecessary surgical procedures, overprescribing, and faulty labeling of the mentally ill and inability to treat them effectively. There is evidence that additional expenditure on medical technology is becoming less productive, and it might be more productive to influence consumers to better utilize the medical care system and to lead healthier lives. There is criticism of the maldistribution of physicians by specialty (i.e., too many surgeons and not enough primary care doctors) and by location (i.e., too many doctors in big cities and not enough in small towns). Increasingly, the public prefers that decisions over resource allocation in the medical care industry be taken out of the hands of physicians. As the organizations in which physicians work increase in size, complexity, and bureaucratization, the power of practicing physicians to allocate resources dwindles compared to that of governing boards, chiefs of services, and key managers.

Despite the influence of physician organizations such as the AMA, the individual doctor is yielding some of his prerogatives to organizational imperatives. Under physician guidance, but with a healthy input from other professions, some medical care tasks have been specified and clustered and are being performed by less trained, less educated, and less expensive, workers. Increasingly, physicians are using physician extenders, even to work in hospitals as extensions of the physician office and under physician supervision. How these extenders relate to nursing is an area of conflict. The division of labor will increasingly be negotiated among physicians, nurses, social workers, pharmacists, and other professionals and evaluated continually and jointly by them. In such negotiations physicians will play a major but not an exclusive part. The responsibility base will shift from the single individual physician to a wider and more shared base.

Part of the idealism of the health care professional is a strong commitment to individual patients as opposed to whole populations or the interests of society. The essence of clinical training is concern for the individual. Customer responsiveness is often ignored within the health care system; patients want professionals to listen more attentively to what they are saying. As a result of competitive pressures, the level of personalized services is expected to improve.

Two major factors eroding physician dominance within HCOs are their increasing employment by those organizations and the professionalization of other health care workers. Salaried physicians increasingly resemble in their work relations salaried professionals in other organizations such as engineers and lawyers. As other health care workers receive more extensive education, they develop organizations that challenge the dominance of physicians. Some groups have claimed to have a mandate and have set up independent licensing and accreditation programs, openly challenging physician control. Nurses, psychologists, and social workers have established independent practices, seeing patients without physician referral and supervision and charging a fee for their services. These kinds of practices have grown.

Fifteen years ago we inaccurately predicted an increasing rationalization of health manpower (Kovner & Martin, 1978). We said that tasks will be specified, clustered—into job categories and career lattices, with corresponding development of educational lattices—implemented, and standardized. This would be reflected in shortened educational programs for many occupations. For example, the psychiatrist may not need the same amount of anatomy and physiology as the specialist in internal medicine. As of early 1994, I do not see these hoped for improvements in the next 5 years either. Nor is there likely to be dramatic changes in education for health care workers, such as increased common core courses cutting across professional and other program boundaries, increased on-the-job and in-service education, and credentialing. There has been increased emphasis on continuing education programs after graduation and to a much lesser extent on relicensing. And the next 5 years will see greater recognition and legitimization given at the work place to the necessity for continuing education programs.

HCOs

The forces described previously are propelling the health care system toward a corporate ethos. Institutionalization is resulting in radical changes in client and provider relations as well as in interpersonal and interprofessional functions. With this has come the development of sophisticated personnel systems, labor relations staff, financing staff, and management information systems. Marketing staffs have been developed not only to aid in recruiting clients but also to plan strategies for new services. These trends will increase.

Greater efforts will be made to integrate care so as to avoid unnecessary and wasteful duplication. Some of this regionalization and franchising will be operated by large HCOs, which will continue to grow larger and more complex. As the pressures for accountability increase, these will focus on top management. To adapt effectively to outside pressures, internal activities will increasingly be organized into responsibility centers, as in business, with subordinate managers held responsible for results. Whether internal activities are grouped by departments, or occupations, or by divisions across occupations or in some combination, that is, matrix management, managers will be held accountable increasingly for results. Private enterprise will continue to expand into the health care industry. Chains will once again increase their hospital operations. Insurance companies will expand their HMO development and growth efforts. The ability of the nonprofit and public organization to survive under increasing competition will be determined by their capability to obtain results. The future will see a massive struggle of solo practitioners and small groups to survive in competition with other organizational forms. There has been no stampede toward multidisciplinary group practice, but there is a solid trend. The concept of group practice will be much more acceptable to the medical student and resident of the 1990s than for those of the 1980s (especially to those in two-career marriages), and many project this as their practice goal. Vigorous competition has developed in some locations between solo practitioners and medical care foundations and between independent and group practice associations and HMOs. The 1990s will see such competition continue.

Hospitals. The hospital has been the focus of organization in the health care field, and hospitals will try to keep this leadership role. The main response of the American Hospital Association (AHA) in the 1970s to public pressures for cost equality control was the development of hospital franchising as a keystone of national health insurance. Under the AHA Ameriplan, hospitals would have been franchised to oversee the delivery of all medical care in a geographic area and would have been held accountable by government for their effectiveness in controlling quality and cost. Of course, the hospital, not the medical society nor the group practice would have been the hub of the system; and competition among hospitals would have decreased, or at least would not have been fostered in a given geographical area. Ameriplan did not come to pass, but has been revived by hospital groups in the form of community care networks.

The next 5 years will see an enormous struggle on the part of hospital leaders to maintain their margin of leadership and to place the health care mandate in the hospital industry. Hospitals will continue to move into prevention and chronic care to supplement their present acute-disease focus.

The traditional primary concerns of hospital governing boards have been not to operate at a deficit and to keep the physicians contented. Under DRG reimbursement and competitive pressures, hospital top management is becoming increasingly concerned with performance in relation to costs. This concern has manifested itself in more formal relationships—both vertically with other providers, such as medical groups and nursing homes, and horizontally with other hospitals to share supporting services (purchasing, public relations, fund raising, data processing) or medical care programs, such as consolidation of obstetrics departments at one hospital and pediatrics departments at another.

The main response to financial problems by several state hospital associations has been to urge transfer payments or special taxes to provide for uncompensated care. State governments, of course, may consider limiting hospital revenues as part of the negotiations. This is what has happened in several northeastern states during the 1970s and 1980s.

Linkages are being developed between major organizations in health care. Hospitals are developing and fostering home care programs and extended-care facilities; they are merging to form larger conglomerates, and contracts with managed care plans. In the absence of mergers, HCOs are collaborating to provide each other with viable services. This has been most evident in the area of obstetrics, where a declining census has motivated closure of services. Shared facilities are also being developed. Thus, there is a major trend for hospitals to develop cooperative arrangements and mergers.

Chronic-Care Organizations. The aging of the population will lead to an increase of chronic disease. Studies have shown that people over 65 have, on the average, four chronic conditions. The needs in chronic care represent the primary future tasks of the health service enterprise. Many think these needs will be too vast for doctors and nurses, and our present "system" will have to be replaced with a better system; and some expect it to be organized primarily on a social rather than a medical model.

In the past 25 years, one approach to responding to these needs has been the integration of chronic-care with acute-care services, thereby enabling some resources to be diverted to chronic care. The establishment in general hospitals of units for the mentally ill and those suffering from additive disease and alcoholism can be viewed in this light, as can the medical supervision by hospitals or group practices of patients in nursing homes and homes for the mentally retarded. Another controversial approach has been the deinstitutionalization of the chronically ill through the development of drug, home, and ambulatory care centers.

The next 5 years are not expected to yield significant and continuing technological advances in chronic care. There will be increasing focus on outcome measures of disability or discomfort and in evaluation of methods for alleviating these conditions. Tasks will increasingly be analyzed and more sensibly allocated so that valuable medical resources will not be squandered and so that providers with less formal education can do valuable work of acceptable quality and be proportionately remunerated. There may be some scaling down of goals where technology is not cost-effective. For example, humane care rather than curative treatment may serve as the official goal of certain chronic care institutions.

There will be additional efforts to employ the chronically ill. During the past 20'years employment opportunities for the mentally retarded have expanded. Traditionally, ex-alcoholics have worked with alcoholics and ex-narcotics addicts with addicts. There may be more emphasis on other approaches in line with innovations on behaviorist therapies. As behavior is modified, many of the chronically ill can become increasingly employable.

There is currently a stigma attached to the chronically ill and dying, which also extends to those who work in such organizations. Whether additional funding and greater integration with the rest of the medical care system has been erasing this stigma is difficult to discern. Clearly, the results achieved by chronic-care organizations will be determined to a greater extent by the cultural values and resource allocations of those who are unlikely to be current clients of the system. Chronic-care organizations cannot respond effectively without additional resources or without scaling down their tasks to do what can realistically be done. More than any other area in health care, chronic care needs additional research support concerning new ways of health care delivery and managerial innovation. It needs to develop and implement successful findings and demonstrations on a large scale. I believe that during the next 5 years such suppprt will increasingly be forthcoming.

HMOs and PPOs. The growth of HMOs and PPOs has been rapid during the 1980s. The number of HMOs and their total enrollment increased from 265 HMOs and 10.8 million enrollees in 1982 to 546 plans and 41.4 million enrollees in 1992. Faster growth has occurred in individual practice association HMOs, which contract with private physicians for services; growth is somewhat slower in staff models in which HMOs contract with or employ physician groups. Enrollment in PPOs grew from 1.3 million Americans in health plans eligible to the PPO services in 1984 to 16.5 million in 1986. Unlike HMOs, PPOs allow patients the freedom to use providers that have not contracted with the PPO. The fundamental strategy is to use financial incentives such as volume discounts to steer patients to cost-effective providers.

What has taken place is regulation of providers by purchasers, with measures such as prior approval screening, use of PPOs and HMOs, and restructuring of benefit plans to shift health costs from employers to employees. Purchasers are beginning to grapple with quality issues as well. In the next 5 years they will be increasingly designing incentives to weigh against the choice of what are perceived to be low-quality providers and assessing the quality of services provided to their beneficiaries. They will attempt to identify outliers—hospitals and physicians that are clearly better or worse than most others in regard to medical outcomes achieved for certain procedures—and they will increasingly steer beneficiaries toward certain providers and away from others.

I believe that more care for more Americans will be purchased by health care purchasing organizations as employers and their agents buy services from fewer providers increasingly organized in local markets. Purchasing alliances or cooperatives have been proposed under the Clinton health plan. The nation will not see the formation of national health care firms with large chunks of the market, as in the auto industry, but in many cities there will be fewer larger groups of providers contracting with purchasers. And the national corporations such as Humana and Kaiser-Permanente and Prudential also will increase in size and have increased market share.

Educational and Credentialing Organizations

Education in the health care professions, particularly in the medical profession, has been directed toward their own interests, with little or no societal responsibility. As Ebert (1985) writes, other than substantial change in distribution of residencies toward primary care, "the medical education establishment has changed little in other ways, except to become increasingly dependent on income from fee-for-service high technology medicine."

Ebert and Ginzberg (1988) assert that "the existing medical educational system is not providing the types of physicians who will be able to meet the health care needs of the public and to function in the newly emerging modes of health care delivery." They recommend shortening medical education by combining the last 2 years of medical school and the first 2 years of graduate medical education as implemented by consortia of medical schools in a geographic area. For specialties other than general medicine, pediatrics, and family medicine, in which education would be completed at the end of medical school, those intending to specialize would spend 3 rather than 4 years in medical school. A stipend would be paid for medical students during the last 2 years of clinical training as it currently exists in graduate medical education. Ebert and Ginzberg note that at present there is no consensus for such reform. Given the median indebtedness of medical school graduates of $55,859 in 1992, and perceptions of oversupply by state and federal legislators, I would expect to see demonstrations funded toward implementing these recommendations in pilot programs over the next 5 years.

Because of higher salaries there has been a decrease in the shortage of nurses, particularly in hospitals. Many are urging (see chapter 5) that nurse practitioners replace primary care physicians as the primary source of care to families, particularly in low-income and rural areas.

Characteristically, health care professionals are educated in separate schools, and there are no career ladders between professions, so it would take less time for a nurse or physical therapist to become a doctor than it would a college graduate. After education in separate schools of medicine, nursing, social work, dentistry, physical therapy, public health, and others, graduates are required to work together taking care of patients. Understandably. there is considerable conflict regarding who is supposed to do what for whom. Productivity is therefore lower than might be the case if expectations took adequate account of which professionals can and should do which tasks and take what responsibilities for the patient at what costs and quality. It is predicted that no significant changes will take place regarding joint training of health professionals, although some pilot programs will be demonstrated.

The direction that medical schools will take in the service area is not clear. Their past record has not always been exemplary as providers of high-quality care, particularly in the ambulatory care area. There has been some outside pressure and a good deal of inside entrepreneurship to make the medical school hospitals the hub of the medical care system as well as the tertiary-care center. The assumption of responsibility for comprehensive medical care for a segment of population has had mixed success when it has been placed in the hands of educational institutions. Leading educators can be found on both sides of the question, but it has become less likely that medical schools will exert leadership in this area as purchasers become more desirous of cheaper prices and more customized services for their beneficiaries.

Credentialing in the health professions has been the province of the professions. It has had little or no governmental or consumer input and has been one more mechanism by which the professional controls access to the professions and the market. This control is being eroded by governmental and consumer forces. Accreditation of educational programs by the educator and the profession without concern for the greater public good will not last much longer. Already, accrediting bodies have nonprofessional representatives, and governmental bodies will begin to demand more consumer concern. During the next 5 years accrediting agencies will still be dominated by providers rather than by consumers.

Licensure should undergo similar shifts. The present restrictions across state lines are archaic. Nursing professions have found methods of breaking down state barriers. I do not see licensing of institutions rather than individuals in the next 5 years. Since institutions are corporate units and can assume responsibility for their practice, it is possible that hospitals, clinics, and groups could be licensed to practice and assume responsibility for their actions. But professional groups have mustered strong forces against accrediting institutions regarding the practice of clinicians within them, rather than the individual clinicians themselves. I predict that the professions will continue to be successful in resisting this change.

Certification has been another area of professional control. There have been no restrictions by government on criteria for certification or on numbers of specialists certified. Certification standards may have been more responsive to physician and hospital needs for inexpensive helping hands than to societal needs for qualified practitioners. Again, governmental and consumer forces outside the profession, as well as forces within the system, have been largely unsuccessful on this issue.

Pressures outside and inside the industry are being directed toward recertification and relicensure to ensure that the health professional continues to maintain a level of competence. This will be implemented in more states during the next 5 years. Unfortunately, there is no assurance that such procedures will result in proper patient care. Undoubtedly, as quality of care becomes of wider concern and measurement capability increases, the work of individual physicians is being scrutinized and the examination of knowledge is giving way to measurement of process and outcome in practice. If quality of process and outcome in practice is measured, relicensure and certification will no longer be necessary. This may be increasingly implemented by state legislators dissatisfied with the pace of private sector improvements.

In the 1900s the AMA had a leadership role in organizing and advocating change in medical care systems. Their position since World War I and particularly in the last 35 years, however, has been to oppose all change that might tend to weaken the physician's autonomy and control over the medical care industry. Such a stance has proved eminently successful, not only in halting or slowing legislation for change but also in channeling whatever change occurred to the massive benefit of the nation's physicians. For example, Medicare, which was bitterly and expensively opposed by the AMA, has resulted in some shift in the delivery of medical services from the under-65 population to those over 65, at a tremendous inflation in medical care prices and at a tremendous increase in physician incomes. Formal AMA opposition to the magnitide and quality of change described here is expected to continue, and lobbying by other professional organizations, such as the American Nurses Association, is expected to increase in order to achieve like rewards for their constituents. Neither organization will achieve the power that the AMA had circa 1950–1975 because of the now increased power of purchaser organizations.

Legislation concerning peer review of physician care has been channeled into control by Peer Review Organizations (PROs) rather than hospitals and other organizations that deliver the care. These organizations seem to have achieved a level of acceptance within medicine and by HCOs and will probably continue to carry out these functions as long as they retain the confidence of government and other purchasers who largely pay their bills. Similar organizations will not be created for other clinicians, such as nurses and social workers, as it is expected that physicians will continue to dominate the decision-making process with respect to diagnosis and treatment, particularly in acute care.

Summary and Conclusions

The author has attempted to predict future directions in the American health care delivery system, not so much because of confidence that they will happen but rather to focus discussion on key issues, the constraints that surround them, and the opportunities for resolving them.

American preferences for pluralism and diversity and distrust of government are likely to continue but universal health care coverage is likely to be enacted in the 1990s. Health care will be provided increasingly by large organizations. Because of cost pressures, Americans will use less medical care per capita on an age-adjusted basis. Government increasingly will regulate the cost of, quality, and access to health care. And the power of physicians to shape and benefit from the delivery system will diminish relative to other providers and to consumers.

Health is the ideal all persons strive for. And health care is the reality which not all persons can afford. The challenge is to gain more of the elusive ideal without forgoing meaningful employment and caring relationships and sufficient food, clothing, and shelter, all of which affect health and are affected by it.

References

Amara, R., Ian, M. J., & Schmid, G., *Looking Ahead at American Health Care.* Washington, DC: McGraw-Hill, 1988.

Arthur Andersen & Co. & American College of Health Care Executives. *The Future of Health Care: Changes & Choices.* Chicago: Author, 1987.

Bender, A. D., Strack, A. E., Ebrigh, G. W., & VanHaunulter, X. X., *A Delphic Study of the Future of Medicine.* Philadelphia: Smith, Kline, and French Laboratories, 1967.

Blendon, R. J., "Three Systems: A Comparative Survey." *Health Management Quarterly, 11*(1), 2, 1989.

Blendon, R. J., & Altman, D. E., "Public Opinion and Health Care Costs." In C. Schramm (ed.), *Health Care and Its Costs.* New York: W. W. Norton, 1987.

Coile, R. C., Jr., "The Promise of Technocracy: A Technoforecast for the 1990s." *Healthcare Executive*, November–December, 1988, p. 22.

Ebert, R. H., "The Medical School Revisited." *Health Affairs, 4*(2), 47, 1985.

Ebert, R. H., & Ginzberg, E., "The Reform of Medical Education." *Health Affairs, 7*, (Suppl. 2), 5, 1988.

Griffith, J., *The Well Managed Community Hospital.* Ann Arbor, MI: Health Administration Press, 1987.

Jonas, S. (Ed.), *Health Care Delivery in the United States* (3d ed.). New York: Springer Publishing Co., 1986.

Kovner, A. R., & Martin S. P. (Eds.), *Community Health and Medical Care.* New York: Grune and Stratton, 1978.

Little, A. D., *The Health Care System in the Mid-1990's.* Boston: 1985.

McLaughlin, C. P., & Sheldon, A., *The Future and Medical Care: A Health Manager's Guide to Forecasting.* Cambridge, MA: Ballinger, 1974.

National Center for Health Services Research and Health Care Technology Assessment. *Research Activities.* Rockville, MD: Department of Health and Human Services (No. 92). 1987.

"Tomorrow's Medicine." *Medical World News,* January 24, 1988, p. 55.

Vladeck, B., *President's Letter.* New York: United Hospital Fund, 1987.

Appendix

Abbreviations

AAMC	Association of American Medical Colleges
AAN	American Academy of Nursing
AARP	American Assocation of Retired Persons
ACHE	American College of Healthcare Executives
ACP	American College of Physicians
ADAMHA	Alcohol, Drug Abuse, and Mental Health Administration
ADC	Aid to Families with Dependent Children
ADL	Activities of Daily Living
ADS	Alternative Delivery Systems
AFDC	Aid to Families with Dependent Children
AHA	American Hospital Association
AHCPR	Agency for Health Policy & Research
AHEC	Area Health Education Center
AHSR	Association for Health Services Research
AIDS	Acquired Immune Deficiency Syndrome
ALOS	Average Length of Stay
AMA	American Medical Association
ANA	American Nurses Assocation
APA	American Psychiatric Association
APHA	American Public Health Association
AUPHA	Association of University Programs in Health Administration
BC/BS	Blue Cross and Blue Shield
BCHS	Bureau of Community Health Services
BHP	Bureau of Health Professions
BLS	Bureau of Labor Statistics
CAT	Computerized Axial Tomography (scanner)
CBO	Congressional Budget Office
CCMC	Committee on the Costs of Medical Care
CCN	Community Care Network
CCU	Coronary Care Unit
CDC	Centers for Disease Control
CEO	Chief Executive Officer
CEU	Continuing Education Unit
CFO	Chief Financial Officer

CFR	Code of Federal Regulations
CHAMPUS	Civilian Health and Medical Program of the Uniformed Services
CHC	Community Health Center
CHP	Comprehensive Health Planning
CME	Continuing Medical Education
CMHC	Community Mental Health Center
CMI	Case Mix Index
COB	Coordination of Benefits
COBRA	Consolidated Budget Reconciliation Act
COGME	Council on Graduate Medical Education
CON	Certificate of Need
COPC	Community-Oriented Primary Care
CORF	Comprehensive Outpatient Rehabilitation Facility
COTH	Council of Teaching Hospitals
CPI	Consumer Price Index
CPR	Cardiopulmonary Resuscitation
CQI	Continuous Quality Improvement
DHHS	Department of Health and Human Services
DME	Durable Medical Equipment
DO	Doctor of Osteopathy
DRG	Diagnosis-Related Group
DVA	Department of Veterans Affairs
EAP	Employee Assistance Program
ECF	Extended Care Facility
EMS	Emergency Medical Services
EPA	Environmental Protection Agency
EPSDT	Early and Periodic Screening, Diagnosis & Treatment
ER	Emergency Room
ERISA	Employee Retirement Income Security Act
ESP	Economic Stabilization Program
ESRD	End Stage Renal Disease
FDA	Food and Drug Administration
FEHBP	Federal Employees Health Benefits Program
FFS	Fee for Service
FHA	Federal Housing Authority
FMC	Foundation for Medical Care
FMG	Foreign Medical Graduate
FTE	Full-time Equivalent
FY	Fiscal Year
GAO	General Accounting Office
GDP	Gross Domestic Product
GHAA	Group Health Association of America

GHI	Group Health Insurance
GMENAC	Graduate Medical Education National Advisory Committee
GNP	Gross National Product
HANES	Health and Nutrition Examination Survey
HCA	Hospital Corporation of America
HCFA	Health Care Financing Administration
HDS	Hospital Discharge Survey
HHS	Health and Human Services (Department of)
HIAA	Health Insurance Association of America
HIS	Health Interview Survey
HIV	Human Immunodeficiency Virus
HMO	Health Maintenance Organization
HPPC	Health Plan Purchasing Cooperative
HRA	Health Resources Administration
HRSA	Health Resources and Services Administration
HSA	Health Systems Agency
ICD	International Classification of Diseases
ICF	Intermediate Care Facility
ICU	Intensive Care Unit
IHS	Indian Health Service
IOM	Institute of Medicine
IPA	Individual Practice Association
IPPB	Intermittent Positive Pressure Breathing
JCAHO	Joint Commission on Accreditation of Healthcare Organizations
LOS	Length of Stay
LPN	Licensed Practical Nurse
LTC	Long-Term Care
MCH	Maternal and Child Health
MD	Medical Doctor
Ml	Myocardial Infarction
MICU	Medical Intensive Care Unit
MRI	Magnetic Resonance Imaging
NAHC	National Association for Home Care
NAMCS	National Ambulatory Care Survey
NCHS	National Center for Health Statistics
NCHSR	National Center for Health Services Research
NHC	Neighborhood Health Center
NHI	National Health Insurance
NHP	National Health Plan
NHS	National Health Service
NHSC	National Health Service Corps

NIH	National Institutes of Health
NIMH	National Institute of Mental Health
NIOSH	National Institute of Occupational Safety and Health
NLM	National Library of Medicine
NLN	National League for Nursing
NMR	Nuclear Magnetic Resonance
OBRA	Omnibus Budget Reconciliation Act
OEO	Office of Economic Opportunity
OHMO	Office of Health Maintenance Organizations
OHTA	Office of Health Technology Assessment
OMB	Office of Management and Budget
OPD	Outpatient Department
OSHA	Occupational Safety and Health Administration
OT	Occupational Therapy
OTA	Office of Technology Assessment
PA	Physician's Assistant
PAC	Political Action Committee
PAS	Professional Activity Study
PAT	Preadmission Testing
PCP	Primary Care Provider
PGP	Prepaid Group Practice
PHS	Public Health Service
PIP	Periodic Interim Payment
PORT	Patient Outcomes Reseach Team
PPO	Preferred Provider Organization
PPRC	Physician Payment Review Commission
PPS	Prospective Payment System
PRO	Peer Review Organization
PROPAC	Prospective Payment Assessment Commission
PSRO	Professional Standards Review Organization
PT	Physical Therapy
QA	Quality Assurance
QOL	Quality of Life
RBRVS	Resource-Based Relative Value Scale
RCC	Ratio of Costs to Charges
RCT	Randomized Clinical Trial
RMP	Regional Medical Program
RN	Registered Nurse
RRA	Registered Records Administrator
RUG	Resource Utilization Group
SCH	Sole Community Hospital
SDS	Same Day Surgery
SHMO	Social Health Maintenance Organization

SICU	Surgical Intensive Care Unit
SNF	Skilled Nursing Facility
SSA	Social Security Administration
STD	Sexually Transmitted Disease
TEFRA	Tax Equity and Fiscal Responsibility Act
Title XVIII	(Medicare)
Title XIX	(Medicaid)
UHDDS	Uniform Hospital Discharge Data Set
UR	Utilization Review
USDA	United States Department of Agriculture
USDHEW	United States Department of Health, Education and Welfare
USDHHS	United States Department of Health and Human Services
USFMG	United States Foreign Medical Graduate
USPHS	United States Public Health Service
VA	Veterans Administration
VNA	Visiting Nurse Association
WC	Workers' Compensation
WHO	World Health Organization
WIC	Women, Infants & Children's Program

Name Index

Aaron, H., 298
Abel-Smith, B., 475
Abramowitz, K. S., 4
Accreditation Association For Ambulatory Health Care, 141
Accreditation Council for Graduate Medical Education (ACGME), 68, 153
Accrediting Commission on Education for Health Services Administration (ACEHSA), 445
Achilles, 26
Addison v. Texas, 257
Administration on Aging, 206
Administration Services Only (ASO), 277
Advance Data, 47, 50
Aetna, 371
Agency for Health Care Policy and Research (AHCPR), 85, 411, 416, 538
Aiken, L., 101
Alcohol Drug Abuse & Mental Health Administration, 273, 331
Altenstetter, C., 460
Altman, D., 540
Amara, R., 535
American Academy of Pediatrics, 87, 513
American Academy of Physician Assistants, 91
American Association of Neuropathologists, 87
American Association of Nurse Anesthetists, 114
American Association of Retired Persons (AARP), 223, 341
American Bar Association (ABA), 260
American Board of Medical Specialties, 69, 88
American Cancer Society (ACS), 364, 366

American College of Healthcare Executives (ACHE), 445–446, 525, 534
American College of Nurse Midwives, 114
American College of Obstetrics & Gynecology, 112, 413
American College of Physicians, 375, 410, 517, 524
American College of Surgeons, 375
American Dietetic Association, 92
American Hospital Association (AHA), 69, 143, 164, 197, 277–278, 375, 425, 428, 445, 489, 524, 546
AMA (American Medical Association), 68–69, 78, 87, 90–91, 95, 148, 152–153, 260, 375, 394, 511, 513, 516, 524, 545, 551
American Nurses Association (ANA), 102, 104, 113, 115, 394, 551
American Occupational Therapy Association, 94
American Physical Therapy Association, 94
American Psychiatric Association (APA), 234, 242–243, 254–255, 256, 260
American Public Health Association (APHA), 445
ARA, 198
American Speech-Language-Hearing Association, 96
Ameriplan, 546–547
Anderson, O., 457, 459
Annas, G., 495
Arthur Andersen and Co., 534
Arthur D. Little & Co., 534
Asklepios, 12
Association of American Medical Colleges (AAMC), 69, 87–88, 148, 394
Association of Operating Room Nurses, 394

Subject Index

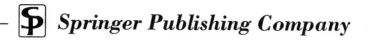

Springer Publishing Company

TUBERCULOSIS
A Sourcebook for Nursing Practice

Felissa L. Cohen, RN, PhD, FAAN, and
Jerry D. Durham, RN, PhD, FAAN, Editors

A hands-on guide for nurses working with persons
with tuberculosis or populations vulnerable to the
disease. A foundation of the most current knowledge
on transmission, diagnosis, treatment and nursing
management is given, followed by in-depth
information on screening and prevention. Information
on HIV/AIDS patients is integrated throughout the
book, as is special handling of drug-resistant TB, and
patients who do not complete therapy. An essential
resource for community and public health nurses, and
acute care nurses in urban areas experiencing the new
resurgence of this ancient disease.

Contents:

I: Background. Introduction. Etiology, Transmission, and Patho-
genesis of Tuberculosis, *M. Shekelton* • The Epidemiology of
Tuberculosis, *F. L. Cohen* **II: Clinical Management of Tuberculosis.**
Symptoms and Diagnosis of TB, *L. Madsen, C. Harriman, F. L. Cohen*
• Medical Treatment of TB, *L. Madsen, C. Harriman, F. L. Cohen* •
Nursing Management of TB, *H. Silbilano* • Adherence to TB Treat-
ment Plan, *E. Sumartojo* **III: Prevention.** Screening for TB: An
Important Prevention Tool, *C. D. Harriman and F. L. Cohen* • Prevent-
ing the Spread of TB in Health Care Facilities and Home Health Care,
J. Otten • Community-Based Strategies for TB Control, *J. A. Boutotte
and S. Etkind* **IV: Special Issues.** TB in Selected Populations HIV/
AIDS Patients, Women, Children, and the Elderly, *A. Kurth, L.
Edwards, E. Peabody, and F. L. Cohen* • TB Among the Homeless: The
Pine Street Inn Experience, *B. McGinnis* • Long-term Inpatient Care:
A Treatment of Last Resort, *L. Singleton and M. Tricarico* • Ethical and
Legal Issues

1994   296pp (est.)   0-8261-8720-X   hardcover

536 Broadway, New York, NY 10012-3955 • (212) 431-4370 • Fax (212) 941-7842

S *Springer Publishing Company*

HEALTH PROMOTION AND AGING

David Haber, PhD

This expertly written text fulfills the need for a broad and integrative perspective on health promotion for the elderly. The author emphasizes individual responsibility for healthy living in collaboration with professionals, as well as through social support. Includes extensive illustrations. For health professionals and educators in aging, as well as for students.

Contents:

Introduction • Health Professionals and Older Clients: A Collaboration • Medical Screenings and Health Assessments • Health Education — Introduction and Exercise • Health Education — Nutrition • Health Education — Other Topics • Social Support • Behavior and Psychological Management • Community Health • Societal Reform

1994   296pp   0-8261-8460-X   hardcover

536 Broadway, New York, NY 10012-3955 • (212) 431-4370 • Fax (212) 941-7842

$\boxed{\textbf{S}}$ *Springer Publishing Company*

INTRODUCTION TO ENVIRONMENTAL HEALTH
2nd Edition

Daniel S. Blumenthal, MD, MPH, and
James Ruttenber, MD, PhD, Editors

This fully revised and updated second edition of a
popular text provides a concise overview of the field
of environmental health, including a unique focus on
health promotion. It serves as a basic resource for
students of medicine, nursing, public and community
health, and other health-related disciplines.

Contents:

The Ecologic Basis of Health and Disease, *J. Ruttenber and
H.L. Ragsdale* • The Pathophysiology of Environmental
Diseases, *J. Ruttenber and R.D. Kimbrough* • Infectious Agents
In The Environment, *D.S. Blumenthal* • Toxic Chemicals in
the Environment, *J. Ruttenber and R.D. Kimbrough* • Ionizing
and Non-Ionizing Radiation, *D. S. Blumenthal and J. Ruttenber*
• Air Pollution, *D.S. Blumenthal and H.L. Ragsdale* • Water
Pollution, *J. Ruttenber* • Environmental Health Law, *A.R. Green*
• Occupational Health, *L.R. Murray* • Environmental Epide-
miology: Assessing Health Risks From Toxic Agents in the
Environment, *J. Ruttenber*

1995   272pp (est.)   0-8261-3901-9   hardcover

536 Broadway, New York, NY 10012-3955 • (212) 431-4370 • Fax (212) 941-7842

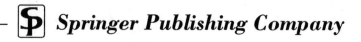
Springer Publishing Company

AN INTRODUCTION TO THE U. S. HEALTH CARE SYSTEM
3rd Edition

Steven Jonas, MD, MPH

"This third edition ... like the system itself, shows further development. Even more than the first two editions, it portrays the 'system as a whole,' complicated but still described and analyzed as a total organism.

"With the sophistication and clarity of Dr. Steven Jonas, this account manages to encompass all the diverse components of the American health system in a relatively short volume. It paints a picture with the necessary highlights and shadows, yet on a canvas within a relatively small frame."

—from the Foreword by Founding Author
Milton Roemer, MD, MPH

Contents:

The US Health Care Delivery System: An Overview • Primary and Ambulatory Care • Hospitals • Personnel • Government • Principles of Health Planning • Financing and Cost Containment • National Health Insurance • National Health Systems Throughout the World • Appendix I: Critical Reports/Analyses of the US Health Care Delivery System, 1927–1983 • Appendix II: Guide to Sources

1992   224pp   0-8261-3984-1   softcover

536 Broadway, New York, NY 10012-3955 • (212) 431-4370 • Fax (212) 941-7842